PROGRESS IN BRAIN RESEARCH

VOLUME 77

PAIN MODULATION

PROGRESS IN BRAIN RESEARCH

VOLUME 77

PAIN MODULATION

EDITED BY

H.L. FIELDS

Department of Neurology, University of California San Francisco, San Francisco, CA 94143, USA

and

J.-M. BESSON

INSERM, U. 161, Unité de Recherches de Neurophysiologie Pharmacologique, 75014 Paris, France

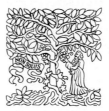

ELSEVIER
AMSTERDAM – NEW YORK – OXFORD
1988

MR

ISBN 0-444-80984-8 (volume)
ISBN 0-444-80104-9 (series)

Published by:
Elsevier Science Publishers B.V. (Biomedical Division)
P.O. Box 211
1000 AE Amsterdam
The Netherlands

Sole distributors for the U.S.A. and Canada:
Elsevier Science Publishing Company, Inc.
52 Vanderbilt Avenue
New York, NY 10017
U.S.A.

LIBRARY OF CONGRESS
Library of Congress Cataloging-in-Publication Data

Pain modulation / edited by H.L. Fields and J.-M. Besson.
      p.   cm. -- (Progress in brain research ; v. 77)
    Based on a conference held in Beaune, France in July 1987.
    Includes bibliographies and index.
    ISBN 0-444-80984-8 (U.S.)
    1. Pain--Pathophysiology--Congresses. 2. Neurophysiology-
  -Congresses. 3. Brain stem--Physiology--Congresses.   I. Fields,
  Howard L. II. Besson, Jean-Marie R. III. Series.
    [DNLM: 1. Brain Stem--physiology--congresses. 2. Neural
  Transmission--congresses. 3. Nociceptors--physiology--congresses.
  4. Pain--physiopathology--congresses.   W1 PR667J v. 77 / WL 704
  P1468 1987]
  QP376.P7 vol. 77
  [RB127]
  612'.82 s--dc19
  [616'.0472]
  DNLM/DLC
  for Library of Congress   88-21289
                                                          CIP

Printed in the Netherlands

List of Contributors

L.C. Abbott, Department of Veterinary and Comparative Anatomy, Pharmacology, and Physiology, Washington State University, College of Veterinarian Medicine, Pullman, WA 99164–6520, USA

N.R.F. Al-Rodhan, Department of Neurology and Pharmacology, Mayo Clinic, Rochester, MN 55905, USA

N.M. Barbaro, Department of Neurological Surgery, 787-M, UCSF, San Francisco, CA 94143, USA

A.I. Basbaum, Department of Anatomy, S-1343, UCSF, San Francisco, CA 94143, USA

M.M. Behbehani, Division of Geriatrics, Office of the Dean, University of Cincinnati College of Medicine, Cincinnati, OH 45267–0555, USA

J.-M. Besson, INSERM, U. 161, Unité de Recherches de Neurophysiologie Pharmacologique, 2 rue d'Alésia, 75014 Paris, France

S. Bourgoin, Neurobiologie Cellulaire et Fonctionnelle, INSERM, U. 288, CHU La Pitié-Salpêtrière, 91 Boulevard de l'Hôpital, 75634 Paris, Cedex 13, France

R.M. Bowker, Department of Veterinary and Comparative Anatomy, Pharmacology, and Physiology, Washington State University, College of Veterinarian Medicine, Pullman, WA 99164–6520, USA

K.L. Casey, University of Michigan Medical Center, Neurology Service, Veterans Administration Medical Center, 2215 Fuller Road, Ann Arbor, MI 48105, USA

B. Caute, Laboratoire de Pharmacie Galénique, Faculté des Sciences Pharmaceutiques, Chemin des Maraîchers, et Laboratoires de Pharmacologie et Toxologie Fondamentales, CNRS, 205 route de Narbonne, 31400 Toulouse, France

F. Cesselin, Neurobiologie Cellulaire et Fonctionnelle, INSERM, U. 288, CHU La Pitié-Salpêtrière, 91 Boulevard de l'Hôpital, 75634 Paris Cedex 13, France

R.E. Chipkin, Department of Pharmacology, Schering/Plough Corporation, Bloomfield, NJ 07003, USA

J.G. Collins, Department of Anesthesiology, Yale University School of Medicine, 333 Cedar Street, New Haven, CT 06510, USA

A. Dickenson, Department of Pharmacology, University College London, Gower Street, London WC1E 6BT, UK

R.P. Dilts, Department of Veterinary and Comparative Anatomy, Pharmacology, and Physiology, Washington State University, College of Veterinarian Medicine, Pullman, WA 99164–6520, USA

J.O. Dostrovsky, Department of Physiology, Faculty of Medicine, University of Toronto, Toronto, Ontario M5S 1A8, Canada

R. Dubner, Neurobiology and Anesthesiology Branch, National Institute of Dental Research, National Institutes of Health, Bldg. 30, Rm. B-18, 9000 Rockville Pike, Bethesda, MD 20892, USA

A.W. Duggan, Department of Pharmacology, John Curtin School of Medical Research, P.O. Box 334, Canberra ACT 2601, Australia

H.L. Fields, Department of Neurology, University of California San Francisco, San Francisco, CA 94143, USA

R.C.A. Frederickson, Searle Research and Development, G.D. Searle and Co., J-1, 4901 Searle Parkway, Skokie, IL 60077, USA

G.F. Gebhart, Department of Pharmacology, College of Medicine, University of Iowa, Iowa City, IA 52242, USA

G. Guilbaud, Unité de Recherches de Neurophysiologie Pharmacologique, INSERM, U. 161, 2 rue d'Alésia, 75014 Paris, France

D.L. Hammond, Department of Central Nervous System Diseases Research, G.D. Searle and Co., Research and Development Division, 4901 Searle Parkway, Skokie, IL 60077, USA

M. Hamon, Neurobiologie Cellulaire et Fonctionnelle, INSERM U. 288, CHU La Pitié-Salpêtrière, 91 Boulevard de l'Hôpital, 75634 Paris Cedex 13, France

M.M. Heinricher, Department of Physiology, University of California San Francisco, San Francisco, CA 94143, USA

A. Herz, Max-Planck-Institut für Psychiatrie, Abteilung für Neuropharmakologie, A. Klopferspitz 18A, D-8033 Planneg-Martinsried, FRG

R.G. Hill, Parke-Davis Research Unit, Addenbrooke's Hospital Site, Hills Road, Cambridge, CB2 2QB, UK

G. Holstege, NASA-Ames Research Center, M.S. 239-7, Moffett Field, CA 94035, USA

Y. Hosobuchi, Section of Functional and Stereotactic Surgery, Department of Neurological Surgery, School of Medicine, 786-M, UCSF, San Francisco, CA 94143, USA

Correspondence to Y.H., MD, c/o The Editorial Office, Department of Neurological Surgery, 1360 Ninth Avenue, Suite 210, San Francisco, CA 94122, USA

T.S. Jensen, Department of Neurology, University of Copenhagen, KAS, Gentofte, 2900 Hellerup, Denmark

S.L. Jones, Department of Physiology, University of North Carolina, Chapel Hill, NC 27514, USA

V. Kayser, Unité de Recherches de Neurophysiologie Pharmacologique, INSERM, U. 161, 2 rue d'Alésia, 75014 Paris, France

G.C. Kwiat, Department of Anatomy, S-1343, UCSF, San Francisco, CA 94143, USA

Y. Lazorthes, Clinique de Neurochirurgie, CHU Rangueil, Chemin du Vallon, 31054 Toulouse, France

D. Le Bars, Unité de Recherches de Neurophysiologie Pharmacologique, INSERM, U. 161, 2 rue d'Alésia, 75014 Paris, France

R. Maranhao, Clinique de Neurochirurgie, CHU Rangueil, Chemin du Vallon, 31054 Toulouse, France

B.A. Meyerson, Department of Neurosurgery, Karolinska Sjukhuset, Box 60500, S-104 01 Stockholm 60, Sweden

M.J. Millan, Max-Planck-Institut für Psychiatrie, Am Klopferspitz 18a, D-8033 Planegg-Martinsried, FRG

C.R. Morton, Department of Pharmacology, John Curtin School of Medical Research, P.O. Box 334, Australian National University, Canberra ACT 2601, Australia

R.M. Murphy, Division of Geriatrics, University of Cincinnati College of Medicine, Cincinnati, OH 45267−0555, USA

J.-L. Oliveras, Unité de Recherches de Neurophysiologie Pharmacologique, INSERM, U. 161, 2 rue d'Alésia, 75014 Paris, France

H.K. Proudfit, Department of Pharmacology, University of Illinois, College of Medicine at Chicago, 901 S. Wolcott Avenue, P.O. Box 6998, Chicago, IL 60680, USA

D.B. Reichling, Department of Anatomy, S-1343, USCF, San Francisco, CA 94143, USA

M.H.T. Roberts, Department of Physiology, University College Cardiff, Cardiff CF1 1XL, UK

M.A. Ruda, Neurobiology and Anesthesiology Branch, National Institute of Dental Research, National Institutes of Health, Bldg. 30, 9000 Rockville Pike, Bethesda, MD 20892, USA

J. Sandkühler, II. Physiologisches Institut, Universität Heidelberg, Im Neuenheimer Feld 326, D-6900 Heidelberg, FRG

B.J. Sessle, Faculty of Dentistry, University of Toronto, 124 Edward Street, Toronto, Ontario M5G 1G6, Canada

M. Tafani, Service de Médecine Nucléaire − Laboratoire des Radio-Isotopes, CHU Purpan, Place du Dr. Baylac, 31052, Toulouse, France

L. Terenius, Department of Pharmacology, University of Uppsala, BMC Box 591, 75124 Uppsala, Sweden

J.-C. Verdié, Clinique de Neurochirurgie, CHU Rangueil, Chemin du Vallon, 31054 Toulouse, France

L. Villanueva, Unité de Recherches de Neurophysiologie Pharmacologique, INSERM U. 161, 2 rue d'Alésia, 75014 Paris, France

W.D. Willis, Jr., Marine Biomedical Institute, 200 University Boulevard, Galveston, TX 77550, USA

T.L. Yaksh, Department of Neurology and Pharmacology, Mayo Clinic, Rochester, MN 55905, USA

F.P. Zemlan, Department of Psychiatry, University of Cincinnati College of Medicine, 231 Bethesda Avenue, Cincinnati, OH 45267−0555, USA

M. Zimmermann, II. Physiologisches Institut, Universität Heidelberg, Im Neuenheimer Feld 326, D-6900 Heidelberg, FRG

Introduction: Pain modulation: past, present and future

The anatomical structures and physiological mechanisms underlying brain stem control of spinal cord dorsal horn interneurons have been under investigation for over three decades (Lundberg, 1982). The relevance of this descending control to nociception was suggested by P.D. Wall's work (1967) revealing tonic supraspinal inhibition of cutaneous inputs of lamina V cells. The subsequent demonstration of stimulation-produced analgesia (SPA) in animals and man provided powerful evidence for a behaviorally relevant, highly selective brain stem control of nociceptive transmission. Concomitantly, the discovery of endogenous opioid peptides and their association, in a variety of species, with brain stem structures involved in antinociception, helped to convince both researchers and physicians of the physiological significance of nociceptive modulating networks.

Since these initial discoveries there has been an explosion of knowledge concerned with the brain stem and spinal mechanisms that underlie nociceptive modulation. A little over a decade ago the first outlines of a nociceptive modulating network had emerged (Liebeskind et al., 1976; Mayer and Price, 1976; Fields and Basbaum, 1978; Basbaum and Fields, 1984). The periaqueductal gray (PAG) was proposed to suppress activity of dorsal horn neurons via serotoninergic neurons in the nucleus raphe magnus (NRM). Since the PAG is sensitive to microinjected opiates, this pathway was also proposed to be involved in opiate analgesia. A second modulatory pathway, probably noradrenergic, from the dorsolateral pons to the dorsal horn was also proposed to play a role in antinociception but its relationship, if any, to the PAG-RVM-dorsal horn pathway was unspecified.

Subsequent research has amply confirmed the basic concept of a PAG-NRM-dorsal horn modulatory network, but has revealed that picture to be both incomplete and oversimplified (see Willis, and Yaksh et al., this volume). For one thing, the brain stem neurons relevant to antinociception are more widely distributed than was originally proposed. For example, at midbrain and medullary levels, inhibition of dorsal horn nociceptive neurons and nociceptive reflexes can be obtained from stimulation of reticular structures lateral to the PAG and NRM, respectively. There is general agreement that the rostral ventromedial medulla (RVM), which includes NRM, is the major relay from the midbrain nociceptive modulating structures PAG to dorsal horn. A significant proportion of the RVM projection to the cord is serotonergic but many non-5HT neurons also contribute to this pathway. Unfortunately, knowing the transmitter content of a medullospinal neuron does not in itself predict what its effect will be. There is a variety of 5HT receptors, some of which may have opposing actions on nociceptive processing at both RVM (Roberts, this volume) and dorsal horn levels

(Zemlan et al., this volume). As if receptor multiplicity were not enough of a complication, many medullospinal 5HT neurons also contain one or more peptide transmitters and there is evidence for heterogeneity in the anatomical distribution of medullary cells containing the different putative transmitters (Bowker et al., this volume). It is also clear that the input to the RVM is complex. There is evidence that RVM receives input from midbrain neurons containing ACh, glutamate, neurotensin and 5HT (Reichling et al., this volume). In addition, RVM receives a noradrenergic input from neurons in the dorsolateral pons, some of which also project to the spinal cord (Holstege, and Reichling et al., this volume).

The PAG is functionally, cytoarchitectonically and hodologically heterogeneous. It receives input from cortex, hypothalamus, locus coeruleus, RVM and spinal cord. Different sub-regions receive different afferent inputs, project to different targets, have different concentrations of various neuropeptides (Reichling et al., this volume) and produce different behavioral effects when electrically stimulated (Oliveras and Besson, this volume). Whether the anatomical and immunocytochemical differences can explain the behavioral differences, remains to be seen.

In addition to the well-studied PAG-RVM-dorsal horn pathway, there are direct projections from diencephalic structures, somatosensory cortex and dorsolateral pons to dorsal horn lamina I (Holstege, this volume). This suggests that there are several nociceptive modulating pathways arising from different levels of the neuraxis. The projection from somatosensory cortex to cord is topographic whereas the PAG-RVM-dorsal horn projection is not somatotopically organized. Whether the various pathways function independently or in concert is not known.

Studies of the physiological properties of neurons in these nociceptive modulating nuclei have also revealed significant complexity. In the RVM and PAG, cells can be divided into three physiological classes based on the correlation of their discharge to tail or paw withdrawal from noxious stimuli (Fields et al., this volume). Cells of one of these classes, the off-cells, are activated by morphine and have a discharge pattern consistent with the role of RVM output inhibitory neuron. Another class, the on-cell (which is suppressed by morphine), has a discharge pattern that suggests it may facilitate nociception.

The possibility of bidirectional, rather than purely inhibitory, control from RVM is a new idea with important conceptual and practical implications. For example, increased responsiveness to noxious stimuli could result from enhancement of facilitation or removal of inhibition; conversely, analgesia could result from enhanced inhibition or reduced facilitation. From an experimental standpoint, if adjacent cells in RVM have opposing actions, any effects of electrical stimulation must be interpreted with caution.

The possibility of bidirectional brain stem control of nociception receives important support from recent work in awake behaving monkeys (Dubner, this volume). In such animals, wide-dynamic range medullary dorsal horn cells show either increases or decreases in firing that can be reliably correlated with some component of a learned behavior. These task-related responses are clearly distinct from responses to noxious stimuli applied in the restricted somatic receptive field of the same cells. The task-related responses could significantly alter the nociceptor-induced responses. It will be of great importance to determine which neural structures generate these task-related responses.

Progress in elucidating the spinal mechanisms underlying the descending antinociceptive actions of brain stem structures has also been made. It is quite clear that there is a postsynaptic inhibitory action of RVM upon dorsal horn nociceptive neurons, including identified spinothalamic tract (STT) cells. Anatomical studies show that STT cells receive a dense direct 5HT input, most likely from RVM (Ruda, this volume). In addition to this direct, presumably inhibitory, 5HT input to STT cells, there is evidence for 5HT inputs to dorsal horn enkephalinergic cells, which could be inhibitory interneurons. Iontophoretic, microinjection and transmitter release studies are consistent with a nociceptive inhibitory role for serotonin, norepinephrine and enkephalin (see chapters by Zemlan et al., Terenius, Hamon et al., Yaksh et al., and Proudfit, this volume). The role, if any, of GABA and other putative transmitters remains to be worked out.

As mentioned above, there is a close association of endogenous opioid peptides with structures implicated in nociceptive control. In view of the sensitivity of these structures to the antinociceptive actions of microinjected exogenous opiates, it is likely that endogenous opioid peptides play an important role in nociceptive modulation. Furthermore, the original concept that the nociceptive modulating networks mediate opiate analgesia is confirmed and extended. It is almost certain that opiate drugs relieve pain by mimicking the action of endogenous opioid peptides. Although the mechanisms underlying the antinociceptive effects of supraspinal microinjection of morphine remain controversial (see chapters by Fields et al., Gebhart and Jones, Dickenson, this volume), morphine injected into the third ventricle of humans induces significant and long-lasting relief from cancer pain (Lazorthes et al., this volume).

There are several different families of opioid peptides, each having a different distribution. β-Endorphin, a cleavage product of pro-opiomelanocortin, is the most potent of the known peptides. It is derived from a discrete cluster of cells in the arcuate nucleus. Herz and Millan (this volume) have presented convincing evidence that, under certain conditions of behavioral stress, these cells can produce antinociception mediated by β-endorphin. A role for the enkephalins is less certain but likely. In contrast, the dynorphins seem to be very weak antinociceptive agents. The interactions of these three families of endogenous opioid peptides present a fascinating challenge for the future.

Human studies have been crucial to the study of nociceptive modulation networks (see chapters by Barbaro, Meyerson, and Hosobuchi, this volume). Ultimately, pain is a subjective experience, and animal studies can provide only inferential data about its relief. The evidence that PAG stimulation can relieve pain in man is of utmost importance. It potentially ties the phenomenon of antinociception in animals to analgesia in man; the fact that a homologous site is effective in both species suggests that a similar neural mechanism is involved. Unfortunately, the human studies are unsatisfactory. To date, there has been no controlled study demonstrating an analgesic effect attributable to stimulation, although a great many neurosurgeons have reported success and electrodes have been implanted in hundreds of patients. The fact that PAG electrodes are only used in cases of chronic pain, while brief cutaneous stimuli are generally used in animal studies, further complicates comparison. Moreover, therapeutic indications for PAG stimulation in humans are vague, thus only a subset of chronic pain patients undergo the procedure. Future studies will hopefully provide more convincing evidence for an analgesic effect in man. Assuming such studies confirm the clinical impression of a potent analgesic effect, an important question will be to what extent SPA in man depends upon descending pathways.

Although there has been significant progress in the past decade and many talented people have been attracted to the field, much remains to be done. We are reaching a level of analysis that will require more sophisticated methods and more systematic investigation. For example, several groups are presently exploring intrinsic brain stem circuitry, and it seems certain that a more accurate picture of excitatory and inhibitory connections will emerge from the current confusion of peptide, biogenic amine and amino-acid transmitters and their various receptors. Similarly, progress can be expected in unraveling the dorsal horn circuitry that underlies nociceptive modulation.

Among the most important questions about descending controls are how and when they are activated. One way is by heterotopic noxious stimulation. This mode of activation requires a complex loop ascending in the anterolateral quadrant and descending in the dorsolateral funiculi (Le Bars and Villanueva, this volume). Other mechanisms of activation of the system need to be studied, particularly in awake animals.

The study of brain stem and dorsal horn neurons in awake, unanesthetized preparations is an area of crucial importance. It is well established that there are important differences in the physiological properties of nociceptive dorsal horn neurons in awake compared to anesthetized animals (see Collins, Dubner, this volume), but it is not clear which brain stem neurons and transmitter systems account for these differences. Answering this question will require recording from putative nociceptive modulating neurons themselves. Such studies will be crucial for understanding the physiological conditions required for activation of the different modulating neurons.

Understanding the physiological function of nociceptive modulation networks is of more than intellectual importance. Once the function is understood it may be possible to ask whether these systems play a role in human disease. Do certain chronic pain patients have some deficiency of pain inhibitory neurons or their transmitters (serotonin, endogenous opioids), or might they have hyperactivity of pain-enhancing neurons? Even if this level of understanding remains in the distant future, accurate analysis of the transmitter systems and receptors involved in the pain-modulating networks is well within reach and offers the possibility of significant advances in the pharmacological management of pain.

References

Basbaum, A.I. and H.L. Fields (1984) Endogenous pain control systems: brainstem spinal pathways and endorphin circuitry. *Annu. Rev. Neurosci.,* 7: 309–338.

Fields, H.L. and A.I. Basbaum (1978) Brainstem control of spinal pain-transmission neurons. *Annu. Rev. Physiol.* 40: 217–248.

Liebeskind, J.C., G.J. Giesler and G. Urca (1976) Evidence pertaining to an endogenous mechanism of pain inhibition in the CNS. In Y. Zotterman (Ed.), *Sensory Functions of the Skin in Primates,* Pergamon Press, London, pp. 561–573.

Lundberg, A. (1982) Inhibitory control from the brain stem of transmission from primary afferents to motoneurons, primary afferent terminals and ascending pathways. In B. Sjölund and A. Björklund (Eds.), *Brain Stem Control of Spinal Mechanisms,* Elsevier Biomedical Press, Amsterdam, pp. 179 – 224.

Mayer, D.J. and D.D. Price (1976) Central nervous system mechanisms of analgesia. *Pain,* 2: 379 – 404.

Wall, P.D. (1967) The laminar organization of dorsal horn and effects of descending impulses. *J. Physiol.,* 188: 403 – 423.

San Francisco   H.L. Fields
and   and
Paris   J.-M. Besson

Acknowledgements

This volume largely represents material that was presented at a conference held in Beaune, France, in July, 1987. The Editors acknowledge the generous financial support of the United States Public Health Service (Grant NS 24527) and l'Institut National de La Santé et de la Recherche Medicale (INSERM). The following pharmaceutical firms also supported this conference: Astra Alab AB, Sweden; Bayer, France; Fidia Research Laboratories, Italy; I.C.I., UK; Janssen, France; McNeil Consumer Products Company, USA; Medtronic Europe; Parke Davis, UK; Rhone-Poulenc Santé, France; Roussel-Uclaf, France; Sandoz, France; Upjohn, France; and Upsa, France. We thank Susan Elliott and Wendy Ng for editorial and administrative support.

H.L. Fields
and
J.-M. Besson

Contents

H.L. Fields and J.-M. Besson (Eds.)
Progress in Brain Research, Vol. 77
© 1988 Elsevier Science Publishers B.V. (Biomedical Division)

CHAPTER 1

Anatomy and physiology of descending control of nociceptive responses of dorsal horn neurons: comprehensive review

Wm. D. Willis, Jr.

Marine Biomedical Institute and Department of Anatomy and Neurosciences, University of Texas Medical Branch, Galveston, TX 77550, USA

Introduction

Descending control of nociceptive transmission

The centrifugal control of sensation is an important theme in sensory physiology (see Willis, 1982). Sensory pathways in vertebrates are generally controlled by descending pathways originating in the central nervous system and projecting to the brain stem and spinal cord or even peripherally to sense organs. This is true for vision, audition, and somatovisceral sensation, including pain. With respect to pain, there has been a considerable interest in the 'analgesia systems' (see Oliveras, this volume) since manipulation of these has promise clinically in the treatment of pain (see Barbaro, Meyerson, and Hosobuchi, this volume). The operation of these 'analgesia systems' is thought to involve inhibition of neurons in the pathways that process nociceptive information. However, in addition there are descending excitatory pathways that enhance sensory transmission, presumably including pain. These might contribute to the mechanism of pain states that results from activity of central neurons (Cassinari and Pagni, 1969).

Nociceptive spinal cord neurons

Function of nociceptive spinal neurons

The initial assumption usually made with respect to nociceptive neurons in the spinal cord is that these cells play some role in pain. However, nociceptive reactions include not only pain sensation, but also somatic and autonomic reflexes as well as a variety of motivational and affective responses. A given spinal cord neuron may respond selectively to noxious stimuli, yet may contribute only to a motor response and not to sensory experience. A prime example of this is the flexor motoneuron, which behaves like a nociceptive neuron when graded intensities of mechanical stimuli are applied to the skin (Fig. 1). When a nociceptive interneuron is encountered during an electrophysiological experiment, it is difficult to be sure of its role unless there is experimental evidence for placing that interneuron into a particular neural circuit, such as a sensory or a reflex pathway.

Similarly, it is difficult to relate the inhibition of a nociceptive spinal neuron by activation of a

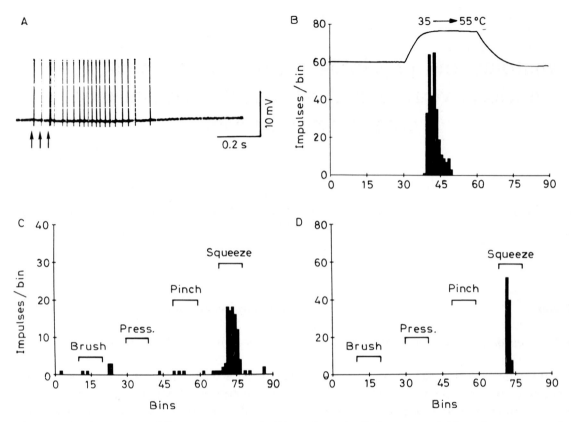

Fig. 1. Nociceptive responses of flexor motoneurons. In (A) are shown the discharges recorded from the motor axon of a flexor motoneuron in response to a brief train of three stimuli (arrows) at an intensity that activated C fibers in the tibial nerve of a cat. The late burst of spikes presumably represents activity that would contribute to a nociceptive flexor reflex. The single pass peristimulus time histogram in (B) shows the response of a flexor motor axon to stimulation of the skin with a noxious heat pulse. (C) and (D) are the responses of two different flexor motor axons to graded intensities of mechanical stimulation of the skin: brushing (BRUSH), a tactile stimulus; pressure (PRESS.) by application of a large arterial clip to a fold of skin, a marginally painful stimulus; pinching (PINCH) with a small arterial clip, a distinctly painful stimulus; and squeezing (SQUEEZE) the skin with serrated forceps, a very painful stimulus. Bin width 1 s. (From Chung et al., 1983a.)

descending pathway to 'analgesia' (the absence of pain sensation) without knowing that the neuron belongs to a sensory pathway. There is now a tendency in the literature to refer to an 'antinociceptive' action when it is unclear if the change in neural responsiveness reflects a change in sensory or motor activity.

Discovery of nociceptive spinal neurons

Spinal cord interneurons responding specifically to noxious stimuli were first described by Kolmodin and Skoglund in 1960. The cells were concentrated in the nucleus proprius of the dorsal horn, in the medial part of laminae VI and VII and in lamina VIII. Kolmodin and Skoglund also described spinal interneurons that had a convergent input from mechanoreceptors and nociceptors. In 1970, Christensen and Perl reported a concentration of neurons in lamina I of the spinal cord dorsal horn that responded specifically to noxious stimuli. Other cells in this same region had convergent inputs from thermoreceptors and nociceptors. Many other laboratories have confirmed the presence of nociceptive-specific neurons in lamina I, although cells with a convergent input from both mechanoreceptors and nociceptors have been found there as well (e.g., Cervero et al., 1976; Light et al., 1986). The functional meaning of neurons with convergent inputs has been one of the puzzles of the pain field.

Problems of nomenclature

Until 1970, experiments on the activity of spinal cord interneurons usually focused on cells that responded to mechanoreceptor input. Investigators concerned chiefly with problems of motor control examined interneurons activated by afferent fibers supplying deep structures, especially muscle (Eccles et al., 1960). Afferent fibers supplying mechanoreceptors in muscle, skin and joints were often found to converge onto the same interneurons, leading to the proposition that these form a special category of 'flexion reflex afferents' (FRA) (R.M. Eccles and Lundberg, 1959a; Holmqvist et al., 1960). A given class of interneurons might receive both a specific input from a particular receptor type (such as group Ia afferents from muscle spindle primary endings or group Ib afferents from Golgi tendon organs) and a convergent input from the FRA (Eccles et al., 1960). Not only interneurons but also ascending tract cells were examined for specific and convergent inputs. For example, several different ascending tracts were found by Lundberg's group to receive input from the FRA (Holmqvist et al., 1960; Lundberg and Oscarsson, 1961, 1962). One of these pathways was undoubtedly a component of the spinocervical tract (SCT). In this case, the specific input was from cutaneous mechanoreceptors. Some SCT cells received just the specific input, whereas others also had a convergent input from the FRA (Lundberg and Oscarsson, 1961).

Recently, Lundberg et al. (1987) have hypothesized that the FRA are activated by movements and that their input sets the appropriate level of excitability in reflex circuits receiving a specific input from particular receptors. A similar arrangement is proposed for ascending pathways (Fig. 2). Ascending tract cells would receive a specific input

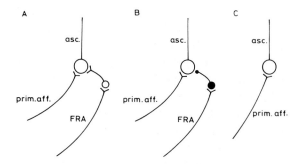

Fig. 2. Circuit arrangements of ascending tract cells receiving a specific input from a particular class of primary afferent fiber (prim. aff.) and a convergent input from the flexion reflex afferents (FRA). In (A), the polysynaptic convergent input from the FRA is excitatory. In (B), the FRA produce inhibition through an inhibitory interneuronal pathway. In (C), there is no FRA input. (From Lundberg et al., 1987.)

from primary afferent fibers. In some cases, the same tract cells will be excited by the FRA through interneuronal pathways (Fig. 2, A); in other cases, the tract cells will be inhibited by the FRA (Fig. 2, B); and in still other cases there is no convergent input from the FRA (Fig. 2, C). Lundberg et al. (1987) propose that the first group of the tract cells will have their activity facilitated and the second group depressed by movements. The third group is suggested to serve as a reference; information provided by these cells will allow brain centers to distinguish between inputs arising during or without accompanying active movements.

Investigators concerned with sensations resulting from stimulation of the skin also described interneurons that responded either to a particular class of cutaneous mechanoreceptor or that received a convergent input from several kinds of receptors; however, by contrast with the cells described above receiving connections from the FRA, the convergence included input from cutaneous nociceptors (Mendell, 1966; Wall, 1960, 1967). Because such interneurons could be excited by a wide range of stimulus intensities, Mendell (1966) called these cells 'wide dynamic range' (WDR) neurons. Neurons with an input from a specific class of cutaneous receptors could be considered 'narrow dynamic range' cells. When the specific input is from nociceptors, these cells are often called 'nociceptive-specific' cells (Price and Dubner, 1977). The term WDR has been criticized, and a number of investigators of the somatosensory system have agreed that it would be better to call WDR cells 'multireceptive' and to specify the nature of the convergent inputs onto a particular neuron (Brown and Rethelyi, 1981).

One of the difficulties of defining response categories of somatosensory neurons is that few laboratories have tried to provide a quantitative description of the characteristic of these cells. LeBars and Chitour (1983) state that 'convergent' cells in the rat spinal cord can usually be activated better by innocuous mechanical stimuli than by noxious heat stimuli, although they respond in an incrementing fashion to graded noxious heat

stimuli. Others define WDR ('multireceptive') cells as those that respond to some extent to innocuous stimuli but best to the most intense stimuli (Chung et al., 1979). However, these descriptions are at best semiquantitative.

Recently, our laboratory has employed multivariate statistical techniques for classifying cells of the primate spinothalamic tract (STT) on the basis of their responses to mechanical and thermal stimuli (Chung et al., 1986; Surmeier et al., 1986a,b). A similar approach has also proven useful for dorsal horn interneurons (Sorkin et al., 1986), and cells of the lateral cervical nucleus and nucleus gracilis (Willis et al., 1987), as well as the ventral posterior lateral nucleus of the thalamus (Chung et al., 1986). Although nociceptors provide an input to most of the classes of these somatosen-

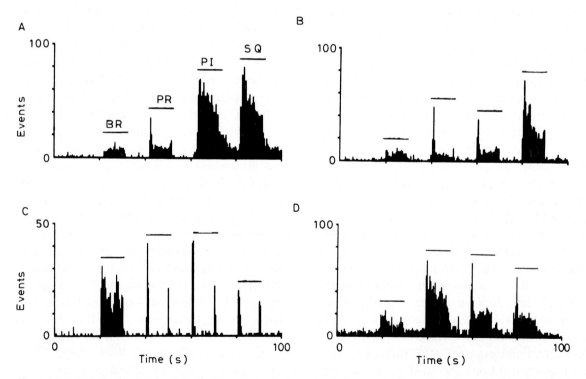

Fig. 3. Responses of primate spinothalamic tract (STT) cells belonging to four different response classes based on an analysis using a multivariate statistical (k means cluster) analysis. Most STT cells are in the classes represented in (A) or (B), which have a dominant input from nociceptors. Some STT cells, such as the one whose responses are shown in (C), belong to a primarily tactile category. Others belong to a group that commonly has no clearly dominant input, although that illustrated in (D) may have received a prominent input from slowly adapting mechanoreceptors. The stimuli used (BR, brush; PR, pressure; PI, pinch; SQ, squeeze) have been described in the legend of Fig. 1.

sory cells that can be recognized on statistical grounds, two classes of STT cells appear to be activated primarily by noxious stimuli (Fig. 3, A and B). Both nociceptive classes generally respond weakly to innocuous stimuli, such as brushing, and to marginally painful stimuli, such as compressing the skin with a large arterial clip. However, cells of one class have a steep stimulus-response curve with respect to intermediate and high-intensity noxious mechanical and thermal stimuli, whereas the other class has a higher threshold and shows a steep stimulus-response curve only for very intense stimuli (Chung et al., 1986; Surmeier et al., 1986b). It was proposed that the cells with a steep input-output curve and lower threshold might serve as an 'early warning system' for painful stimuli and that the higher threshold group might signal damage (Surmeier et al., 1986b).

At least two other classes of STT cells were recognized (Fig, 3, C and D). One of these had a dominant input from rapidly adapting mechanoreceptors (Fig. 3, C). The other had a convergent input from many types of receptors, and it was difficult to determine what was the dominant input (although it may have been slowly adapting mechanoreceptors for the case shown in Fig. 3, D). Left out of consideration in Fig. 3 is the input to STT cells from muscle receptors. Foreman et al. (1979a,b) showed that many STT cells receive an input from large and small muscle afferents. A similar finding has been reported by Kniffki et al. (1977) for SCT cells.

If much of the input to STT cells from muscle, along with that from cutaneous mechanoreceptors, is considered to represent an FRA input, then the scheme of Lundberg et al. (1987) might be inter-

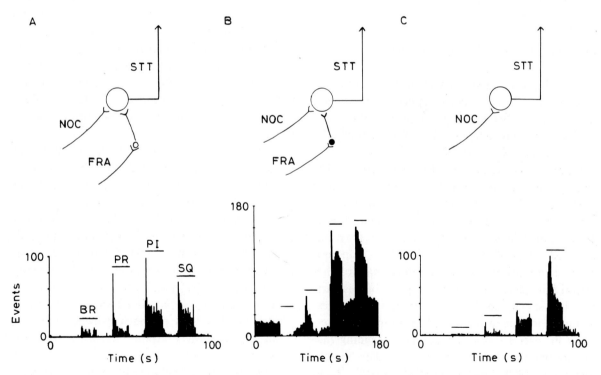

Fig. 4. Interpretation of responses of STT cells in the framework of the FRA hypothesis of Lundberg et al. (1987). In (A) is shown a circuit arrangement in which an STT cell receives a dominant input from nociceptors (NOC.), and an excitatory polysynaptic convergent input from the FRA. The histogram shows the activity of an STT cell that could be interpreted to belong to such a circuit. In (B), the STT cell receives an excitatory input from nociceptors and an inhibitory one from the FRA. In (C), the STT cell receives a purely nociceptive input.

preted with respect to the STT in the way shown in Fig. 4. The dominant and specific primary afferent input to most STT cells would be from nociceptors. Many of the STT cells also receive a convergent input from the FRA that would facilitate the activity of these cells during active movements (Fig. 4, A), whereas other STT cells receive only a nociceptive input and hence would signal nociceptive input in the same way regardless of a concurrent movement (Fig. 4, C). Some STT cells are inhibited by mechanoreceptor input (Fig. 4, B). These appear to be more common in the thoracic and sacral cord than in the lumbar enlargement (Blair et al., 1981; Milne et al., 1981) and may represent the third of the arrangements proposed by Lundberg et al. (1987). This application of the concept of Lundberg et al. (1987) to nociceptive pathways has a strong appeal given the well-recognized aggravation of pain by reflex activity and movement.

Locations of nociceptive spinal neurons

Since 1970, nociceptive-specific and WDR ('multireceptive') cells have been found to be widely distributed in the spinal cord gray matter, including not only lamina I but also laminae II, IV – VIII, and X (reviewed in Willis, 1985).

Parallel studies have revealed that many of the cells giving rise to ascending sensory tracts are nociceptive. The proportion of nociceptive neurons varies with the particular tract (Willis et al., 1987). Ascending tracts that seem to play an especially important role in signalling pain are those whose axons are in the ventral part of the lateral funiculus, since the interruption of this part of the spinal cord by cordotomy produces analgesia in humans and a reduction in pain reactivity in several species of animals, including the rat and monkey (White and Sweet, 1969; Vierck and Luck, 1979; Peschanski et al., 1986). These pathways include the spinothalamic, spinoreticular and spinomesencephalic tracts. All have substantial nociceptive components (see Willis, 1985). It has recently been demonstrated that spinothalamic

tract neurons of lamina I have axons that ascend in the dorsal part of the lateral funiculus (Jones et al., 1987). Most lamina I spinothalamic tract cells are nociceptive (Craig and Kniffki, 1985; Ferrington et al., 1987). Other pathways ascending in the dorsal part of the spinal cord that have a nociceptive component include the spinocervical tract, the postsynaptic dorsal column pathway (Willis, 1985), and the lamina I component of the spinomesencephalic tract (Hylden et al., 1986).

Cells of origin of one or more of these sensory tracts can be found in all of the laminae that contain nociceptive neurons (Willis, 1985).

Tonic descending inhibition

Flexion reflex

Some of the experimental work on the flexion reflex has been summarized previously (Willis, 1982). There are at least two forms of flexion reflex: one is a component of rhythmic motor behaviors, such as locomotion, and the other is the flexor withdrawal reflex, a nociceptive reaction (Sherrington, 1910). Unfortunately, most modern investigations do not make a clear distinction between these.

Both forms of the flexion reflex have been found to be subject to tonic inhibition by pathways descending from the brain stem. Sherrington and Sowton (1915) first demonstrated that the flexion reflex is under tonic inhibitory control by the brain stem. They found that the flexion reflex in a limb evoked by electrical stimulation of a peripheral nerve in a decerebrate cat is enhanced following transection of the spinal cord. Presumably the reflex was analogous to a flexor withdrawal reflex. Liddell et al. (1932) provided evidence that the brain stem pathways responsible for the tonic inhibition of the flexor withdrawal reflex in the cat descend primarily ipsilaterally in both the dorsolateral and ventral white matter. They presumed that the pathways interrupted included both reticulospinal and vestibulospinal tracts. However, Holmqvist and Lundberg (1959) showed that the inhibitory fibers affecting the FRA pathways descend bilaterally in the dorsal part of the lateral funiculi. Neither the cerebellum nor the vestibular nuclei contributed to the tonic inhibition of the FRA paths. A tonic inhibitory system was found to affect not only the flexion reflexes in limbs but also other forms of the flexion reflex, such as the tail flick reflex in the rat, which is a nociceptive reflex that is increased following spinal transection (Irwin et al., 1951). An analysis of many of the details of the flexion reflexes of the hindlimb in decerebrate and spinalized preparations using monosynaptic reflex testing can be found in papers by R.M. Eccles and Lundberg (1959b) and Kuno and Perl (1960).

The brain-stem centers responsible for the tonic descending inhibition of the flexion reflex evoked by the FRA were examined in ablation experiments by Holmqvist and Lundberg (1961). They found that the inhibitory system could be interrupted by lesions in the medial part of the brain stem. There was independent control of the FRA pathways to flexor and extensor muscles, since release of inhibition of extensors occurred after a low pontine lesion, whereas release of excitation of flexors required a lesion in the caudal medulla. Inhibition of flexor motoneurons was enhanced after low pontine lesions. Engberg et al. (1968a) made extensive lesions of the pontine and medullary raphe and found that the inhibition was only partly eliminated (mainly that affecting inhibitory pathways to extensor motoneurons), indicating that at least a component of tonic descending inhibition is produced by neurons located lateral to the raphe.

Lundberg's group also examined the source of the inhibition of the reflex pathways receiving input from the FRA by experiments using focal electrical stimulation of the brain stem. Inhibition of the reflex actions of the FRA resulted from stimulation within the nucleus raphe magnus and the magnocellular part of the nucleus reticularis gigantocellularis (Engberg et al., 1968b). The axons responsible for the inhibitory actions descended in the dorsal part of the lateral funiculus, and the inhibitory system was named the 'dorsal

reticulospinal system', since no anatomical substrate for a direct reticulospinal pathway descending in the dorsolateral funiculus was known at that time. It should be noted that in these experiments the spinal cord was interrupted except for the dorsal quadrant contralateral to the side tested and the stimulus strength was kept low in order to confine the inhibitory actions to interneuronal pathways. The inhibition was attributed to inhibitory postsynaptic potentials that could be recorded from at least some interneurons in the flexion reflex pathways in response to stimulation in the medial brain stem or of the dorsolateral funiculus (Engberg et al., 1968c).

When only one ventral quadrant of the spinal cord was left intact, inhibitory actions conveyed by ventral pathways could also be produced by stimulation in the same region of the brain stem, but in this case the inhibition affected motoneurons directly (Jankowska et al., 1968). Both dorsal and ventral pathways can also produce primary afferent depolarization of large muscle and cutaneous afferent fibers (Carpenter et al., 1966; Engberg et al., 1968b).

Tonic descending inhibition of nociceptive spinal cord neurons

A very useful method for producing a reversible cold block of tonic descending inhibition was introduced by Brown (1971). A number of investigators have demonstrated the presence of tonic descending inhibition of nociceptive spinal cord interneurons using cold block or spinal cord lesions. The locations of the recording sites for the nociceptive neurons examined have included lamina I (Cervero et al., 1976; Necker and Hellon, 1978) and IV – VI (Wall, 1967; Hillman and Wall, 1969; Besson et al., 1975; Handwerker et al., 1975; Duggan et al., 1977, 1981).

Cervero et al. (1979) found that neurons of the substantia gelatinosa are not subject to tonic descending inhibition. These interneurons could be inhibited phasically by stimulation of the dorsolateral funiculus, and it was suggested that inhibitory interneurons of lamina II might mediate tonic inhibition of dorsal horn neurons in other laminae.

Holmqvist et al. (1960) showed that there is tonic descending inhibition of several ascending tracts by recordings of mass discharges from the spinal cord white matter before and during cold block of the dorsal part of the lateral funiculus. Brown (1971) reported that cold block of the spinal cord at a thoracic level enhanced the responses of SCT cells to peripheral stimuli, some of which became clearly nociceptive. Cervero et al. (1977) found that most SCT cells (84%) respond in some fashion, by excitation or inhibition or both, to noxious stimuli during cold block of the cord (Fig. 5).

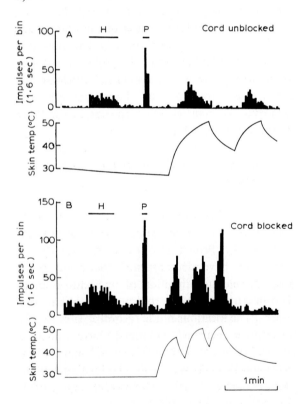

Fig. 5. Responses of a spinocervical tract (SCT) neuron to mechanical and thermal stimuli before and during cold block of tonic descending inhibitory pathways. In (A), the responses to hair movement (H), pressure (P) and noxious heating are seen with the cord unblocked and in (B) with the cord blocked. (From Cervero et al. 1977.)

Apart from this work on the SCT, it is not certain how widespread the tonic control of nociceptive ascending tracts is. Some evidence that STT cells are tonically inhibited has been reported (Willis et al., 1977; Hori et al., 1984), but so far reversible cold block has not been done while recordings have been made from these neurons. One problem with such experiments is that STT cells cannot be identified with certainty in decerebrate animals, and tonic descending inhibition is less pronounced in anesthetized animals than in decerebrate, unanesthetized ones.

Source of tonic descending inhibition of nociceptive dorsal horn neurons

Lesions of the pontine and medullary raphe do not eliminate or even reduce tonic descending inhibition of nociceptive dorsal horn neurons (Hall et al., 1981, 1982; see Duggan, this volume). Nor do lesions of the periaqueductal gray, nucleus reticularis gigantocellularis, paramedian reticular nucleus, inferior olivary nucleus or several cranial nerve nuclei (Hall et al., 1982). On the other hand, tonic descending inhibition of nociceptive dorsal horn neurons can be eliminated by bilateral lesions of the ventrolateral medulla in the region of the lateral reticular nucleus (Fig. 6; Hall et al., 1982; Morton et al., 1983). Lesions just rostral or medial to this area had no effect, suggesting that the cells responsible for the tonic inhibition were destroyed by the lesions, rather than a descending pathway. However, these lesions were not complete enough to rule this possibility out. Hall et al. (1982) point out that their experiments differ from those of Engberg et al. (1968a) in which a lesion of the medullary raphe decreased (but did not eliminate) tonic descending inhibition of the FRA pathways, since the tonic inhibition from the region of the lateral reticular nucleus was tested using responses to volleys in C fibers, whereas the FRA are myelinated axons. However, the FRA may also include unmyelinated axons (Lundberg, personal communication). Stimulation in the same region of the lateral medulla caused a potent and selective in-

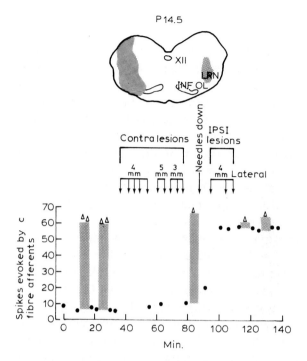

Fig. 6. Elimination of tonic descending inhibition of a nociceptive dorsal horn neuron by lesions placed in the ventrolateral medulla. The locations of the lesions are shown in the drawing of a transverse section of the medulla of a cat just caudal to the obex. The graph shows the number of spikes in the responses of a dorsal horn neuron to volleys in C fibers of a peripheral nerve before any lesions, after several lesions of the contralateral medulla, and after additional lesions of the ipsilateral medulla. The hatched vertical bars indicate tests for tonic descending inhibition by blocking the cord with cold. When the inhibitory path was blocked, the responses to C fiber volleys were enhanced initially. Bilateral lesions of the ventral lateral medulla enhanced the responses to C fiber volleys and occluded the effects of cold block. (From Hall et al., 1982.)

jections of a GABA agonist to inhibit neuronal cell bodies were employed to localize the inhibitory neurons to an area just ventral to the facial nucleus. It was concluded that the elimination of tonic descending inhibition by more caudal lesions was in fact due to interruption of descending projections.

Tonic descending inhibition in awake animals

Recent experiments done on awake, behaving cats show a paucity of spontaneous activity in dorsal horn neurons (Sorkin, 1983; Collins, 1984). However, this does not appear to be due to the presence of tonic descending inhibition, since spinal cord transection does not enhance the spontaneous activity (Collins et al., 1987). However, WDR ('multireceptive') neurons are much less common in awake, behaving cats than in either barbiturate anesthetized or spinal cord transected animals (Collins and Ren, 1987; Collins et al., 1987), suggesting that tonic descending inhibition suppresses nociceptive responses of dorsal horn neurons in awake, behaving animals and that this inhibition is prevented by anesthesia as well as by interruption of descending inhibitory pathways (cf., also Frank and Ohta, 1971 and Mori et al., 1981).

Effect of tonic descending inhibition on intensity coding

The stimulus-response curves of dorsal horn neurons to graded noxious heat stimuli were generally found to undergo a parallel shift (change in set point or threshold), rather than a change in slope (change in gain) following cold block of the spinal cord (Dickhaus et al., 1985). This type of change resembled that produced by stimulation within the lateral midbrain reticular formation (and also nucleus raphe magnus and medullary reticular formation; Gebhart et al., 1983a,b) rather than in the periaqueductal gray (PAG) (Carstens et al., 1980a), supporting the hypothesis that tonic descending inhibition of nociceptive dorsal horn

hibition of the responses of dorsal horn neurons to C-fiber input (Morton et al., 1983). Perhaps the tonic descending inhibition of the nociceptive withdrawal reflex originates from this same lateral reticular area.

Recently, Foong and Duggan (1986) did further lesioning experiments and found evidence that tonic inhibition might in fact originate further rostrally at a level between the facial nucleus and the middle of the inferior olivary nucleus. Microin-

neurons may originate from a separate population of neurons than the system involving the PAG (see above).

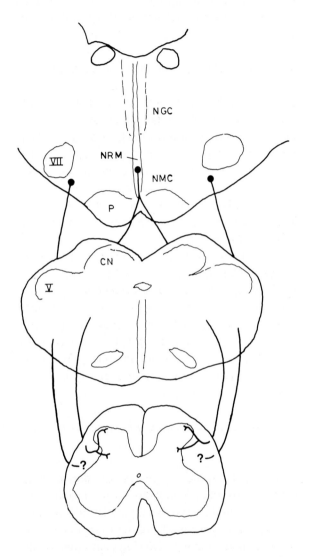

Fig. 7. Schematic diagram showing some of the sources of tonic descending inhibition. The NRM (and presumably adjacent reticular formation) contributes to the tonic inhibitory control of FRA pathways. The NRM projects bilaterally dorsal to the inferior olivary nuclei, through the region of the lateral reticular nuclei, and caudally through the dorsolateral funiculi. Some of the endings are in laminae I and V, as shown. Tonic descending inhibition of nociceptive dorsal horn neurons appears to arise from neurons in the vicinity of the facial nuclei.

Comment

The experiments by Lundberg's and Duggan's groups on tonic descending inhibition suggest that there may be separate control systems for FRA and for nociceptive pathways. The anatomical bases of these systems are incompletely understood, but evidently at least part of the FRA control system involves the region of the raphe, whereas the nociceptive control system involves the ventral lateral medulla (Fig. 7). Both of these systems are likely to be important for the control of pain, if the model suggested in Fig. 4 is correct. According to this model the FRA would facilitate activity in nociceptive neurons during reflex activity and movements, and so inhibition of FRA pathways by the control system originating from the raphe and vicinity would reduce the total excitatory drive on-to nociceptive neurons with a convergent FRA input. Inhibition of nociceptive input by the system originating in the ventral lateral medulla would, of course, also contribute to pain relief, but in a more direct fashion by interfering with the specific input from nociceptors. It is of interest that both pathways traverse the same region in the caudal ventral lateral medulla, since the nucleus raphe magnus (NRM) projection to the spinal cord passes laterally over the inferior olivary nucleus and then caudally adjacent to the lateral reticular nucleus (Fig. 7; Basbaum et al., 1978).

Stimulation-evoked inhibition of nociceptive transmission

Flexion reflex

As discussed earlier, the flexor withdrawal reflex is one of a number of pain reactions. There is often a correspondence between the presence of a nociceptive flexion reflex in humans and the perception of pain (Willer, 1977), although the two can be dissociated (Willer et al., 1979). The most dramatic dissociation results from spinal cord transection, which increases the tail flick reflex in the rat (Irwin et al., 1951) while obviously eliminating pain sensation. Willer (1977) can also record a short latency flexion reflex in humans in response to lower intensity stimulation that is associated with a tactile sensation and not with pain. Presumably this flexion reflex can be attributed to the FRA.

Nociceptive flexion reflexes have often been used to test for stimulation-produced analgesia (see Oliveras, this volume). Here, emphasis will be placed on the use of the flexor withdrawal reflex as a test of stimulation-evoked inhibition of nociceptive transmission.

Iwamoto et al. (1980), using an anesthetized cat preparation, found that stimulation in the NRM (or nucleus raphe obscurus) could inhibit the nociceptive flexion reflex evoked by volleys in C fibers of a cutaneous nerve. The tail flick reflex of the rat has also been shown to be powerfully inhibited in anesthetized animals by stimulation in the NRM (Zorman et al., 1981). A calculation has been made that direct activation of only some 30 neurons in the NRM can completely eliminate the tail flick response (Hentall et al., 1984).

A systematic mapping study in lightly anesthetized rats by Sandkuhler and Gebhart (1984) has shown that the tail flick reflex can be inhibited from sites in several areas of the midbrain and medulla, including not only the PAG and NRM, but also the nucleus cuneiformis, substantia nigra, red nucleus, central midbrain tegmentum, nucleus reticularis gigantocellularis, and nucleus paragigantocellularis (Fig. 8). Gebhart and Ossipov (1986) added the lateral reticular nucleus of the ventral caudal medulla to this list.

A reduction in a flexor withdrawal reflex can in principle be produced by any combination of the following: (1) postsynaptic inhibition of flexor motoneurons, (2) presynaptic inhibition of nociceptive primary afferent fibers, (3) postsynaptic inhibition of interneurons in the flexion reflex pathway, (4) presynaptic inhibition of the terminals of interneurons in the flexion reflex path. Nothing can be said about the last mechanism, since this possibility has not been investigated. The others will be discussed in turn.

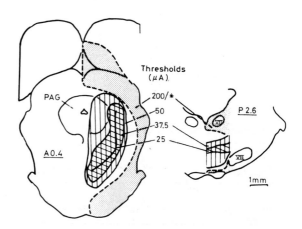

Fig. 8. Distribution of some of the sites within the midbrain (left) and rostral medulla (right) which when stimulated cause inhibition of the tail flick reflex in lightly anesthetized animals. (From Sandkuhler and Gebhart, 1984.)

Postsynaptic inhibition of flexor motoneurons

As mentioned earlier, Jankowska et al. (1968) showed that stimulation in the nucleus raphe magnus and adjacent nucleus reticularis magnocellularis caused postsynaptic inhibition of flexor (and also extensor) motoneurons (Fig. 9). They suggested that this region corresponds to Magoun's inhibitory center (Magoun and Rhines, 1946). Postsynaptic inhibition was demonstrated by intracellular recordings of inhibitory postsynaptic potentials (IPSPs) and by an increase in membrane conductance following repetitive stimulation in the medial medulla.

It appears that no studies have been done to determine if stimulation at other sites evoking stimulation-produced analgesia (SPA) have a postsynaptic inhibitory action on motoneurons. In the case of the tail flick reflex, little is known of the details of the reflex pathway. Recordings have recently been made from axons of some of the motoneurons responsible for the tail flick (Cargill et al., 1985), but no intracellular recordings have been made to date from these cells. Therefore, the role of postsynaptic inhibition of tail flick motoneurons in the powerful suppression of the tail flick reflex following stimulation in the nucleus

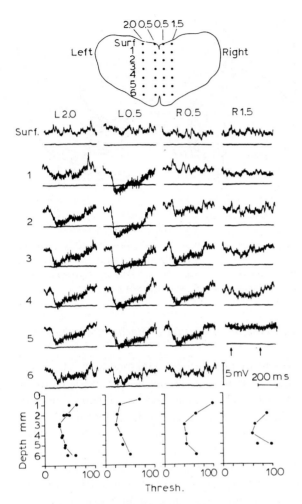

Fig. 9. Sites within the medial medulla that evoke inhibitory postsynaptic potentials (IPSPs) in motoneurons of the lumbar spinal cord. The drawing shows a grid of stimulus sites, and the recordings show motoneuron membrane potential changes resulting from stimulation of corresponding points within the grid. Thresholds for evoking IPSPs at different locations are shown by the graphs below. (From Jankowska et al., 1968.)

raphe magnus (Zorman et al., 1981; Hentall et al., 1984), the PAG or other sites (Sandkuhler and Gebhart, 1984), is unknown.

Presynaptic inhibition of nociceptive afferent fibers

Presynaptic inhibition in mammals has been studied in detail only with respect to group Ia af-

ferent fibers (Eccles, 1964; Schmidt, 1971). The evidence to date indicates that presynaptic inhibition involves a reduction in the release of synaptic transmitter from presynaptic terminals as a result of their depolarization by interneuronal pathways. The exact biophysical mechanism by which depolarization reduces transmitter release is still unclear. Nevertheless, there is an association between depolarization of synaptic terminals and presynaptic inhibition. With respect to primary afferent fibers, this depolarization (called 'primary afferent depolarization' or PAD) can be detected in any of several ways. Populations of terminals may produce positive field potentials that can be recorded from the dorsal surface of the spinal cord and a slow negative potential that can be recorded from the dorsal root. These events reflect chiefly PAD of large axons, since these produce the largest extracellular currents. Other methods that can be used to detect PAD include excitability testing and intrafiber recording. The latter is useful only for afferent fibers large enough to be impaled by a microelectrode (dorsal root ganglion cells are at too great an electrotonic distance from the afferent terminals to make recordings of PAD from these feasible). Excitability testing can be used for the analysis of PAD in populations of primary afferent fibers or in individual fibers. The general presumption is that an increase in excitability of the preterminals of an afferent fiber reflects PAD. Conversely, a reduction in excitability may indicate primary afferent hyperpolarization (PAH); alternatively, terminal excitability could be lowered by an increased membrane conductance without a shift in membrane potential.

As mentioned earlier, stimulation in the medullary reticular formation can produce PAD in large myelinated axons (Carpenter et al., 1966; Engberg et al., 1968b). In addition, Martin et al. (1979) have shown by excitability testing that stimulation in either the nucleus raphe magnus (NRM) or nucleus reticularis gigantocellularis (NGc) produces PAD in both large cutaneous mechanoreceptor afferents and in Aδ fibers, including mechanical nociceptors (Fig. 10, I). This

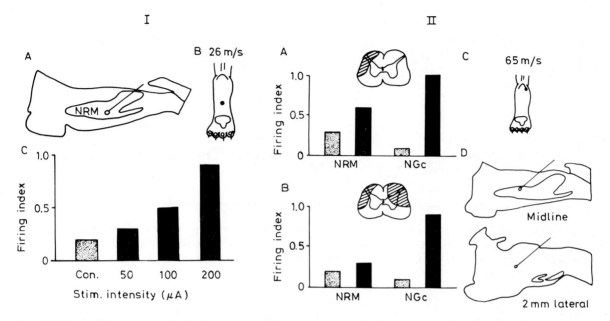

Fig. 10. Primary afferent depolarization of cutaneous afferents evoked by stimulation in the medial medulla. In (I), stimulation in the NRM increased the excitability of an Aδ mechanical nociceptor. The stimulus site is shown in (A), the receptive field and conduction velocity of the afferent in (B), and the firing index for control responses (hatched bar) and following conditioning stimulation in the NRM at several different intensities in (C) (black bars). In (II), the excitability increases produced in an Aβ afferent fiber from stimulation in the NRM and nucleus gigantocellularis (NGc) are shown in (A) after a lesion of one dorsolateral funiculus and in (B) after bilateral lesions. Note that the effect from the NRM is markedly reduced while that from the NGc is unchanged. (C) shows the receptive field and conduction velocity of the afferent fiber and (D) the stimulation sites. (From Martin et al., 1979.)

was true in both the cat and the monkey. PAD from stimulation in the cat NRM was blocked by lesions of the dorsolateral funiculus bilaterally, whereas PAD from stimulation in the NGc persisted after such lesions (Fig. 10, II).

The terminals of single nociceptive afferent C fibers have also been tested for excitability changes in response to stimulation in the NRM (Hentall and Fields, 1979). Both C polymodal and C high threshold mechanoreceptors (as well as C mechanoreceptors) showed an increased threshold due to stimulation in the NRM (Fig. 11). Since NRM stimulation reduces the responses of spinal cord neurons to volleys in C fibers, it was suggested that this change might reflect either presynaptic inhibition due to an increased conductance in the terminal (without depolarization) or a presynaptic facilitation of input to inhibitory interneurons.

Interestingly, there is a reduction in terminal excitability of C fibers when the spinal cord is transected or blocked by cold (Calvillo et al., 1982). Apparently, there is a tonic descending control system affecting C fibers, and this may act by producing a maintained depolarization of the terminals of these afferents; presumably this would result in tonic presynaptic inhibition of C fiber pathways. This observation is not inconsistent with the report by Hentall and Fields (1979), since tonic inhibition of C fiber pathways presumably originates from the lateral medulla (Hall et al., 1981, 1982), rather than from the NRM.

Inhibition of nociceptive dorsal horn interneurons

As pointed out earlier, none of the many studies of brain stem inhibition of nociceptive dorsal horn neurons have demonstrated whether the neurons

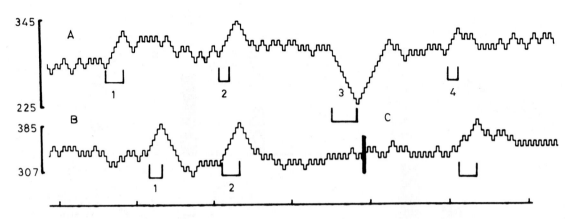

Fig. 11. Modulation of presynaptic excitability of C fibers by stimulation in the NRM. The vertical axis shows thresholds for antidromic activation of single C fibers. The fiber in (A) was a C mechanoreceptor, and those in (B) and (C) were C polymodal nociceptors. Stimulation in the NRM at 1, 2 and 4 in (A), at 1 in (B) and at the bracket in (C) caused an elevation in C fiber thresholds. (From Hentall and Fields, 1979.)

belong to reflex or sensory pathways. Such a detailed demonstration has been attempted with respect to only a few types of spinal interneurons involved in motor control, such as group I interneurons (e.g., Jankowska and Roberts, 1972a,b; Jankowska and Lindstrom, 1972). Since descending controls can operate independently on the nociceptive flexion reflex and on pain (Willer et al., 1979), it cannot be assumed that inhibition of a given interneuron would affect both motor and sensory transmission.

Nucleus raphe magnus and periaqueductal gray

The earliest study of inhibition of nociceptive dorsal horn neurons that was related to 'analgesia' systems was concerned with the effects of stimulation in the PAG in the cat (Liebeskind et al., 1973; Oliveras et al., 1974). The inhibition affected chiefly WDR ('multireceptive') neurons, although some neurons responsive just to innocuous mechanical stimuli were also inhibited. A specifically inhibitory system seemed to be involved, since PAG stimulation produced excitation of less than 5% of the interneurons examined.

The Besson group soon extended their investigation of descending 'analgesia' systems to the NRM and showed that stimulation in the NRM causes inhibition of nociceptive dorsal horn neurons (Guilbaud et al., 1977). Fields et al. (1977) demonstrated comparable effects. Both groups found that the inhibitory actions were most apparent for WDR ('multireceptive') neurons, and Fields et al. also observed inhibition of high threshold cells of lamina I. Tactile and proprioceptive neurons were less likely to be affected. Inhibition was considerably reduced after a lesion of the ipsilateral dorsolateral funiculus (Fields et al., 1977), indicating that the main inhibitory pathway descends on the ipsilateral side. However, in a recent report Sandkuhler et al. (1987) conclude, based on experiments using lidocaine blocks of different parts of the spinal cord white matter, that the inhibition produced by NRM stimulation depends chiefly on the contralateral rather than on the ipsilateral dorsolateral funiculus.

Numerous reports have confirmed a predominantly inhibitory action of stimulation in the PAG and NRM on nociceptive dorsal horn interneurons, although inhibition of other types of interneurons and excitatory actions have also been seen (Willis et al., 1977; Belcher et al., 1978; Bennett and Mayer, 1979; Carstens et al., 1979, 1980a,b, 1981; Duggan and Griersmith, 1979;

Rivot et al., 1980; Griffith and Gatipon, 1981; Edeson and Ryall, 1983; Gebhart et al., 1983a; Gray and Dostrovsky, 1983; Morton et al., 1984; Mokha et al., 1985; Light et al., 1986).

Duggan and Griersmith (1979) found that the inhibition of WDR ('multireceptive') cells in the nucleus proprius from the PAG was unselective (see also Carstens et al., 1980a), whereas that from the NRM reduced responses to noxious but not to tactile stimuli. However, Carstens et al. (1981) observed that PAG stimulation had at least partially specific effects in that nociceptive responses were inhibited more powerfully than were responses to innocuous stimuli. Light et al. (1986) recorded intracellularly from neurons in laminae I and II and found that stimulation in the NRM or in PAG often produced inhibitory postsynaptic potentials (IPSPs) in nociceptive-specific neurons and either IPSPs or excitatory postsynaptic potentials (EPSPs) followed by IPSPs in many WDR ('multireceptive') neurons (Fig. 12). Low threshold cells were more often excited than were nociceptive neurons. The difference from the study of Duggan and Griersmith (1979) was suggested by Light et al. (1986) to be due to the location of the population of neurons sampled (or possibly to technical differences).

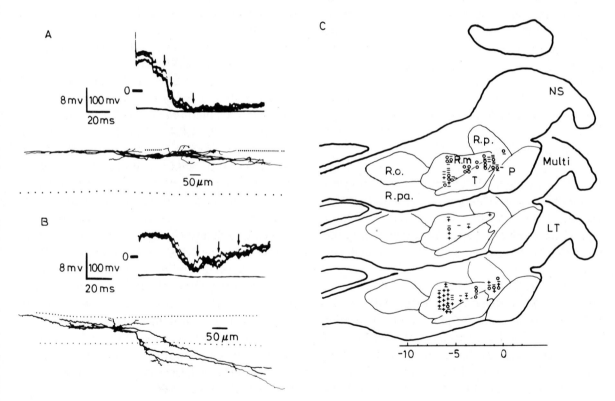

Fig. 12. Inhibitory postsynaptic potentials (IPSPs) generated in nociceptive dorsal horn neurons following stimulation in the nucleus raphe magnus. In (A) is an IPSP that was recorded from a WDR ('multireceptive') cell in lamina I. Arrows indicate successive increments in the IPSP. The cell was injected with horseradish peroxidase, and the drawing shows its appearance after histological reconstruction. (B) shows a similar IPSP recorded from a nociceptive-specific neuron in lamina II; the reconstructed cell is shown below. The drawings of midsagittal sections of the lower brain stem in (C) show sites within the raphe complex from which IPSPs (−), excitatory postsynaptic potentials followed by IPSPs (+) or no effect (○) were produced in dorsal horn neurons of the nociceptive-specific (NS), multireceptive (Multi) or low threshold (LT) varieties. Abbreviations: P, pons; R.m., raphe magnus; R.p., raphe pontis; R.pa., raphe pallidus; R.o., raphe obscurus; T, trapezoid body. (From Light et al., 1986.)

Other inhibitory sites

Areas of the brain stem besides the PAG and NRM that when stimulated produce inhibition of nociceptive dorsal horn neurons include the region of the lateral reticular nucleus (Morton et al., 1983), the nucleus reticularis magnocellularis and lateral tegmental field in the cat medulla (Edeson and Ryall, 1983), the lateral midbrain reticular formation (Carstens et al., 1980b), the locus coeruleus region (Hodge et al., 1981, 1983; Mokha et al., 1985, 1986; Jones and Gebhart, 1986), including the Kölliker-Fuse nucleus (Hodge et al., 1986), and the anterior pretectal nucleus (Rees and Roberts, 1987). In addition, a number of diencephalic and telencephalic sites, such as the hypothalamus (Carstens, 1982) and medial preoptic and septal regions (Carstens et al., 1982) have been shown to be effective sites for stimulation-evoked inhibition of nociceptive dorsal horn neurons.

Inhibition of identified ascending tract cells

Spinothalamic tract

The STT is thought to be one of the main pathways responsible for mediating pain sensation (White and Sweet, 1969; Willis, 1985). Therefore, inhibition of nociceptive STT cells by stimulation in the brain stem would presumably reflect an analgesic action.

Nociceptive STT cells are inhibited by stimulation in the NRM (Beall et al., 1976; Willis et al., 1977; McCreery et al., 1979; Gerhart et al., 1981a; Giesler et al., 1981a; Yezierski et al., 1982b; Ammons et al., 1984), medullary reticular formation (McCreery and Bloedel, 1975; Haber et al., 1978, 1980; McCreery et al., 1979; Gerhart et al., 1981a), periaqueductal gray and adjacent midbrain reticular formation (Hayes et al., 1979; Gerhart et al., 1984), subcoeruleus-parabrachial region (Girardot et al., 1987), periventricular gray (Ammons et al., 1986) and ventrobasal complex of the thalamus (Gerhart et al., 1981b, 1983).

Stimulation in the NRM produces inhibition of WDR ('multireceptive') and nociceptive-specific STT cells; inhibition is seen of STT cells in lamina I and in laminae IV – VI (Beall et al., 1976; Willis et al., 1977; Gerhart et al., 1981a; Ammons et al., 1984). The responses of WDR ('multireceptive') STT cells to both innocuous and noxious cutaneous stimuli are generally inhibited from the NRM, although the inhibition is sometimes selective for responses to noxious stimuli (Gerhart et al., 1981a; Ammons et al., 1984). Inhibition of responses of STT cells to volleys in C fibers is more powerful than of responses to A fibers (Gerhart et al., 1981a; Ammons et al., 1984) and of responses to volleys in Aδ fibers than in Aβ fibers (Willis et al., 1977). Responses to visceral stimuli, as well as to somatic ones, are inhibited by NRM stimulation (Fig. 13; Ammons et al., 1984). Excitation of primate STT cells following NRM stimulation has rarely been observed (Willis et al., 1977; Gerhart et al., 1981a; Ammons et al., 1984), although NRM stimulation often produced a transient excitation (followed by inhibition) of STT cells in the cat (McCreery et al., 1979). NRM inhibition of STT cells depends largely on pathways descending in the dorsolateral funiculi (Willis et al., 1977), although some inhibition can be demonstrated even after bilateral dorsolateral funiculus lesions (McCreery et al., 1979; Gerhart et al., 1984).

Several mechanisms can be proposed for the inhibition from the NRM. Stimulation in the NRM often produces inhibitory postsynaptic potentials in STT cells (Giesler et al., 1981a). In addition, as mentioned earlier, NRM stimulation results in PAD in Aδ mechanical nociceptors (Martin et al., 1979) and exerts presynaptic control of C nociceptors (Hentall and Fields, 1979). Another possibility is inhibition of interneurons in polysynaptic excitatory pathways to STT cells.

Inhibition of STT cells is also produced by stimulation in the medullary reticular formation (McCreery and Bloedel, 1975; McCreery et al., 1979; Haber et al., 1979, 1980; Gerhart et al., 1981a). The inhibition could be produced by stimulation on either side of the midline. Responses to innocuous and noxious stimuli were

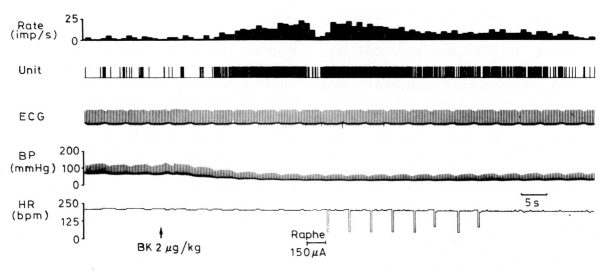

Fig. 13. Inhibition of a primate spinothalamic tract (STT) neuron activated by stimulation of visceral receptors of the heart with bradykinin. The firing rate of the STT cell is shown in the upper histogram and in the chart recording below it. The electrocardiogram (ECG), systemic blood pressure (BP) and heart rate (HR) records are also shown. Bradykinin (BK) was injected into the right atrium at the time indicated by the arrow, and stimulation in the raphe magnus nucleus was done at the time shown by the bar. (From Ammons et al., 1984.)

reduced in a non-selective fashion, but the inhibition reduced responses to volleys in C fibers more than to those in A fibers (Gerhart et al., 1981a) and to volleys in Aδ fibers than in Aβ fibers (Haber et al., 1980). An inhibitory 'wind-up' was sometimes seen with repetitive stimulation (Haber et al., 1980). Inhibition persisted following bilateral lesions of the dorsolateral funiculus, indicating that the inhibitory pathway descends in the ventral part of the cord (Haber et al., 1980; however, cf., McCreery et al., 1979, who stimulated more rostrally in the reticular formation).

Stimulation at some sites within the medullary reticular formation produces an excitation of primate STT cells projecting to the ventral posterior lateral nucleus of the thalamus (Haber et al., 1980). Presumably such excitation could contribute to the aversive responses that can be associated with stimulation in the reticular formation (Casey, 1971). In addition, it is conceivable that in pathological conditions excitatory pathways to STT cells might contribute to central pain (Cassinari and Pagni, 1969). With repetitive stimulation, wind-up of the excitation could be

seen (Haber et al., 1980). An excitatory point for one STT cell might produce inhibition of other STT cells, and so it was unclear what the anatomical difference was for the source of the different effects (Haber et al., 1980). The excitatory pathway, like the inhibitory one, descends in the ventral part of the spinal cord, since excitation persisted after bilateral lesions of the dorsolateral funiculus (Haber et al., 1980; however, cf., McCreery et al., 1979, who stimulated more rostrally in the reticular formation).

Reticular formation stimulation can also excite STT cells projecting to the central lateral nucleus (Giesler et al., 1981b). The excitation in this case contributes to the receptive fields of these cells, as shown by the reduction in receptive field size from the entire surface of the body and face to just the ipsilateral hindlimb following a lesion interrupting the spinal cord at an upper cervical level. A looping pathway from the spinal cord to the reticular formation and back to the spinal cord has also been shown to contribute to the receptive fields of spinal cord neurons responding to visceral input (Cervero and Wolstencroft, 1984).

STT cells could also be inhibited by stimulation in the PAG and adjacent midbrain reticular formation (Hayes et al., 1979; Gerhart et al., 1984). Both WDR ('multireceptive') and nociceptive-specific STT cells were inhibited, whether located in lamina I or in laminae IV – V. Usually, the inhibition of WDR cells was non-selective, reducing the responses to both innocuous and noxious stimuli; however, sometimes a selective inhibition of nociceptive responses was observed (Gerhart et al., 1984). The inhibition was more effective in reducing responses to volleys in C fibers than in A fibers. Bilateral lesions of the spinal cord white matter indicated that the inhibitory pathways descended in part in the dorsolateral funiculus. However, part of the inhibition was mediated through more ventral pathways.

Stimulation in the region of the subcoeruleus-parabrachial complex has recently been shown to produce inhibition of STT cells projecting from the upper thoracic spinal cord to either the ventral posterior lateral (VPL) nucleus, the CL nucleus or both (Girardot et al., 1987). Inhibition was found whether the STT cells were of the WDR ('multireceptive') or nociceptive-specific type and without regard to laminar location. Inhibition was found for responses to either innocuous or noxious stimuli.

Another inhibitory site affecting STT cells is the periventricular gray (Ammons et al., 1986). The most effective inhibitory loci were within 0.5 mm of the ventricle. The inhibited STT cells included ones that projected to the VPL nucleus, the CL nucleus or both, WDR ('multireceptive') and nociceptive-specific cells, and STT cells in laminae, I, IV – V and VII. Responses to innocuous and noxious cutaneous stimuli and to noxious stimulation of the heart (with bradykinin) were inhibited. Bilateral lesions of the dorsolateral funiculus did not change the inhibition.

Stimulation on either side in the ventral posterior lateral (VPL; and also ventral posterior medial) nucleus of the thalamus causes inhibition of STT cells (Gerhart et al., 1981b; 1983). Both WDR ('multireceptive') and nociceptive-specific cells are affected, and there is inhibition of responses to innocuous as well as noxious stimuli. Responses to volleys in C fibers were more affected than those to volleys in A fibers. The descending pathway appeared to be diffusely distributed in the spinal cord white matter. One explanation for the inhibition is antidromic activation of STT cells, with subsequent excitation of neurons in the medial brain stem that in turn produces inhibition in the spinal cord. Evidence in favor of this explanation is recordings of excitation of raphe-spinal neurons by stimulation in the VPL nucleus (Tsubokawa et al., 1981; Willis et al., 1984).

Spinocervicothalamic and dorsal column pathways

The spinocervicothalamic pathway, including SCT cells and cells of the lateral cervical nucleus, is unlikely to serve normally as a major pathway for pain in primates, including man, but it may contribute to pain sensation in cats (Brown and Franz, 1969; Cervero et al., 1977), and it is possible that nociceptive transmission in man could occur through this pathway in pathological states (Willis, 1985).

Stimulation in the brain stem has been shown to inhibit SCT cells (Taub, 1964), as has stimulation in the dorsolateral and ventral funiculi of the spinal cord (Brown et al., 1973). The NRM and PAG were found to inhibit non-nociceptive responses of SCT cells (Hong et al., 1979; Gray and Dostrovsky, 1983; Kajander et al., 1984) and of cells in the lateral cervical nucleus (LCN) (Dostrovsky, 1984). Dostrovsky (1984) also showed that stimulation in the nucleus gigantocellularis, nucleus magnocellularis and nucleus cuneiformis inhibited cells of the lateral cervical nucleus. Most of the inhibitory effects on LCN cells could have been indirect ones, mediated by reducing the responsiveness of SCT cells. NRM and PAG stimulation also inhibit the responses of neurons in the dorsal column nuclei to non-nociceptive stimulation (Dostrovsky, 1980; Gerhart et al., 1981a). Evidently, the descending 'analgesia' systems regulate transmission in a variety of somatosensory pathways, not just those related to pain.

Other somatosensory pathways

Little is known about the effects of brain stem stimulation on cells of the spinoreticular, spinomesencephalic, and postsynaptic dorsal column pathways, although some of the STT cells to which reference has already been made projected also to the reticular formation or midbrain. A recent abstract by Yezierski and McDonald (1986) indicates that spinomesencephalic tract cells are subject to complex descending controls.

Candidate descending pathways

Direct and indirect pathways and the fibers of passage problem

It would clearly be of great interest to know which pathways are responsible for tonic descending inhibition or are activated by stimulation in the brain stem at sites that result in inhibition or excitation of nociceptive spinal cord neurons. Identification of the responsible pathways could lead to identification of the neurotransmitters involved and possibly result in new strategies for therapeutic interventions. The pathways that are the easiest to investigate are the long tracts that directly connect the brain stem with the spinal cord. These can be readily studied with retrograde and anterograde tracing techniques, and neuroactive substances contained in these neurons can be identified by immunocytochemistry. However, it should be kept in mind that indirect pathways either through descending or ascending connections to other brain stem sites could mediate effects produced by stimulation at a particular location in the brain stem. Another major problem is that electrical stimulation can activate not only cell bodies in a particular nucleus but also fibers of passage originating from nuclei that may be quite distant from the one being stimulated. One way around

this problem is through chemical stimulation, such as microinjection of neurotransmitter or agonist, either excitatory or inhibitory, into a nucleus in order to activate or depress cell bodies specifically (e.g., Behbehani and Fields, 1979; Jones and Gebhart, 1986; Foong and Duggan, 1986).

Medial medulla and pons

The most prominent pathways originating in the medial part of the medulla and pons that are likely to contribute to the descending inhibitory (and excitatory) control of nociceptive spinal neurons include the raphe- and reticulospinal tracts. The cells of origin of these tracts have been mapped in retrograde labelling studies and include cells of the nuclei raphe magnus, pallidus and obscurus and nuclei reticularis gigantocellularis, magnocellularis and pontis caudalis (Carlton et al., 1985; Kneisley et al., 1978; Kuypers and Maisky, 1975, 1977; Tohyama et al., 1979a,b; Zemlan et al., 1984).

The medullary raphe nuclei project to the spinal cord through the lateral and ventral funiculi. Studies attempting to assign particular projections to different parts of the spinal cord white matter have been done, using either labeling of particular white matter components or injections of label caudal to a lesion of part of the spinal white matter (see Holstege, this volume). These experiments indicate that the rostral part of the NRM projects chiefly through the dorsolateral funiculi, whereas the caudal NRM, raphe obscurus and raphe pallidus project mostly in the ventral lateral or ventral funiculi (Fig. 14; Basbaum and Fields, 1979; Carlton et al., 1985; Kuypers and Maisky, 1977; Leichnetz et al., 1978; Martin et al., 1978; Tohyama et al., 1979b). Anterograde labelling experiments (Basbaum et al., 1978; see also Holstege, this volume) have shown that the spinal projections from the NRM pass caudally just superficial to the inferior olivary nuclei, then traverse the region just medial and then caudal to the lateral reticular nuclei and finally descend bilaterally in the dorsolateral funiculi (Fig. 7). The termination zones include laminae I, II, and V – VII.

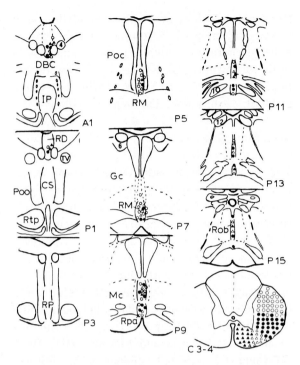

Fig. 14. Locations of raphe neurons in the cat labeled retrogradely from various parts of the spinal cord white matter at C3 – 4. Cells labeled from the dorsolateral funiculus are indicated by open circles; those from progressively more ventral sites are shown successively by filled circles, open triangles and filled triangles. Abbreviations: CS, central superior nucleus; DBC, decussation of the brachium conjunctivum; Gc, nucleus gigantocellularis; IP, interpeduncular nucleus; Mc, nucleus magnocellularis; Poc, Poo, nuclei pontis caudalis and oralis; RD, raphe dorsalis; RM, raphe magnus; Rob, raphe obscurus; Rpa, raphe pallidus; Rtp, reticularis tegmenti pontis. (From Tohyama et al., 1979b.)

The nucleus magnocellularis projects mostly ipsilaterally in both the dorsolateral funiculus and in the ventral part of the lateral funiculus (Basbaum et al., 1978; Tohyama et al., 1979a; Zemlan et al., 1984); the projection in the dorsolateral funiculus follows a course similar to that of the NRM projection, and the termination zone is comparable, but unilateral (Basbaum et al., 1978), except that no endings were seen in laminae I and II in the rat (Zemlan et al., 1984). The nucleus gigantocellularis projects bilaterally by way of the medial longitudinal fasciculi; the fibers descend through the spinal cord in the lateral and ventral funiculi ipsilaterally and in the ventral funiculus contralaterally (Basbaum et al., 1978; Zemlan et al., 1984). The spinal cord terminations are largely in laminae VI, VII and VIII.

Lateral medulla and pons

The lateral part of the medulla and pons contain many neurons that project to the spinal cord. The nuclei giving rise to the most prominent projections include the ventral part of the central nucleus of the medulla, the nucleus of the lateral medulla (which is near the lateral reticular nucleus), and several groups of cells extending through the pons from just dorsal to the superior olivary nucleus,

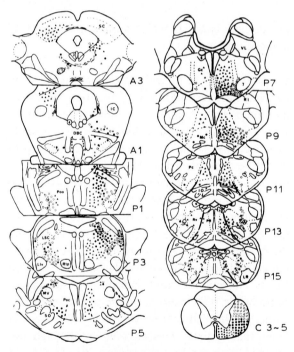

Fig. 15. Reticular formation neurons projecting through different parts of the spinal cord white matter in the cat labeled retrogradely by horseradish peroxidase injections at C3 – 4. See legend of Fig. 14 for use of symbols and for some of the abbreviations. Additional abbreviations: Cun, nucleus cuneiformis; IC, intercollicular nucleus; LC, LSC, nuclei locus coeruleus and subcoeruleus; LR, lateral reticular nucleus; MV, motor nucleus of V; SC, superior colliculus. (From Tohyama et al., 1979a.)

along the lateral lemniscus to the locus coeruleus-subcoeruleus complex, the Kölliker-Fuse nucleus and parabrachial region (Fig. 15; Carlton et al., 1985; Hancock and Fougerousse, 1976; Kneisley et al., 1978; Tohyama et al., 1979a,b; Westlund and Coulter, 1980). There is also a prominent group of spinally projecting neurons just ventral to the facial nucleus (Fig. 15).

Descending projections from the locus coeruleus-subcoeruleus complex were traced by Westlund and Coulter (1980) both through the medial longitudinal fasciculus region and through the lateral tegmentum of the brain stem. Most of the descending axons travel in the ventrolateral funiculus, although some are in the dorsolateral funiculus. Terminals were in laminae I, II, IV – X. A discrete group of neurons in the lateral pontine tegmentum have also been shown to project to laminae I, II, V and VI of the spinal cord (Tan and Holstege, 1986).

PAG and midbrain reticular formation

Only a few neurons of the PAG or midbrain reticular formation project to the spinal cord (Carlton et al., 1983; Castiglioni et al., 1978; Tohyama et al., 1979a; however, cf., Mantyh and Peschanski, 1982), although a larger number project to the upper cervical spinal cord than more caudally (Castiglioni et al., 1978), and so it has been suggested that the inhibitory effects of stimulating in the PAG are produced by activation of bulbospinal neurons in the medulla (Basbaum and Fields, 1978). Candidate neurons for relaying the inhibition include neurons of the NRM. Evidence for this includes a projection from the PAG (and adjacent nucleus cuneiformis) to the NRM (Abols and Basbaum, 1981; Carlton et al., 1983; Chung et al., 1983a,b; Fardin et al., 1984; Gallagher and Pert, 1978; Mantyh, 1983; Shah and Dostrovsky, 1980; Yezierski et al., 1982a) and recordings from NRM neurons, including raphe-spinal cells, that can be excited by stimulation in the PAG (Behbehani and Fields, 1979; Behbehani

and Zemlan, 1986; Fields and Anderson, 1978; Lovick et al., 1978; Pomeroy and Behbehani, 1979; Willis et al., 1984). However, there is also a projection from the PAG to the reticular formation adjacent to the NRM, including the nuclei gigantocellularis and magnocellularis (Abols and Basbaum, 1981), and neurons in this part of the reticular formation are also excited following stimulation in the PAG (Mohrland and Gebhart, 1980; Willis et al., 1984). Furthermore, there are connections between several nuclei of the reticular formation, including the nucleus magnocellularis, and the NRM (Abols and Basbaum, 1981; Fardin et al., 1984). The PAG projections to the NRM and to the adjacent reticular formation originate from different neurons (Beitz et al., 1983).

Experiments involving injections of local anesthetic to block activity in small volumes of neural tissue have shown that both the NRM and the medullary reticular formation are involved in mediating the inhibitory effects of PAG stimulation on nociceptive dorsal horn neurons (Gebhart et al., 1983b). In addition, there is likely to be a pathway from the PAG to neurons projecting through the region of the lateral reticular nucleus other than the NRM, since PAG inhibition of responses of nociceptive dorsal horn neurons to volleys in C fibers is reduced by only one quarter following extensive lesions of the raphe and adjacent reticular formation, whereas it is reduced much more by bilateral lesions in the area of the lateral reticular nucleus (Morton et al., 1984).

The descending pathways from the PAG and the lateral midbrain reticular formation and from the medial medulla appear to be separate or a transformation of information processing occurs, since the inhibition produced by stimulation in these areas is different (Carstens et al., 1980b). Stimulation in the PAG causes a reduction in the slope of the stimulus-response curve (gain change) of nociceptive dorsal horn cells activated by graded noxious heat stimuli. On the other hand, stimulation in the lateral midbrain reticular formation (Carstens et al., 1980b), the NRM or the medullary reticular formation (Gebhart et al., 1983a,b) causes a parallel shift in the curve (changed set-point or threshold).

Not all of the neurons in the NRM and adjacent reticular formation are excited by activation of neurons in the PAG. Some are instead inhibited and others unaffected. This suggests a functional heterogeneity of the NRM. Fields and his associates (this volume) have reported further evidence about this. Although flexion reflexes are enhanced following spinal cord transection, they may normally be triggered by circuits involving ascending connections to brain stem neurons and descending pathways. An example of this is the tail flick reflex (Fields and Heinricher, 1985). In animals with an intact neuraxis, certain neurons in the raphe nuclei discharge just prior to a tail flick ('on-cells'), whereas other raphe cells cease discharging ('off-cells'). In fact, noxious stimuli excite 'on-cells' and inhibit 'off-cells' no matter where the noxious stimuli are applied. It is hypothesized that the 'off-cells' are inhibitory and that their pause permits the beginning of the tail flick. The fact that 'off-cells' are inhibited by noxious stimuli indicates that they are not part of a simple negative feed-back circuit (cf., Basbaum and Fields, 1978). Electrical stimulation in the PAG excites both 'on-' and 'off-cells', but morphine injections in the PAG (or systemically) excite 'off-' and inhibit 'on-cells'. Recently, 'on-' and 'off-cells' have also been found in the PAG (Heinricher et al., 1987).

Periventricular gray

There is a direct hypothalamospinal tract arising from the paraventricular nucleus (Hancock, 1976; Kuypers and Maisky, 1975; Swanson and Kuypers, 1980). In addition, descending fibers from the hypothalamus reach the PAG (Conrad and Pfaff, 1976; Saper et al., 1979). Thus, several routes are available for the mediation of inhibit or effects on spinal cord nociceptive neurons from the PVG.

Conclusions

The delineation of neural systems that control nociceptive transmission in the spinal cord has continued to be an active field. More effort is needed in several areas, including detailed studies of the neural circuits responsible for spinal cord processing of descending commands, assessment of the roles of pre- and postsynaptic inhibition, assignment of the effects of stimulation in different brain stem areas to particular pathways, and analysis of the neurotransmitters used in the various control systems. It can be anticipated that such investigations will be useful not only for a better understanding of antinociception but also for centrifugal sensory control in general.

Acknowledgements

The author thanks his scientific and technical colleagues for their contributions to the work cited done in his laboratory and Phyllis Waldrop for typing. The work in the author's laboratory is supported by NIH grants NS 09743 and NS 11255.

References

Abols, I.A. and Basbaum, A.I. (1981) Afferent connections of the rostral medulla of the cat: a neural substrate for midbrain-medullary interactions in the modulation of pain. *J. Comp. Neurol.,* 201: 285 – 297.

Ammons, W.S., Blair, R.W. and Foreman, R.D. (1984) Raphe magnus inhibition of primate T1 – T4 spinothalamic cells with cardiopulmonary visceral input. *Pain,* 20: 247 – 260.

Ammons, W.S., Girardot, M.N. and Foreman, R.D. (1986) Periventricular gray inhibition of thoracic spinothalamic cells projecting to medial and lateral thalamus. *J. Neurophysiol.,* 55: 1091 – 1103.

Basbaum, A.I. and Fields, H.L. (1978) Endogenous pain control mechanisms: review and hypothesis. *Ann. Neurol.,* 4: 451 – 462.

Basbaum, A.I. and Fields, H.L. (1979) The origin of descending pathways in the dorsolateral funiculus of the spinal cord of the cat and rat: further studies on the anatomy of pain modulation. *J. Comp. Neurol.,* 187: 513 – 532.

Basbaum, A.I., Clanton, C.H. and Fields, H.L. (1978) Three bulbospinal pathways from the rostral medulla of the cat: an autoradiographic study of pain modulating systems. *J. Comp. Neurol.,* 1978: 209 – 224.

Beall, J.E., Martin, R.F., Applebaum, A.E. and Willis, W.D. (1976) Inhibition of primate spinothalamic tract neurons by stimulation in the region of the nucleus raphe magnus. *Brain Res.,* 114: 328 – 333.

Behbehani, M.M. and Fields, H.L. (1979) Evidence that an excitatory connection between the periaqueductal gray and nucleus raphe magnus mediates stimulation produced analgesia. *Brain Res., 170:* 85 – 93.

Behbehani, M.M. and Zemlan, F.P. (1986) Response of nucleus raphe magnus neurons to electrical stimulation of nucleus cuneiformis: role of acetylcholine. *Brain Res.,* 369: 110 – 118.

Beitz, A.J., Mullett, M.A. and Weiner, L.L. (1983) The periaqueductal gray projections to the rat spinal trigeminal, raphe magnus, gigantocellular pars alpha and paragigantocellular nuclei arise from separate neurons. *Brain Res.,* 288: 307 – 314.

Belcher, G., Ryall, R.W. and Schaffner, R. (1978) The differential effects of 5-hydroxytryptamine, noradrenaline and raphe stimulation on nociceptive and non-nociceptive dorsal horn interneurones in the cat. *Brain Res.,* 151: 307 – 321.

Bennett, G.J. and Mayer, D.J. (1979) Inhibition of spinal cord interneurons by narcotic microinjection and focal electrical stimulation in the periaqueductal central gray matter. *Brain Res.,* 172: 243 – 257.

Besson, J.M., Guilbaud, G. and LeBars, D. (1975) Descending inhibitory influences exerted by the brain stem upon the activities of dorsal horn lamina V cells induced by intra-arterial injection of bradykinin into the limbs. *J. Physiol. (Lond.),* 248: 725 – 739.

Blair, R.W., Weber, R.N. and Foreman, R.D. (1981) Characteristics of primate spinothalamic tract neurons receiving viscerosomatic convergent inputs in T3 – T5 segments. *J. Neurophysiol.,* 46: 797 – 811.

Brown, A.G. (1971) Effects of descending impulses on transmission through the spinocervical tract. *J. Physiol. (Lond.),* 219: 103 – 125.

Brown, A.G. and Franz, D.N. (1969) Responses of spinocervical tract neurones to natural stimulation of identified cutaneous receptors. *Exp. Brain Res.,* 7: 231 – 249.

Brown, A.G. and Rethelyi, M. (Eds.) (1981) In: *Spinal Cord Sensation.* Scottish Academic Press, Edinburgh, pp. 332 – 333.

Brown, A.G., Kirk, E.J. and Martin, H.F. (1973) Descending and segmental inhibition of transmission through the spinocervical tract. *J. Physiol. (Lond.),* 230: 689 – 705.

Calvillo, O., Madrid, J. and Rudomin, P. (1982) Presynaptic depolarization of unmyelinated primary afferent fibers in the spinal cord of the cat. *Neuroscience,* 7: 1389 – 1400.

Cargill, C.L., Steinman, J.L. and Willis, W.D. (1985) A fictive tail flick reflex in the rat. *Brain Res.,* 345: 45 – 53.

Carlton, S.M., Leichnetz, G.R., Young, E.G. and Mayer, D.J. (1983) Supramedullary afferents of the nucleus raphe magnus in the rat: a study using the transcannula HRP gel and autoradiographic techniques. *J. Comp. Neurol.,* 214: 43 – 58.

Carlton, S.M., Chung, J.M., Leonard, R.B. and Willis, W.D. (1985) Funicular trajectories of brainstem neurons projecting to the lumbar spinal cord in the monkey (*Macaca fascicularis*): a retrograde labeling study. *J. Comp. Neurol.,* 241: 382 – 404.

Carpenter, D., Engberg, I. and Lundberg, A. (1966) Primary afferent depolarization evoked from the brain stem and the cerebellum. *Arch. Ital. Biol.,* 104: 73 – 85.

Carstens, E. (1982) Inhibition of spinal dorsal horn neuronal responses to noxious skin heating by medial hypothalamic stimulation in the cat. *J. Neurophysiol.,* 48: 808 – 822.

Carstens, E., Yokota, T. and Zimmermann, M. (1979) Inhibition of spinal neuronal responses to noxious skin heating by stimulation of mesencephalic periaqueductal gray in the cat. *J. Neurophysiol.,* 42: 558 – 568.

Carstens, E., Klumpp, D. and Zimmermann, M. (1980a) Time course and effective sites for inhibition from midbrain periaqueductal gray of spinal dorsal horn neuronal responses to cutaneous stimuli in the cat. *Exp. Brain Res.,* 38: 425 – 430.

Carstens, E., Klumpp, D. and Zimmermann, M. (1980b) Differential inhibitory effects of medial and lateral midbrain stimulation on spinal neuronal discharges to noxious skin heating in the cat. *J. Neurophysiol.,* 43: 332 – 342.

Carstens, E., Bihl, H., Irvine, D.R.F. and Zimmermann, M. (1981) Descending inhibition from medial and lateral midbrain of spinal dorsal horn neuronal responses to noxious and nonnoxious cutaneous stimuli in the cat. *J. Neurophysiol.,* 45: 1029 – 1042.

Carstens, E., MacKinnon, J.D. and Guinan, M.J. (1982) Inhibition of spinal dorsal horn neuronal responses to noxious skin heating by medial preoptic and septal stimulation in the cat. *J. Neurophysiol.,* 48: 981 – 991.

Casey, K.L. (1971) Escape elicited by bulboreticular stimulation in the cat. *Int. J. Neurosci.,* 2: 29 – 34.

Cassinari, V. and Pagni, C.A. (1969) *Central Pain. A Neurosurgical Survey.* Harvard University Press, Cambridge.

Castiglioni, A.J., Gallaway, M.C. and Coulter, J.D. (1978) Spinal projections from the midbrain in monkey. *J. Comp. Neurol.,* 178: 329 – 346.

Cervero, F. and Wolstencroft, J.H. (1984) A positive feed-back loop between spinal cord nociceptive pathways and antinociceptive areas of the cat's brain stem. *Pain,* 20: 125 – 138.

Cervero, F., Iggo, A. and Ogawa, H. (1976) Nociceptor-driven dorsal horn neurones in the lumbar spinal cord of the cat. *Pain,* 2: 5 – 24.

Cervero, F., Iggo, A. and Molony, V. (1977) Responses of spinocervical tract neurones to noxious stimulation of the skin. *J. Physiol. (Lond.),* 267: 537 – 558.

Cervero, F., Molony, V. and Iggo, A. (1979) Supraspinal linkage of substantia gelatinosa neurones: effects of descending impulses. *Brain Res.,* 175: 351 – 355.

Christensen, B.N. and Perl, E.R. (1970) Spinal neurons

specifically excited by noxious or thermal stimuli: marginal zone of the dorsal horn. *J. Neurophysiol.*, 33: 293 – 307.

Chung, J.M., Kenshalo, D.R., Jr., Gerhart, K.D. and Willis, W.D. (1979) Excitation of primate spinothalamic neurons by cutaneous C-fiber volleys. *J. Neurophysiol.*, 42: 1354 – 1369.

Chung, J.M., Fang, Z.R., Cargill, C.L. and Willis, W.D. (1983a) Prolonged, naloxone-reversible inhibition of the flexion reflex in the cat. *Pain*, 15: 35 – 53.

Chung, J.M., Kevetter, G.A., Yezierski, R.P., Haber, L.H., Martin, R.F. and Willis, W.D. (1983b) Midbrain nuclei projecting to the medial medulla oblongata in the monkey. *J. Comp. Neurol.*, 214: 93 – 102.

Chung, J.M., Surmeier, D.J., Lee, K.H., Sorkin, L.S., Honda, C.N., Tsong, Y. and Willis, W.D. (1986) Classification of primate spinothalamic and somatosensory thalamic neurons based on cluster analysis. *J. Neurophysiol.*, 56: 308 – 327.

Collins, J.G. (1984) Neuronal activity recorded from the spinal dorsal horn of physiologically intact, awake, drug-free, restrained cats: a preliminary report. *Brain Res.*, 322: 301 – 304.

Collins, J.G. and Ren, K. (1987) WDR response profiles of spinal dorsal horn neurons may be unmasked by barbiturate anesthesia. *Pain*, 28: 369 – 378.

Collins, J.G., Ren, K. and Tang, J. (1987) Lack of spontaneous activity of cutaneous spinal dorsal horn neurons in awake, drug-free, spinally transected cats. *Exp. Neurol.*, 96: 299 – 306.

Conrad, L.C.A. and Pfaff, D.W. (1976) Afferents from medial basal forebrain and hypothalamus in the rat. II. An autoradiographic study of the anterior hypothalamus. *J. Comp. Neurol.*, 169: 221 – 262.

Craig, A.D. and Kniffki, K.D. (1985) Spinothalamic lumbosacral lamina I cells responsive to skin and muscle stimulation in the cat. *J. Physiol. (Lond.)*, 365: 197 – 221.

Dickhaus, H., Pauser, G. and Zimmermann, M. (1985) Tonic descending inhibition affects intensity coding of nociceptive responses of spinal dorsal horn neurones in the cat. *Pain*, 23: 145 – 158.

Dostrovsky, J.O. (1980) Raphe and periaqueductal gray induced suppression of non-nociceptive neuronal responses in the dorsal column nuclei and trigeminal sub-nucleus caudalis. *Brain Res.*, 200: 184 – 189.

Dostrovsky, J.O. (1984) Brainstem influences on transmission of somatosensory information in the spinocervicothalamic pathway. *Brain Res.*, 292: 229 – 238.

Duggan, A.W. and Griersmith, B.T. (1979) Inhibition of the spinal transmission of nociceptive information by supraspinal stimulation in the cat. *Pain*, 6: 149 – 161.

Duggan, A.W., Hall, J.G., Headley, P.M. and Griersmith, B.T. (1977) The effect of naloxone on the excitation of dorsal horn neurones of the cat by noxious and non-noxious cutaneous stimuli. *Brain Res.*, 138: 185 – 189.

Duggan, A.W., Griersmith, B.T. and Johnson, S.M. (1981) Supraspinal inhibition of the excitation of dorsal horn

neurones by impulses in unmyelinated primary afferents: lack of effect by strychnine and bicuculline. *Brain Res.*, 210: 231 – 241.

Eccles, J.C. (1964) *The Physiology of Synapses.* Springer, New York.

Eccles, J.C., Eccles, R.M. and Lundberg, A. (1960) Types of neurons in and around the intermediate nucleus of the lumbosacral cord. *J. Physiol. (Lond.)*, 154: 89 – 114.

Eccles, R.M. and Lundberg, A. (1959a) Synaptic actions in motoneurones by afferents which may evoke the flexion reflex. *Arch. Ital. Biol.*, 97: 199 – 221.

Eccles, R.M. and Lundberg, A. (1959b) Supraspinal control of interneurones mediating spinal reflexes. *J. Physiol. (Lond.)*, 147: 565 – 584.

Edeson, R.O. and Ryall, R.W. (1983) Systematic mapping of descending inhibitory control by the medulla of nociceptive spinal neurones in cats. *Brain Res.*, 271: 251 – 262.

Engberg, I., Lundberg, A. and Ryall, R.W. (1968a) Is the tonic decerebrate inhibition of reflex paths mediated by monoaminergic pathways? *Acta Physiol. Scand.*, 72: 123 – 133.

Engberg, I., Lundberg, A. and Ryall, R.W. (1968b) Reticulospinal inhibition of transmission in reflex pathways. *J. Physiol. (Lond.)*, 194: 201 – 223.

Engberg, I., Lundberg, A. and Ryall, R.W. (1968c) Reticulospinal inhibition of interneurones. *J. Physiol. (Lond.)*, 194: 225 – 236.

Fardin, V., Oliveras, J.L. and Besson, J.M. (1984) Projections from the periaqueductal gray matter to the B3 cellular area (nucleus raphe magnus and nucleus reticularis paragigantocellularis) as revealed by the retrograde transport of horseradish peroxidase in the rat. *J. Comp. Neurol.*, 223: 483 – 500.

Ferrington, D.G., Sorkin, L.S. and Willis, W.D. (1987) Responses of spinothalamic tract cells in the superficial dorsal horn of the primate lumbar spinal cord. *J. Physiol. (Lond.)*, 388: 681 – 703.

Fields, H.L. and Anderson, S.D. (1978) Evidence that raphespinal neurons mediate opiate and midbrain stimulation-produced analgesias. *Pain*, 5: 333 – 349.

Fields, H.L. and Heinricher, M.M. (1985) Anatomy and physiology of a nociceptive modulatory system. *Phil. Trans. Roy. Soc. Lond. B*, 308: 361 – 374.

Fields, H.L., Basbaum, A.I., Clanton, C.H. and Anderson, S.D. (1977) Nucleus raphe magnus inhibition of spinal cord dorsal horn neurons. *Brain Res.*, 126: 441 – 453.

Foong, F.W. and Duggan, A.W. (1986) Brainstem areas tonically inhibiting dorsal horn neurons: studies with microinjection of the GABA analogue piperidine-4-sulphonic acid. *Pain*, 27: 361 – 372.

Foreman, R.D., Kenshalo, D.R., Jr., Schmidt, R.F. and Willis, W.D. (1979a) Field potentials and excitation of primate spinothalamic neurones in response to volleys in muscle afferents. *J. Physiol. (Lond.)*, 286: 197 – 213.

Foreman, R.D., Schmidt, R.F. and Willis, W.D. (1979b) Effects of mechanical and chemical stimulation of fine muscle afferents upon primate spinothalamic tract cells. *J. Physiol. (Lond.),* 286: 215 – 231.

Frank, G.B. and Ohta, M. (1971) Blockade of the reticulospinal inhibitory pathway by anesthetic agents. *Br. J. Pharmacol.,* 42: 328 – 342.

Gallagher, D.W. and Pert, A. (1978) Afferents to brain stem nuclei (brain stem raphe, nucleus pontis caudalis and nucleus gigantocellularis) in the rat as demonstrated by microiontophoretically applied horseradish peroxidase. *Brain Res.,* 144: 257 – 275.

Gebhart, G.F. and Ossipov, M. (1986) Characterization of inhibition of the spinal nociceptive tail flick reflex in the rat from the medullary lateral reticular nucleus. *J. Neurosci.,* 6: 701 – 713.

Gebhart, G.F., Sandkuhler, J., Thalhammer, J.G. and Zimmermann, M. (1983a) Quantitative comparison of inhibition in spinal cord of nociceptive information by stimulation in periaqueductal gray or nucleus raphe magnus of the cat. *J. Neurophysiol.,* 50: 1433 – 1445.

Gebhart, G.F., Sandkuhler, J., Thalhammer, J.G. and Zimmermann, M. (1983b) Inhibition of spinal nociceptive information by stimulation in the midbrain of the cat is blocked by lidocaine microinjected in nucleus raphe magnus and the medullary reticular formation. *J. Neurophysiol.,* 50: 1446 – 1457.

Gerhart, K.D., Wilcox, T.K., Chung, J.M. and Willis, W.D. (1981a) Inhibition of nociceptive and nonnociceptive responses of primate spinothalamic cells by stimulation in medial brain stem. *J. Neurophysiol.,* 45: 121 – 136.

Gerhart, K.D., Yezierski, R.P., Wilcox, T.K., Grossman, A.E. and Willis, W.D. (1981b) Inhibition of primate spinothalamic tract neurons by stimulation in ipsilateral or contralateral ventral posterior lateral (VPLc) thalamic nucleus. *Brain Res.,* 229: 514 – 519.

Gerhart, K.D., Yezierski, R.P., Fang, Z.R. and Willis, W.D. (1983) Inhibition of primate spinothalamic tract neurons by stimulation in ventral posterior lateral (VPLc) thalamic nucleus: possible mechanisms. *J. Neurophysiol.,* 49: 406 – 423.

Gerhart, K.D., Yezierski, R.P., Wilcox, T.K. and Willis, W.D. (1984) Inhibition of primate spinothalamic tract neurons by stimulation in periaqueductal gray or adjacent midbrain reticular formation. *J. Neurophysiol.,* 51: 450 – 466.

Giesler, G.J., Gerhart, K.D., Yezierski, R.P., Wilcox, T.K. and Willis, W.D. (1981a) Postsynaptic inhibition of primate spinothalamic neurons by stimulation in nucleus raphe magnus. *Brain Res.,* 204: 184 – 188.

Giesler, G.J., Yezierski, R.P., Gerhart, K.D. and Willis, W.D. (1981b) Spinothalamic tract neurons that project to medial and/or lateral thalamic nuclei: evidence for a physiologically novel population of spinal cord neurons. *J. Neurophysiol.,* 46: 1285 – 1308.

Girardot, M.N., Brennan, T.J., Martindale, M.E. and Fore-

man, R.D. (1987) Effects of stimulating the subcoeruleus-parabrachial region on the non-noxious and noxious responses of T1 – T5 spinothalamic tract neurons in the primate. *Brain Res.,* 409: 19 – 30.

Gray, B.G. and Dostrovsky, J.O. (1983) Descending inhibitory influences from periaqueductal gray, nucleus raphe magnus, and adjacent reticular formation. I. Effects on lumbar spinal cord nociceptive and nonnociceptive neurons. *J. Neurophysiol.,* 49: 932 – 947.

Griffith, J.L. and Gatipon, G.B. (1981) A comparative study of selective stimulation of raphe nuclei in the cat inhibiting dorsal horn neuron responses to noxious stimulation. *Brain Res.,* 229: 520 – 524.

Guilbaud, G., Oliveras, J.L., Giesler, G. and Besson, J.M. (1977) Effects induced by stimulation of the centralis inferior nucleus of the raphe on dorsal horn interneurons in cat's spinal cord. *Brain Res.,* 126: 355 – 360.

Haber, L.H., Martin, R.F., Chatt, A.B. and Willis, W.D. (1978) Effects of stimulation in nucleus reticularis gigantocellularis on the activity of spinothalamic tract neurons in the monkey. *Brain Res.,* 153: 163 – 168.

Haber, L.H., Martin, R.F., Chung, J.M. and Willis, W.D. (1980) Inhibition and excitation of primate spinothalamic tract neurons by stimulation in region of nucleus reticularis gigantocellularis. *J. Neurophysiol.,* 43: 1578 – 1593.

Hall, J.G., Duggan, A.W., Johnson, S.M. and Morton, C.R. (1981) Medullary raphe lesions do not reduce descending inhibition of dorsal horn neurones of the cat. *Neurosci. Lett.,* 25: 25 – 29.

Hall, J.G., Duggan, A.W., Morton, C.R. and Johnson, S.M. (1982) The location of brainstem neurones tonically inhibiting dorsal horn neurones of the cat. *Brain Res.,* 244: 215 – 222.

Hamilton, B.L. (1973) Projections of the nuclei of the periaqueductal gray matter in the cat. *J. Comp. Neurol.,* 152: 45 – 58.

Hancock, M.B. (1976) Cells of origin of hypothalamo-spinal projections in the rat. *Neurosci. Lett.,* 3: 179 – 184.

Hancock, M.B. and Fougerousse, C.L. (1976) Spinal projections from the nucleus locus coeruleus and nucleus subcoeruleus in the cat and monkey as demonstrated by the retrograde transport of horseradish peroxidase. *Brain Res. Bull.,* 1: 229 – 234.

Handwerker, H.O., Iggo, A. and Zimmermann, M. (1975) Segmental and supraspinal actions on dorsal horn neurons responding to noxious and non-noxious skin stimuli. *Pain,* 1: 147 – 165.

Hayes, R.L., Price, D.D., Ruda, M.A. and Dubner, R. (1979) Suppression of nociceptive responses in the primate by electrical stimulation of the brain or morphine administration: behavioral and electrophysiological comparisons. *Brain Res.,* 167: 417 – 421.

Heinricher, M.M., Cheng, Z.F. and Fields, H.L. (1987) Evidence for two classes of nociceptive modulating neurons in the periaqueductal gray. *J. Neurosci.,* 7: 271–278.

Hentall, I.D. and Fields, H.L. (1979) Segmental and descending influences on intraspinal thresholds of single C-fibers. *J. Neurophysiol.,* 42: 1527–1537.

Hentall, I.D., Zorman, G., Kansky, S. and Fields, H.L. (1984) An estimate of minimum number of brain stem neurons required for inhibition of a flexion reflex. *J. Neurophysiol.,* 51: 978–985.

Hillman, P. and Wall, P.D. (1969) Inhibitory and excitatory factors influencing the receptive fields of lamina 5 spinal cord cells. *Exp. Brain Res.,* 9: 284–306.

Hodge, C.J., Apkarian, A.V., Stevens, R., Vogelsang, G. and Wisnicki, H.J. (1981) Locus coeruleus modulation of dorsal horn unit responses to cutaneous stimulation. *Brain Res.,* 204: 415–420.

Hodge, C.J., Apkarian, A.V., Stevens, R.T., Vogelsang, G.D., Brown, O. and Frank, J.I. (1983) Dorsolateral pontine inhibition of dorsal horn cell responses to cutaneous stimulation: lack of dependence on catecholaminergic system in cat. *J. Neurophysiol.,* 50: 1220–1235.

Hodge, C.J., Apkarian, A.V. and Stevens, R.T. (1986) Inhibition of dorsal-horn cell responses by stimulation of the Kolliker-Fuse nucleus. *J. Neurosurg.,* 65: 825–833.

Holmqvist, B. and Lundberg, A. (1959) On the organization of the supraspinal inhibitory control of interneurones of various spinal reflex arcs. *Arch. Ital. Biol.,* 97: 340–356.

Holmqvist, B. and Lundberg, A. (1961) Differential supraspinal control of synaptic actions evoked by volleys in the flexion reflex afferents in alpha motoneurones. *Acta Physiol. Scand.,* 54, Suppl. 186: 1–51.

Holmqvist, B., Lundberg, A. and Oscarsson, O. (1960) Supraspinal inhibitory control of transmission of three ascending spinal pathways influenced by the flexion reflex afferents. *Arch. Ital. Biol.,* 98: 60–80.

Hong, S.K., Kniffki, K.D., Mense, S., Schmidt, R.F. and Wendisch, M. (1979) Descending influences on the responses of spinocervical tract neurones to chemical stimulation of fine muscle afferents. *J. Physiol. (Lond.),* 290: 129–140.

Hori, Y., Lee, K.H., Chung, J.M., Endo, K. and Willis, W.D. (1984) The effects of small doses of barbiturate on the activity of primate nociceptive tract cells. *Brain Res.,* 307: 9–15.

Hylden, J.L.K., Hayashi, H. and Bennett, G.J. (1986) Lamina I spinomesencephalic neurons in the cat ascend via the dorsolateral funiculi. *Somatosens. Res.,* 4: 31–41.

Irwin, S., Houde, R.W., Bennett, D.R., Hendershot, L.C. and Steevers, M.H. (1951) The effects of morphine, methadone and meperidine on some reflex responses of spinal animals to nociceptive stimulation. *J. Pharmacol. Exp. Ther.,* 101: 132–143.

Iwamoto, G.A., Ryu, H. and Wagman, I.H. (1980) Effects of stimulation of the caudal brain stem on late ventral root reflex discharge elicited by high threshold sural nerve afferents. *Brain Res.,* 183: 193–199.

Jankowska, E. and Lindstrom, S. (1972) Morphology of in-

terneurones mediating Ia reciprocal inhibition of motoneurones in the spinal cord of the cat. *J. Physiol. (Lond.),* 226: 805–823.

Jankowska, E. and Roberts, W.J. (1972a) An electrophysiological demonstration of the axonal projections of single spinal interneurones in the cat. *J. Physiol. (Lond.),* 222: 597–622.

Jankowska, E. and Roberts, W.J. (1972b) Synaptic actions of single interneurones mediating reciprocal Ia inhibition of motoneurones. *J. Physiol. (Lond.),* 222: 623–642.

Jankowska, E., Lund, S., Lundberg, A. and Pompeiano, O. (1968) Inhibitory effects evoked through ventral reticulospinal pathways. *Arch. Ital. Biol.,* 106: 124–140.

Jones, M.W., Apkarian, A.V., Stevens, R.T. and Hodge, C.J. (1987) The spinothalamic tract: an examination of the cells of origin of the dorsolateral and ventral spinothalamic pathways in cats. *J. Comp. Neurol.,* 260: 349–361.

Jones, S.L. and Gebhart, G.F. (1986) Quantitative characterization of ceruleospinal inhibition of nociceptive transmission in the rat. *J. Neurophysiol.,* 56: 1397–1410.

Kajander, K.C., Ebner, T.J. and Bloedel, J.R. (1984) Effects of periaqueductal gray and raphe magnus stimulation on the responses of spinocervical and other ascending projection neurons to non-noxious inputs. *Brain Res.,* 291: 29–37.

Kneisley, L.W., Biber, M.P. and Lavail, J.H. (1978) A study of the origin of brain stem projections to monkey spinal cord using the retrograde transport method. *Exp. Neurol.,* 60: 367–378.

Kniffki, K.D., Mense, S. and Schmidt, R.F. (1977) The spinocervical tract as a possible pathway for muscular nociception. *J. Physiol. (Paris),* 73: 359–366.

Kolmodin, G.M. and Skoglund, C.R. (1960) Analysis of spinal interneurons activated by tactile and nociceptive stimulation. *Acta Physiol. Scand.,* 50: 337–355.

Kuno, M. and Perl, E.R. (1960) Alteration of spinal reflexes by interaction with suprasegmental and dorsal root activity. *J. Physiol. (Lond.),* 151: 103–122.

Kuypers, H.G.J.M. and Maisky, V.A. (1975) Retrograde axonal transport of horseradish peroxidase from spinal cord to brain stem cell groups in the cat. *Neurosci. Lett.,* 1: 9–14.

Kuypers, H.G.J.M. and Maisky, V.A. (1977) Funicular trajectories of descending brain stem pathways in cat. *Brain Res.,* 136: 159–165.

LeBars, D. and Chitour, D. (1983) Do convergent neurones in the spinal dorsal horn discriminate nociceptive from nonnociceptive information? *Pain,* 17: 1–19.

Leichnetz, G.R., Watkins, L., Griffin, G., Murfin, R. and Mayer, D.J. (1978) The projection from nucleus raphe magnus and other brainstem nuclei to the spinal cord in the rat: a study using the HRP blue-reaction. *Neurosci. Lett.,* 8: 119–124.

Liebeskind, J.C., Guilbaud, G., Besson, J.M. and Oliveras, J.L. (1973) Analgesia from electrical stimulation of the periaqueductal gray matter in the cat: behavioral observations and inhibitory effects on spinal cord interneurons. *Brain Res.*, 50: 441–446.

Liddell, E.G.T., Matthes, K., Oldberg, E. and Ruch, T.C. (1932) Reflex release of flexor muscles by spinal section. *Brain*, 55: 239–246.

Light, A.R., Casale, E.J. and Menetrey, D.M. (1986) The effects of focal stimulation in nucleus raphe magnus and periaqueductal gray on intracellularly recorded neurons in spinal laminae I and II. *J. Neurophysiol.*, 56: 555–571.

Lovick, T.A., West, D.C. and Wolstencroft, J.H. (1978) Responses of raphe spinal and other bulbar raphe neurones to stimulation of the periaqueductal gray in the cat. *Neurosci. Lett.*, 8: 45–49.

Lundberg, A. and Oscarsson, O. (1961) Three ascending spinal pathways in the dorsal part of the lateral funiculus. *Acta Physiol. Scand.*, 51: 1–16.

Lundberg, A. and Oscarsson, O. (1962) Two ascending spinal pathways in the ventral part of the cord. *Acta Physiol. Scand.*, 54: 270–286.

Lundberg, A., Malmgren, K. and Schomburg, E.D. (1987) Reflex pathways from group II muscle afferents. 3. Secondary spindle afferents and the FRA: a new hypothesis. *Exp. Brain Res.*, 65: 294–306.

Magoun, H.W. and Rhines, R. (1946) An inhibitory mechanism in the bulbar reticular formation. *J. Neurophysiol.*, 9: 165–171.

Mantyh, P.W. (1983) Connections on midbrain periaqueductal gray in the monkey. II. Descending efferent projections. *J. Neurophysiol.*, 49: 582–594.

Mantyh, P.W. and Peschanski, M. (1982) Spinal projections from the periaqueductal grey and dorsal raphe in the rat, cat and monkey. *Neuroscience*, 7: 2769–2776.

Martin, R.F., Jordan, L.M. and Willis, W.D. (1978) Differential projections of cat medullary raphe neurons demonstrated by retrograde labelling following spinal cord lesions. *J. Comp. Neurol.*, 182: 77–88.

Martin, R.F., Haber, L.H. and Willis, W.D. (1979) Primary afferent depolarization of identified cutaneous fibers following stimulation in medial brain stem. *J. Neurophysiol.*, 42: 779–790.

McCreery, D.B. and Bloedel, J.R. (1975) Reduction of the response of cat spinothalamic neurons to graded mechanical stimuli by electrical stimulation of the lower brain stem. *Brain Res.*, 97: 151–156.

McCreery, D.B., Bloedel, J.R. and Hames, E.G. (1979) Effects of stimulating in raphe nuclei and in reticular formation on response of spinothalamic neurons to mechanical stimuli. *J. Neurophysiol.*, 42: 166–182.

Mendell, L.M. (1966) Physiological properties of unmyelinated fiber projection to the spinal cord. *Exp. Neurol.*, 16: 316–332.

Milne, R.J., Foreman, R.D., Giesler, G.J. and Willis, W.D. (1981) Convergence of cutaneous and pelvic visceral nociceptive inputs onto primate spinothalamic neurons. *Pain*, 11: 163–183.

Mohrland, J.S. and Gebhart, G.F. (1980) Effects of focal electrical stimulation and morphine microinjection in the periaqueductal gray of the rat mesencephalon on neuronal activity in the medullary reticular formation. *Brain Res.*, 201: 23–37.

Mokha, S.S., McMillan, J.A. and Iggo, A. (1985) Descending control of spinal nociceptive transmission. Actions produced on spinal multireceptive neurones from the nuclei locus coeruleus (LC) and raphe magnus (NRM). *Exp. Brain Res.*, 58: 213–226.

Mokha, S.S., McMillan, J.A. and Iggo, A. (1986) Pathways mediating descending control of spinal nociceptive transmission from the nuclei locus coeruleus (LC) and raphe magnus (NRM) in the cat. *Exp. Brain Res.*, 61: 597–606.

Mori, K., Komatsu, T., Tomemori, N., Shingu, K., Urabe, N., Seo, N. and Hatano, Y. (1981) Pentobarbital anesthetized and decerebrate cats reveal different physiological responses in anesthetic-induced anesthesia. *Acta Anaesthesiol. Scand.*, 25: 349–354.

Morton, C.R., Johnson, S.M. and Duggan, A.W. (1983) Lateral reticular regions and the descending control of dorsal horn neurones of the cat: selective inhibition by electrical stimulation. *Brain Res.*, 275: 13–21.

Morton, C.R., Duggan, A.W. and Zhao, Z.Q. (1984) The effects of lesions of medullary midline and lateral reticular areas on inhibition in the dorsal horn produced by periaqueductal grey stimulation in the cat. *Brain Res.*, 301: 121–130.

Necker, R. and Hellon, R.F. (1978) Noxious thermal input from the rat tail: modulation by descending inhibitory influences. *Pain*, 4: 231–242.

Oliveras, J.L., Besson, J.M., Guilbaud, G. and Liebeskind, J.C. (1974) Behavioral and electrophysiological evidence of pain inhibition from midbrain stimulation in the cat. *Exp. Brain Res.*, 20: 32–44.

Peschanski, M., Kayser, V. and Besson, J.M. (1986) Behavioral evidence for a crossed ascending pathway for pain transmission in the anterolateral quadrant of the rat spinal cord. *Brain Res.*, 376: 164–168.

Pomeroy, S.L. and Behbehani, M.M. (1979) Physiologic evidence for a projection from periaqueductal gray to nucleus raphe magnus in the rat. *Brain Res.*, 176: 143–147.

Price, D.D. and Dubner, R. (1977) Neurons that subserve the sensory-discriminative aspects of pain. *Pain*, 3: 307–338.

Rees, H. and Roberts, M.H.T. (1987) Anterior pretectal stimulation alters the responses of spinal dorsal horn neurones to cutaneous stimulation in the rat. *J. Physiol. (Lond.)*, 385: 415–436.

Rivot, J.P., Chaouch, A. and Besson, J.M. (1980) Nucleus raphe magnus modulation of response of rat dorsal horn neurons to unmyelinated fiber inputs: partial involvement of serotonergic pathways. *J. Neurophysiol.*, 44: 1039–1057.

Sandkuhler, J. and Gebhart, G.F. (1984) Characterization of

28

inhibition of a spinal nociceptive reflex by stimulation medially and laterally in the midbrain and medulla in the pentobarbital-anesthetized rat. *Brain Res.,* 305: 67 – 76.

Sandkuhler, J., Maisch, B. and Zimmermann, M. (1987) Raphe magnus-induced descending inhibition of spinal nociceptive neurons is mediated through contralateral spinal pathways in the cat. *Neurosci. Lett.,* 76: 168 – 172.

Saper, C.B., Swanson, L.W. and Cowan, W.M. (1979) Some efferent connections of the rostral hypothalamus in the squirrel monkey (*Saimiri sciureus*) and cat. *J. Comp. Neurol.,* 184: 205 – 242.

Schmidt, R.F. (1971) Presynaptic inhibition in the vertebrate central nervous system. *Ergeb. Physiol.,* 63: 20 – 101.

Shah, Y. and Dostrovsky, J.O. (1980) Electrophysiological evidence for a projection of the periaqueductal gray matter to nucleus raphe magnus in cat and rat. *Brain Res.,* 193: 534 – 538.

Sherrington, C.S. (1910) Flexion-reflex of the limb, crossed extension-reflex and reflex stepping and standing. *J. Physiol (Lond.),* 50: 28 – 121.

Sherrington, C.S. and Sowton, S.C.M. (1915) Observations on reflex responses to single break-shocks. *J. Physiol. (Lond.),* 49: 331 – 348.

Sorkin, L.S. (1983) *Spinal Cord Unit Activity in the Awake Cat.* Doctoral dissertation, University of Michigan.

Sorkin, L.S., Ferrington, D.G. and Willis, W.D. (1986) Somatotopic organization and response characteristics of dorsal horn neurons in the cervical spinal cord of the cat. *Somatosens. Res.,* 3: 323 – 338.

Surmeier, D.J., Honda, C.N. and Willis, W.D. (1986a) Responses of primate spinothalamic neurons to noxious thermal stimulation of glabrous and hairy skin. *J. Neurophysiol.,* 56: 328 – 350.

Surmeier, D.J., Honda, C.N. and Willis, W.D. (1986b) Temporal features of the responses of primate spinothalamic neurons to noxious thermal stimulation of hairy and glabrous skin. *J. Neurophysiol.,* 56: 351 – 369.

Swanson, L.W. and Kuypers, H.G.J.M. (1980) The paraventricular nucleus of the hypothalamus: cytoarchitectonic subdivisions and organization of projections to the pituitary, dorsal vagal complex, and spinal cord as demonstrated by retrograde fluorescence double-labeling methods. *J. Comp. Neurol.,* 194: 555 – 570.

Tan, J. and Holstege, G. (1986) Anatomical evidence that the pontine lateral tegmental field projects to lamina I of the caudal spinal trigeminal nucleus and spinal cord and to the Edinger-Westphal nucleus in the cat. *Neurosci. Lett.,* 64: 317 – 322.

Taub, A. (1964) Local, segmental, and supraspinal interaction with a dorsolateral spinal cutaneous afferent system. *Exp. Neurol.,* 10: 357 – 374.

Tohyama, M., Sakai, K., Salvert, D., Touret, M. and Jouvet, M. (1979a) Spinal projections from the lower brain stem in the cat as demonstrated by the horseradish peroxidase techni-

que. I. Origins of the reticulospinal tracts and their funicular projections. *Brain Res.,* 173: 383 – 403.

Tohyama, M., Sakai, T., Touret, M., Salvert, D. and Jouvet, M. (1979b) Spinal projections from the lower brain stem in the cat as demonstrated by the horseradish peroxidase technique. II. Projections from the dorsolateral pontine tegmentum and raphe nuclei. *Brain Res.,* 176: 215 – 231.

Tsubokawa, T., Yamamoto, T., Katayama, Y. and Moriyasu, N. (1981) Diencephalic modulation of activities of raphe-spinal neurons in the cat. *Exp. Neurol.,* 74: 561 – 572.

Vierck, C.J. and Luck, M.M. (1979) Loss and recovery of reactivity to noxious stimuli in monkeys with primary spinothalamic cordotomies, followed by secondary and tertiary lesions of other cord sectors. *Brain,* 102: 233 – 248.

Wall, P.D. (1960) Cord cells responding to touch, damage, and temperature of skin. *J. Neurophysiol.,* 23: 197 – 210.

Wall, P.D. (1967) The laminar organization of dorsal horn and effects of descending impulses. *J. Physiol. (Lond.),* 188: 403 – 423.

Westlund, K.N. and Coulter, J.D. (1980) Descending projections of the locus coeruleus and subcoeruleus/medial parabrachial nuclei in monkey: axonal transport studies and dopamine-beta-hydroxylase immunocytochemistry. *Brain Res. Rev.,* 2: 235 – 264.

White, J.C. and Sweet, W.H. (1969) *Pain and the Neurosurgeon.* Thomas, Springfield.

Willer, J.C. (1977) Comparative study of perceived pain and nociceptive flexion reflex in man. *Pain,* 3: 69 – 80.

Willer, J.C., Boureau, F. and Albe-Fessard, D. (1979) Supraspinal influences on nociceptive flexion reflex and pain sensation in man. *Brain Res.,* 179: 61 – 68.

Willis, W.D. (1982) Control of nociceptive transmission in the spinal cord. In: D. Ottoson (Ed.), *Progress in Sensory Physiology, 3,* Springer-Verlag, Berlin.

Willis, W.D. (1985) *The Pain System. The Neural Basis of Nociceptive Transmission in the Mammalian Nervous System,* Karger, Basel.

Willis, W.D., Haber, L.H. and Martin, R.F. (1977) Inhibition of spinothalamic tract cells and interneurons by brain stem stimulation in the monkey. *J. Neurophysiol.,* 40: 968 – 981.

Willis, W.D., Gerhart, K.D., Willcockson, W.S., Yezierski, R.P., Wilcox, T.K. and Cargill, C.L. (1984) Primate raphe- and reticulospinal neurons: effects of stimulation in periaqueductal gray or VPLc thalamic nucleus. *J. Neurophysiol.,* 51: 467 – 480.

Willis, W.D., Surmeier, D.J., Chung, J.M., Ferrington, D.G., Honda, C.N., Downie, J.W. and Sorkin, L.S. (1987) Classification of somatosensory tract cells by cluster analysis. In *Role of Fine Afferent Nerve Fibers in Somatovisceral Sensation,* pp. 377 – 389.

Yezierski, R.P. and McDonald, E.A. (1986) The effects of brainstem stimulation and spinal lesions on the response and receptive field properties of spinomesencephalic tract (SMT) cells in the cat. *Neurosci. Abstr.,* 12: 375.

Yezierski, R.P., Bowker, R.M., Kevetter, G.A., Westlund, K.N., Coulter, J.D. and Willis, W.D. (1982a) Serotonergic projections to the caudal brain stem: a double label study using horseradish peroxidase and serotonin immunocytochemistry. *Brain Res.,* 239: 258 – 264.

Yezierski, R.P., Wilcox, T.K. and Willis, W.D. (1982b) The effects of serotonin antagonists on the inhibition of primate spinothalamic tract cells produced by stimulation in nucleus raphe magnus or the periaqueductal gray. *J. Pharmacol. Exp. Ther.,* 220: 266 – 277.

Zemlan, F.P., Behbehani, M.M. and Beckstead, R.M. (1984) Ascending and descending projections from nucleus reticularis magnocellularis and nucleus reticularis gigantocellularis: an autoradiographic and horseradish peroxidase study in the rat. *Brain Res.,* 292: 207 – 220.

Zorman, G., Hentall, I.D., Adams, J.E. and Fields, H.L. (1981) Naloxone-reversible analgesia produced by microstimulation in the medulla. *Brain Res.,* 219: 137 – 148.

H.L. Fields and J.-M. Besson (Eds.)
Progress in Brain Research, Vol. 77
© 1988 Elsevier Science Publishers B.V. (Biomedical Division)

CHAPTER 2

Anatomy, physiology and pharmacology of the periaqueductal gray contribution to antinociceptive controls

David B. Reichling, Geoffrey C. Kwiat and Allan I. Basbaum

Departments of Anatomy and Physiology and Division of Neurosciences, University of California San Francisco, San Francisco, CA 94143, USA

Introduction

Many studies have emphasized the multiplicity of the bulbospinal antinociceptive control systems that are activated by electrical stimulation of or microinjection of opiates into the midbrain periaqueductal gray (PAG; Basbaum and Fields, 1978, 1984; Basbaum et al., 1983) In addition to a 5-hydroxytryptamine (5HT) descending connection, there are important noradrenergic controls (see Proudfit, this volume; Gebhart, this volume) and a wide variety of peptide-containing bulbospinal neurons (Menetrey and Basbaum, 1987; Bowker, this volume). Comparatively little is known about the mechanisms through which the descending controls are initiated. This review will summarize recent studies which have clarified the cytochemistry of the afferent and efferent connections of the PAG and some of the intrinsic circuits within the PAG through which the controls are activated.

How to produce analgesia

Most studies of the antinociceptive function of the PAG have used techniques of electrical stimulation

or drug microinjection. Since these two manipulations do not affect PAG neural circuitry in the same way, they yield somewhat different results. Electrical stimulation simultaneously activates all classes of neuron (excitatory, inhibitory, local and projection). In addition, afferents to and efferents from the PAG, as well as axons that course through the PAG, are both antidromically and orthodromically stimulated. This complicated and highly artificial pattern of evoked neural activity makes it difficult to characterize the underlying circuitry in the PAG using electrical stimulation.

Drug injection is more selective. Microinjection of glutamate activates cell bodies, but not axons, which avoids some of the pitfalls of electrical stimulation. Nevertheless, as with electrical stimulation, neuronal cell bodies are indiscriminately activated. Diffusion of the drug is also very difficult to control. Opiate microinjection might more closely mimic a 'normal' mode of physiological activation of PAG antinociceptive circuitry. Unfortunately, the opiate most commonly used, morphine, although relatively selective for the μ-receptor, almost certainly generates effects through multiple opiate receptor classes. Even when the opioid peptides themselves, or other neurotransmitters, are used, the concentrations are not physiological. Moreover, it is likely that opioid peptide neurotransmitters act in concert with mul-

Please address all communication to Dr. Allan Basbaum, Department of Anatomy, UCSF, San Francisco, CA 94143, USA; 415-476-5270.

tiple other compounds to produce a phar-macological pattern of neurotransmitter release that is impossible to reproduce in the laboratory.

Subdivisions of the PAG

Although early cytoarchitectural studies recogniz-ed a variety of cell types in the PAG, its regional differentiation was not emphasized until Hamilton identified three major subdivisions, based on com-bined cytoarchitectural and tracing studies in the

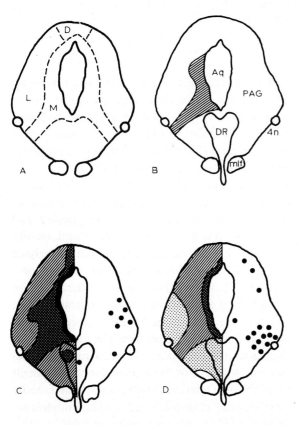

Fig. 1. This illustrates the parcellation of the PAG based on the cytoarchitectural characterization of Hamilton (A) and the distribution of immunoreactive β-endorphin (B), enkephalin (C) and dynorphin (D) cells and terminals in the PAG of the rat. The density of the terminal staining is indicated by the density of cross-hatching; cells are indicated by black dots. It is clear that the densest concentration of the three different opioid pep-tides is found in the region which corresponds to the nucleus medialis (M). L and D refer to the nucleus lateralis and the nucleus dorsalis, respectively.

cat (Hamilton, 1973; Liu and Hamilton, 1980) (see Fig. 1). The 'nucleus medialis' forms an annulus around the aqueduct and has a prominent exten-sion into the ventrolateral PAG. It contains relatively sparsely distributed, small cell bodies. The 'nucleus dorsalis' lies dorsal to the aqueduct and contains mostly medium-sized cell bodies. The 'nucleus lateralis' constitutes the remainder and largest component of the PAG. It is a cell-rich region that contains many larger neurons. Al-though some recent studies concluded that the PAG is largely homogenous, both with respect to its cellular makeup and connectivity (Mantyh, 1982; Gioia et al., 1984), studies by Beitz (1985a,b) in the rat support the Hamilton scheme. According to Beitz the medial subdivision does not extend in-to the ventrolateral PAG, and he recognized a separate dorsolateral subdivision. Since the nucleus medialis overlaps extensively with areas from which electrical stimulation and opiate microinjection most effectively evoke analgesia, this region is probably the most relevant to an-tinociception. As described below, the nucleus medialis also corresponds to the region containing the densest opioid peptide immunoreactivity.

The nucleus raphe dorsalis (RD) is embedded in the ventral PAG, but it is logically considered a component of the serotonin-rich brain stem raphe system (Dahlström and Fuxe, 1964; Wiklund et al., 1981). Rostrally, the RD is replaced by neurons of the Edinger-Westphal (EW) nucleus. The projec-tion pattern and the peptide content of neurons within EW is significantly different from that of the RD. Unfortunately, some authors fail to make the distinction between the two regions, a fact which has led to considerable confusion about the source of descending projections and controls that arise from the ventral PAG.

Endogenous opioid peptides in the PAG

In light of the differential actions of electrical stimulation and drug microinjection described above, it is critical to identify the source of opioid peptide terminals in the PAG. β-Endorphin ter-

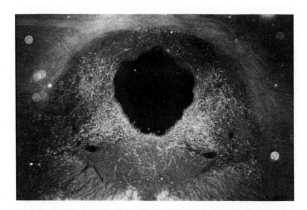

Fig. 2. Photomicrograph of the distribution of immunoreactive β-endorphin through the caudal part of the PAG of the rat. Note that the densest staining is found in the ventrolateral region of the PAG, in the region which corresponds to the nucleus medialis of Hamilton.

minals arise from neurons of the arcuate nucleus (Bloom et al., 1978). They are particularly dense in a band that extends ventrolaterally from the aqueduct (Figs. 1, 2), i.e. in the lateral extension of the nucleus medialis. The RD also contains moderate numbers of immunoreactive β-endorphin terminals. Enkephalin cells outnumber dynorphin cells in the PAG (Khatchaturian et al., 1982; Kawashima and Basbaum, 1984). Both are concentrated caudally and laterally; the population of dynorphin cells lies somewhat ventral to the group of enkephalin cells. In the most rostral PAG of both the rat and cat, there is another cluster of enkephalin cells in the nucleus dorsalis (Beitz 1982; Moss et al., 1983). The terminal distribution of the two peptides is similar but the density of enkephalin staining is much greater. Although it was generally assumed that PAG enkephalin terminals derived exclusively from PAG interneurons, Yamano et al. (1986) recently demonstrated a hypothalamic source of PAG enkephalin terminals. In summary, the highest concentration of opioid peptides is in the zone that is equivalent to the nucleus medialis of Hamilton, which is the region surrounding the aqueduct and its ventrolateral extension. These regions correspond to those areas from which analgesia is best elicited by

opiate microinjection (Yaksh et al., 1976; Lewis and Gebhart, 1977).

Paradoxically, although the densest concentration of opioid peptide is in the ventrolateral PAG, the highest concentration of opiate binding sites, as revealed by binding of tritiated naloxone to tissue sections, is in the dorsolateral sector of the PAG, i.e. precisely where the endogenous opioid peptides are in lowest abundance (Herkenham and Pert, 1982). Even more puzzling are the results of recent studies which used more specific opioid receptor ligands to map the distributions of receptor subtypes within the PAG (Mansour et al., 1987). Kappa binding, revealed by binding of tritiated bremazocine in the presence of cold μ and δ blockers, was the *most* extensive. Since there is little evidence for a κ-mediated analgesia in the PAG, this result is unexpected. Significant μ binding was only found in the rostral, dorsal and dorsolateral PAG. Delta binding was negligible. These data have been confirmed by Leslie et al. (personal communication).

These results are difficult to reconcile with pharmacological data which suggest that supraspinal opiate analgesia is largely mediated through a μ or δ receptor. Based on the fact that the apparent pA_2 values for naloxone antagonism of δ or μ ligand-evoked analgesia were identical when the latter drugs were administered intracerebroventricularly (i.c.v.), Fang et al. (1980) concluded that δ ligand-evoked analgesic effects are, in fact, generated through a μ receptor. In contrast, Porreca and colleagues (1987) concluded that both μ and δ supraspinal receptor subtypes contribute to analgesia and referred to the possibility raised by Heyman et al. (1986) that the similarity of the pA_2 value was coincidental. In the Porreca study, mice were made acutely μ tolerant by systemically injecting large doses of morphine. That treatment shifted the dose response curve to i.c.v. morphine and to other traditional μ ligands, but did *not* change the dose response curve to the δ-specific ligand, [D-Pen²,D-Pen⁵]enkephalin (DPDPE). Furthermore, the analgesia produced by DPDPE, but not by morphine, was blocked by the δ antagonist ICI 174,864. More recently, Mathiasen and Vaught (1987) reported that i.c.v. injection of δ ligands exerts an analgesic effect in 'jimpy' mice, a mutant strain that is deficient in μ receptors; μ ligands were without effect in the jimpy mouse.

Another interpretation to the different conclusions in the cross-tolerance and pA$_2$ studies depends on the fact that the test drug is typically administered in the presence of the drug used to make the animal tolerant; i.e. in a 'μ' tolerant animal, the μ ligand is on board when the δ ligand is being tested. This is certainly the case in studies of acute tolerance where the test drug is administered within hours of injection of the 'tolerizing' drug. Conceivably the test drug 'reactivates' the drug to which the animal was made tolerant, i.e. it might reduce tolerance. The resultant analgesia might, therefore, be due to the same receptor subtype which mediated the analgesic response to the tolerizing drug.

Which ligand for which receptor

Recent studies by Herz and colleagues (this volume) also support the idea that a μ receptor is important in the analgesia evoked from the PAG. These authors concluded that β-endorphin, one of the most potent endogenous ligands of the μ receptor, is the most important opioid peptide for PAG-initiated antinociception. Disruption of the hypothalamic arcuate nucleus significantly reduces stimulation-produced analgesia (SPA) from the PAG (Millan et al., 1986). Since β-endorphin axons all derive from cell bodies outside of the PAG, these studies imply that a critical feature of electrical stimulation within the PAG is the stimulation of β-endorphinergic axons. The contribution of the enkephalin neurons in the PAG to μ-mediated analgesia is not clear. Studies directed at the interactions between enkephalin and β-endorphin terminals in the PAG may help answer that question.

The function of PAG dynorphin neurons is more confusing. As described above, κ binding predominates in the PAG, and dynorphin is the putative endogenous κ ligand (Chavkin et al., 1982). Nevertheless, κ agonists are not considered good analgesics, whether administered supraspinally or spinally. In fact, in the naive mouse, dynorphin antagonizes the analgesia evoked by a variety of μ agonists, including β-endorphin and morphine (Tulunay et al., 1981). Interestingly, dynorphin does not affect the analgesia evoked by δ ligands. The antagonism does not appear to result from changes in the affinity of the μ ligand for the μ-opiate binding site. A somewhat comparable antagonism was reported at the level of the spinal cord, in both behavioral (Schmauss and Herz, 1987) and electrophysiological studies (Dickenson and Knox, 1987). Conceivably, dynorphin neurons provide an opposing, excitatory input to the neurons which are inhibited by β-endorphin and/or enkephalin. It is, in fact, possible that some of the dynorphin terminals in the PAG derive from spinal and trigeminal dynorphin containing neurons, some of which send axons rostrally (Standaert et al., 1986). Taken together with the observed presence of dynorphin in some primary afferent fibers (Botticelli et al., 1981; Sweetnam et al., 1982; Weihe et al., 1985; Basbaum et al., 1986), these data suggest that dynorphin is associated more with the transmission than the control of nociceptive messages.

The target of the PAG opioid peptide

Despite the evidence for involvement of the μ opioid receptor, and the differential contributions of the different opioid peptides, little is known about the neuronal circuitry *within* the PAG through which antinociceptive effects are generated. In this section, we address possible targets of the endogenous opioid peptides. Since electrical stimulation of or glutamate injection into the PAG does produce analgesia, and since electrolytic lesion of the PAG does not (Dostrovsky and Deakin, 1977), it has been concluded that to initiate descending antinociceptive controls, the PAG neuron that projects to the medullary nucleus raphe magnus (NRM) must be excited. Opioidergic synapses, however, are believed to be exclusively inhibitory (Nicoll and Alger, 1979). Thus, for opiates to excite the PAG output neuron, it has been proposed that opioid peptides inhibit an interneuron that tonically inhibits the output neuron (Yaksh et al., 1976). In other words, opiates *disinhibit* the PAG output neuron (see Fig. 3). Pharmacological, physiological and anatomical evidence is consistent with the idea that the tonically active inhibitory interneuron is GABAergic (Basbaum and Fields, 1984; Fields, this volume).

If there were a tonically active GABAergic control, blockade of that control should produce analgesia, and increasing the GABAergic control should counteract opiate analgesia. Although there are reports that systemic administration of GABA agonists antagonize morphine analgesia, most studies report that *analgesia* is produced (DeFeudis, 1983; Retz and Holaday, 1986). This apparent paradox might reflect a direct spinal antinociceptive action of systemic GABA agonists. In fact, when supraspinal levels of GABA are selective-

ly increased, opiate analgesia is usually antagonized. For example, the analgesia evoked by i.c.v. enkephalin is blocked by coadministration of GABA (Izumi et al., 1980). Furthermore, microinjection of the GABA agonist muscimol into the PAG or RD antagonizes the analgesia produced by systemic (Zambotti et al., 1982; Romandini and Samanin, 1984) or PAG morphine (Moreau and Fields, 1986) or β-endorphin (Zonta et al., 1981). Conversely, manipulations which decrease the effectiveness of supraspinal GABAergic synapses produce analgesia. For example, intracisternal (Ueda et al., 1987) or PAG (Moreau and Fields, 1986) microinjection of the GABA A antagonist bicuculline produces a potent analgesia. In addition, microinjection of either bicuculline or picrotoxin into the PAG has the same effect as morphine on the firing of identified neurons of the NRM (Moreau and Fields, 1986; Fields, this volume).

We have recently addressed the anatomical substrate for this GABAergic effect (Reichling and Basbaum, 1987). Immunoreactive GABA cell bodies are very common in the PAG, particularly in regions where opioid terminals are most dense,

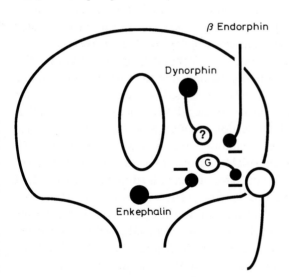

Fig. 3. This schematic outlines the proposed synaptic interaction between the opioid peptides and GABAergic interneurons in the PAG. Both enkephalin terminals (deriving from local interneurons) and β-endorphin terminals, deriving from the hypothalamus, are presumed to inhibit a GABAergic interneuron (G) which tonically inhibits PAG neurons which project to the NRM. The influence of the dynorphin interneuron in the PAG is unclear.

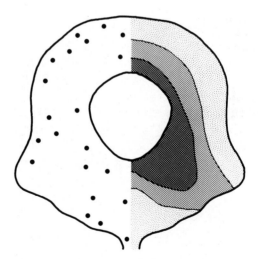

Fig. 4. Scheme of the distribution of immunoreactive GABA cells and terminals in the PAG of the rat. The cells are rather evenly distributed; the terminals decrease in density as one moves from the aqueduct laterally.

i.e. the ventrolateral extension of the nucleus medialis (Fig. 4). Immunoreactive GABA terminals are also widely distributed; they are most dense in the region around the aqueduct but are found in a relatively high concentration through the lateral regions of the PAG. Thus, GABAergic elements are well-situated to intercede between opioid terminals and the PAG output neuron. In fact, we established that there are GABAergic synaptic contacts onto some PAG neurons which project to the NRM. The latter were identified after injection of the colloidal gold labelled retrograde tracer, WGAapoHRP-Au (Basbaum and Menetrey, 1987) into the NRM. PAG sections containing retrogradely labelled cells were processed for GABA immunocytochemistry and then observed at the the EM level. Fig. 5 illustrates an example of a synaptic contact between an immunoreactive GABA terminal and a PAG neuron which was retrogradely labelled from the NRM. These data indicate that the PAG to NRM output cell is likely to be under inhibitory GABAergic control. We are presently investigating the target of the PAG opioid terminal by combined immunocytochemical localization of GABA and

enkephalin or β-endorphin. Since the majority of enkephalin terminals in the PAG form axodendritic synapses (Moss and Basbaum, 1983), we hypothesize that enkephalin neurons postsynaptically inhibit the GABAergic interneuron. Other studies have reported GABAergic interactions with the 5HT-containing neurons of the RD (Gallagher and Aghajanian, 1976; Pujol et al., 1981; Nishikawa and Scatton, 1983; Lee et al., 1987). The relationship of the RD neurons to neurons in the NRM has, however, not been established. Thus, the GABA-5HT synaptic interaction in the RD may not be relevant to descending controls. On the other hand, it might be involved in the ascending controls evoked from the PAG (see below).

The PAG output neuron: target and cytochemistry

That the PAG sends axons to the ventromedial medulla is well established (Ruda, 1976; Gallagher and Pert, 1978; Abols and Basbaum, 1981; Mantyh, 1983b). Both anterograde and retrograde tracing studies have identified this projection. Electrophysiological studies have also demonstrated that electrical stimulation of the PAG (Fields and Anderson, 1978; Vanegas et al., 1984) or microinjection of glutamate into the PAG (Behbehani and Fields, 1979) has a predominantly excitatory effect on neurons of the NRM. Other studies found that microinjection of morphine into the PAG produces excitation, inhibition or no effect on different NRM neurons. (The effects of PAG morphine injection are described in detail by Fields et al., this volume.) The importance of the PAG-NRM connection in the generation of descending antinociception has been confirmed in many other studies including: the contribution of 5HT to PAG antinociceptive controls (Basbaum et al., 1983; Roberts, 1984); the fact that lesions of the dorsolateral funiculus (DLF), through which raphespinal axons course (Basbaum et al., 1978), block the antinociceptive effects of PAG stimulation (Basbaum et al., 1977); and the fact that surgical (Prieto et al., 1984), or anesthetic blockade (Gebhart et al., 1983; Aimone and Gebhart, 1986) of

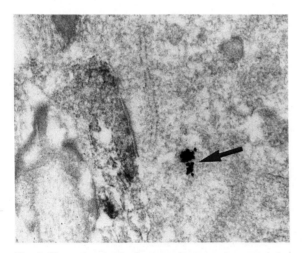

Fig. 5. Photomicrograph of a synaptic contact between an immunoreactive GABA terminal in the PAG that is presynaptic to a neuron retrogradely labeled after injection of the retrograde tracer, WGAapoHRP-Au into the NRM. The dark staining (arrow) in the cell body identifies the silver retrograde deposit.

the raphe and adjacent reticular formation interrupt PAG-evoked analgesia.

These observations demonstrate that some elements within the ventromedial medulla are implicated in PAG controls, but do not identify the target of the PAG projection. It is not known, for example, whether there is a direct connection between the PAG and the 5HT raphe-spinal or non-5HT spinally projecting neurons. To address this question directly, we recently performed an electron microscopic triple label study (Lakos and Basbaum, 1988). The approach is illustrated in Fig. 6 A. All rats underwent an electrolytic lesion of the PAG so that degenerating PAG axon terminals in the raphe could be identified. To identify the raphe spinal neuron, we injected the retrograde tracer, WGAHRP, into the spinal cord of rats.

The subpopulation of those labelled neurons which contained 5HT was simultaneously characterized immunocytochemically, using an electron dense chromogen, benzidine dihydrochloride (BDHC). BDHC generates a precipitate that can be distinguished from the reaction product that identified the spinally projecting, retrogradely labelled neurons (Lakos and Basbaum, 1986). We found that there are indeed direct, monosynaptic, connections from the PAG to both 5HT and non-5HT spinally projecting neurons of the ventromedial medulla. The 5HT neurons receive PAG inputs onto proximal and distal dendrites (Fig. 7). Non-5HT projection neurons receive both axosomatic and axodendritic synaptic contacts from the PAG. These data provide the first definitive evidence that electrical stimulation of the PAG is likely to direct-

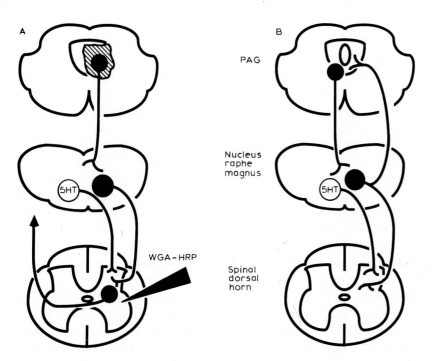

Fig. 6. The circuitry involved in descending controls generated from the PAG. (A) illustrates the method used to identify the target of the PAG projection neuron. First, a lesion of the PAG is made (hatched lines). In the same animal, there is an injection of the retrograde tracer, WGAHRP, into the spinal cord. The latter is taken up and transported to neurons of the medulla, including some that can be stained with antisera against serotonin (5HT) and others which cannot (see Fig. 8 for example of results from such an experiment). (B) summarizes the results of studies of the collateralization of neurons in the nucleus raphe magnus. We found that there are cells in the NRM which send axon collaterals to the spinal cord and also to the PAG; however, these could not be stained with an antiserum against 5HT. Therefore, the 5HT neurons of the NRM do not project to the PAG and thus would not be antidromically activated by electrical stimulation in the PAG.

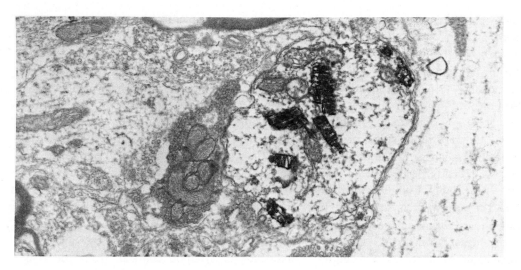

Fig. 7. This photomicrograph illustrates results from an experiment outlined in Fig. 6 (A). Specifically, a 5HT-immunoreactive dendrite in the NRM (labelled by dense crystalline BDHC reaction product) is postsynaptic to a dark, degenerating terminal. The latter was induced by making an electrolytic lesion in the PAG.

ly affect spinally projecting neurons of the medulla that have been implicated in the inhibitory control of spinal nociceptive neurons. Taken together with our recent demonstration that almost all of the immunoreactive serotonin axons in the DLF are unmyelinated (Basbaum et al., 1987), these data indicate that the electrophysiological studies of spinally projecting raphe neurons which conduct between 10 and 50 ms have almost certainly missed the 5HT raphe-spinal neurons.

A large number of peptides have been identified in PAG neurons, but only a few have been localized in neurons that project to the NRM. (For review, see Beitz, 1985.) Double-labelled neurotensin cells were found in the ventrolateral and dorsal PAG; these predominated in the rostral PAG (Beitz, 1982). The neurotensin population is of particular interest because Behbehani and Pert (1984) have demonstrated excitation of NRM neurons by iontophoresis of neurotensin. Injection of neurotensin into the NRM also produces a dose-dependent antinociceptive effect (Fang et al., 1987). Since the PAG contains a rich complement of neurotensin terminals as well as cells, it is likely that the PAG output cells collateralize within the PAG. More recently, it was demonstrated that

there is also a large population of glutamate-positive neurons in the PAG (Clements et al., 1987); some of these send an axon to the NRM (Beitz, personal communication). A significant number of 5HT neurons was also retrogradely labelled. Finally, in preliminary studies we found that no more than 1% of the immunoreactive GABA cells of the PAG could be retrogradely labelled from the NRM (Reichling and Basbaum, 1987). The majority are likely to be interneurons which influence the outflow of the projection neuron.

The PAG-noradrenaline connection

In addition to the contribution of PAG-activated descending serotonergic systems that arise in the NRM, there is considerable evidence for an equal, if not greater, contribution of descending noradrenergic systems to the analgesic action of electrical brain stimulation and opiate injection. Details of the latter are outlined in the article by Proudfit in this volume. In this review we wish to discuss the relationship of the PAG to the likely sites of origin of the descending noradrenergic (NE) systems and report on some data which demonstrate that the extensive collateralization of noradrenergic neurons can significantly complicate the interpretation of electrical stimulation studies.

That there is a PAG projection to the different brain stem NE cell groups has, in fact, never been unequivocally established. Brain stem cell groups containing noradrenergic neurons that project to the spinal cord include those in the dorsolateral pontine tegmentum (locus coeruleus, subcoeruleus, Kölliker-Fuse nucleus and parabrachial nuclei) and the more caudal A5 cell group which is situated between the superior olive and exiting branch of the VIIth cranial nerve (Westlund et al., 1983, 1984; Stevens et al., 1982). Although anterograde tracing studies (Mantyh, 1983; Ruda, 1976) and earlier retrograde tracing studies (Sakai et al., 1977; Cederbaum and Aghajanian, 1978) reported a projection from the PAG to the locus coeruleus and parabrachial region, other retrograde studies could not confirm the PAG projection to the locus coeruleus (Aston-Jones et al., 1986) or to the parabrachial region (Milner et al., 1986). In fact, it has been demonstrated that the locus coeruleus receives a restricted input, almost exclusively from the nucleus reticularis paragigantocellularis lateralis of the ventral medulla and from the prepositus hypoglossi nucleus (Aston-Jones et al., 1986; Guyenet and Young, 1987). A recent study of afferents of the A5 cell group (Byrum and Guyenet, 1987) found a projection from rostral levels of the PAG; levels through the caudal, ventrolateral PAG, from which NE-mediated stimulation-produced analgesia is elicited, were not described. Taken together, these data do not permit a definitive conclusion that the noradrenergic neurons of the dorsolateral pontine tegmentum or A5 cell groups, considered to be potential sources of descending noradrenergic controls of spinal neurons, are directly activated from the PAG.

Clearly, a multisynaptic, indirect activation of these NE controls from the PAG is possible, and likely. It is also conceivable that electrical stimulation of the PAG excites spinally projecting NE cell bodies by antidromically activating branches of their axons in the PAG. Therefore, we designed an experiment to test whether there are noradrenergic neurons in the brain stem that send divergent collaterals to the PAG and to the spinal cord. To identify as many spinally projecting brain stem neurons as possible, we first made a large injection of the retrograde tracer, True Blue, into the cervical enlargement of the spinal cord. Several days later, to identify the afferent connections of the PAG, a localized injection of a second, gold-labelled, retrograde tracer, WGAapoHRP-Au, was made into the PAG. Sections that contained double-labelled neurons were then processed immunocytochemically to localize tyrosine hydroxylase, a marker for noradrenergic neurons (Kwiat and Basbaum, 1987).

The results from this study established that there are indeed noradrenergic neurons that send axon branches both to the spinal cord and to the PAG. Consistent with previous studies of the afferent connections of the PAG (Beitz, 1982; Meller and Dennis, 1986), most of these were found in the A5 cell group, which lies adjacent to the superior olive, in the locus coeruleus and in the A7/Kölliker-Fuse group (Fig. 8). These projections probably contribute to the extensive noradrenergic innervation of the PAG (Dahlström and Fuxe, 1965; Swanson and Hartman, 1975; Levitt and Moore, 1979). We conclude that electrical stimulation of the PAG might activate bulbospinal noradrenergic controls via antidromic activation of the noradrenergic axons which project to the PAG, and subsequent orthodromic activation of the spinally projecting collaterals of the NE cells in A5, locus coeruleus, subcoeruleus and A7/Kölliker-Fuse.

To test for a comparable bifurcation of the bulbospinal 5HT neurons located in the NRM and adjacent reticular formation, some sections were immunostained for 5HT. We, in fact, found that many neurons in the region of the NRM projected both to the cord and to the PAG; however, we were rarely able to triple-label the cells with an antiserum to serotonin. This indicates that those cells at the origin of the bulbospinal 5HT projection are

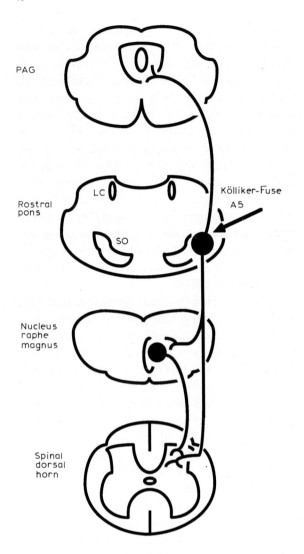

PAG

LC

Rostral
pons

Kölliker-Fuse
A5

SO

Nucleus
raphe
magnus

Spinal
dorsal
horn

Fig. 8. Scheme of the results from studies of the collateralization of immunoreactive tyrosine hydroxylase (TH) neurons of
the brain stem of the rat. In these studies, one retrograde tracer
was placed either in the NRM or in the PAG; a second tracer
was placed in the spinal cord. Sections containing labelled
neurons were then stained for norepinephrine (NE), using an
antibody directed against TH. Cells which send axons to the
NRM and cord, or to the PAG and cord were concentrated in
the A5 cell group and in the A7/Kölliker-Fuse cell group
located near the superior olive (SO). The Fig. implies that a
single cell projects to all three sites; however, this was not
directly established. Some collateralizing cells (not shown) were
also found in the locus coeruleus (LC). Electrical stimulation in
either the PAG or the NRM might evoke the release of
noradrenaline in the spinal cord via antidromic activation of the
collaterals of the NE-positive cells.

not the source of a 5HT input to the PAG (Fig. 6
B). The latter conclusion is at odds with recent
data from Beitz et al. (1986) who performed a
similar study and reported that greater than 50%
of the NRM neurons retrogradely labelled from
the NRM could be immunostained with an antibody to serotonin. On the other hand, Bowker
(1986) studied the labelling pattern in the NRM
after injections of the somewhat insensitive
retrograde tracer, HRP, into the ascending MLF.
Although many neurons in the NRM were
retrogradely labelled, none of these were
serotonin-immunostained. Since the distribution
of retrogradely labelled cells was comparable in the
three studies it is difficult to reconcile the different
results. One possibility is that the injection site using WGAHRP, the tracer used in the Beitz et al.
(1986) study, could not be restricted to the PAG.
The 5HT neurons in the NRM which were retrogradely labelled may have projected to regions adjacent to but not in the PAG. In addition, since
WGAHRP is readily taken up by axons of passage,
it is possible that the results from the Beitz et al.
(1986) study reflect transport via serotonergic axons originating in the NRM that course through,
but do not terminate within the PAG.

The complexity of the catecholamine contribution to descending control is underscored by the
observation of Hammond et al. (1985) that electrical stimulation of the NRM evokes the release of
both 5HT and NE in the spinal cord CSF. Since
there are no catecholamine cell bodies in the raphe
magnus (Dahström and Fuxe, 1964), this observation raises the interesting possibility that NRM
stimulation activates an excitatory link to the cells
at the origin of the bulbospinal NE projection.
Alternatively, there may be antidromic activation
of a noradrenergic input to the NRM (one which
presumably exerts an inhibitory control on the bulbospinal 5HT neurons (Hammond, this volume).
To address this issue we used the triple-label approach once again (Basbaum and Menetrey, unpublished observations). In this case True Blue was
injected into the spinal cord and the tracer,
WGAapoHRP-Au was injected into the NRM.

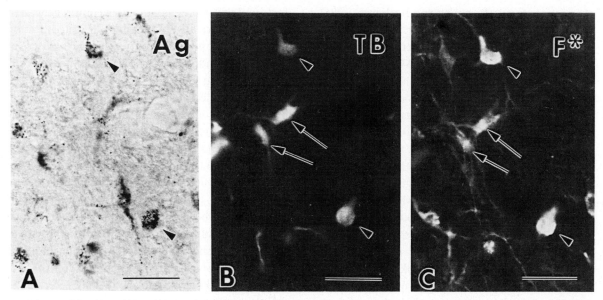

Fig. 9. Triple labelling of neurons in the A5 cell group adjacent to the superior olive. One retrograde tracer, WGAapoHRP-Au, was injected into the NRM. The bright-field photomicrograph in (A) illustrates silver-enhanced (Ag) retrogradely labelled cells in the A5 cell group. A second retrograde tracer, True Blue (TB), was injected into the spinal cord. Epifluorescent illumination of the same section as (A) reveals TB-containing retrogradely labelled neurons (B). The section containing these cells was stained with an antiserum to TH followed by a fluorescein-coupled second antibody. Fluorescein (F*)-positive cells are illustrated in (C). The arrowheads in (A), (B) and (C) identify triple-labelled cells. The arrows indicate cells that are TB- and TH-positive, but which do not project to the NRM. (From Basbaum and Menetrey, 1987.)

Double-labelled cells were found in many parts of the brain stem, which demonstrates that many brain stem neurons that project to the cord also send a collateral to the NRM. More importantly, some of the double-labelled cells in the A5 cell group and in the Kölliker-Fuse nucleus stained positively with antisera directed against tyrosine hydroxylase (TH) (Fig. 9). These data provide an anatomical basis for the spinal release of nor-adrenaline by electrical stimulation in the NRM. Fig. 8 illustrates the divergence of the noradrenergic projection from the A5 and Kölliker-Fuse cell groups and suggests the possibility that a single catecholaminergic neuron might collateralize to the cord, PAG and NRM. Our data, of course, do not rule out an orthodromic activation of bulbospinal NE neurons from the raphe, however, they emphasize the care that must be taken when drawing pharmacological circuit diagrams that are based exclusively on results from studies using electrical stimulation.

PAG ascending connections

Although most studies of the antinociceptive function of the PAG have focussed on the contribution of its descending projections to the medulla, there are also extensive rostrally directed projections (Mantyh, 1983a). Electrical stimulation of several of the rostral targets of the PAG, including specific zones within the hypothalamus, thalamus, amygdala and frontal cortex, produces analgesia (see Oliveras, this volume). To investigate the relationship between PAG neurons that project rostrally and caudally, we performed double-label retrograde tracing studies of PAG efferents in the rat. We injected the fluorescent tracer, True Blue, into the NRM and WGAapoHRP-Au into one of the rostral targets (Reichling and Basbaum, 1986).

Approximately 20% of PAG neurons that project to the parafascicular nucleus (PF) of the thalamus also project to the NRM; about 13% of PAG neurons labelled from injections in the medial hypothalamus were labelled from the NRM. These double-labelled neurons are most common in the dorsal and ventrolateral PAG. In contrast, PAG projections to the ventrobasal thalamus (VB), lateral hypothalamus (LH), amygdala and frontal cortex orginate almost exclusively from the midline RD. Most of the latter stained positively for serotonin, but only a few per cent of the 5HT neurons that projected rostrally also sent a collateral to the NRM. From these data we concluded that analgesia evoked by electrical stimulation of the PF and medial hypothalamus, but not of the VB, amygdala, LH or frontal cortex, might result from antidromic activation of PAG neurons which have axons that collateralize to the NRM. This, of course, would result in analgesia that bypasses the synaptic circuitry of the PAG, although it would be interrupted by a lesion of the PAG (see Rhodes, 1979). Importantly, the pharmacology of analgesia evoked from these rostral sites would not be determined by the intrinsic circuitry of the PAG, but rather might be more dependent on the neurotransmitters released by PAG axons in the NRM.

Since electrical stimulation of the RD decreases noxious stimulus-evoked activity of PF neurons (Andersen and Dafny, 1983a,b), the possibility that a component of the antinociceptive controls generated by electrical stimulation of, or drug microinjection into the PAG results from an ascending modulation of nociceptive inputs must also be considered (see Andersen, 1986). The inhibition of nociceptive neurons in the ventrobasal and medial thalamus by systemic (Guilbaud et al., 1983) or PAG injection of morphine (Kayser et al., 1983) might similarly result from activation of an ascending inhibitory RD/PAG control. Since there are significant numbers of PAG neurons that send collaterals to both the PF and the NRM, it is, in

fact, quite possible that antinociception, generated either by electrical stimulation of or drug injection into the PAG, is mediated by simultaneous activation of ascending and descending projections, perhaps arising from the same PAG neurons. The ascending projection from the PAG to the medial hypothalamus might also provide a feedback control of the β-endorphin-containing neurons that, in turn, project to the PAG. In fact, microinjection of morphine into the PAG depresses neuronal activity in the ventromedial hypothalamus (Lakosi and Gebhart, 1984) and electrical stimulation of the PAG has been shown to excite or inhibit the firing of medial hypothalamic neurons (Pittman et al., 1979). It should be pointed out that in all of these studies the possibility that the controls exerted in the PF are secondary to inhibition of the spinal ascending transmission, was not tested. It would be of interest, for example, to study the effect of PAG stimulation (or of microinjection of narcotics into the PAG) on the firing of PF neurons in an animal which had bilateral lesions of the DLF.

The studies outlined in this review illustrate the complexity of antinociceptive controls exerted from the midbrain PAG. Anatomically and functionally, the PAG is heterogeneous. There is evidence that β-endorphin, enkephalin, dynorphin, GABA and neurotensin neurons contribute to the controls generated from the PAG. Electrical stimulation of or microinjection of drugs into the PAG activates multiple stages of this circuitry. Because of the extensive collateralization of neuronal elements within this descending control system, interpretation of data from electrical stimulation studies is particularly difficult. The complex interaction of narcotics, such as morphine, with the multiple opioid receptor sites in the PAG makes interpretation of drug injection studies equally complicated. Taken together, these observations emphasize the critical need for detailed anatomical data as a basis for characterizing the functional circuitry of the descending controls activated from the PAG.

Acknowledgements

We thank Ms. Allison Gannon and Simona Ikeda for photographic assistance. This work was supported by PHS grants NS 14627 and 21445.

References

Abols, I.A. and Basbaum, A.I. (1981) Afferent connections of the rostral medulla of the cat: a neural substrate for mid-brain-medullary interactions. *J. Comp. Neurol.,* 201: 285 – 297.

Aimone, L.D. and Gebhart, G.F. (1986) Stimulation-produced spinal inhibition from the midbrain in the rat is mediated by an excitatory amino acid neurotransmitter in the medial medulla. *J. Neurosci.,* 6: 1803 – 1813.

Andersen, E. (1986) Periaqueductal gray and cerebral cortex modulate responses of medial thalamic neurons to noxious stimulation. *Brain Res.,* 375: 30 – 36.

Andersen, E. and Dafny, N. (1983a) An ascending serotonergic pain modulation pathway from the dorsal raphe nucleus to the parafascicularis nucleus of the thalamus. *Brain Res.,* 269: 57 – 67.

Andersen, E. and Dafny, N. (1983b) Dorsal raphe stimulation reduces responses of parafascicular neurons to noxious stimulation. *Pain,* 15: 323 – 331.

Aston-Jones, G., Ennis, M., Pieribone, V.A., Nickell, W.T., and Shipley, M.T. (1986) The brain nucleus locus coeruleus: restricted afferent control of a broad efferent network. *Science,* 234: 734 – 737.

Basbaum, A.I. and Fields, H.L. (1978) Endogenous pain control mechanisms: review and hypothesis. *Ann. Neurol.,* 4: 451 – 462.

Basbaum, A.I. and Fields, H.L. (1984) Endogenous pain control systems: brainstem spinal pathways and endorphin circuitry. *Annu. Rev. Neurosci.,* 7: 309 – 338.

Basbaum, A.I. and Menétrey, D. (1987) Wheat germ agglutinin-apoHRP gold: a new retrograde tracer for light- and electron-microscopic single- and double-label studies. *J. Comp. Neurol.,* 261: 306 – 318.

Basbaum, A.I., Marley, N., O'Keefe, J. and Clanton, C.H. (1977) Reversal of opiate and stimulus-produced analgesia by subtotal spinal cord lesions. *Pain,* 3: 43 – 56.

Basbaum, A.I., Clanton, C.H. and Fields, H.L. (1978) Three bulbospinal pathways from the rostral medulla of the cat: an autoradiographic study of pain modulating systems. *J. Comp. Neurol.,* 178: 209 – 224.

Basbaum, A.I., Moss, M.M. and Glazer, E.J. (1983) Opiate and stimulation-produced analgesia: the contribution of the monoamines. *Adv. Pain Res. Ther.,* 5: 323 – 339.

Basbaum, A.I., Cruz, L. and Weber, E. (1986) Immunoreactive dynorphin B in sacral primary afferent fibers of the cat. *J. Neurosci.,* 6: 127 – 133.

Basbaum, A.I., Zahs, K., Lord, B.A.P. and Lakos, S. (1988) The fiber caliber of 5HT immunoreactive axons in the dorsolateral funiculus of the spinal cord of the rat and cat. *Somatosens. Res.,* 5: 177 – 185.

Behbehani, M.M. and Fields, H.L. (1979) Evidence that an excitatory connection between the periaqueductal gray and the nucleus raphe magnus mediates stimulation-produced analgesia. *Brain Res.,* 170: 85 – 93.

Behbehani, M.M. and Pert, A. (1984) A mechanism for the analgesic effect of neurotensin as revealed by behavioral and electrophysiological techniques. *Brain Res.,* 324: 35 – 42.

Beitz, A.J. (1982a) The organization of afferent projections to the midbrain periaqueductal gray of the rat. *Neuroscience,* 7: 133 – 159.

Beitz, A.J. (1982b) The sites of origin of brainstem neurotensin and serotonin projections to the rodent nucleus raphe magnus. *J. Neurosci.,* 2: 829 – 842.

Beitz, A.J. (1985a) The midbrain periaqueductal gray in the rat. I. Nuclear volume, cell number, density, orientation, and regional subdivisions. *J. Comp. Neurol.,* 237: 445 – 459.

Beitz, A.J. (1985b) The midbrain periaqueductal gray in the rat. II. A Golgi analysis. *J. Comp. Neurol.,* 237: 460 – 475.

Beitz, A.J. (1985c) Reticular formation, central gray and related nuclei. In G. Paxinos (Ed.), *The Rat Central Nervous System,* Vol. 2, Academic Press, New York, pp. 1 – 28.

Beitz, A.J., Clements, J.R., Mullet, M.A. and Ecklund, L.J. (1986) Differential origin of brainstem serotoninergic projections to the midbrain periaqueductal gray and superior colliculus of the rat. *J. Comp. Neurol.,* 250: 498 – 509.

Bloom, F., Battenberg, E., Rossier, J., Ling, N. and Guillemin, R. (1978) Neurons containing beta endorphin in rat brain exist separately from those containing enkephalin: immunocytochemical studies. *Proc. Natl. Acad. Sci. USA,* 75: 1591 – 1595.

Botticelli, L.H., Cox, B.M. and Goldstein, A. (1981) Immunoreactive dynorphin in mammalian spinal cord and dorsal root ganglia. *Proc. Natl. Acad. Sci. USA,* 78: 7783 – 7786.

Bowker, R.M. (1986) The relationship between descending serotonin projections and ascending projections in the nucleus raphe magnus: a double labeling study. *Neurosci. Lett.,* 70: 348 – 353.

Byrum, C.E. and Guyenet, P.G. (1987) Afferent and efferent connections of the A5 noradrenergic cell group in the rat. *J. Comp. Neurol.,* 261: 529 – 542.

Cedarbaum, J.M. and Aghajanian, G.K. (1978) Afferent projections to the rat locus coeruleus as determined by a retrograde tracing technique. *J. Comp. Neurol.* 178: 1 – 16.

Chavkin, D., James, I.F. and Goldstein, A. (1982) Dynorphin is a specific endogenous ligand of the kappa opioid receptor. *Science,* 215: 413 – 415.

Dahlström, A. and Fuxe, K. (1964) Evidence for the existence of monoamine neurons in the central nervous system. I.

Demonstration of monoamines in the cell bodies of brain stem neurons. *Acta Physiol. Scand.,* Suppl 232, 62: 1 – 55.

Dahlström, A. and Fuxe, K. (1965) Evidence for the existence of monoamine neurons in the central nervous system. The distribution of monoamine terminals in the central nervous system. *Acta Physiol. Scand.,* Suppl. 247, 64: 37 – 84.

Defeudis, F.V. (1983) Central GABAergic systems and analgesia. *Drug Dev. Res.,* 3: 1 – 15.

Dickenson, A.H. and Knox, R.J. (1987) Antagonism of μ-opioid receptor mediated inhibitions of nociceptive neurones by U50488H and dynorphin-A$_{1-13}$ in the rat dorsal horn. *Neurosci. Lett.,* 75: 229 – 234.

Dostrovsky, J.O. and Deakin, J.F.W. (1977) Periaqueductal gray lesions reduce morphine analgesia in the rat. *Neurosci. Lett.,* 4: 99 – 103.

Fang, F.G., Fields, H.L. and Lee, N.M. (1986) Action at the mu receptor is sufficient to explain the supraspinal analgesic effect of opiates. *J. Pharmacol. Exp. Ther.,* 238: 1039 – 1044.

Fang, F.G., Moreau, J.O. and Fields, H.L. (1987) Dose-dependent antinociceptive action of neurotensin microinjected into the rostroventromedial medulla of the rat. *Brain Res.,* 426: 171 – 174.

Fields, H.L. and Anderson, S.D. (1978) Evidence that raphe spinal neurons mediate opiate and midbrain stimulation-produced analgesia. *Pain,* 5: 333 – 349.

Gallagher, D.W. and Aghajanian, G.W. (1976) Effect of antipsychotic drugs on the firing of dorsal raphe cells. II. Reversal by picrotoxin. *Eur. J. Pharmacol.,* 39: 357 – 364.

Gallagher, D.W. and Pert, A. (1978) Afferents to brainstem nuclei (brainstem raphe, n. reticularis pontis caudalis and n. gigantocellularis) in the rat as demonstrated by microiontophoretically applied horseradish peroxidase. *Brain Res.,* 144: 257 – 275.

Gebhart, G.F., Sandkühler, J., Thalhammer, J.G. and Zimmerman, M. (1983) Inhibition of spinal nociceptive information by stimulation in midbrain of the cat is blocked by lidocaine microinjections in nucleus raphe magnus and medullary reticular formation. *J. Neurophysiol.,* 50: 1446 – 1459.

Gioia, M., Bianchi, R. and Tredici, G. (1984) Cytoarchitecture of the periaqueductal gray matter in the cat: a quantitative Nissl study. *Acta Anat.,* 119: 113 – 117.

Guilbaud, G., Kayser, V., Benoist, J.M. and Gautron, M. (1983) Depressive effects of morphine and of an enkephalinase inhibitor on responses of ventrobasal thalamic neurons to noxious stimuli. *Life Sci.,* 33: 545 – 547.

Guyenet, P.G. and Young, B.S. (1987) Projections of nucleus paragigantocellularis lateralis to locus coeruleus and other structures in rat. *Brain Res.,* 406: 171 – 184.

Hamilton, B.L. (1973) Cytoarchitectural subdivisions of the periaqueductal gray matter in the cat. *J. Comp. Neurol.,* 149: 1 – 28.

Hammond, D.L, Tyce, G.M. and Yaksh, T.L. (1985) Efflux of 5-hydroxytryptamine and noradrenaline into spinal cord during stimulation of the rat medulla. *J. Physiol. (Lond.),* 359: 151 – 162.

Herkenham, M. and Pert, C.B. (1982) Light microscopic localization of brain opiate receptors: A general autoradiographic method which preserves tissue quality. *J. Neurosci.* 2: 1129 – 1149.

Heyman, J.S., Koslo, R.J., Mosber, H.I., Tallarida, R.J. and Porreca, F. (1987) Estimation of the affinity of naloxone at supraspinal and spinal opioid receptors *in vivo*: studies with receptor selective agonists. *Life Sci.,* 39: 1795 – 1803.

Izumi, K., Munekata, E., Yamamoto, H., Nakanishi, T. and Barbeau, A. (1980) Effects of taurine and gamma aminobutyric acid on akinesia and analgesia induced by D-Ala-metenkephalinamide in rats. *Peptides,* 1: 139 – 146.

Kawashima, Y. and Basbaum, A.I. (1984) Distribution of different endogenous opioid peptide families in the rat periaqueductal grey. *Pain,* Suppl. 2: S325.

Kayser, V., Benoist, J.M. and Guilbaud, G. (1983) Low dose of morphine microinjected in the ventral periaqueductal grey matter of the rat depresses responses of nociceptive ventrobasal thalamic neurons. *Neurosci. Lett.,* 37: 193 – 198.

Khatchaturian, H., Watson, S.J., Lewis, M.E., Coy, D., Goldstein, A. and Akil, H. (1982) Dynorphin immunocytochemistry in the rat central nervous system. *Peptides,* 3: 941 – 954.

Kwiat, G. and Basbaum, A.I. (1987) Organization and cytochemistry of brainstem neurons with divergent collaterals to the midbrain periqueductal gray and the spinal cord. *Neurosci. Abst.,* 13: 302.

Lakos, S. and Basbaum, A.I. (1986) Benzidine dihydrochloride as a chromogen for single- and double-label light and electron microscopic immunocytochemical studies. *J. Histochem. Cytochem.,* 34: 1047 – 1056.

Lakos, S. and Basbaum, A.I. (1988) An ultrastructural study of the projections from the midbrain periaqueductal gray to spinally projecting, serotonin-immunoreactive neurons of the medullary nucleus raphe magnus in the rat. *Brain Res.,* 443: 383 – 388.

Lakoski, J.M. and Gebhart, G.F. (1984) Depression of neuronal activity in the hypothalamic ventromedial nucleus of the rat following microinjection of morphine in the amygdala or the periaqueductal gray. *Neuroscience,* 12: 255 – 266.

Lee, E.H.Y., Wang, F.B., Tang, Y.P. and Geyer, M.A. (1987) GABAergic interneurons in the dorsal raphe mediate the effects of apomorphine on serotonergic system. *Brain Res. Bull.,* 18: 345 – 353.

Levitt, P. and Moore, R.Y. (1979) Origin and organization of brainstem catecholamine innervation in the rat. *J. Comp. Neurol.,* 186: 505 – 528.

Lewis, V.A. and Gebhart, G.F. (1977) Evaluation of the periaqueductal gray as a morphine-specific locus of action and examination of morphine-induced and stimulation-produced analgesia at coincident PAG loci. *Brain Res.,* 124: 283 – 303.

Liu, R.P.C. and Hamilton, B.L. (1980) Neurons of the periaqueductal gray matter as revealed by Golgi study. *J. Comp. Neurol.*, 189: 403–418.

Mansour, A., Khatchaturian, H., Lewis, M.E., Akil, H. and Watson, S.J. (1987) Autoradiographic differentiation of mu, delta and kappa opioid receptors in the rat forebrain and midbrain. *J. Neurosci.*, 7: 2445–2464.

Mantyh, P.W. (1982) The midbrain periaqueductal gray of the rat, cat and monkey: a Nissl, Weil and Golgi analysis. *J. Comp. Neurol.*, 204: 349–363.

Mantyh, P.W. (1983a) Connections of the midbrain periaqueductal gray in the monkey. I. Ascending efferent projections. *J. Neurophysiol.*, 49: 567–581.

Mantyh, P.W. (1983b) Connections of the midbrain periaqueductal gray in the monkey. II. Descending efferent projections. *J. Neurophysiol.*, 49: 582–594.

Mathiasen, J.R. and Vaught, J.L. (1987) [D-Pen^2,L-Pen^5]enkephalin-induced analgesia in the jimpy mouse: in vivo evidence for delta-receptor-mediated analgesia. *Eur. J. Pharmacol.*, 136: 405–407.

Meller, S.T. and Dennis, B.J. (1986) Afferent projections to the periaqueductal gray in the rabbit. *Neuroscience*, 19: 927–964.

Menétrey, D. and Basbaum, A.I. (1987) The distribution of substance P, enkephalin and dynorphin immunoreactive neurons in the medulla of the rat and their contribution to bulbospinal pathways. *Neuroscience*, 23: 173–188.

Millan, M.H., Millan, M.J. and Herz, A. (1986) Depletion of central beta endorphin blocks midbrain stimulation-produced analgesia in the freely-moving rat. *Neuroscience*, 18: 641–649.

Milner, T.A., Joh, T.H. and Pickel, V.M. (1986) Tyrosine hydroxylase in the rat parabrachial region: ultrastructural localization and extrinsic sources of immunoreactivity. *J. Neurosci.*, 6: 2585–2603.

Moreau, J.L. and Fields, H.L. (1986) Evidence for GABA involvement in midbrain control of medullary neurons that modulate nociceptive transmission. *Brain Res.*, 397: 37–46.

Moss, M.M. and Basbaum, A.I. (1983) The fine structure of the caudal periaqueductal grey of the cat: morphology and synaptic organization of normal and immunoreactive enkephalin-labelled profiles. *Brain Res.*, 289: 27–43.

Moss, M.M., Glazer, E.J. and Basbaum, A.I. (1983) The peptidergic organization of the cat periaqueductal grey. I. The distribution of immunoreactive enkephalin. *J. Neurosci.*, 3: 603–616.

Nicoll, R.A. and Alger, B.E. (1979) Enkephalin blocks inhibitory pathways in the vertebrate CNS. *Nature*, 287: 22–25.

Nishikawa, T. and Scatton, B. (1983) Evidence for a GABAergic inhibitory influence on serotonergic neurons originating from the dorsal raphe. *Brain Res.*, 279: 325–329.

Pittman, Q.J., Blume, H.W., Kearney, R.E. and Renaud, L.P. (1979) Influence of midbrain stimulation on the excitability of neurons in the medial hypothalamus of the rat. *Brain Res.*, 174: 39–53.

Porreca, F., Heyman, J.S. Mosberg, H.I., Ominaas, J.R. and Vaught, J.L. (1987) Role of mu and delta receptors in the supraspinal and spinal analgesic effects of [D-Pen^2,D-Pen^5]enkephalin in the mouse. *J. Pharmacol. Exp. Ther.*, 241: 393–400.

Prieto, G.F., Cannon, J.T. and Liebeskind, J.C. (1983) Nucleus raphe magnus lesions disrupt stimulation-produced analgesia from ventral but not dorsal midbrain areas in the rat. *Brain Res.*, 261: 53–57.

Pujol, J.F., Belin, M.F., Gamrani, H., Aguera, M. and Calas, A. (1981) Anatomical evidence for GABA-5HT interaction in serotonergic neurons. In Haber et al. (Eds.) *Serotonin: Current Aspects of Neurochemistry*, Plenum Press, New York, pp. 67–79.

Reichling, D. and Basbaum, A.I. (1986) Some periaqueductal gray neurons of rat which project to the nucleus raphe magnus have ascending collaterals. *Neurosci. Abst.*, 12: 616.

Reichling, D. and Basbaum, A.I. (1987) Anatomical evidence that GABA influences the projection from the periaqueductal gray matter to the NRM. *Pain*, Suppl. 4: S40.

Retz, K.C. and Holaday, L.M. (1986) Analgesia and motor activity following administration of THIP into the periaqueductal gray and lateral ventricle of rats. *Drug Dev. Res.*, 9: 133–142.

Rhodes, D.L. (1979) Perventricular system lesions in stimulation-produced analgesia. *Pain*, 7: 31–51.

Roberts, M.H.T. (1984) 5-Hydroxytryptamine and antinociception. *Neuropharmacology*, 23: 1529–1536.

Romandini, S. and Samanin, R. (1984) Muscimol injections in the nucleus raphe dorsalis block the antinociceptive effects of morphine in rats: apparent lack of 5-hydroxytryptamine involvement in muscimol's effect. *Br. J. Pharmacol.*, 81: 25–29.

Ruda, M.A. (1976) Autoradiographic study of the efferent projections of the midbrain central gray in the cat. Doctoral Thesis, University of Pennsylvania.

Sakai, K., Touret, M., Salvert, D., Leger, L. and Jouvet, M. (1977) Afferent projections to the cat locus coeruleus as visualized by the horseradish peroxidase technique. *Brain Res.*, 119: 21–41.

Schmauss, C. and Herz, A. (1987) Intrathecally administered dynorphin-(1-17) modulates morphine-induced antinociception differently in morphine-naive and morphine-tolerant rats. *Eur. J. Pharmacol.*, 135: 429–431.

Standaert, D.G., Watson, S.J., Houghten, R.A. and Saper, C.B. (1986) Opioid peptide immunoreactivity in spinal and trigeminal dorsal horn neurons projecting to the parabrachial nucleus in the rat. *J. Neurosci.*, 6: 1220–1226.

Stevens, R.T., Hodge, C.J. and Apkarian, A.V. (1982) Kölliker-Fuse nucleus: the principle source of pontine catecholamine cells projecting to the lumbar spinal cord of cat. *Brain Res.,* 239: 589 – 594.

Swanson, L.W. and Hartman, B.K. (1975) The central adrenergic system. An immunofluorescence study of the location of cell bodies and their efferent connections in the rat utilizing dopamine-β-hydroxylase as a marker. *J. Comp. Neurol.,* 163: 467 – 506.

Sweetnam, P.M., Neale, J.H., Barker, J.L. and Goldstein, A. (1982) Localization of immunoreactive dynorphin in neurons cultured from spinal cord and dorsal root ganglia. *Proc. Natl. Acad. Sci. USA,* 79: 6742 – 6746.

Tulunay, F.C., Jen, M.-F., Chang, J.-K., Loh, H.H. and Lee, N.M. (1981) Possible regulatory role of dynorphin on morphine- and β-endorphin-induced analgesia. *J. Pharmacol. Exp. Ther.,* 219: 296 – 298.

Ueda, H., Ming, G., Satoh, M. and Takagi, H. (1987) Subconvulsive doses of intracisternal bicuculline methiodide, a GABA receptor antagonist, produce potent analgesia as measured in the tail pinch test in mice. *Eur. J. Pharmacol.,* 136: 129 – 131.

Vanegas, H., Barbaro, N.M. and Fields, H.L. (1984) Midbrain stimulation inhibits tail-flick only at currents sufficient to excite rostral medullary neurons. *Brain Res.,* 321: 127 – 133.

Weihe, E., Hartschuh, W. and Weber, E. (1985) Prodynorphin opioid peptides in small somatosensory primary afferents of guinea pig. *Neurosci. Lett.,* 58: 347 – 352.

Westlund, K.N., Bowker, R.M., Ziegler, M.G. and Coulter, J.D. (1983) Noradrenergic projections to the spinal cord of the rat. *Brain Res.,* 263: 15 – 31.

Westlund, K.N., Bowker, R.M., Ziegler, M.G. and Coulter, J.D. (1984) Origins and terminations of descending noradrenergic projections to the spinal cord of monkey. *Brain Res.,* 292: 1 – 16.

Wiklund, L., Leger, L., and Persson, M. (1981) Monoamine cell distribution in the cat brainstem. A fluorescence histochemical study with quantification of indolaminergic and locus coeruleus cell groups. *J. Comp. Neurol.,* 203: 613 – 649.

Yaksh, T.L., Yeung, J.C. and Rudy, T.A. (1976) Systematic examination in the rat of brain sites sensitive to the direct application of morphine: observation of differential effects within the periaqueductal gray. *Brain Res.,* 114: 83 – 103.

Yamano, M., Inagaki, S., Kito, S., Takashi, S., Matsuzaki, T., Shinohara, Y. and Tohyama, M. (1986) Enkephalinergic projections from the ventromedial hypothalamic nucleus to the midbrain central gray matter in the rat: an immunocytochemical analysis. *Brain Res.,* 398: 337 – 346.

Zonta, N., Zambotti, F., Vicentini, L., Tammiso, R. and Montegazza, P. (1981) Effects of some GABA-mimetic drugs on the antinociceptive activity of morphine and beta-endorphin in rats. *Naunyn-Schmiedebergs Arch. Pharmacol.,* 316: 231 – 234.

Zambotti, F., Zonta, N., Parenti, N., Tommasi, R. Vicentini, L., Conci, F., and Montegazza, P. (1982) Periaqueductal gray matter involvement in the muscimol-induced decrease of morphine antinociception. *Naunyn-Schmiedebergs Arch. Pharmacol.,* 318: 368 – 369.

H.L. Fields and J.-M. Besson (Eds.)
Progress in Brain Research, Vol. 77
© 1988 Elsevier Science Publishers B.V. (Biomedical Division)

CHAPTER 3

Direct and indirect pathways to lamina I in the medulla oblongata and spinal cord of the cat

Gert Holstege

Department of Anatomy, University of California San Francisco Medical School, San Francisco, CA 94143, USA

Introduction

Physiological studies (Christensen and Perl, 1970; Cervero et al., 1976) have indicated that in the dorsal horn of the spinal cord neurons exist that can only be activated by nociceptive stimuli. These neurons can be subdivided into two groups. The first group contains nociceptive specific or high-threshold neurons (Price and Dubner, 1977; Chung et al., 1979) and the second group contains nociceptive non-specific or wide dynamic range neurons (Mendell, 1966). The first group of neurons is exclusively activated by nociceptive stimulation, mechanical and/or thermal, whereas the second group receives both nociceptive and non-nociceptive inputs. The nociceptive specific neurons are located mainly in the superficial zones of the spinal cord (Rexed's lamina I and the upper part of lamina II (Rexed, 1954)), whereas the nociceptive non-specific neurons predominate in laminae IV to VI of Rexed but most densely in lamina V (see Willis, 1982 and Besson and Chaouch, 1987, for reviews). However, nociceptive non-specific neurons are also numerous in the superficial laminae of the dorsal horn (Woolf and Fitzgerald, 1983), while nociceptive specific neurons can also be found in deep laminae of the dorsal horn (Willis et al., 1974) or in more ventral

areas of the spinal gray (Fields et al., 1977a). Lamina I contains few neurons that respond exclusively to innocuous stimuli. Except for some non-nociceptive thermoreceptive neurons (Christensen and Perl, 1970), lamina I and the outer part of lamina II do not contain low-threshold mechanoreceptor neurons. According to a study, using intraaxonal injection of horseradish peroxidase (HRP), high-threshold $A\delta$ fibers terminate mainly in lamina I, the outer part of II, the lateral part of V and in the dorsal periependymal zone (Light and Perl, 1979; Ralston and Ralston, 1979). By contrast, low-threshold A fibers mainly terminate in lamina III and not in laminae I and II (Light and Perl, 1979). Intraaxonal staining of C fibers in the guinea pig demonstrates terminations mainly in outer lamina II and in lamina I (Sugiura et al., 1986). In conclusion, the great majority of lamina I neurons receive $A\delta$ and C fiber input and are likely involved in nociception. This means that studies on the anatomy of supraspinal projections to lamina I of the spinal cord most probably reveal pathways directly related to supraspinal control of nociception.

In this report only the brain stem and cortical regions giving rise to descending pathways to lamina I will be discussed. The brain stem areas projecting to the spinal cord, but not to lamina I (e.g., the vestibular nuclei, the dorsal medullary and pontine reticular nuclei, the red nucleus and the superior colliculus) will not be reviewed,

Correspondence: G. Holstege, NASA/Ames Research Center, Mail Stop 239-7, Moffett Field, CA 94043, USA.

although it must be emphasized that this does not rule out the possibility that these structures play a role in supraspinal nociception control. Furthermore, the structures in mes-, di- and telencephalon, providing strong afferent connections to lamina I projecting brain stem structures, will be examined. The various structures and pathways will be presented on the basis of retrograde HRP and anterograde autoradiographic tracing findings obtained by the author (see also Hopkins and Holstege, 1978; Holstege and Kuypers, 1982; Holstege et al., 1985 and Holstege, 1987a) and compared with the anatomical tracing and physiological results of others. The histochemical aspects of many of these pathways will be dealt with by several other authors in this volume and will only be discussed briefly.

Materials and methods

HRP injections in the spinal cord

In five cats, horseradish peroxidase (HRP) was injected unilaterally into various levels of the spinal cord; in Case 1602 at the level of C2, in Case 1320 at the level of T1, in Case 1740 at the level of L6, and in Cases 1313 and 1786 at the level of S1. In one case (1320) 50 μl of 30% HRP dissolved in water was injected and in Case 1786 20 μl of 30% HRP was injected. Since HRP is transported both from terminals and from damaged axons (Kristensson and Olsson, 1974), multiple needle penetrations were made in the spinal gray and white matter (Kuypers and Maisky, 1975). This resulted in retrograde transport through fibers that terminate in the injected segments as well as through fibers of passage. In order to verify that the retrogradely labeled neurons in the brain stem distributed their axons only through the funiculi of the injected half of the spinal cord, contralateral spinal hemisections were made prior to the HRP injections in three cases. In the case with a T1 injection (1320), a hemisection was made at the level of C1 – C2 and in one case with an S1 injection (1786) at the level of L2. However, the hemisections in these two cases spared the most medial

part of the ventral funiculus. In Cases 1602 and 1740, hemi-infiltrations of HRP were made at the levels of C2 and L6, respectively. This was done after a dorsal approach by placing a piece of HRP slow-release gel (Griffin et al., 1979) in the ventromedial funiculus. The pia mater between the ipsilateral and contralateral ventral funiculi was left intact to prevent spread of HRP into the contralateral side as much as possible. The remaining parts of the ipsilateral half of the spinal cord in these cases were filled with approximately 15 μl of 30% HRP dissolved in saline. In both cases, however, the injection site extended somewhat into the contralateral side and the resulting distribution pattern of HRP-labeled neurons in the mesencephalon was, in one case (1740), almost completely bilateral.

HRP injections in the brain stem

In three cats (1508, 1694 and 1708), after a ventral approach and retraction of the basilar artery, a small deposit of HRP slow release gel (Griffin et al., 1979) was implanted in the caudal pontine and upper medullary medial tegmentum, including the nucleus raphe magnus (NRM) and the most rostral portion of the nucleus raphe pallidus (NRP).

All HRP-injected cases survived 3 days, after which each animal was deeply anesthetized with nembutal and perfused transcardially with: (1) 2 l of 0.9% saline at room temperature, (2) 4 l of a solution containing 0.1 M phosphate buffer (pH 7.2 – 7.4) with 1% paraformaldehyde and 1.25% glutaraldehyde, also at room temperature, and (3) 2 l of 0.2 M phosphate buffer containing 20% sucrose at 4°C. Each whole brain and spinal cord was removed and stored overnight in 20% sucrose in buffered phosphate at 4°C. When fully impregnated, each brain was frozen and sectioned transversely at 30 μm. Every fourth section was collected from phosphate buffer and incubated according to the tetramethyl benzidine (TMB) method of Mesulam (1978). The resulting pattern and number of HRP-labeled neurons in the brain stem and ventral parts of di- and telencephalon was plotted.

Tritiated leucine injections

Since the retrograde HRP-labeling of brain stem and forebrain neurons did not indicate specifically where the axons terminated within the spinal gray or brain stem, a number of cats were prepared using the anterograde autoradiographic tracing technique. Areas within the brain stem and forebrain, which contained HRP-filled neurons, were injected with radioactive tracer.

In 47 cats L-[4,5-^{3}H]leucine, specific activity > 100 Ci/mmol, in distilled water, was injected into the brain stem and the forebrain. In all cases except four, 0.5 μl was injected over a period of 5 min, after which the needle was left in place for an additional 30 min to prevent the spread of the ^{3}H-leucine along the needle track. Four cases (1465, 1468 with injections in the somatosensory cortex and 1653 and 1654 with hypothalamic injections) were injected with 1.0 μl of a ^{3}H-leucine solution containing approximately 100 μCi. All cats, except two, survived for 6 weeks. Cat 746, with an injection in the amygdala, survived for 2 weeks and cat 1707, with an injection in the bed nucleus of the stria terminalis, survived for 4 weeks. The 6-week survival time for all the other cats was chosen because earlier findings by Holstege et al. (1979) indicated that in cases with ^{3}H-leucine injections in the pontine tegmentum a 6-week survival time resulted in a much more pronounced autoradiographic labeling in lumbosacral and coccygeal segments than did a survival of 2 weeks. In the same study (Holstege et al., 1979), it was demonstrated that this pronounced enhancement of the terminal distribution pattern using ^{3}H-leucine is not due to transneuronal transport (see also Elam et al., 1987).

In all 47 cats the injections were placed stereotaxically using a Hamilton microsyringe fitted with a 22-gauge needle. After the survival period the animals were deeply anesthetized and perfused with saline followed by 10% formalin. The brains and spinal cords were postfixed in 10% formalin for at least 1 week, after which they were cut into transverse 25-μm frozen sections. One series of every 10th section was mounted (Hendrickson et al., 1972), coated with Ilford G5 emulsion by dipping (Kopriwa and Leblond, 1962) and stored in the dark at 5°C for 3 months. Subsequently, the material was developed with Kodak D19 at 16°C, fixed and counterstained with cresyl violet. The sections were studied with a Wild-Heerbrugg M7S darkfield stereomicroscope, and low-magnification brightfield and darkfield photomicrographs were taken of representative brain stem and spinal cord sections.

The injection sites showed a dense accumulation of silver grains in the area around the end of the needle track. In the central zone of the injection the silver grains were located over cell bodies of neurons and glia and over the neuropil. This zone was surrounded by a second zone in which the silver grains were located mainly over the neuropil. The injection area in the various experiments was defined as that area in which the silver grains over the cell bodies were either as numerous as or more numerous than those over the surrounding neuropil (Holstege et al., 1977, 1979). Light microscopic autoradiographic data do not allow the verification of actual fiber terminations. Therefore, it was assumed that labeled fibers clearly surrounding neurons represented fibers with terminals on these cells.

Results

Medulla oblongata

The medulla oblongata in the cat contains several different reticular and raphe nuclei. Rostrally in the medulla, at levels rostral to the hypoglossal nucleus, the gigantocellular reticular nucleus (Taber, 1961) occupies the dorsal two thirds of the medial reticular formation and the magnocellular reticular nucleus the ventral one third (Berman, 1968). Both areas are laterally bounded by the parvocellular reticular nucleus (Taber, 1961). Medially, at the level of the hypoglossal nucleus, the interfascicular nucleus is present (Taber, 1961) and laterally the dorsal and ventral subnuclei of the central nucleus of the medulla oblongata (Taber, 1961). These last two nuclei, together with the par-vocellular reticular nucleus and the rostrally ad-joining area h of Meessen and Olszewski (1949) and ventral parabrachial nuclei, are also called the bulbar lateral tegmental field (Holstege et al., 1977; Holstege and Kuypers, 1982). This area con-tains many neurons that serve as interneurons for the motoneurons in the caudal brain stem and up-per cervical cord (Holstege et al., 1977; Holstege and Kuypers, 1982), in the same way as neurons in the spinal intermediate zone serve as interneurons for the motoneurons in the spinal cord (Sterling and Kuypers, 1967; Rustioni et al., 1971; Molenaar, 1978). The medullary midline raphe consists of three nuclei. The nucleus raphe magnus (NRM) in the rostral medulla is bounded ventrally and caudally by the nucleus raphe pallidus (NRP). Located dorsally and caudally to the NRM and NRP is the nucleus raphe obscurus which contains only a limited number of neurons (Taber, 1960).

Caudal raphe nuclei and adjoining reticular forma-tion

Retrograde HRP results (Fig. 1) clearly indicate that a great number of neurons in the medulla oblongata project to the spinal cord. Strikingly, no major differences were found between the cases with hemi-infiltrations of HRP in the C2, T1, L6 or S1 levels, except that the number of labeled neurons was higher in the cases with injections in the rostral than in the caudal spinal cord. This in-dicates that many of the medullary neurons project throughout the length of the spinal cord. This con-clusion is in agreement with the findings of others (Martin et al., 1981b; Hayes and Rustioni, 1981 and Huisman et al., 1982), who have demonstrated by means of a retrograde double labeling tracing technique that many of the neurons, especially in the ventral part of the medulla, project to cervical as well as lumbar levels of the spinal cord and to the caudal spinal trigeminal nucleus (Lovick and Robinson, 1983). Retrograde tracing studies, however, do not give insight in the actual termina-tions of the neurons projecting to the spinal cord.

In this respect the autoradiographic tracing techni-que is a more appropiate tool, and a large portion of what is known about these pathways has been obtained by means of this technique.

The most well-known structure in the medulla oblongata giving rise to descending projections to lamina I of the spinal cord is the nucleus raphe magnus (NRM). Basbaum and coworkers (1978) were the first to demonstrate in the cat that ^{3}H-leucine injections involving the NRM revealed pro-jections to the marginal layer of the caudal spinal trigeminal nucleus and in the spinal cord to laminae I and II, more deeply to laminae V, VI and VII and to the thoracolumbar intermediolateral cell column. In the cat the raphe nuclei contain many serotonergic neurons (Wiklund et al., 1981), some of which also contain substance P and leucine-enkephalin (see Bowker, this volume). In-terestingly, Basbaum et al. (1978) found similar projections from the reticular formation adjoining the NRM, i.e. the ventral part of the medial reticular formation at the level of the facial nuclei, also called the nucleus reticularis magnocellularis, or in humans the nucleus reticularis gigan-tocellularis (Olszewski and Baxter, 1954). In this part of the reticular formation serotonergic neurons are scarce (Wiklund et al., 1981), in-dicating that the projections from these regions are not serotonergic. A possible neurotransmitter can-didate for these pathways is acetylcholine (Bowker et al., 1983; Jones et al., 1986). The results of Basbaum et al. (1978) were confirmed by the fin-dings of Martin et al. (1979, 1985) in the opossum and rat and by Holstege et al. (1979) and Holstege and Kuypers (1982) in the cat (see also Fig. 3, left; Fig 4, upper left; and Fig. 5, lower left). Holstege and Kuypers (1982) also demonstrated that the rostral portion of the NRM and adjoining reticular formation (Cases 1201 and 1293; Fig 2, R, S) does not project specifically to laminae I and V but to all laminae of the dorsal horn, and in some sec-tions the impression was gained that the main pro-jection was to the inner part of lamina II and to laminae III and IV (Fig. 4, upper right). Another very important finding was that the nucleus raphe

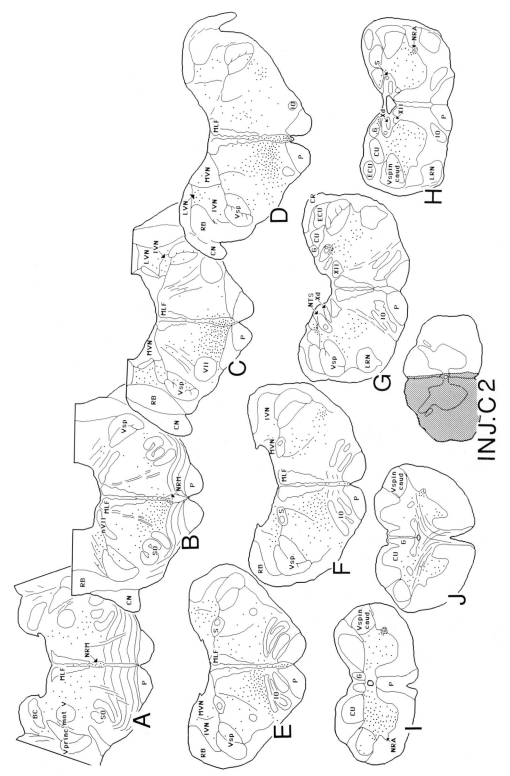

Fig. 1. Schematic drawings of HRP-labeled neurons in the caudal pontine and medullary tegmentum in Case 1602 (HRP hemi-infiltration in the C2 segment). (N.B: For abbreviations in the Figures, see p. 87.)

52

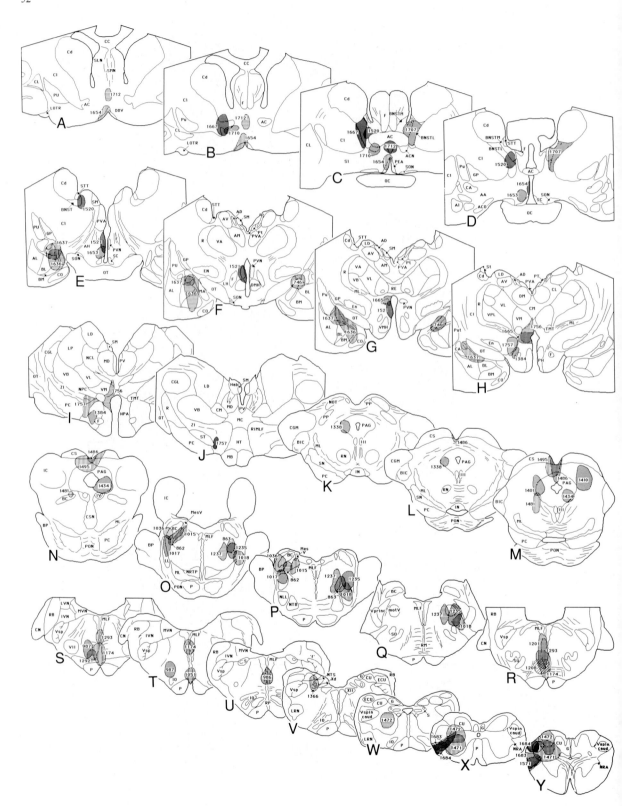

Fig. 2. Schematic drawings of the sites of injection of ³H-leucine in the various parts of the brain stem, hypothalamus, amygdala and bed nucleus of the stria terminalis.

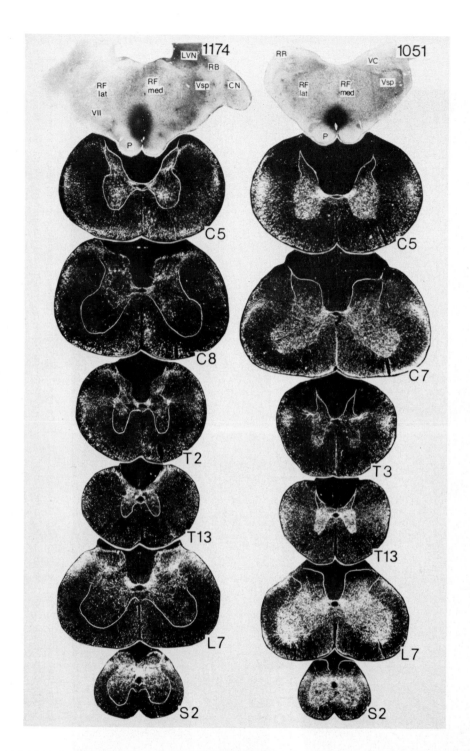

Fig. 3. Bright-field photomicrographs of the autoradiographs showing the tritiated leucine injection sites, and dark-field photomicrographs showing the spinal distributions of the labeled fibers in Cases 1174 (on the left) and 1051 (on the right). In Case 1174, with an injection in the caudal NRM and adjoining reticular formation, labeled fibers are distributed mainly to the dorsal horn (lamina I, the upper part of laminae II and V), the intermediate zone and the autonomic motoneuronal cell groups. In Case 1051, with an injection in the NRP and immediately adjoining tegmentum, labeled fibers are not distributed to the dorsal horn, but very strongly to the ventral horn (intermediate zone and autonomic and somatic motoneuronal cell groups. (From Holstege and Kuypers, 1982; Progress in Brain Research, Vol. 57, p. 158.)

54

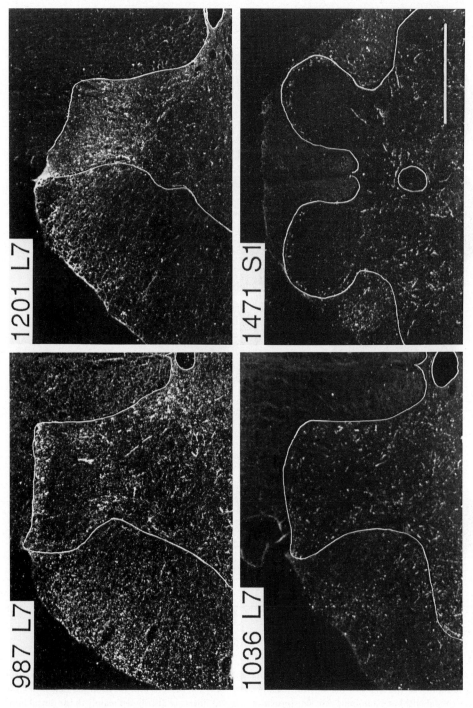

Fig. 4. Dark-field photomicrographs of the dorsal horn of the level of L7 in Cases 987 (injection in the rostral medullary medial reticular formation; upper left), 1201 (injection in the caudal pontine medial tegmental field, involving the rostral NRM; upper right) and 1036 (injection in the dorsolateral pontine tegmental field, including the lateral nucleus subcoeruleus and the ventral parabrachial nuclei; lower left). Lower right shows a dark-field photomicrograph of the dorsal horns of the S1 segment of Case 1471 (injection in the most caudal medullary tegmentum). Note that the medial tegmentum next to the NRM projects also to lamina I of the dorsal horn (upper left), but the rostral NRM mainly to other parts of the dorsal horn (upper right). Note further that the dorsolateral pontine tegmentum (probably the noradrenergic neurons in this area) projects very diffusely to the dorsal horn, while a slight, but clear projection to lamina I is derived from the caudal medulla (lower right). Bar represents 1 mm.

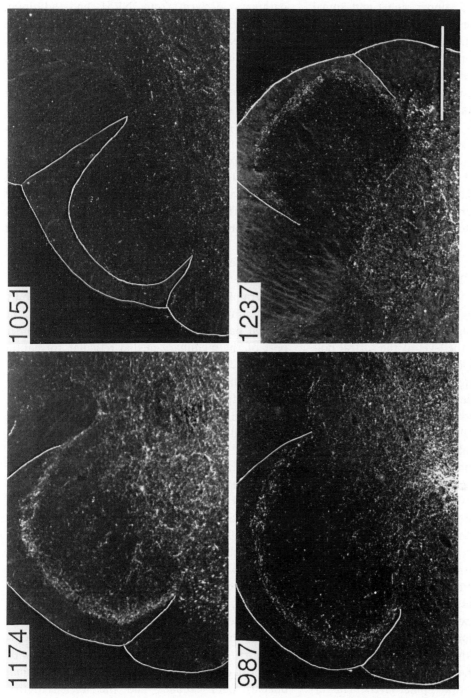

Fig. 5. Dark-field photomicrographs of the caudal spinal trigeminal nucleus of Case 1174, with an injection of ³H-leucine in the NRM (upper left), Case 1051 (injection in the NRP; upper right), Case 987 (injection in the ventral part of the upper medullary medial tegmental field; lower left) and Case 1237 (injection in the paralemniscal tegmental field; lower right). Note that labeled fibers are abundant in the marginal layer of the caudal spinal trigeminal nucleus after an injection in the NRM, upper medullary medial tegmentum and paralemniscal tegmental field, but absent in this nucleus after an injection in the NRP. Note further that the projection from the paralemniscal tegmentum is contralateral. Bar represents 1 mm.

pallidus (NRP) and its adjoining reticular formation did not project to the dorsal horn of the caudal medulla (Fig. 5, upper right) and spinal cord (Fig. 3, right), but to all other parts of the spinal grey matter including the somatic and autonomic motoneuronal cell groups (Martin et al., 1981a; Holstege et al., 1979; Holstege and Kuypers, 1982; Fig. 3, right). Further caudally, at the level of the rostral pole of the hypoglossal nucleus, the medullary medial reticular formation projects to only the somatic motoneuronal cell groups (Case 1166; Fig. 2, V). Interestingly in the cases in which labeled fibers were distributed to lamina I (Cases 987, 1174, 1208 and 1292; Fig. 2, R, S, T), labeled fibers were also present in the autonomic (sympathetic and parasympathetic) preganglionic cell groups (Fig. 3). These projections were also found in the rostral NRP injected cases (986 and 1051; Fig. 2, T, U), but not when the injections included only the rostral NRM and adjacent reticular formation (Cases 1201 and 1293; Fig. 2, R, S) or the ventral part of the medullary medial reticular formation at the level of the rostral pole of the hypoglossal nucleus (Case 1166). In conclusion, a strong heterogeneity exists in the projections of the ventral part of the medullary medial reticular formation and the caudal raphe nuclei, in which (1) the rostral NRM and adjoining reticular formation project to all parts of the dorsal horn (possibly with an emphasis on the projections to laminae II to IV), (2) the caudal NRM and adjoining reticular formation project to mainly laminae I and V and the autonomic motoneuronal cell groups, (3) the NRP and adjoining reticular formation project to the intermediate zone and the ventral horn including the autonomic and somatic motoneuronal cell groups and (4) the ventral part of the medial reticular formation at the level of rostral pole of the hypoglossal nucleus projects to the somatic motoneuronal cell groups. A very important feature of all these projections is that they descend throughout the length of the spinal cord, giving off collaterals to all spinal levels. This indicates that these projection systems are diffuse, i.e. not topographically organized.

For the most part, physiological studies are consistent with the anatomy of the descending pathways derived from NRM and adjoining reticular formation to the dorsal horn of the spinal cord. Electrical stimulation in the NRM inhibits neurons in the caudal spinal trigeminal nucleus (Hu and Sessle, 1979; Lovick and Wolstencroft, 1979; Sessle et al., 1981) and spinal dorsal horn (Engberg et al., 1968; Fields et al., 1977b; Willis et al., 1977). More recently, Light et al. (1986), stimulating the NRM, produced an inhibitory postsynaptic potential (IPSP) in neurons in laminae I and II at a latency consistent with a monosynaptic connection. Stimulation in the NRP is less effective and stimulation in the nucleus raphe obscurus is ineffective (Griffith and Gatipon, 1981). Fields et al. (1977b) have also shown that the inhibition caused by stimulation is mediated by a pathway descending in the dorsolateral funiculus of the spinal cord. Not only NRM stimulation, but stimulation in the adjacent ventral part of the caudal pontine and/or upper part of the medullary medial reticular formation (the nucleus reticularis gigantocellularis or magnocellularis) also produces inhibition of neurons in the dorsal horn (Fields et al., 1977; Akaike et al., 1978). These findings are in full agreement with the anatomical data (see above).

Reticular formation of the caudal medulla

A hitherto unknown projection to lamina I of the spinal cord is derived from the lateral part of the dorsal subnucleus of the central nucleus (Taber, 1961), located in the most caudal part of the medulla oblongata. In five cases, ^{3}H-leucine injections were made in this part of the medulla and in two of them (Cases 1471 and 1472; Fig. 2, W, X, Y), labeled fibers were distributed to lamina I. In Case 1471, the injection site occupied large parts of the reticular formation, including the ventral horn, and extended laterally into all parts of the most caudal portion of the spinal trigeminal nucleus pars caudalis and the nucleus retroambiguus. In Case 1472 the injection site was located more dorsally and involved dorsal parts of the reticular formation, the lateral part of the cuneate nucleus and the dorsomedial portion of the caudal spinal trigeminal nucleus. The injection in this case did not extend into the nucleus retroambiguus proper. In both cases labeled fibers descended in the dorsolateral funiculus, from where they were distributed to lamina I throughout the length of the spinal cord, but they were scarce at cervical and thoracic levels and only present ipsilaterally. At lumbosacral levels they were more numerous and were found on both sides of the spinal cord (Fig. 4, lower right). The nucleus retroambiguus seems not to be involved in this projection, because it is not injected in Case 1472, and lamina I projections were not observed in Cases 1571, 1683 and 1684 (Fig. 2, X, Y), with injections involving this nucleus. The HRP cases showed a few HRP-labeled neurons just medially to the caudal spinal trigeminal nucleus. Since this area is injected in both cases (1471 and 1472), these neurons may give rise to the lamina I projections. The function of this limited but circumscribed projection is unclear.

Dorsal column nuclei

Another possible source of projections to lamina I are the dorsal column nuclei (Burton and Loewy, 1977). The HRP spinal cord hemi-infiltration cases revealed HRP-labeled neurons in the dorsal column nuclei (Fig. 1, G, H). In the lumbosacral cord injected cases, the labeled neurons were found laterally in the rostral gracile nucleus while after T1 and C2 hemi-infiltrations labeled neurons were found rostrally in both the gracile and cuneate nuclei. They were most numerous ventrally in the lateral part of the gracile and in the medial part of the cuneate nucleus at levels just rostral to the obex. These results correspond with the findings of Kuypers and Maisky (1975) and Burton and Loewy (1977). In one case (1366; Fig. 2, V), an injection of ^{3}H-leucine was made just rostrally to the obex in the area of the lateral solitary nucleus, but extended ventrally into the dorsal part of the lateral reticular formation (parvocellular reticular nucleus) and dorsally into the transition zone between

the gracile and cuneate nucleus. This latter area, according to the HRP results, contains many neurons projecting to the spinal cord. In Case 1366 a strong bilateral projection of labeled fibers was observed to the phrenic nucleus, derived from neurons in the lateral solitary nucleus. More interesting for this report, another contingent of labeled fibers descended ipsilaterally in the dorsal and dorsolateral funiculi close to the dorsal horn throughout the length of the spinal cord to terminate in lamina IV and, to a limited extend, in the lower portion of lamina III of the dorsal horn. Only at cervical and upper thoracic levels labeled fibers were also distributed to the intermediate zone (laminae V, VI and VII), but they probably represent short propriobulbospinal pathways derived in the lateral reticular formation of the caudal medulla travelling in more ventral parts of the dorsolateral funiculus (see also Holstege and Kuypers, 1982). Importantly, no labeled fibers were distributed to the lateral cervical nucleus or lamina I. Burton and Loewy (1977), in an autoradiographic tracing study, also observed fibers derived from the dorsal column nuclei terminating in lamina IV, but their finding of projections to the lateral cervical nucleus and 'possibly' lamina I could not be confirmed. This would indicate that the descending projections of the dorsal column nuclei to the spinal cord are most likely not involved in supraspinal control of nociception.

Pons

The HRP spinal cord injected cases revealed many labeled neurons in the pontine tegmentum. These neurons can be subdivided into three groups: (a) the pontine medial tegmental field, (b) the dorsolateral pontine tegmental field and (c) the contralateral pontine lateral tegmental field or paralemniscal pontine reticular formation. Neurons of group (a), which does not include the NRM and adjacent area, do not project to lamina I (Martin et al., 1979; Holstege and Kuypers, 1982) and will not be discussed further.

The dorsolateral pontine tegmental field

In this area several different structures are present subserving different functions. These structures are (a) the micturition control centers, (b) the pneumotaxic center, (c) the pontine taste area and (d) the noradrenergic neurons in the locus coeruleus, nucleus subcoeruleus and parabrachial nuclei. Micturition centers are located in the medial part of the dorsolateral pontine tegmentum (Barrington's nucleus (Barrington, 1925), or M-region of Holstege et al., 1986) and in the lateral part of this region (L-region of Holstege et al., 1986). The pneumotaxic center is located in the parabrachial nuclei (Bertrand and Hugelin, 1971; Bertrand et al., 1974), the lateral part of which sends fibers to the phrenic nucleus and the T1 – T3 intermediolateral cell column (Holstege and Kuypers, 1982). The parabrachial nuclei also serve as relay for the solitary nucleus and the caudal brain stem lateral tegmental field (parvocellular reticular nucleus) to the limbic system (hypothalamus, amygdala and bed nucleus of the stria terminalis) and thalamus (paraventricular, intralaminar and ventromedial basal nucleus), (Saper and Loewy, 1980). This indicates that not only information about taste (Norgren, 1976) but also about many other visceral functions such as respiration (Bertrand and Hugelin, 1971) and cardiovascular control (Wang and Ranson, 1939) are conveyed in these nuclei. Furthermore, there is increasing evidence that the ventral parabrachial nuclei may play an important role in nociception control (Hayes et al., 1984; Hayes and Katayama, 1985).

In relation to the descending pathways to the dorsal horn, the neurons in the nucleus subcoeruleus and ventral part of the parabrachial nuclei are of interest. According to the HRP spinal cord injected cases a large number of labeled neurons in this area project to the spinal cord (Fig. 6, I, J). In four cases ³H-leucine injections were made in this area. In Case 1015, the injection involved the nucleus subcoeruleus, extending into the medial tegmentum, the locus coeruleus and the adjoining part of the periaqueductal gray (PAG)

and slightly into the medial parabrachial area. In Case 862, the injection was located slightly more rostrally and involved the nucleus subcoeruleus and the dorsally adjoining brachium conjunctivum. The injection did not extend into the ventral and lateral parabrachial nuclei or in the nucleus Kölliker-Fuse. In the other two cases (1017 and 1036) the injections were more laterally placed, sparing the medial nucleus subcoeruleus, but involving the ventral parabrachial nuclei and the nucleus Kölliker-Fuse. In all four cases labeled fibers were diffusely distributed throughout the ventral and lateral tegmentum of the caudal brain stem, including some to the NRM and the rostral NRP. In Case 1015, (Fig. 7, right), in which the injection extended into the pontine medial tegmentum, labeled fibers were also distributed to dorsomedial parts of the caudal brain stem tegmentum. In all four cases a diffuse distribution pattern of labeled fibers was also observed in the spinal cord. Labeled fibers descended in the dorsolateral and ventrolateral funiculi to terminate in all parts of the spinal gray, including lamina I and other parts of the dorsal horn throughout the length of the spinal cord (Fig. 4, lower left; Fig. 8, left). In the two cases with lateral injections (1017 and 1036), a large stream of labeled fibers descended through and terminated in the lateral tegmental field of pons and medulla. From this lateral fiber stream, at caudal pontine levels, many labeled fibers branched off to pass ventrally and medially to terminate in the NRM and adjacent tegmentum, but not in the nucleus raphe pallidus (NRP) (Fig. 7, left). These results indicate that this specific pathway to the NRM and adjacent tegmentum originates in the ventral parabrachial nuclei and/or the nucleus Kölliker-Fuse, but not in the nucleus subcoeruleus (Holstege, 1988). Another, contralaterally descending fiber stream was also found in all four cases. From the injection site these labeled fibers ascended, gradually passing medially and crossed the midline in the ventral part of the rostral pontine tegmentum. Subsequently, many of these fibers turned caudally to terminate in the ventral part of the caudal pontine and upper medullary

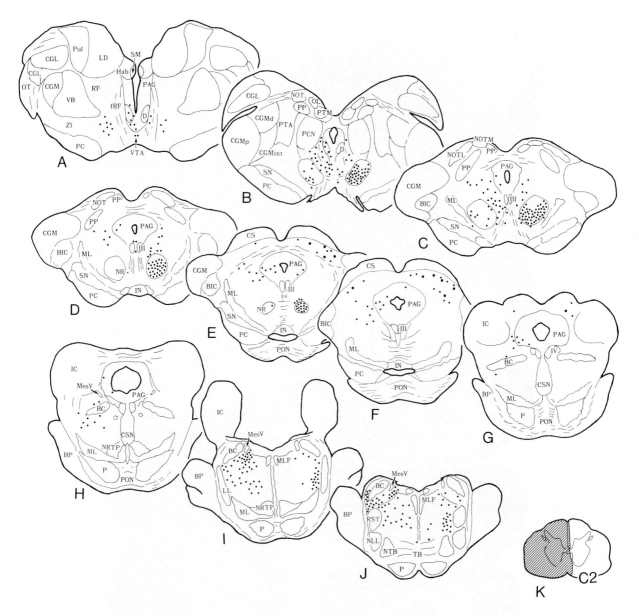

Fig. 6. Schematic drawings of HRP-labeled neurons in the mesencephalic and pontine tegmentum in Case 1602 (HRP hemi-infiltration in the C2 segment).

medial tegmental field at the contralateral side (Fig. 7, left A – C). The impression was gained that in the laterally injected cases (1017 and 1036) some labeled fibers were distributed from this contralateral pathway to the NRM (Holstege, 1988).

Wide projections from the nucleus subcoeruleus to the caudal brain stem tegmentum and limited projections to the NRM have also been reported in the rat by Jones and Yang (1985) and by Westlund and Coulter (1980) in the monkey. The spinal cord projections have also been demonstrated in the opossum (Martin et al., 1979), cat (Holstege et al.,

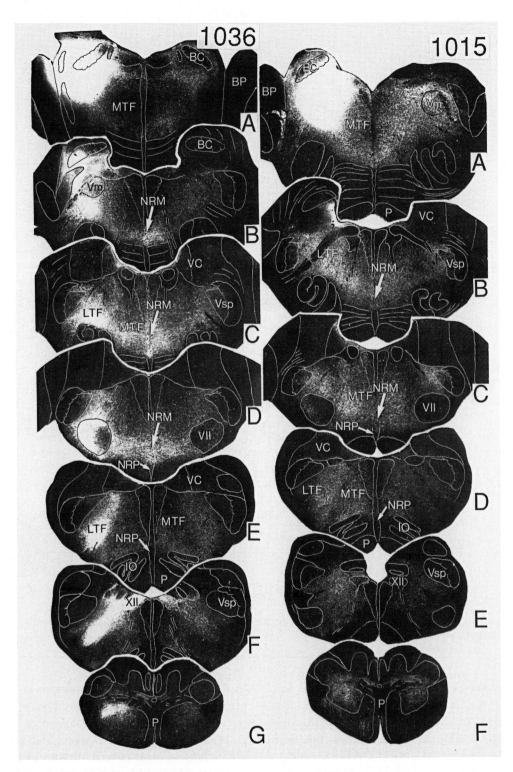

Fig. 7. Dark-field photomicrographs of seven sections of the caudal brain stem of Case 1036 (on the left) and six sections of Case 1015 (on the right). Note the wide projections in both cases but the dense projections to the bulbar lateral tegmental field and to the NRM and adjacent tegmentum in Case 1036. (From Holstege, 1988; Brain Res., 447: 154–158.)

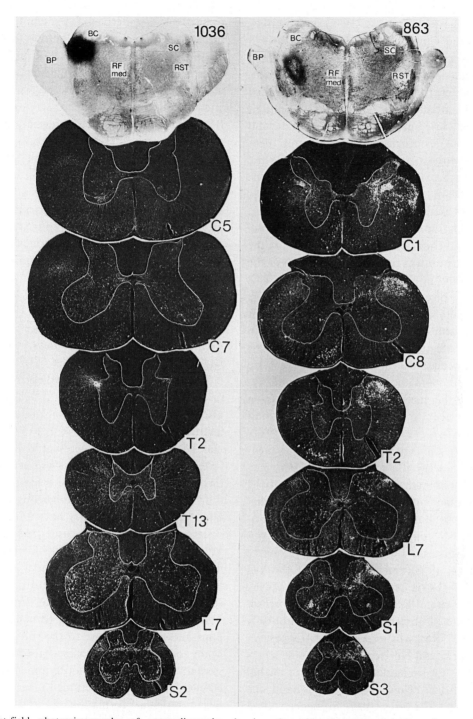

Fig. 8. Bright-field photomicrographs of autoradiographs showing the tritiated leucine injection sites and dark-field photomicrographs showing the spinal distributions of the labeled fibers in Case 1036 (on the left) and Case 863 (on the right). Note that in Case 1036, with an injection in the ventral parabrachial nuclei, the nucleus Kölliker-Fuse and the lateral part of the nucleus subcoeruleus, labeled fibers are distributed to all parts of the spinal gray including all parts of the dorsal horn and the motoneuronal cell groups. Note in Case 863, with an injection in the lateral part of the pontine tegmentum, the pronounced projection to the dorsal horn (mainly laminae I and V) throughout the spinal cord. Note also the strong projection to the lateral cervical nuclei and the nuclei of Onuf in the sacral cord. (From Holstege and Kuypers, 1982; Progress in Brain Research, Vol. 57, pp. 151 and 153.)

1979; Holstege and Kuypers, 1982) and monkey (Westlund and Coulter, 1980). Many neurons in the nucleus subcoeruleus and the parabrachial nuclei contain noradrenaline (Jones and Friedman, 1983). However, the NRM contains only a limited number of noradrenergic fibers and terminals (Jones and Friedman, 1983; Westlund and Coulter, 1980), evidence that noradrenergic neurons do not project strongly to the NRM. On the other hand, the widely distributed fibers to the spinal cord are probably noradrenergic, since Nygren and Olson (1977) have demonstrated that, after lesioning the dorsolateral pontine tegmental field, the number of noradrenergic terminals in the spinal grey matter was reduced by 25 – 50% in the dorsal horn and by 95% in the ventral horn. This noradrenergic projection is probably not a specific nociception inhibitory pathway, because in all four autoradiographic cases labeled fibers terminated in both the dorsal and the ventral horn. Nevertheless there is evidence that in the rat noradrenergic fibers derived from the locus coeruleus and descending via the ventrolateral funiculus, have an inhibitory effect on nociception (Jones and Gebhart, 1987).

Strong projections to the bulbar lateral tegmental field, with a specific contingent of fibers passing to and terminating in the ventral part of the caudal pontine and upper medullary medial tegmentum, do not only originate in the parabrachial nuclei, but also in the lateral hypothalamus (Holstege, 1987a), amygdala (Hopkins and Holstege, 1978) and lateral part of the bed nucleus of the stria terminalis (Holstege et al., 1985). These lateral limbic structures also project strongly to the parabrachial nuclei, but not or only weakly to the NRM, which receives its strongest input not from lateral but from medial limbic structures, such as the periaqueductal gray and medial hypothalamus (see below). On the other hand, the lateral limbic structures may influence NRM neurons indirectly (via the parabrachial nuclei and/or the PAG). The parabrachial nuclei not only receive afferent connections from the lateral limbic system, but also from the spinal cord. Many of these fibers are derived from lamina I cells and probably represent collaterals from the spinothalamic tract (Hylden et al., 1986).

In conclusion, the parabrachial nuclei receive many fibers from the limbic system and spinal cord and send many (possibly cholinergic) fibers to the NRM and adjacent reticular formation, which explains its involvement in nociception control. In this respect, electrical stimulation (DeSalles et al., 1985) or injections of carbachol, a cholinergic agonist (Hayes et al., 1984; Hayes and Katayama, 1985), in the ventral part of the parabrachial nuclei produced profound nociceptive suppression. Systemically administered naloxone (an opiate antagonist) did not reliably attenuate carbachol-produced analgesia, indicating that opiate mechanisms are not involved in this type of analgesia.

Pontine lateral tegmental field (paralemniscal reticular formation)

The HRP spinal cord injected cases revealed that in the lateral pontine tegmental field or paralemniscal reticular formation a contralateral cluster of neurons was present (Fig. 6, I, J). This paralemniscal cell group was also present in the S1 HRP injected case, suggesting that these neurons project throughout the length of the spinal cord. According to retrograde double-labeling findings of Huisman et al. (1982), they have a high degree of collateralization. In four cases (863, 1018, 1235, 1237; Fig. 2, O, P, Q), ^{3}H-leucine injections were made in this pontine area and, in all cases, labeled fibers were observed crossing from the injection site just beneath the floor of the IVth ventricle to descend in the lateral reticular formation of caudal pons and medulla, close to the rubrospinal tract. Many of these fibers passed through the dorsolateral facial nucleus, not terminating there. No labeled fibers were distributed to the NRM and adjacent reticular formation. In the spinal cord, labeled fibers descended in the dorsolateral funiculus throughout its length (Fig. 8, right). In the brain stem, caudally to the obex labeled fibers were distributed to the marginal layer of the caudal spinal trigeminal nucleus (Fig. 5, lower left) and at the level of C1 – C2 a very strong bilateral projection was observed to the lateral cervical nucleus (Fig. 8, right C1), a small group of cells lying just laterally to the dorsal horn of the C1 – C2 spinal cord (Westman, 1968). Throughout the length of the spinal cord, labeled fibers were distributed to especially lamina I, the outer part of II and the lateral parts of V and VI. This pathway in the brain stem was first reported by Busch (1961). The projections to the spinal cord were also found by Martin et al. (1979, 1982), Holstege et al. (1979), Holstege and Kuypers (1982), Carlton et al. (1985) and Tan and Holstege (1986). Afferents to this pontine area include a large number of fibers ascending in the ventrolateral funiculus of the upper cervical cord, which might represent collaterals from the spinothalamic tract (Mehler et al., 1960; Mehler, 1962, 1969). The spinothalamic tract, which is largely derived from neurons in laminae I, V, VII and VIII, is almost completely crossed (Carstens and Trevino, 1978). As already mentioned, the neurons in the pontine lateral tegmental or paralemniscal cell group also project contralaterally and may terminate, (although not exclusively) on neurons from which the spinothalamic tract originates. This paralemniscal cell cluster area also receives strong afferent projections from the limbic system (PAG, lateral hypothalamus, amygdala and bed nucleus of the stria terminalis, see later). Physiological studies of Carstens et al. (1980) indicated that stimulation in the area of this paralemniscal cell group generated a more powerful descending inhibition of nociception than stimulation in the PAG. Carstens et al. (1981) indicated that serotonin plays a role in the mediation of the PAG-induced inhibition of nociception, but that was not the case for the paralemniscal cell group. The anatomical findings correspond completely with these results, since the paralemniscal cell group projects directly to the spinal cord and does not maintain connections with the NRM and adjacent reticular formation.

The projection of the lateral pontine cell group to the lateral cervical nucleus (LCN) is of interest, because this nucleus may play a role in the conveyance of nociceptive information. The LCN receives afferents from the so-called spinocervical tract neurons, which are located in lamina IV throughout the length of the spinal cord. These spinocervical neurons receive afferent input from cutaneous hair follicles, but a significant proportion of them can also be excited by nociceptive cutaneous and muscle afferents (Brown and Franz, 1969; Hong et al., 1979). However, only a small number of the LCN neurons responds to noxious stimuli (Oswaldo-Cruz and Kidd, 1964; Craig and Tapper, 1978). Dostrovsky (1984) and Kajander et al. (1984) demonstrated that electrical stimulation of the PAG, NRM, nucleus cuneiformis and nuclei reticularis gigantocellularis and magnocellularis was very effective in inhibiting the responses of the LCN neurons evoked by electrical and tactile stimulation of the skin. The inhibition took place at the level of the spinal cord (spinocervical neurons) and not directly on LCN neurons. This observation corresponds with the anatomical findings, that do not show any projections from the PAG, NRM with adjacent reticular formation, or nucleus cuneiformis to the LCN. It would, therefore, be very interesting to study electrophysiologically the direct projections from the lateral pontine tegmentum to the LCN.

In summary, the pontine dorsolateral and lateral tegmentum contains three areas, that are involved in nociception control: (1) the locus coeruleus and/or the nucleus subcoeruleus, (2) the parabrachial nuclei and (3) the lateral pontine tegmental field or paralemniscal reticular formation. The locus coeruleus/nucleus subcoeruleus projects to all parts of the caudal brain stem reticular formation and spinal gray matter, and has direct access to dorsal as well as ventral horn neurons. This noradrenergic projection may, therefore, not be a specific nociception inhibitory pathway. The parabrachial nuclei project strongly to the NRM and adjoining reticular formation and exert their inhibitory effects on the dorsal horn via this indirect pathway. Finally, the paralemniscal cell group projects directly to the contralateral marginal layer of the caudal spinal trigeminal nucleus and laminae I, V and VI of the spinal cord dorsal horn and may be considered as involved in modulation of the spinothalamic tract.

Mesencephalon

The periaqueductal gray (PAG) and adjacent areas
The PAG is, together with the NRM, the most well-known structure involved in supraspinal control of nociception. Stimulation in the PAG as well as in the NRM produces analgesia (see Willis, 1982; and Besson and Chaouch, 1987, for reviews). The caudal NRM projects directly to nociceptive neurons in the spinal cord (see above), but the PAG does not. The C2 spinal cord injected HRP case reveals only a few labeled neurons in the lateral PAG and adjacent mesencephalic tegmentum (Fig. 6, C – G), but not in other parts of the PAG. After HRP injections in the upper thoracic cord, HRP-labeled neurons were very scarce in the PAG and they were almost absent after HRP injections in the lumbosacral cord. On the other hand, HRP injections in the NRM, rostral NRP and adjacent reticular formation resulted in an enormous number of HRP-labeled neurons in the PAG and laterally and ventrolaterally adjoining areas (Fig. 9, A – E). All portions of the PAG, except its dorsolateral part, contained HRP-labeled neurons. The autoradiographic tracing technique gave more precise results. All injections of ^{3}H-leucine in different parts of the PAG show the same basic projection pattern to the caudal brain stem. After injections in the dorsal (Cases 1486 and 1495; Fig. 2, L – N), lateral (Cases 1338 and 1401; Fig. 2, K – M), ventrolateral PAG (Case 1434; Fig. 2, M, N) and ventrolaterally adjacent tegmentum and cuneiform nucleus (Case 1481; Fig. 2, M, N), a large stream of labeled fibers was observed passing from the PAG ventrolaterally to descend through the pontine lateral tegmental field. From this fiber stream labeled fibers were distributed to the locus coeruleus and nucleus subcoeruleus and to the pontine lateral tegmental or paralemniscal cell group. At caudal pontine levels the PAG descend-

ing fiber stream gradually shifted ventrally and medially to terminate in the ventral part of the medullary reticular formation and in the NRM (Figs. 10, 11). Only when the injection site involved the ventrolateral PAG or the mesencephalic tegmentum ventrolateral to it (Cases 1434 and 1481), labeled fibers were also distributed to the NRP (Fig. 10, left; Fig. 11, lower left and right). This projection pattern is reminiscent of the caudal brain stem projections derived from more rostral parts of the limbic system (see below). In the cases with the most medially located injections (1486 and 1495), the projections to the medially located NRM were stronger than the projections to the laterally adjoining reticular formation (Fig. 11, upper left). By contrast, in one case (1410), in which the injection site did not involve the PAG but only the laterally adjoining mesencephalic tegmentum and the intermediate and deep layers of the superior colliculus (Fig. 2, M), a less pronounced and more laterally located ipsilateral fiber stream to pons and medulla was observed. Labeled fibers were distributed to the lateral pontine tegmentum and laterally to the ventral part of the caudal pontine and upper medullary medial tegmentum. No labeled fibers terminated in the NRM (Fig. 11, upper right). In Case 1401, in which the injection involved the most lateral part of the lateral PAG and its laterally adjoining tegmentum, only a limited number of labeled fibers were distributed to the NRM, but many more to the adjacent medial tegmentum (Fig. 11, lower left). These findings suggest that a mediolateral organization exists in the projections from PAG and adjacent tegmentum to the caudal brain stem.

In cases with injections in the lateral PAG, but only to a very limited extent in cases with dorsal PAG injections, labeled fibers were distributed to the nucleus retro-ambiguus (see also Holstege, 1987b), but not to the dorsal group of the nucleus ambiguus, containing motoneurons innervating the pharynx and soft palate muscles (Holstege et al., 1983). As already indicated by the HRP results, only limited projections to the spinal cord were observed. In two cases (1401 and 1434), with

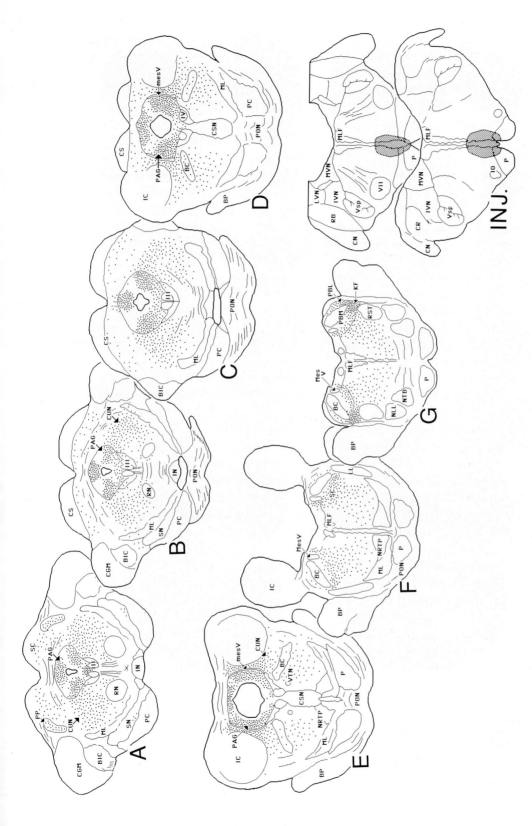

Fig. 9. Schematic drawings of HRP-labeled neurons in mesencephalon and pons after injection of HRP in the NRM/NRP region. Note the dense distribution of labeled neurons in the PAG (except its dorsolateral part) and the tegmentum ventrolateral to it. Note also the distribution of labeled neurons in the area of the ventral parabrachial nuclei and the nucleus Kölliker-Fuse.

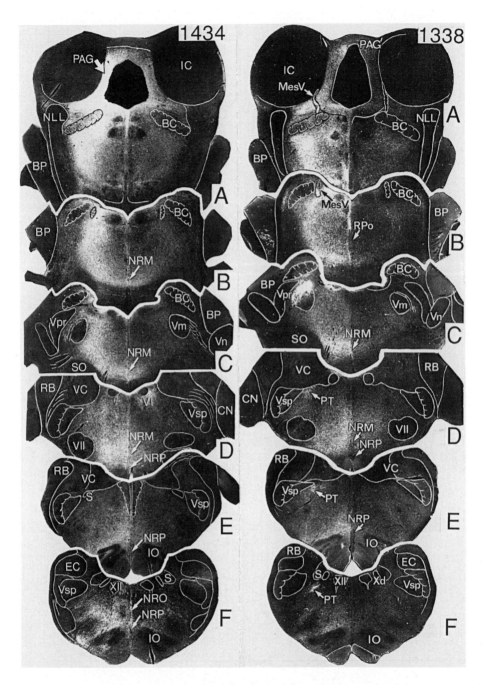

Fig. 10. Dark-field photomicrographs of the brain stem in the Cases 1434 and 1338 with injections in, respectively, the ventrolateral PAG and more rostrally in the lateral PAG. Note the strong projections to the NRM and the ventral part of the medial tegmentum of caudal pons and medulla in both cases. Note that in Case 1434, but not in Case 1338 labeled fibers were also distributed to the NRP.

67

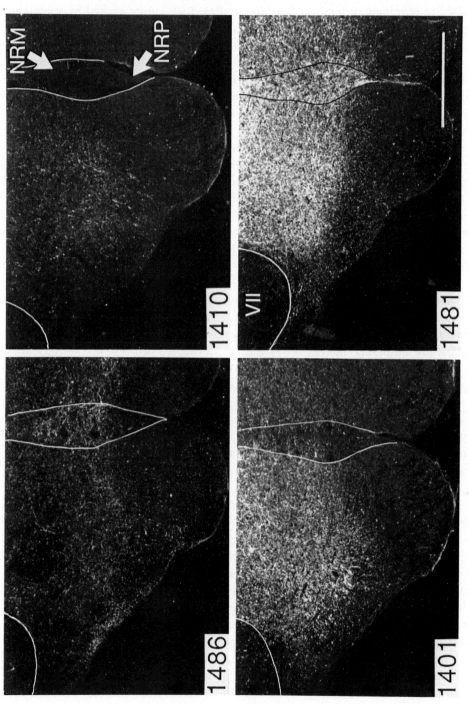

Fig. 11. Dark-field photomicrographs of the NRM and adjoining medullary medial tegmentum in Case 1486 (injection in the dorsal PAG; upper left), Case 1410 (injection in the intermediate and deep layers of the superior colliculus and the mesencephalic tegmentum just ventral to it; upper right), Case 1401 (injection in the lateral PAG and laterally adjoining tegmentum just ventral to it; upper right), Case 1401 (injection in the lateral PAG and laterally adjoining tegmentum; lower left and Case 1481 (injection in the tegmentum ventrolateral to the PAG, extending slightly into the ventrolateral PAG; lower right). Note that the dorsal PAG projects mainly to the medial part of this area (NRM), while the lateral PAG and the area next to it project mainly to more lateral parts of this region and not (Case 1410), or only slightly (Case 1401), to the NRM. Note further that the strongest projection is derived from the tegmentum ventrolateral to the PAG and that this area projects to NRM, NRP and the adjoining medial tegmentum. Bar represents 1 mm.

injections in the lateral PAG, labeled fibers descended through the ipsilateral ventral funiculus of the cervical spinal cord to terminate in lamina VIII and the adjoining part of lamina VII (Fig. 12) (see also Martin et al., 1979). A very few fibers descended ipsilaterally in the lateral funiculus to terminate in the T1 – T2 intermediolateral cell column (Fig. 12). The projection to the medial part of the intermediate zone of the cervical cord is more suggestive to be involved in head movement than in nociception control. Thus, no labeled fibers were distributed to lamina I or other laminae, containing nociception-involved neurons. A more detailed report on the projections of the PAG and adjacent areas is in preparation. The anatomical results are in general agreement with other autoradiographic tracing studies (Mantyh, 1983; Jürgens and Pratt, 1979) in the monkey, although some differences exist. For example, no direct connections to the dorsal group of the nucleus ambiguus were observed, and projections to the NRP were only derived from the ventral part of the PAG and the ventrolaterally adjoining mesencephalic tegmentum. On the other hand, all anatomical reports agree that the PAG does not have direct access to the nociception-related neurons in the spinal cord or caudal spinal trigeminal nucleus. The strong impact of the PAG on nociception therefore must go indirectly, probably via the NRM and adjacent reticular formation. This corresponds with the physiological finding that in cases with reversible blocks of the NRM and adjacent reticular formation, PAG stimulation results in only reduced analgesic effects (Gebhart et al., 1983; Sandkuhler and Gebhart, 1984). In this respect the PAG projections to the pontine lateral tegmental cell group must be taken into account. Part of the antinociceptive action of the PAG may be exerted through this pathway. It must be emphasized that the PAG and especially the adjoining cuneiform nucleus not only project to those caudal brain stem areas, involved in nociception, but also to the NRP and adjoining areas, in turn projecting to the ventral horn, including the somatic motoneuronal cell groups

(Holstege and Kuypers, 1982; see also Fig. 3, right). These projections might play a role in the lordosis reflex, that can be elicited by stimulating the PAG (Sakuma and Pfaff, 1979a,b). They also may form the anatomical framework for the facilitation of the medullary reticulospinal activation of axial muscle EMG and lateral vestibulospinal activation of back muscle EMG in the rat observed after PAG stimulation (Cottingham et al., 1987; Cottingham and Pfaff, 1987). The PAG projections to the nucleus retroambiguus may account for the vocalization responses observed during PAG stimulation (Holstege, 1987b).

Nucleus Edinger-Westphal

All HRP spinal cord injected cases, including the S1 injected cases, showed HRP-labeled neurons in the nucleus of Edinger-Westphal. From early clinical studies, this nucleus was thought to contain parasympathetic preganglionic neurons innervating the sphincter pupillae and ciliary muscle. In the cat, however, neurons in the nucleus of Edinger-Westphal project to the spinal cord, while the parasympathetic neurons are located in surrounding areas dorsal (PAG) and ventral (ventral tegmental area) to it (Toyoshima et al., 1980). Autoradiographic tracing data of Loewy and Saper (1978) in the cat indicated that neurons in the Edinger-Westphal nucleus projected to the marginal layer of the caudal spinal trigeminal nucleus and to laminae I and V of the upper three cervical segments. They could not follow this projection further caudally, probably because they injected only small amounts of tracer and used a short survival time (see Holstege, 1987a). The spinally projecting Edinger-Westphal neurons use substance P and cholecystokinin as neurotransmitters (Maciewicz et al., 1983, 1984), and some physiological studies (Innis et al., 1979; Innis and Aghajanian, 1986) indicate that this nucleus plays a role in nociception control. Notably, the Edinger-Westphal nucleus projects to the lateral pontine or paralemniscal cell group, in turn projecting to laminae I, V and VI of the spinal cord

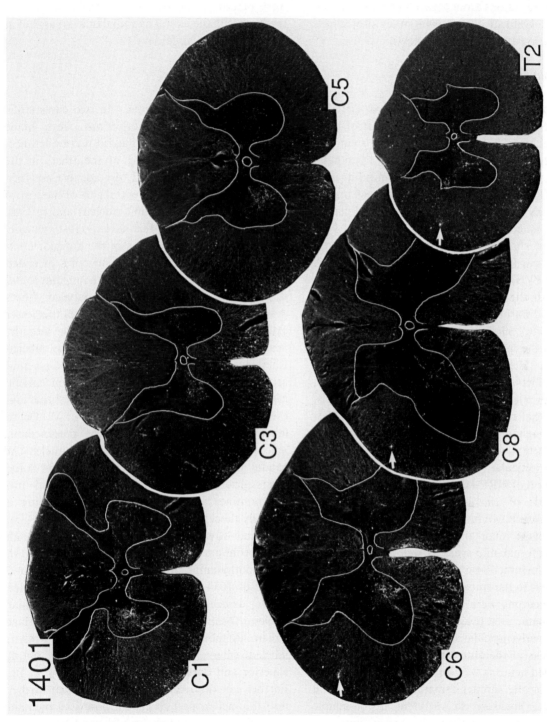

Fig. 12. Dark-field photo-micrographs of cervical and upper thoracic sections of the spinal cord in Case 1401, with an injection in the lateral PAG, its adjacent tegmentum and the deep collicular layers. Note that labeled fibers descend ipsilaterally through the ventral and ventrolateral funiculi to terminate in the medial part of the cervical and upper thoracic intermediate zone. Note also that a small contingent of labeled fibers descends in the ipsilateral dorsolateral funiculus (see arrows). These fibers probably terminate in the upper thoracic intermediolateral cell group (see section T2). Contralaterally, a few tectospinal fibers descend in the ventral funiculus of the upper cervical cord to terminate in the lateral part of the upper cervical intermediate zone.

(Graybiel 1977; Loewy and Saper, 1978), and it receives projections from this cell group (Tan and Holstege, 1986). It also receives many projections from the hypothalamus (see below).

Hypothalamus

The hypothalamus consists of several different structures, with different functions. Part of these structures project to the caudal brain stem and spinal cord. At the level of the caudal hypothalamus, in all spinal cord HRP hemi-infiltration cases, HRP-labeled neurons were present mainly ipsilaterally in the posterior, dorsal and lateral hypothalamic areas (Fig. 13).

Further rostrally, numerous labeled neurons were present in the paraventricular hypothalamic nucleus (PVN). These results are in general agreement with the findings of Kuypers and Maisky (1975) and Basbaum et al. (1978) in the cat, Saper et al. (1976), Hosoya (1980) and Watkins et al. (1981) in the rat, and Crutcher et al. (1978) in the opossum. The finding that the distribution of labeled fibers was approximately the same in all cases with injections at different spinal cord levels, suggests that many hypothalamospinal fibers descend throughout the length of the spinal cord. The HRP injections involving NRM, rostral NRP and adjacent reticular formation showed a similar distribution of HRP-labeled neurons in the caudal two thirds of the hypothalamus, but labeled neurons were much more numerous. Many labeled neurons were found in the posterior, lateral and dorsal hypothalamic areas as well as in the PVN and the dorsomedial hypothalamic area (Fig. 13). In contrast to the spinal cord injected cases, many labeled neurons were also found in the anterior hypothalamic area (except in its medial part), the anterior periventricular hypothalamic nucleus and the nucleus of the anterior commissure (Fig. 13). No labeled neurons were present in the supraoptic nucleus or the suprachiasmatic nucleus. To find out where precisely the different hypothalamic structures project to in the brain stem, in nine cases ^{3}H-leucine injections were made in various parts of the hypothalamus. In six cases the injections were placed in the medial hypothalamus and in three cases in the lateral hypothalamic areas, but at different rostrocaudal levels.

Medial hypothalamus

Anterior hypothalamic area. In two cases (1654 and 1712), ^{3}H-leucine injections were made bilaterally, but with an ipsilateral preponderance, at the level of the crossing of the fibers in the anterior commissure (Fig. 2, A–D). In Case 1654 the injection involved the ventral part of the rostral periventricular hypothalamic nucleus and in Case 1712 the dorsal part of this nucleus, just ventrally to the crossing of the fibers in the anterior commissure. In this same case the injection extended rostrally into the ventral part of the medial septal nucleus. In both cases, many labeled fibers descended via a medial fiber stream and, to a lesser extent, via the medial forebrain bundle into the brain stem. In the mesencephalon many labeled fibers were distributed to the ventral tegmental area of Tsai (VTA), the rostral mesencephalic raphe nuclei, the nucleus of Edinger-Westphal and the inner parts of the PAG (Fig. 14, A). Dense labeling was also observed in the paramedian, apical and posterior interpeduncular nuclei. At caudal mesencephalic levels in Case 1654 some fibers gradually shifted laterally to descend into the pontine lateral tegmental field, forming a laterally descending fiber stream (Fig. 14, A–D). This fiber stream was also present and even much more pronounced in cases with lateral injections in the hypothalamus, which will be described below. In Cases 1654 and 1712, the bulk of the labeled fibers descended next to the interpeduncular nuclei, forming a medially descending fiber stream. At pontine levels, from this fiber stream, labeled fibers were distributed to the central superior and dorsal raphe nuclei (Fig. 14, A, B). Further caudally, labeled fibers descended further into the medial part of caudal pons and medulla immediately adjacent to the NRM and NRP and a few descended in the dorsomedial portion of the

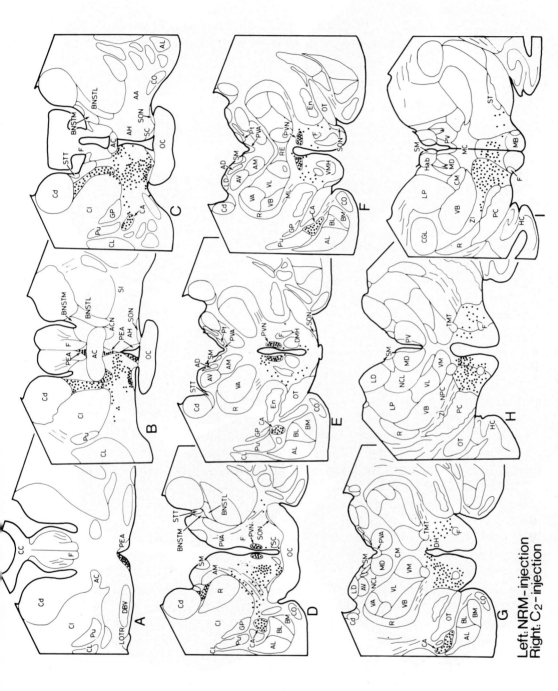

Fig. 13. Schematic drawing of HRP neurons in the hypothalamus, amygdala and bed nucleus of the stria terminalis. On the left, the pattern of distribution of labeled neurons in Case 1508 (HRP injection of the NRM, rostral NRP and adjoining tegmentum) is indicated. On the right, the pattern of distribution of HRP-labeled neurons in Case 1602 (hemi-infiltration in the C2 segment) is shown. (From Holstege, 1987; J. Comp. Neurol., 260: 102.)

Left: NRM - injection
Right: C₂ - injection

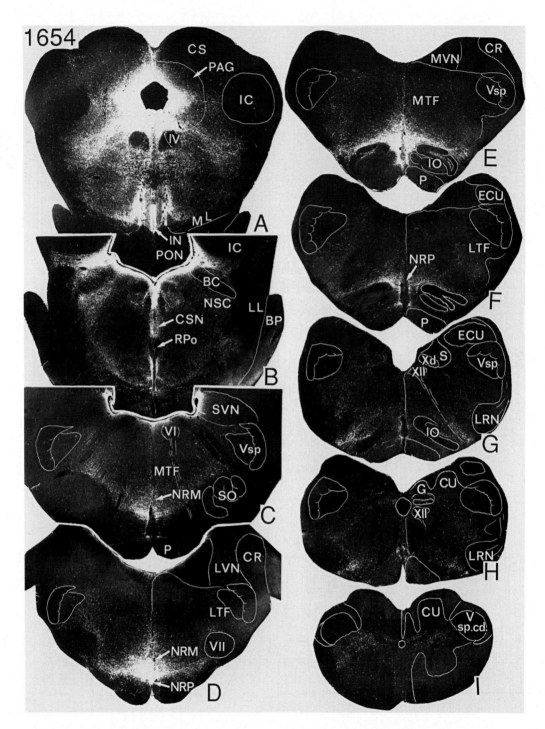

Fig. 14. Dark-field photomicrographs of the brain stem in Case 1654 with an injection in the medial part of the anterior hypothalamic area. Note the strong projections to the medially located NRM/NRP and to the ventral part of the upper medullary medial tegmental field. Note also that only the most rostral part of the NRP receives labeled fibers. (From Holstege, 1987; J. Comp. Neurol., 260: 109.)

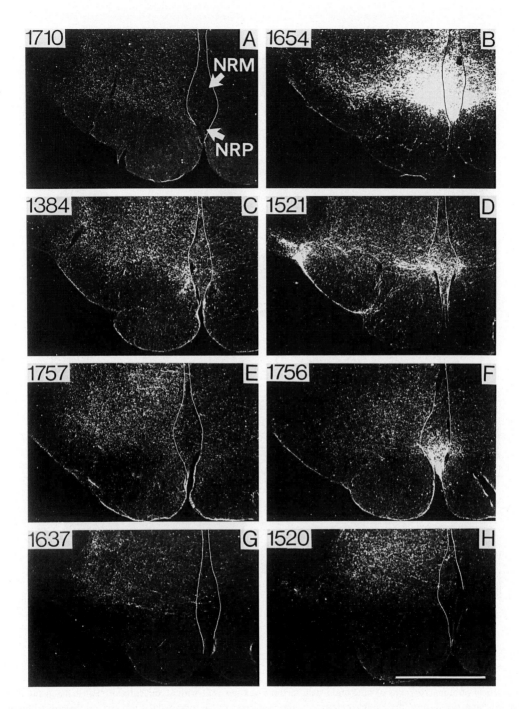

Fig. 15. Dark-field photomicrographs of the NRM, rostral NRP and adjoining tegmental field at the level of the facial nucleus in eight cases with injections in the lateral hypothalamic area (Cases 1710, 1384 and 1757), the medial part of the anterior hypothalamic area (1654), the PVN of the hypothalamus (1521), the medial part of the caudal hypothalamus (1756), the central nucleus of the amygdala (1637) and bed nucleus of the stria terminalis (1520). Note the relatively small number of labeled fibers in the NRM/NRP after lateral injections in the limbic system (Cases 1520, 1637, 1710 and 1757) and the strong projections to the NRM/NRP after medial injections in the limbic system. The injection in Case 1384 involved the lateral hypothalamus but extended slightly into the medial hypothalamus, which explains the labeled fibers in NRM/NRP in this case. Bar represents 2 mm.

74

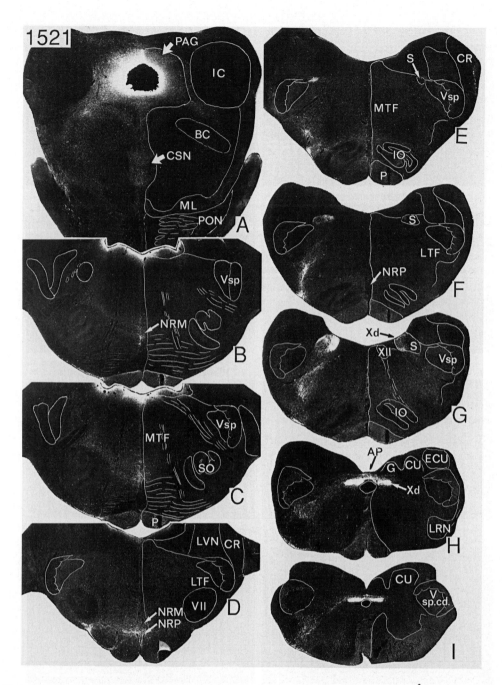

Fig. 16. Dark-field photomicrographs of nine brain-stem sections of Case 1521 with an injection of ^{3}H-leucine in the PVN of the hypothalamus. Note the distinct descending pathway in the area next to the pyramidal tract and its fiber distribution to the NRM/NRP, dorsal vagal nucleus, area postrema and rostral solitary complex. (From Holstege, 1987; J. Comp. Neurol., 260: 115.)

pyramidal tract. From this fiber stream labeled fibers were distributed to NRM and rostral NRP, but many were also distributed to the reticular formation next to the NRM and NRP (Fig. 14, C – F; Fig. 15, upper row right).

The strong projections from the anterior hypothalamus to the PAG, (see also Conrad and Pfaff, 1976a,b; Saper et al., 1978, 1979a; Swanson et al., 1978; Anderson and Shen, 1980), and to the NRM and the adjoining reticular formation, suggest an involvement of this part of the hypothalamus in nociception control. Indeed, stimulation in the anterior hypothalamus inhibited dorsal horn unit heat-evoked responses (Carstens, 1982). In a later study, Carstens et al. (1983) showed that systemic administration of the opiate antagonist naloxone did not consistently affect this inhibition, indicating that endogeneous opioid peptides are not primarily involved in the mediation of this inhibition. Application of cholinergic drugs in the anterior hypothalamus results in an emotional aversive response, including defense posture and cardiovascular and other autonomic manifestations (Brudzynski and Eckersdorff, 1984; Tashiro et al., 1985). This corresponds with the finding that cardiovascular and nociception regulatory mechanisms are often coordinated (see Zamir and Maixner, 1986, for a review).

Paraventricular hypothalamus nucleus (PVN). In three cases, ^{3}H-leucine injections were made in this nucleus. In Case 1653, the injection involved the rostral PVN, but extended rostrally into the anterior hypothalamic area and ventrally into the ventral part of the medial hypothalamus (Fig. 2, D, E). In Case 1521 the rostral and medial portions of the PVN and surrounding areas were injected (Fig. 2, E – G) and the most caudally located injection was made in Case 1665, involving the caudal part of PVN and the dorsal and posterior hypothalamic areas and the parvicellular hypothalamic nucleus (Fig. 2, G, H). At mesencephalic levels, the same distribution of labeled fibers was observed as in the two cases with injections in the medial part of the anterior

hypothalamic area, and also the same medial descending fiber stream was present, distributing fibers to the NRM, the ventral part of the rostral NRP and the adjacent reticular formation. However, in all three PVN-injected cases a well-defined lateral fiber stream was observed, which descended through the medial forebrain bundle, shifted laterally in the mesencephalon and passed further caudally in the most lateral part of the caudal mesencephalic and upper pontine tegmentum (Fig. 16, A). At that level they shifted ventromedially, filtering through (but not terminating in) the pontine nuclei to arrive in a very peripheral position lateral to the pyramidal tract (Fig. 16, E – I). This lateral stream continued into the lateral and dorsolateral funiculus of the spinal cord throughout its total length. At caudal pontine and upper medullary levels, labeled fibers filtered from this lateral stream through the pyramidal tract and ventral part of the reticular formation to terminate in the NRM and rostral NRP (Fig. 15, second row right; Fig. 16, B – D). Labeled fibers were also distributed to an area just ventral to the facial nucleus and to all parts of the dorsal vagal nucleus, the rostral solitary nucleus, the area postrema and to specific parts of the caudal medullary lateral reticular formation. This latter distribution may represent a PVN projection to the parasympathetic neurons located in this area (Kalia and Mesulam, 1980) and perhaps to the noradrenergic nuclei A1 and A2. Labeled fibers were also distributed to the marginal layer of the caudal spinal trigeminal nucleus (Fig. 17, upper left) (not observed in Case 1665). In the spinal cord, labeled fibers were distributed to lamina X next to the central canal, to the thoracolumbar (T1 – T4) intermediolateral (sympathetic) cell group and to the sacral (S2 – S3) intermediomedial and intermediolateral cell groups (Fig. 18). In Cases 1653 and 1521, but not in Case 1665, labeled fibers were also present in lamina I throughout the length of the spinal cord (Fig. 18, C8, T2, L7). This projection was continuous with the projection to the marginal layer of the caudal spinal trigeminal nucleus. In all three cases labeled fibers

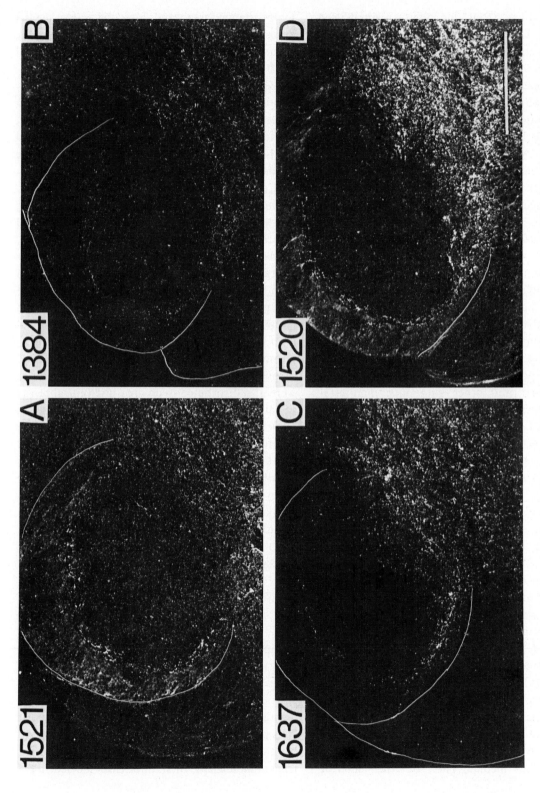

Fig. 17. Dark-field photomicrographs of the caudal spinal trigeminal nucleus in Cases 1521 (with an injection in the PVN of the hypothalamus; upper left), 1384 (injection in the lateral hypothalamus; upper right), 1637 (injection in the central nucleus of the amygdala; lower left) and 1520 (injection in the bed nucleus of the stria terminalis; lower right). Only in Case 1521 this projection extended caudally into lamina I throughout the length of the spinal cord. Bar represents 1 mm.

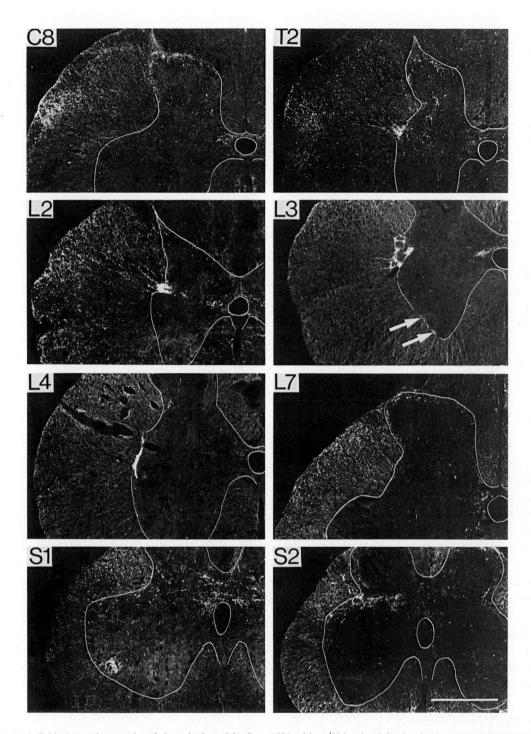

Fig. 18. Dark-field photomicrographs of the spinal cord in Case 1521 with a ³H-leucine injection in the area of the PVN of the hypothalamus. Note the projection to lamina I (C8, T2 and L7), the sympathetic intermediolateral cell group (T2, L2, L3 and L4), the nucleus of Onuf (S1) and the parasympathetic intermediomedial and intermediolateral cell group (S2). The arrows in L3 probably indicate projections to distal dendrites of the motoneurons located in the sympathetic intermediolateral cell group. (From Holstege, 1987; J. Comp. Neurol., 260: 118.)

were also found in the so-called nucleus of Onuf, located in the upper sacral cord (Fig. 18, S1). This cell group contains somatic (however, see Holstege and Tan, 1987) motoneurons innervating the striated muscles of the pelvic floor including those of the urethral and anal sphincters (Sato et al., 1978).

The autoradiographic tracing results, indicating direct pathways from the PVN to lamina I of the caudal spinal trigeminal nucleus and spinal cord, suggest strong involvement of this part of the hypothalamus in nociception control. Swanson (1977) and Nilaver (1980) traced a neurophysin (a carrier protein for oxytocin and vasopressin) pathway to laminae I and X of the spinal cord. Since most neurophysin-containing neurons are present in the PVN, it was assumed that this pathway originated in the PVN. The same pathway also distributed fibers to the dorsal vagal nucleus, solitary nucleus and the thoracic intermediolateral cell column, which projections were also found in the anterograde tracing study. It indicates a strong connection between nociception and autonomic system control. Interestingly, Swanson (1977) and Nilaver (1980) did not report neurophysin projections to the NRM/NRP. This is in agreement with the findings of Holstege and Van Leeuwen (unpublished results), who did not observe either vasopressinergic or oxytocinergic fibers or terminals in the NRM/NRP. Apparently, non-oxytocin and non-vasopressin PVN neurons (only 20% of the PVN neurons, projecting to caudal brain stem and spinal cord, contain vasopressin and neurophysin (Sawchenko and Swanson, 1982)) project to NRM/NRP. Carstens (1982) observed, after stimulating in the medial hypothalamus, a strong inhibition of dorsal horn neuronal responses to noxious skin heating, but his stimulation area was not limited to the PVN.

Posterior hypothalamus. In one case (1756) a ^{3}H-leucine injection was made in the caudal hypothalamus not involving the PVN. In this case the distribution of labeled fibers was the same as in Case 1665, except that the lateral well-defined

pathway and its fiber distribution was not present. Another difference was that in this case the distribution of labeled fibers to the NRM was much weaker than in the previous cases, but the projection to the NRP (Fig. 15, third row right) was stronger and involved not only the ventral part of the rostral NRP, but also its caudal parts. In this same case (1756), a few labeled fibers descended ipsilaterally in the lateral funiculus throughout the length of the spinal cord and distributed fibers to the upper thoracic intermediolateral cell group and to lamina X. The strong projection to the NRP was also observed by Hosoya (1985) in the rat. The finding that the emphasis of the posterior hypothalamus/caudal brain stem projections is on the NRP and not on the NRM suggests that this part of the hypothalamus is not strongly involved in nociception control. This idea is further corroborated by the results of Carstens (1982) who, stimulating the caudal hypothalamus, found less inhibition of dorsal horn neuronal responses to noxious skin heating than after stimulating more anterior regions of the hypothalamus.

In summary, the medial hypothalamus projects strongly to the PAG, the NRM/NRP and the directly adjoining reticular formation. The anterior part of the medial hypothalamus projects most strongly to the NRM, while the caudal part of the medial hypothalamus projects mainly to the NRP. The PVN gives rise to a well-defined pathway, giving off fibers to the NRM/rostral NRP, dorsal vagal nucleus, rostral solitary nucleus, lamina I of the spinal cord and caudal spinal trigeminal nucleus, the thoracolumbar and sacral intermediolateral cell column, lamina X of the spinal cord and to the nucleus of Onuf in the sacral cord.

The lateral hypothalamic area

In three cases, ^{3}H-leucine injections were made in this part of the hypothalamus. In Case 1710 (Fig. 2, B, C) the injection was present in the anterior hypothalamus just ventral to the anterior commissure and it involved the so-called nucleus of the anterior commissure (Berman and Jones,

1982). In Cases 1384 and 1757, the injection sites were located at the level just rostral to the mammillary bodies (Fig. 2, H – J). The injection in Case 1757 extended into the medial portion of the subthalamic nucleus. In all three cases labeled fibers descended in the medial forebrain bundle, but shifted laterally at mesencephalic levels and descended further in the pontine and medullary lateral reticular formation. Only in Cases 1384 and 1757 some fibers continued in the lateral and dorsolateral funiculus of the spinal cord. In Case 1384 these fibers could not be observed beyond the C2 level, but in Case 1757 they traveled throughout the length of the cord. In the rostral mesencephalon, via medial fiber streams, labeled fibers were distributed to the ventral tegmental area of Tsai, the rostral mesencephalic raphe nuclei, the nucleus Edinger-Westphal, the rostral PAG and to the dorsal part of the substantia nigra. In Cases 1384 and 1757, labeled fibers were found in the intermediate and deep layers of the superior colliculus. Further caudally, labeled fibers were traced to the intermediate and posterior interpeduncular nuclei, to the superior central and dorsal raphe nuclei and to the locus coeruleus. From the lateral descending fiber stream, labeled fibers were distributed to the lateral mesencephalic tegmentum, the PAG, except its dorsolateral part, and the subependymal layer, the cuneiform nucleus, the pontine lateral tegmental or paralemniscal cell group, the parabrachial nuclei, the nucleus subcoeruleus and, especially in Case 1710, to the area just ventral and medial to the mesencephalic trigeminal tract, possibly representing Barrington's (1925) nucleus or the M-region of Holstege et al. (1986). In the caudal brain stem in all three cases labeled fibers were distributed to area h of Meessen and Olszewski (1949), located around the motor trigeminal nucleus and throughout the caudal pontine and medullary lateral reticular formation (parvocellular reticular nucleus). Many labeled fibers were also traced to the rostral half of the solitary nucleus and to the dorsal vagal nucleus, but mainly to its peripheral parts and the area immediately surrounding it. At levels just

rostral to the motor trigeminal nucleus, a separate contingent of labeled fibers branched off from the lateral fiber stream, passed ventromedially to terminate in the ventral part of the caudal pontine and upper medullary medial reticular formation and, but only to a limited extent, to the NRM and NRP (Fig. 15, upper three rows left). This projection is interesting, because it involves only those reticular areas that project to the spinal cord dorsal horn, and not the reticular areas that project to the ventral horn. In Cases 1384 and 1757, but not in Case 1710, labeled fibers were distributed to the marginal layer of the rostral portion of the caudal spinal trigeminal nucleus (Fig. 17, upper right). No labeled fibers were found in the caudal part of the caudal spinal trigeminal nucleus or in the spinal cord. In Case 1757, labeled fibers descended throughout the length of the spinal cord to distribute fibers to the intermediate zone, lamina X and the thoracolumbar sympathetic intermediolateral cell column.

With the exception of the ones to the spinal cord, the caudal brain stem projections from the lateral hypothalamus are very similar to the ones derived from the amygdala and the bed nucleus of the stria terminalis (see below). Carstens et al. (1983) showed that stimulation in the lateral hypothalamus of the cat results in inhibition of dorsal horn neuronal responses to noxious skin heating. It has always been difficult to study the function of the lateral hypothalamus by means of lesion or stimulation techniques, because the medial forebrain bundle passes through this area and this fiber bundle contains many fibers derived from other than lateral hypothalamic areas (see Nieuwenhuys et al., 1982, for review). For example, the PVN fibers descending to the spinal cord pass through the lateral hypothalamus as do the fibers from amygdala and bed nucleus of the stria terminalis on their way to the brain stem. Part of the findings of Carstens et al. (1983) may, therefore, be due to stimulation of fibers derived from these nuclei. On the other hand, the lateral hypothalamus projects to the PAG (except its dorsolateral part), the lateral pontine tegmental or paralemniscal cell group, the parabrachial nuclei and to the caudal pontine and upper medullary medial reticular formation, which in turn projects to the dorsal horn (Holstege and Kuypers, 1982; and this paper). Carstens et al. (1983) also demonstrated that administration of methysergide, an antagonist of serotonin, gave a partial reduction of the inhibitory effect. This would indicate that the NRM, which contains spinal cord projecting serotonergic neurons (Wiklund et al., 1981; Bowker et al., 1982), plays a role in this inhibitory effect. As indicated above, the lateral hypothalamus has, at most, a very limited direct projection to the NRM, which would emphasize the importance in nociception control of the indirect projections of the lateral hypothalamus (via PAG and/or parabrachial nuclei) to the NRM.

Amygdala and bed nucleus of the stria terminalis

The HRP results indicated that the medial part of the central nucleus of the amygdala and the lateral part of the bed nucleus of the stria terminalis (BNST) project to the area of the NRM and adjoining reticular formation, but not directly to the spinal cord (with the exception of the C1 segment, see below). As has already been pointed out by Johnston (1923), the central and medial amygdaloid nuclei and the BNST can be considered as one anatomical entity (see De Olmos et al., 1985; Holstege et al., 1985, for reviews). Also the projections from the amygdala and the BNST to the caudal brain stem are identical (Hopkins and Holstege, 1978; Holstege et al., 1985). Therefore, the pathways from these structures to the brain stem will be described together. In three cases ^{3}H-leucine injections were made in the central nucleus of the amygdala. In Case 1637 the injection extended slightly into the lateral part of the medial and ventrally into the basolateral amygdaloid nucleus (Fig. 2, E – H). The injection in Case 1636 was made slightly more medially, but extended ventrally into the basolateral and basomedial amygdaloid nuclei (Fig. 2, E – G). The injection in Case 746 was the most medially located and involv-

ed the medial part of the central amygdaloid nucleus and adjacent parts of the medial, basolateral and basomedial amygdaloid nuclei (Fig. 2, F, G). In three other cases injections were made in the BNST. In Case 1667 the most rostrally located injection was made and involved the rostral part of the lateral BNST and the medial part of the medial BNST (Fig. 2, B, C). In Case 1707 a relatively large injection was present, involving both parts of the BNST (Fig. 2, C, D). The injection in Case 1520 was relatively small, but extended further caudally than in the other two cases. It involved the dorsal parts of the lateral and medial BNST (Fig. 2, C – E). In all six cases the descending labeled fibers joined the medial forebrain bundle by passing ventrally (BNST fibers) or medially via the ventral amygdalofugal pathway (amygdala fibers). At mesencephalic levels the labeled fibers in the medial forebrain bundle gradually shifted laterally and descended further in the lateral mesencephalic, pontine and medullary lateral tegmental field. From this fiber stream, at mesencephalic levels, labeled fibers were distributed to the dorsal part of the substantia nigra, the ventral tegmental area of Tsai and to the mesencephalic midline raphe nuclei. They were also distributed to the nucleus of the posterior commissure, the mesencephalic lateral tegmentum and to the PAG including its laterally and ventrolaterally adjoining tegmentum (Fig. 19, A). Labeled fibers could not be traced to the dorsolateral PAG or its subependymal layer. Further caudally some labeled fibers were found in the dorsal raphe nucleus but almost none in the raphe centralis superior. At pontine levels, labeled fibers were distributed to the pontine lateral tegmental field including the paralemniscal nucleus, the locus coeruleus, the nucleus subcoeruleus, the parabrachial nuclei, and the area h of Meessen and Olszewski (1949) surrounding the motor trigeminal nucleus (Fig. 19, B, C). At the level just rostral to the motor trigeminal nucleus, labeled fibers branched off from the lateral fiber stream to pass ventrally and medially to terminate in the ventral part of the caudal pontine and upper medullary reticular formation (Fig. 19, C – E).

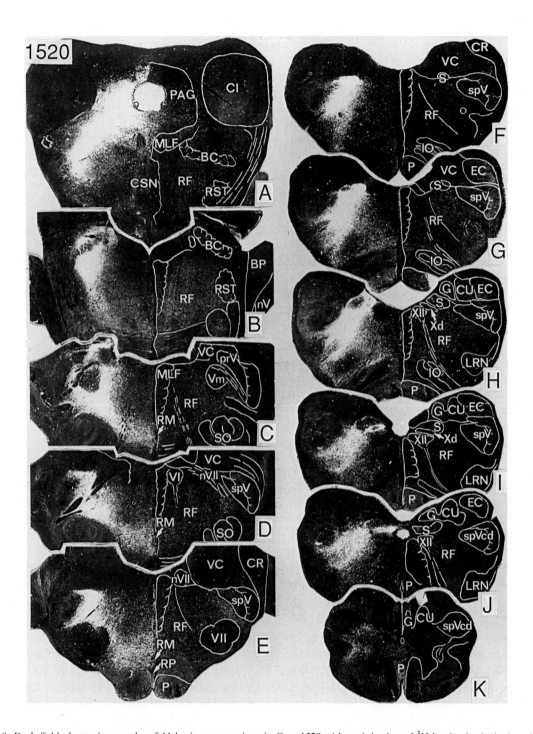

Fig. 19. Dark-field photomicrographs of 11 brain stem sections in Case 1520 with an injection of ^{3}H-leucine in the bed nucleus of the stria terminalis. Note the strong projection to the bulbar lateral tegmental field and the specific projection to the ventral part of the caudal pontine and upper medullary medial tegmentum. (From Holstege et al., 1985; Exp. Brain Res., 58: 385.)

82

Neurons in this area in turn project to the dorsal, but not the ventral horn of the spinal cord.

In the medulla many labeled fibers were distributed to the lateral reticular formation, to the dorsal vagal nucleus (mainly its peripheral and immediately surrounding parts), to the solitary nucleus (mainly to the rostral half of it) (Fig. 19, F – K) and to the marginal layer of the rostral part of the caudal spinal trigeminal nucleus (Fig. 17, lower row left and right). A few labeled fibers were observed in the intermediate zone of the first cervical segment of the spinal cord, but not beyond that level.

It is clear that, with only a few exceptions, the brain stem projections from the amygdala and BNST are almost identical to the ones derived from the lateral hypothalamus. It is not surprising, therefore, that stimulation in the amygdala results in inhibition of dorsal horn neuronal responses to noxious heat stimulation in the same way as stimulation in the lateral hypothalamus (Carstens, 1986). It is predictable that stimulation in the BNST will also have this effect.

Cortex

Direct projections from the cortex to the spinal cord in the cat originate in the motor (area 4) and somatosensory cortex (areas 3a, 3b, 1, 2 and 5; Gross et al., 1978). In two cats ³H-leucine injections were made in the somatosensory cortex. In the first cat (Case 1465), the injection was located in the lateral part of the pericruciate area (foreleg area of Woolsey, Woolsey, 1958), involving not only area 3, but also area 4 (Fig. 20). In Case 1468, the injection was present in the medial part of the postcruciate sulcus (hindleg area of Woolsey, Woolsey, 1958) and involved areas 3 and 1 (Fig. 20). Both injection sites involved all cortical laminae. In both cases all labeled corticospinal fibers crossed in the pyramidal decussation and descended contralaterally in the dorsolateral funiculus of the spinal cord. In both cases labeled fibers were distributed to all laminae of the dorsal horn (I to IV), except their most lateral parts. In

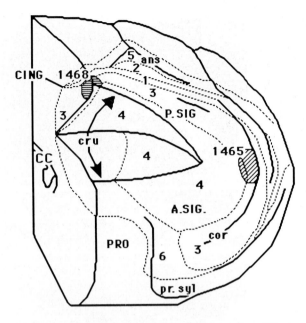

Fig. 20. Diagrammatic representation of the location of the injections in the cat pericruciate cortex of the two Cases 1465 and 1468. The cruciate sulcus is shown opened. The cytoarchitectonic areas have been delineated according to Hassler and Mühs-Clement (1964).

Case 1465, with an injection in the lateral pericruciate area, this distribution was present in C7 and the rostral half of C8 (Fig. 21), and in Case 1468, with an injection in the medial pericruciate area, in caudal L5, L6 and rostral L7. In Case 1465, in which the injection extended into area 4, an additional distribution was present to the lateral intermediate zone, i.e. the lateral parts of laminae V and VI and the dorsal part of VII at the levels C5 – T1 (Fig. 21). In Case 1468 no labeled fibers were observed in the intermediate zone. In both cases an additional projection could be traced to the medial parts of laminae V and VI at the levels C1 – T7 (Case 1465) and L4 – S3 (Case 1468). In the caudal brain stem, many labeled fibers were distributed to the contralateral cuneate nucleus (Case 1465) and to the contralateral gracile nucleus (Case 1468). No labeled fibers could be traced to the NRM or other brain stem structures giving rise to direct projections to lamina I of the medullary and spinal dorsal horn. These findings are in keep-

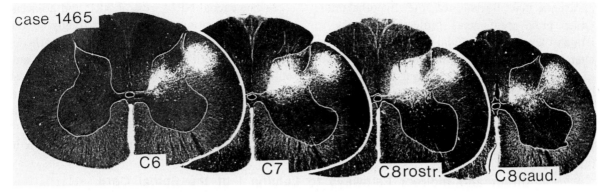

Fig. 21. Dark-field photomicrographs of the C6–C8 spinal segments in Case 1465 with an injection in the lateral part of the pericruciate cortex, involving areas 3 and 4. Note the very dense and localized projection in C7 and rostral C8 to all parts of the dorsal horn except its most lateral part. (From Armand et al., 1985; Brain Res., 343: 354.)

ing with the lesion-degeneration findings of Nyberg-Hansen and Brodal (1963), who demonstrated somatotopically organized projections from the somatosensory cortex to lamina IV and the medial parts of laminae V and VI of the spinal cord dorsal horn. The autoradiographic tracing results (see also Armand et al., 1985) demonstrate that these dorsal horn projections are not limited to these laminae (IV, V and VI), but also involve laminae I, II and III. Cheema et al. (1984), using the anterograde HRP technique, also observed direct projections from the somatosensory cortex to the superficial dorsal horn in cat and monkey. Electrophysiological findings of Yezierski et al. (1983) provide additional evidence that the somatosensory cortex exerts a direct influence on nociception control. They found that in the monkey intermediate and long-duration stimulus trains in the somatosensory cortex reduced the responses of spinothalamic cells. These responses were evoked by noxious mechanical or thermal stimuli and by A- and C-fiber volleys in the sural nerve. Short-duration stimulus trains only produced inhibition of spinothalamic cell responses to innocuous stimuli (Coulter et al., 1974). It is important to recall that the cortical projections are somatotopically organized, while the projections originating in the brain stem (NRM, its adjacent reticular formation and the paralemniscal nuclei) project diffusely throughout the length of the

spinal cord.

In the rat, projections from the infralimbic cortex to the spinal cord have been reported by Hurley-Gius et al. (1986). After WGA-HRP injections in this part of the cortex, they observed labeled fibers descending contralaterally in the base of the dorsal colum and bilaterally in the dorsolateral funiculi. These fibers terminated in laminae I and IV–V throughout the length of the spinal cord and a few in the intermediolateral cell column. Descending projections from the prefrontal cortex to the locus coeruleus and the dorsal and central superior raphe regions have been demonstrated by Arnsten and Goldman-Rakic (1984) in the monkey, to the solitary nucleus by Van der Kooy et al. (1984) in the rat, and by Willett et al. (1986) in the cat. Projections from the prefrontal cortex to the NRM and adjacent tegmentum have not been described.

Conclusions

1. The anatomical results show clearly that, in the cat, the NRM and adjacent caudal pontine and upper medullary reticular formation are not the only regions maintaining direct projections to lamina I of the spinal cord. The most important other structures are the pontine lateral tegmental or paralemniscal cell group, projecting contralaterally to laminae I, V and VI, and the

paraventricular nucleus of the hypothalamus. Other brain stem areas projecting directly to lamina I are the most caudal part of the medullary lateral reticular formation, the nucleus sub-coeruleus and the nucleus Edinger-Westphal.

2. The NRM and adjoining reticular formation projects not only to lamina I, the outer part of II and the lateral part of V, but especially its rostral part also to the other parts of the dorsal horn.

3. The caudal NRM, rostral NRP and adjacent reticular formation also project strongly to the autonomic (sympathetic and parasympathetic) preganglionic cell groups in caudal brain stem and spinal cord. A similar picture can also be observed in the descending projections from the nucleus subcoeruleus and paraventricular hypothalamic nucleus.

4. There exists a mediolateral organization in

Direct and Indirect Pathways to Lamina I of the Spinal Cord

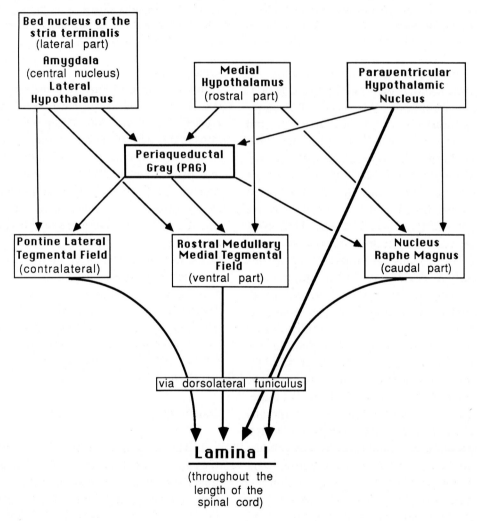

Fig. 22. Schematic representation of the strongest direct and indirect projections to lamina I of the caudal medulla and the spinal cord. Note that the minor projections, such as those derived from the nucleus Edinger-Westphal and the parabrachial nuclei are not indicated in this scheme.

the projections from the PAG to the medulla. The medially located cells in the dorsal PAG project heavily to the NRM and less strongly to the adjacent reticular formation. Conversely, the neurons located just lateral to the PAG project only to the lateral part of the ventral caudal pontine and upper medullary medial reticular formation and not to the NRM. Neurons in the lateral PAG project only to a limited extent to the NRM, but strongly to its adjacent reticular formation. These findings also indicate that not only PAG cells, but also neurons located next to the PAG take part in the projections to the medial medulla.

5. The PAG projects not only to caudal pontine and upper medullary regions that are connected with the medullary and spinal dorsal horn, but also to more caudal parts of the medial reticular formation which in turn project to the ventral horn. Moreover, the ventrolateral PAG and ventrally adjoining mesencephalic tegmentum also project to the rostral NRP, which gives rise to very strong (serotonergic) fiber projections to all parts of the ventral horn throughout the length of the spinal cord. This indicates that the PAG is not only involved in nociceptive or non-nociceptive, but also in motor control. The same is true for the medial hypothalamus (anterior part and PVN).

6. The NRM not only receives a large number of afferents from the PAG, but also from the parabrachial nuclei, the mesencephalic tegmentum ventrolateral to the PAG, the paraventricular hypothalamic nucleus (PVN) and the medial part of the hypothalamus, with the exception of its most caudal portion (Fig. 22). All structures

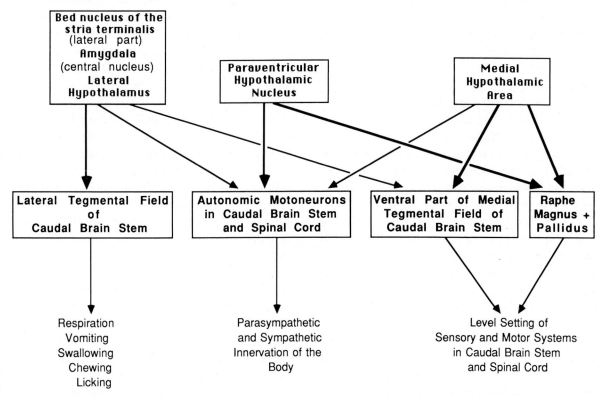

Descending Pathways from Limbic System to Caudal Brain Stem and Spinal Cord

Fig. 23. Representation of the mediolateral organization of the limbic system pathways to brain stem and spinal cord and its possible functional implications. The strongest projections are indicated by thick arrows.

belong to the limbic system or are closely associated with it.

7. The reticular formation, adjacent to the PAG, not only receives afferents from the structures mentioned in '6', but also from the lateral parts of the limbic system: the mesencephalic tegmentum lateral to the PAG, the lateral hypothalamus, the central nucleus of the amygdala and the lateral part of the bed nucleus of the stria terminalis. These structures also project strongly to the paralemniscal cell group.

8. The somatosensory cortex projects directly to all parts of the dorsal horn, including lamina I. In contrast to the diffuse projections originating in the brain stem structures, the cortical projections are strictly somatotopically organized.

The anatomical data emphasize the importance of the limbic system or emotional brain in relation to the nociception inhibitory areas in the brain stem. Limbic structures also have strong access to the medullary areas (NRP and adjacent reticular formation), that project to all the autonomic preganglionic and somatic motoneuronal cell groups throughout the length of the spinal cord. The diffuse organization of these brain stem efferent pathways suggests that they do not steer specific motor activities such as movements of distal (arm, hand or leg) or axial parts of the body, but have a more global effect on the level of activity of the motoneurons in general by changing its membrane excitability (see McCall and Aghajanian, 1979; White and Neuman, 1980; Hounsgaard et al., 1986; Fung and Barnes, 1987). The same is probably true for the nociception inhibitory areas in the brain stem, which produce a global modulatory influence on nociception. The lamina I projections originating in the somatosensory cortex function in a different framework. They are somatotopically organized and are not under direct limbic control.

As a final conclusion one could say that the emotional brain has a great impact on the sensory as well as on the motor system (Fig. 23). In both systems it sets the level of functioning of the neurons. This level reflects the emotional state of the individual. For example it is well known that many forms of stress, such as aggression, fear and sexual arousal induce analgesia, while the motor system is set at a 'high' level and motoneurons can easily be excited. In this concept the brain stem nociception inhibitory systems can be considered as tools for the limbic system controlling spinal cord activity.

Summary

In this study the projections to lamina I of the spinal cord cord were investigated by means of the retrograde HRP and anterograde autoradiographic tracing technique. The HRP findings indicated that several neuronal cell groups in the brain stem and hypothalamus project to the spinal cord throughout its total length. The autoradiographic tracing results demonstrated that the strongest projections to lamina I are derived from four areas: (1) the caudal nucleus raphe magnus (NRM), (2) the ventral part of the caudal pontine and medullary medial tegmental field, adjoining the NRM, (3) the contralaterally projecting lateral pontine or paralemniscal tegmentum, and (4) the paraventricular nucleus (PVN) of the hypothalamus. A limited, especially at lumbosacral levels, distinct projection to lamina I originated in the most caudal part of the medullary tegmentum. In addition, although not demonstrated in my own experiments, neurons in the nucleus Edinger-Westphal seem to project to lamina I of the spinal cord. A diffuse projection to all parts of the spinal gray, including lamina I, was derived from the (probably noradrenergic) neurons in the dorsolateral pontine tegmentum. All these brain stem and hypothalamic cell groups projected throughout the length of the spinal cord. This was not the case with the projections derived from the sensory cortex, which were somatotopically organized. For example, neurons in the medial portion of the pericruciate cortex projected to the lumbosacral cord dorsal horn, while those in the lateral pericruciate cortex projected to the dorsal horn of the lower cervical cord. These projections not only involved the deeper layers of the dorsal horn, but all parts of them, including lamina I.

The next step was to determine which areas control the brain stem areas that project to lamina I. HRP experiments demonstrated that the major input to NRM and adjoining tegmentum is derived from the ventral parabrachial nuclei (including the nucleus Kölliker-Fuse), the periaqueductal gray (PAG), the nucleus cuneiformis and more medial parts of the mesencephalic tegmentum, the hypothalamus, the central nucleus of the amygdala and the bed nucleus of the stria terminalis. The autoradiographical tracing experiments showed that from these structures, the ones located medially such as the dorsal PAG and the medial hypothalamic areas project preferentially to the medially located NRM, and to a lesser extent to the more laterally located ventral part of the caudal pontine and upper medullary medial tegmental field. The reverse is true for the laterally located structures, such as the lateral PAG and adjacent tegmentum, the lateral hypothalamus, the central nucleus of the amygdala and the bed nucleus of the stria terminalis. They project mainly to the tegmentum adjacent to the NRM, but to a much lesser degree to the NRM itself. They also project strongly to the paralemniscal cell group. These findings suggest a mediolateral organization within the indirect projections to lamina I. The results demonstrate the importance of limbic structures in the direct and indirect pathways to lamina I neurons in the spinal cord. The importance of the limbic system in supraspinal control of nociception as well as motor systems is discussed.

Acknowledgements

The author thanks Mr. A.M. Vreugdenhil, Mr. R.C. Boer and Mrs. C.M. Bijker-Biemond for their technical help. This work was supported by NASA Grant NCC 2-491 to the Department of Anatomy of the School of Medicine of the University of California San Francisco.

Abbreviations

AA	anterior amygdaloid nucleus
AC	anterior commissure
ACN	nucleus of the anterior commissure
AD	anterodorsal nucleus of the thalamus
AH	anterior hypothalamic area
AL	lateral amygdaloid nucleus
AM	anteromedial nucleus of the thalamus
ans	ansate sulcus
AP	area postrema
A. SIG.	anterior sigmoid gyrus
AV	anteroventral nucleus of the thalamus
BC	brachium conjunctivum
BIC	brachium of the inferior colliculus
BL	basolateral amygdaloid nucleus
BM	basomedial amygdaloid nucleus
BNSTL	lateral part of the bed nucleus of stria terminalis
BNSTM	medial part of the bed nucleus of the stria terminalis
BP	brachium pontis
CA	central nucleus of the amygdala
CC	corpus callosum
Cd	caudate nucleus
CGL	lateral geniculate body
CGM	medial geniculate body
CGMd	medial geniculate body, dorsal part
CGMint	medial geniculate body, interior division
CGMp	medial geniculate body, principal part
cing.	cingulate sulcus
CI	capsula interna
CL	claustrum
CM	centromedian thalamic nucleus
CN	cochlear nuclei
CO	cortical amygdaloid nucleus
cor.	coronal sulcus
cru	cruciate sulcus
CS	superior colliculus
CSN	nucleus centralis superior
CU	nucleus cuneatus
CUN	cuneiform nucleus
D	nucleus of Darkschewitsch
DBV	nucleus of the diagonal band of Broca

DH	dorsal hypothalamic area	NR	red nucleus
DMH	dorsomedial hypothalamic nucleus	NRA	nucleus retroambiguus
EC	external cuneate nucleus	NRM	nucleus raphe magnus
ECU	external cuneate nucleus	NRP	nucleus raphe pallidus
En	entopeduncular nucleus	NRTP	nucleus reticularis tegmenti pontis
F	fornix	NSC	nucleus subcoeruleus
fRF	fasciculus retroflexus	NTB	nucleus of the trapezoid body
G	nucleus gracilis	NTS	nucleus tractus solitarius
GP	globus pallidus	nV	trigeminal nerve
Hab	habenular nucleus	nVII	facial nerve
HC	hippocampus	OC	optic chiasm
HPA	posterior hypothalamus area	OL	olivary pretectal nucleus
HT	hypothalamus	OT	optic tract
IC	inferior colliculus	P	pyramidal tract
IN	interpeduncular nucleus	PAG	periaqueductal gray
IO	inferior olive	PBL	lateral parabrachial nucleus
IVN	inferior vestibular nucleus	PBM	medial parabrachial nucleus
KF	nucleus Kölliker-Fuse	PC	pedunculus cerebri
LD	nucleus lateralis dorsalis of the thalamus	PCN	nucleus of the posterior commissure
		PEA	anterior part of periventricular hypothalamic nucleus
LGN	lateral geniculate nucleus		
LH	lateral hypothalamic area	PON	pontine nuclei
LL	lateral lemniscus	PP	posterior pretectal nucleus
LOTR	lateral olfactory tract	PRO.	proreate gyrus
LP	lateral posterior nucleus of the thalamus	pr. syl	presylvian sulcus
		P. SIG.	posterior sigmoid gyrus
LRN	lateral reticular nucleus	Pt	parataenial nucleus of the thalamus
LTF	lateral tegmental field	PT	Probst tract
LVN	lateral vestibular nucleus	PTM	medial pretectal nucleus
MB	mammillary body	PVA	paraventricular nucleus of the thalamus (anterior part)
MC	nucleus medialis centralis of the thalamus		
		PVN	paraventricular hypothalamic nucleus
MD	nucleus medialis dorsalis of the thalamus	Pu	putamen
		PUL	pulvinar nucleus of the thalamus
MesV	mesencephalic trigeminal tract	PV	posterior paraventricular nucleus of the thalamus
ML	medial lemniscus		
MLF	medial longitudinal fasciculus	R	reticular nucleus of the thalamus
motV	motor trigeminal nucleus	RB	restiform body
MTF	medial tegmental field	RE	nucleus reuniens of the thalamus
MVN	medial vestibular nucleus	RF	reticular formation
NCL	nucleus centralis lateralis	RFmed	medial reticular formation
NLL	nucleus of the lateral lemniscus	RFlat	lateral reticular formation
NOT	nucleus of the optic tract	RiMLF	rostral interstitial nucleus of the MLF
NOTM	medial nucleus of the optic tract	RM	nucleus raphe magnus
NPC	nucleus parencentralis of the thalamus	RN	red nucleus

RP	nucleus raphe pallidus
Rpo	nucleus raphe pontis
RST	rubrospinal tract
S	solitary complex
SC	suprachiasmatic nucleus
SC	nucleus subcoeruleus (Figs. 8, 9)
SI	substantia innominata
SLN	lateral septal nucleus
SM	stria medullaris
SMN	medial septal nucleus
SN	substantia nigra
SO	superior olivary complex
SON	supraoptic nucleus
ST	subthalamic nucleus
STT	stria terminalis
SVN	superior vestibular nucleus
TB	trapezoid body
TMT	mammillothalamic tract
VA	ventroanterior nucleus of the thalamus
VB	ventrobasal complex of the thalamus
VC	vestibular complex
VL	ventrolateral nucleus of the thalamus
VM	ventromedial nucleus of the thalamus
Vn	trigeminal nerve
VTA	ventral tegmental area of Tsai
VTN	ventral tegmental nucleus
ZI	zona incerta
III	oculomotor nucleus
IV	trochlear nucleus
Vm	motor trigeminal nucleus
Vpr	principal trigeminal nucleus
Vsp	spinal trigeminal complex
Vsp.cd.	caudal part of spinal trigeminal complex
VI	abducens nucleus
VII	facial nucleus
Xd	dorsal vagal nucleus
VII	hypoglossal nucleus

References

Akaike, A., Shibata, T., Satoh, M. and Takagi, H. (1978) Analgesia induced by microinjection of morphine into and electrical stimulation of the nucleus paragigantocellularis of rat medulla oblongata. *Neuropharmacology,* 17: 775 – 778.

Anderson, C.H. and Chen, C.L. (1980) Efferents of the medial preoptic area in the guinea pig: an autoradiographic study. *Brain Res. Bull.,* 5: 257 – 265.

Armand, J., Holstege, G. and Kuypers, H.G.J.M. (1985) Differential corticospinal projections in the cat. An autoradiographic tracing study. *Brain Res.,* 343: 351 – 355.

Arnsten, A.F.T. and Goldman-Rakic, P.S. (1984) Selective prefrontal cortical projections to the region of the locus coeruleus and raphe nuclei in the Rhesus monkey. *Brain Res.,* 306: 9 – 18.

Barrington, F.J.F. (1925) The effect of lesion of the hind- and midbrain on micturition in the cat. *Quart. J. Exp. Physiol.,* 15: 81 – 102.

Basbaum, A.I., Clanton, C.H. and Fields, H.I. (1978) Three bulbospinal pathways from the rostral medulla of the cat: an autoradiographic study of pain modulating systems. *J. Comp. Neurol.,* 178: 209 – 224.

Berman, A.L. (1968) *The Brain Stem of the Cat.* University of Wisconsin Press, 175 pp.

Berman, A.L. and Jones, E.G. (1982) *The Thalamus and the Basal Telencephalon of the Cat.* A cytoarchitectonic atlas with stereotaxic coordinates. University of Wisconsin Press, Madison.

Bertrand, F. and Hugelin, A. (1971) Respiratory synchronizing function of nucleus parabrachialis medialis: pneumotaxic mechanisms. *J. Neurophysiol.,* 34: 189 – 207.

Bertrand, F., Hugelin, A and Vibert, J.F. (1974) A stereological model of pneumotaxic oscillator based on spatial and temporal distributions of neuronal bursts. *J. Neurophysiol.,* 37: 91 – 107.

Besson, J.-M. and Chaouch, A. (1987) Peripheral and spinal mechanisms of nociception. *Physiol. Rev.,* 67: 67 – 186.

Blomqvist, A. and Berkley, K.J. (1987) A spino-diencephalic relay through the parabrachial nucleus in the cat. *Soc. Neurosci. Abstr.,* Vol. 13, part 1: 114.

Bowker, R.M., Westlund, K.N., Sullivan, M.C. and Coulter, J.D. (1982) Organization of descending serotonergic projections to the spinal cord. In H.G.J.M. Kuypers and G.F. Martin (Eds.), *Descending Pathways to the Spinal Cord, Progressin Brain Research, Vol. 57,* Elsevier, Amsterdam, pp. 239 – 265.

Bowker, R.M., Westlund, K.N., Sullivan, M.C., Wilber, J.F. and Coulter, J.D. (1983) Descending serotonergic, peptidergic and cholinergic pathways from the raphe nuclei: a multiple transmitter complex. *Brain Res.,* 288: 33 – 48.

Brown, A.G. and Franz, D.N. (1969) Responses of spinocervical tract neurons to natural stimulation of identified cutaneous receptors. *Exp. Brain Res.,* 7: 231 – 249.

Brudzynski, S.M. and Eckersdorf, B. (1984) Inhibition of

locomotor activity during cholinergically-induced emotional aversive response in the cat. *Behav. Brain Res.,* 14: 247–253.

Burton, H. and Loewy, A.D. (1977) Projections to the spinal cord from medullary somatosensory relay nuclei. *J. Comp. Neurol.,* 173: 773–792.

Busch, H.F.M. (1961) *An Anatomical Analysis of the White Matter in the Brain Stem of the Cat.* Van Gorcum, Assen.

Carlton, S.M., Chung, J.M., Leonard, R.B. and Willis, W.D. (1985) Funicular trajectories of brain stem neurons projecting to the lumbar spinal cord in the monkey (*Macaca fascicularis*): a retrograde labeling study. *J. Comp. Neurol.,* 241: 382–404.

Carstens, E. (1982) Inhibition of spinal dorsal horn neuronal responses to noxious skin heating by medial hypothalamic stimulation in the cat. *J. Neurophysiol.* 48: 808–822.

Carstens, E. (1986) Hypothalamic inhibition of rat dorsal horn neuronal responses to noxious skin heating. *Pain,* 25: 95–107.

Carstens, E. and Trevino, D.L. (1978) Laminar origins of spinothalamic projections in the cat as determined by the retrograde transport of horseradish peroxidase. *J. Comp. Neurol.,* 182: 151–166.

Carstens, E., Klumpp, D. and Zimmermann, M. (1980) Differential inhibitory effects of medial and lateral midbrain stimulation on spinal neuronal discharges to noxious skin heating in the cat. *J. Neurophysiol.,* 43: 332–342.

Carstens, E., Fraunhoffer, M. and Zimmermann, M. (1981) Serotonergic mediation of descending inhibition from midbrain periaqueductal gray, but not reticular formation, of spinal nociceptive transmission in the cat. *Pain,* 10: 149–167.

Carstens, E., Fraunhoffer, M. and Suberg, S.N. (1983a) Inhibition of dorsal horn neuronal responses to noxious skin heating by lateral hypothalamic stimulation in the cat. *J. Neurophysiol.,* 50: 192–204.

Carstens, E., Guinan, M.J. and MacKinnon, J.D. (1983b) Naloxone does not consistently affect inhibition of spinal nociceptive transmission produced by medial diencephalic stimulation in the cat. *Neurosci. Lett.,* 42: 71–76.

Cervero, F., Iggo, A. and Ogawa, H. (1976) Nociceptor driven dorsal horn neurons in the lumbar spinal cord of the cat. *Pain,* 2: 5–24.

Cheema, S.S., Rustioni, A. and Whitsel, B.L. (1984) Light and electron microscopic evidence for a direct corticospinal projection to superficial laminae of the dorsal horn in cats and monkeys. *J. Comp. Neurol.,* 225: 276–290.

Christensen, B.N. and Perl, E.R. (1970) Spinal neurons specifically excited by noxious and thermal stimuli: marginal zone of the dorsal horn. *J. Neurophysiol.,* 33: 293–307.

Chung, J.M., Kenshalo, Jr. D.R., Gerhart, K.D. and Willis, W.D. (1979) Excitation of primate spinothalamic neurons by cutaneous C-fiber volleys. *J. Neurophysiol.,* 42: 1354–1369.

Conrad, L.C.A. and Pfaff, D.W. (1976a) Efferents from medial basal forebrain and hypothalamus in the rat. I. An autoradiographic tracing study of the medial preoptic area. *J. Comp. Neurol.,* 169: 185–220.

Conrad, L.C.A. and Pfaff, D.W. (1976b) Efferents from medial basal forebrain and hypothalamus in the rat. II. An autoradiographic study of the anterior hypothalamus. *J. Comp. Neurol.,* 169: 221–262.

Cottingham, S.L. and Pfaff, D.W. (1987) Electrical stimulation of the midbrain central gray facilitates lateral vestibulospinal activation of back muscle EMG in the rat. *Brain Res.,* 421: 397–400.

Cottingham, S.L., Femano, P.A. and Pfaff, D.W. (1987) Electrical stimulation of the midbrain central gray facilitates reticulospinal activation of axial muscle EMG. *Exp. Neurol.,* 97: 704–724.

Coulter, J.D., Maunz, R.A. and Willis, W.D. (1974) Effects of stimulation of sensorimotor cortex on primate spinothalamic neurons. *Brain Res.,* 65: 351–356.

Craig, Jr., A.D. and Tapper, D.N. (1978) Lateral cervical nucleus in the cat: functional organization and characteristics. *J. Neurophysiol.,* 41: 1511–1534.

De Olmos, J., Alheid, G.F. and Beltramino, C.A. (1985) Amygdala. In G. Paxinos (Ed.), *The Rat Nervous System, Vol. I,* Academic Press, Syndey, Tokyo, pp. 223–334.

DeSalles, A.A., Katayama, Y., Becker, D.P. and Hayes, R.L. (1985) Pain suppression induced by electrical stimulation of the pontine parabrachial region. Experimental study in cats. *J. Neurosurg.,* 62: 397–407.

Dostrovsky, J.O. (1984) Brain stem influences on transmission of somatosensory information in the spinocervicothalamic pathway. *Brain Res.,* 292: 229–238.

Elam, J.S., Contos, N. and Berkley, K.J. (1987) Differences in the efficiency and pattern of incorporation of [^{3}H]leucine and [^{3}H]proline into proteins of adult cat brains. *Brain Res.,* 413: 129–134.

Engberg, I., Lundberg, A. and Ryall, R.W. (1968) Reticulospinal inhibition of interneurons. *J. Physiol. (London),* 194: 225–236.

Fields, H.L., Clanton, C.H. and Anderson, S.D. (1977a) Somatosensory properties of spinoreticular neurons in the cat. *Brain Res.,* 120: 49–66.

Fields, H.L., Basbaum, A.I., Clanton, C.H. and Anderson, S.D. (1977b) Nucleus raphe magnus inhibition of spinal cord dorsal horn neurons. *Brain Res.,* 126: 441–453.

Fung, S.J. and Barnes, C.D. (1987) Membrane excitability changes in hindlimb motoneurons, induced by stimulation of the locus coeruleus in cats. *Brain Res.,* 402: 230–242.

Gebhart, G.F., Sandkühler, J., Thalhammer, J.G. and Zimmermann, M. (1983) Inhibition of spinal nociceptive information by stimulation in midbrain of the cat is blocked by lidocaine microinjected in nucleus raphe magnus and medullary reticular formation. *J. Neurophysiol.,* 50:

1446 – 1459.

Graybiel, A. (1977) Direct and indirect preoculomotor pathways of the brain stem: an autoradiographic study of the pontine reticular formation in the cat. *J. Comp. Neurol.,* 175, 37 – 78.

Griffin, G., Watkins, L.R. and Mayer, D.J. (1979) HRP pellets and slow release-gels: two new techniques for greater localization and sensitivity. *Brain Res.,* 168: 595 – 601.

Griffith, J.L. and Gatipon, G.B. (1981) A comparative study of selective stimulation of raphe nuclei in the cat in inhibiting dorsal horn neuron responses to noxious stimulation. *Brain Res.,* 229: 520 – 524.

Gross, W.P., Ewing, L.K., Carter, C.M. and Coulter, J.D. (1978) Organization of corticospinal neurons in the cat. *Brain Res.,* 143: 393 – 419.

Hassler, R. and Mühs-Clement, K. (1964) Architektonischer Aufbau des sensomotorischen und parietalen Cortex der Katze. *J. Hirnforsch.,* 6: 377 – 420.

Hayes, N.L. and Rustioni, A. (1981) Descending projections from brain stem and sensorimotor cortex to spinal enlargements in the cat. *Exp. Brain Res.,* 41: 89 – 107.

Hayes, R.L. and Katayama, Y. (1985) Range of environmental stimuli producing nociceptive suppression: implications for neural mechanisms. *Ann. NY Acad. Sci.,* 467: 1 – 13.

Hayes, R.L., Katayama, Y., Watkins, L.R. and Becker, D.P. (1984) Bilateral lesions of the dorsolateral funiculus of the cat spinal cord: effects on basal nociceptive reflexes and nociceptive suppression produced by cholinergic activation of the pontine parabrachial region. *Brain Res.,* 311: 267 – 280.

Hendrickson, A., Moe, L. and Noble, B. (1972) Staining for autoradiography of the central nervous system. *Stain Technol.,* 47: 283 – 290.

Holstege, G. (1987a) Some anatomical observations on the projections from the hypothalamus to brain stem and spinal cord: an HRP and autoradiographic tracing study in the cat. *J. Comp. Neurol.,* 260: 98 – 126.

Holstege, G. (1987b) The final common pathway in vocalization in the cat. *Soc. Neurosci. Abstr.,* Vol. 13, part 2, p. 855.

Holstege, G. (1988) Anatomical evidence for a strong ventral parabrachial projection to nucleus raphe magnus and adjacent tegmental field. *Brain Res.,* 447: 154 – 158.

Holstege, G. and Kuypers, H.G.J.M. (1982) The anatomy of brain stem pathways to the spinal cord in cat. A labeled amino acid tracing study. In H.G.J.M. Kuypers and G.F. Martin (Eds.), *Descending Pathways to the Spinal Cord, Progress in Brain Research, Vol. 57,* Elsevier, Amsterdam, pp. 145 – 175.

Holstege, G. and Tan, J. (1987) Supraspinal control of motoneurons innervating the striated muscles of the pelvic floor including urethral and anal sphincters in the cat. *Brain,* 110: 1323 – 1344.

Holstege, G., Kuypers, H.G.J.M. and Dekker, J.J. (1977) The organization of the bulbar fibre connections to the trigeminal, facial and hypoglossal motor nuclei. *Brain,* 100: 265 – 286.

Holstege, G., Kuypers, H.G.J.M. and Boer, R.C. (1979) Anatomical evidence for direct brain stem projections to the somatic motoneuronal cell groups and autonomic preganglionic cell groups in cat spinal cord. *Brain Res.,* 171: 329 – 333.

Holstege, G., Graveland, G., Bijker-Biemond, C.M. and Schuddeboom, I. (1983) Location of motoneurons innervating soft palate, pharynx and esophagus. Anatomical evidence for a possible swallowing center in the pontine reticular formation. An HRP and autoradiographic tracing study. *Brain Behav. Evol.,* 23: 47 – 62.

Holstege, G., Meiners, L. and Tan, K. (1985) Projections of the bed nucleus of the stria terminalis to the mesencephalon, pons, and medulla oblongata in the cat. *Exp. Brain Res.,* 58: 379 – 391.

Holstege, G., Griffiths, D., De Wall, H. and Dalm, E. (1986) Anatomical and physiological observations on supraspinal control of bladder and urethral sphincter muscles in the cat. *J. Comp. Neurol.,* 250: 449 – 461.

Hopkins, D.A. and Holstege, G. (1978) Amygdaloid projections to the mesencephalon, pons and medulla oblongata in the cat. *Exp. Brain Res.,* 32: 529 – 547.

Hong, S.K., Kniffki, K.D., Mense, S., Schmidt, R.F. and Wendisch, M. (1979) Descending influences on the responses of spinocervical tract neurones to chemical stimulation of fine muscle afferents. *J. Physiol. (Lond.),* 290: 129 – 140.

Hosoya, Y. (1985) Hypothalamic projections to the ventral medulla oblongata in the rat, with special reference to the nucleus raphe pallidus: a study using autoradiographic and HRP techniques. *Brain Res.,* 344: 338 – 350.

Hounsgaard, J., Hultborn, H. and Kiehn, O. (1986) Transmitter-controlled properties of α-motoneurons causing long-lasting motor discharge to brief excitatory inputs. In H.-J. Freund, U. Büttner, B. Cohen and J. Noth (Eds.), *The Oculomotor and Skeletalmotor Systems: Differences and Similarities, Progress in Brain Research., Vol. 64,* Elsevier, Amsterdam, pp. 39 – 50.

Hu, J.W. and Sessle, B.J. (1979) Trigeminal nociceptive and non nociceptive neurons: brain stem intranuclear projections and modulation by orofacial, periaqueductal and nucleus raphe magnus stimuli. *Brain Res.,* 170: 547 – 552.

Huisman, A.M., Kuypers, H.G.J.M. and Verburgh, C.A. (1982) Differences in collateralization of the descending spinal pathways from red nucleus and other brain stem cell groups in cat and monkey. In H.G.J.M. Kuypers and G.F. Martin (Eds.), *Descending Pathways to the Spinal Cord, Progress in Brain Research, Vol. 57,* Elsevier, Amsterdam, pp. 185 – 217.

Hurley-Gius, K.M., Cechetto, D.F. and Saper, C.B. (1986) Spinal connections of the infralimbic autonomic cortex. *Soc.*

Neurosci. Abstr., Vol. 12, Part 1, p. 538.

Hylden, J.L.K., Hayashi, H., Dubner, R. and Bennett, G.J. (1986) Physiology and morphology of the lamina I spinomesencephalic projection. *J. Comp. Neurol.,* 247: 505 – 515.

Innis, R.B. and Aghajanian, G.K. (1986) Cholecystokinin-containing and nociceptive neurons in rat Edinger-Westphal nucleus. *Brain Res.,* 363: 230 – 238.

Innis, R.B., Correa, F.M., Uhl, G.R., Schneider, B. and Snyder, S.H. (1979) Cholecystokinin octapeptide-like immunoreactivity: histochemical localization in rat brain. *Proc. Natl. Acad. Sci. USA,* 76: 521 – 525.

Johnston, J.B. (1923) Further contributions to the study of the evolution of the forebrain. *J. Comp. Neurol.,* 35: 337 – 481.

Jones, B.E. and Friedman, L. (1983) Atlas of catecholamine perikarya, varicosities and pathways in the brain stem of the cat. *J. Comp. Neurol.,* 215: 382 – 396.

Jones, B.E. and Yang, T-Z (1985) The efferent projections from the reticular formation and the locus coeruleus studied by anterograde and retrograde axonal transport in the rat. *J. Comp. Neurol.,* 242: 56 – 92.

Jones, B.E., Pare, M. and Beaudet, A. (1986) Retrograde labeling of neurons in the brain stem following injections of ^{3}H-choline into the rat spinal cord. *Neuroscience,* 18: 901 – 916.

Jones, S.L. and Gebhart, G.F. (1987) Spinal pathways mediating tonic, coeruleospinal, and raphe-spinal descending inhibition in the rat. *J. Neurophysiol.,* 58: 138 – 159.

Jürgens, U. and Pratt, R. (1979) Role of the periaqueductal grey in vocal expression. *Brain Res.,* 167: 367 – 378.

Kajander, K.C., Ebner, T.J. and Bloedel, J.R. (1984) Effects of the periaqueductal gray and raphe magnus stimulation on the responses of spinocervical and other ascending projection neurons to noxious inputs. *Brain Res.,* 291: 29 – 30.

Kalia, M. and Mesulam, M.-M. (1980) Brain stem projections of sensory and motor components of the vagus complex in the cat. II. Laryngeal, tracheobronchial, pulmonary, cardiac and gastrointestinal branches. *J. Comp. Neurol.,* 193: 467 – 508.

Kopriwa, B.M. and LeBlond, C.P. (1962) Improvements in the coating technique for autoradiography. *J. Histochem. Cytochem.,* 10: 269 – 284.

Kristensson, K. and Olsson, Y. (1974) Retrograde transport of horseradish peroxidase in transected axons. I Time relationships between transport and induction of chromatolysis. *Brain Res.,* 79: 101 – 109.

Kuypers, H.G.J.M. and Maisky, V.A. (1975) Retrograde transport of horseradish peroxidase from spinal cord to brain stem cell groups in the cat. *Neurosci. Lett.,* 1: 9 – 14.

Light, A.R. and Perl, E.R. (1979) Spinal termination of functionally identified primary afferent neurons with slowly conducting myelinating fibers. *J. Comp. Neurol.,* 186: 133 – 150.

Light, A.R., Casale, E.J. and Menetrey, D.M. (1986) The effects of focal stimulation in nucleus raphe magnus and periaqueductal gray on intracellularly recorded neurons in spinal laminae I and II. *J. Neurophysiol.,* 56: 555 – 571.

Loewy, A.D. and Saper, C.B. (1978) Edinger-Westphal nucleus: projections to the brain stem and spinal cord in the cat. *Brain Res.,* 150: 1 – 27.

Lovick, T.A. and Wolstencroft, J.H. (1979) Inhibitory effects of nucleus raphe magnus on neuronal responses in the spinal trigeminal nucleus to nociceptive compared with non-nociceptive inputs. *Pain,* 7: 135 – 145.

Lovick, T.A. and Robinson, J.P. (1983) Bulbar raphe neurones with projections to the trigeminal nucleus caudalis and the lumbar cord in the rat: a fluorescence double labeling study. *Exp. Brain Res.,* 50: 299 – 309.

Maciewicz, R., Phipps, B.S., Foote, W.E., Aronin, N. and DiFiglia, M. (1983) The distribution of substance P-containing neurons in the cat Edinger-Westphal nucleus: relationship to efferent projection systems. *Brain Res.,* 270: 217 – 230.

Maciewicz, R., Phipps, B.S., Grenier, J. and Poletti, C.E. (1984) Edinger-Westphal nucleus: cholecystokinin immunocytochemistry and projections to spinal cord and trigeminal nucleus in the cat. *Brain Res.,* 299: 139 – 145.

Mantyh, P.W. (1983) Connections of midbrain periaqueductal gray in the monkey. II. Descending efferent projections. *J. Neurophysiol.,* 49: 582 – 594.

Martin, G.F., Humbertson, A.O., Laxson, L.C., Panneton, W.M. and Tschismadia, I. (1979) Spinal projections from the mesencephalic and pontine reticular formation in the North American opossum: a study using axonal transport techniques. *J. Comp. Neurol.,* 187: 373 – 401.

Martin, G.F., Cabana, T., Humbertson, Jr., A.O., Laxson, L.C. and Panneton, W.M. (1981a) Spinal projections from the medullary reticular formation of the North American opossum: evidence for heterogeneity. *J. Comp. Neurol.,* 196: 663 – 682.

Martin, G.F., Cabana, T. and Humbertson, Jr., A.O. (1981b) Evidence for collateral innervation of the cervical and lumbar enlargements of the spinal cord by single reticular and raphe neurons. Studies using fluorescent markers in double-labeling experiments on the North American opossum. *Neurosci. Lett.,* 24: 1 – 6.

Martin, G.F., Cabana, T., Ditirro, F.J., Ho, R.H. and Humbertson, A.O. (1982) Reticular and raphe projections to the spinal cord of the North American opossum. Evidence for connectional heterogeneity. In H.G.J.M. Kuypers and G.F. Martin (Eds.), *Descending Pathways to the Spinal Cord, Progress in Brain Research, Vol. 57,* Elsevier, Amsterdam, pp. 109 – 144.

Martin, G.F., Vertes, R.P. and Waltzer, R. (1985) Spinal projections of the gigantocellular reticular formation in the rat. Evidence for projections from different areas to laminae I and II and lamina IX. *Exp. Brain Res.,* 58: 154 – 162.

McCall, R.B. and Aghajanian, G.K. (1979) Serotonergic excitation of facial motoneuron excitation. *Brain Res.,* 169: 11–27.

Meessen, H. and Olszewsi, J. (1949) *Cytoarchitektonischer Atlas der Rautenhirn des Kaninchens.* Karger, Basel.

Mehler, W.R. (1962) The anatomy of the so-called 'pain tract' in man: an analysis of the course and distribution of the ascending fibers of the fasciculus anterolateralis. In J.D. French and R.W. Porter (Eds.), *Basic Research in Paraplegia,* Charles C Thomas, Springfield, IL, pp. 26–55.

Mehler, W.R. (1969) Some neurological species differences – a posteriori. *Ann. NY Acad. Sci.,* 167: 424–468.

Mehler, W.R., Feferman, M.E. and Nauta, W.J.H. (1960) Ascending axon degeneration following anterolateral cordotomy. An experimental study in the monkey. *Brain,* 83: 718–750.

Mendell, L.M. (1966) Physiological properties of unmyelinated fiber projection to the spinal cord. *Exp. Neurol.,* 16: 316–332.

Mesulam, M.-M. (1978) Tetramethyl benzidine for horseradish peroxidase neurohistochemistry: a non-carcinogenic blue reaction-product with superior sensitivity for visualizing neural afferents and efferents. *J. Histochem. Cytochem.,* 26: 106–117.

Molenaar, I. and Kuypers, H.G.J.M. (1978) Cells of origin of propiospinal fibers and of fibers ascending to supraspinal levels. An HRP study in cat and rhesus monkey. *Brain Res.,* 152: 429–450.

Nieuwenhuys, R., Geeraedts, L.M.G. and Veening, J.G. (1982) The medial forebrain bundle of the rat. I. General introduction. *J. Comp. Neurol.,* 206: 49–81.

Nilaver, G., Zimmerman, E.A., Wilkins, J., Michaels, J., Hoffman, D. and Silverman, A.J. (1980) Magnocellular hypothalamic projections to the lower brain stem and spinal cord of the rat. *Neuroendocrinology,* 30: 150–158.

Norgren, R. (1976) Taste pathways to hypothalamus and amygdala. *J. Comp. Neurol.,* 166: 17–33.

Nyberg Hansen, R. and Brodal, A. (1963) Sites of termination of corticospinal fibers in the cat. An experimental study with silver impregnation methods. *J. Comp. Neurol.,* 120: 369–391.

Nygren, L.-G. and Olson, L. (1977) A new major projection from locus coeruleus: the main source of noradrenergic nerve terminals in the ventral and dorsal columns of the spinal cord. *Brain Res.,* 132: 85–93.

Olszewski, J. and Baxter, D. (1954) *Cytoarchitecture of the Human Brain Stem.* Karger, Basel.

Oswaldo-Cruz, E. and Kidd, C. (1964) Functional properties of neurons in the lateral cervical nucleus of the cat. *J. Neurol.,* 27: 1–14.

Price, D.D. and Dubner, R. (1977) Neurons that subserve the sensoridiscriminative aspects of pain. *Pain,* 3: 307–338.

Ralston, H.J., III. and Ralston, D.D. (1979) The distribution of dorsal root axons in laminae I, II and III of the Macaque spinal cord: a quantitative electron microscope study. *J. Comp. Neurol.,* 184: 643–684.

Rexed, B.A. (1954) A cytoarchitectonic atlas of the spinal cord in the cat. *J. Comp. Neurol.,* 100: 297–380.

Rustioni, A., Kuypers, H.G.J.M. and Holstege, G. (1971) Propiospinal projections from the ventral and lateral funiculi to the motoneurons of the lumbosacral cord of the cat. *Brain Res.,* 35: 255–275.

Sakuma, Y. and Pfaff, D.W. (1979a) Facilitation of female reproductive behavior from mesencephalic central gray in the rat. *Am. J. Physiol. (Regulatory and Integrative Comp. Physiol. 6),* 237: R278–R284.

Sakuma, Y. and Pfaff, D.W. (1979b) Mesencephalic mechanisms for integration of female reproductive behavior in the rat. *Am. J. Physiol. (Regulatory and Integrative Comp. Physiol. 6),* 237: R285–R290.

Sandkühler, J. and Gebhart, G.F. (1984) Relative contribution of the nucleus raphe magnus and adjacent medullary reticular formation to the inhibition by stimulation in the periaqueductal gray of a spinal nociceptive reflex in the pentobarbital-anesthetized rat. *Brain Res.,* 305: 77–87.

Saper, C.B. and Loewy, A.D. (1980) Efferent connections of the parabrachial nucleus in the rat. *Brain Res.,* 197: 291–317.

Saper, C.B., Swanson, L.W. and Cowan, W.M. (1978) The efferent connections of the anterior hypothalamic area of the rat, cat and monkey. *J. Comp. Neurol.,* 182: 575–600.

Saper, C.B., Swanson, L.W. and Cowan, W.M. (1979) An autoradiographic study of the efferent connections of the lateral hypothalamic area in the rat. *J. Comp. Neurol.,* 183: 689–706.

Sato, M., Mizuno, N. and Konishi, A. (1978) Localization of motoneurons innervating perineal muscles: an HRP study in cat. *Brain Res.,* 140: 149–154.

Sawchenko, P.E. and L.W. Swanson (1982) Immunohistochemical identification of neurons in the paraventricular nucleus of the hypothalamus that project to the medulla or to the spinal cord in the rat. *J. Comp. Neurol.,* 205: 260–272.

Sessle, B.J., Hu, J.W., Dubner, R. and Lucier, G.E. (1981) Functional properties of neurons in cat trigeminal subnucleus caudalis (medullary dorsal horn). II. Modulation of responses of noxious and nonnoxious stimuli by periaqueductal gray, nucleus raphe magnus, cerebral cortex, and afferent influences, and effect of naloxone. *J. Neurophysiol.,* 45: 193–207.

Steedman, W.M., Molony, V. and Iggo, A. (1985) Nociceptive neurons in the superficial dorsal horn of cat lumbar spinal cord and their primary afferent inputs. *Exp. Brain Res.,* 58: 171–182.

Sterling, P. and Kuypers, H.G.J.M. (1968) Anatomical organization of the brachial spinal cord of the cat. III. The propiospinal connections. *Brain Res.*, 7: 419–443.

Sugiura, Y., Lee, C.L. and Perl, E.R. (1986) Central projections of identified, unmyelinated (C) fibers innervating mammalian skin. *Science*, 234: 358–361.

Swanson, L.W. (1977) Immunohistochemical evidence for a neurophysin-containing autonomic pathway arising in the paraventricular nucleus of the hypothalamus. *Brain Res.*, 128: 346–353.

Swanson, L.W., Kucharczyk, J. and Mogenson, J. (1978) Autoradiographic evidence for pathways from the medial preoptic area to the midbrain involved in drinking response to Angiotensine II. *J. Comp. Neurol.*, 178: 645–660.

Taber, E. (1961) The cytoarchitecture of the brain stem of the cat. I. Brain stem nuclei of the cat. *J. Comp. Neurol.*, 116: 27–69.

Taber, E., Brodal, A. and Walberg, F. (1960) The raphe nuclei of the brain stem in the cat. I. Normal topography and cytoarchitecture and general discussion. *J. Comp. Neurol.*, 114: 161–187.

Tan, J. and Holstege, G. (1986) Anatomical evidence that the pontine lateral tegmental field projects to lamina I of the caudal spinal trigeminal nucleus and spinal cord and to the Edinger-Westphal nucleus in the cat. *Neurosci. Lett.*, 64: 317–322.

Tashiro, N., Tanaka, T., Fukumoto, T., Hirata, K. and Nakao, H. (1985) Emotional behavior and arrhythmias induced in cats by hypothalamic stimulation. *Life Sci.*, 36: 1087–1094.

Toyoshima, K., Kawana, E. and Sakai, H. (1980) On the neuronal origin of the afferents to the ciliary ganglion in cat. *Brain Res.*, 185: 67–76.

Van der Kooy, D., Koda, L.Y., McGinty, J.F., Gerfen, C.R. and Bloom, F.E. (1984) The organization of projections from the cortex, amygdala, and hypothalamus to the nucleus of the solitary tract in rat. *J. Comp. Neurol.*, 224: 1–24.

Wang, S.C. and Ranson, S.W. (1939) Autonomic responses to electrical stimulation of the lower brain stem. *J. Comp. Neurol.*, 71: 437–455.

Watkins, L.R., Griffin, G., Leichnetz, G.R. and Mayer, D.J. (1981) Identification and somatotopic organization of nuclei projecting via the dorsolateral funiculus in rats: a retrograde tracing study using HRP slow-release gels. *Brain Res.*, 223: 237–255.

Westlund, K.N. and Coulter, J.D. (1980) Descending projections of the locus coeruleus and subcoeruleus/medial parabrachial nuclei in monkey: axonal transport studies and dopamine-β-hydroxylase immunocytochemistry. *Brain Res. Rev.*, 2: 235–264.

Westman, J. (1968) The lateral cervical nucleus in the cat. I. A Golgi study. *Brain Res.*, 10: 352–368.

White, R.S. and Neuman, R.S. (1980) Facilitation of spinal motoneurone excitability by 5-hydroxytryptamine and noradrenaline. *Brain Res.*, 188: 119–127.

Wiklund, L., Léger, L. and Persson, M. (1981) Monoamine cell distribution in the cat brain stem. A fluorescence histochemical study with quantification of indolaminergic and locus coeruleus cell groups. *J. Comp. Neurol.*, 203: 613–647.

Willett, C.J., Gwyn, D.G., Rutherford, J.G. and Leslie, R.A. (1986) Cortical projections to the nucleus of the tractus solitarius: an HRP study in the cat. *Brain Res. Bull.*, 16: 497–505.

Willis, W.D. (1982) Control of nociceptive transmission in the spinal cord. In *Progress of Sensory Physiology, Vol. 3*, Berlin, Springer Verlag.

Willis, W.D., Trevino, D.L., Coulter, J.D. and Maunz, R.A. (1974) Responses of primate spinothalamic tract neurons to natural stimuli of hindlimb. *J. Neurophysiol.*, 37: 358–372.

Willis, W.D., Haber, L.H. and Martin, R.F. (1977) Inhibition of spinothalamic tract cells and interneurons by brain stem stimulation in the monkey. *J. Neurophysiol.*, 40: 968–981.

Woolf, C.J. and Fitzgerald, M. (1983) The properties of neurones recorded in the superficial dorsal horn of the rat spinal cord. *J. Comp. Neurol.*, 221: 313–328.

Woolsey, C.N. (1958) Organization of somatic sensory and motor areas of cerebral cortex. In H.F. Harlow and C.N. Woolsey (Eds.), *Biological and Biochemical Basis of Behaviour.* University of Wisconsin Press, Madison, pp. 63–81.

Yezierski, R.P., Gerhart, K.D., Schrock, B.J. and Willis, W.D. (1983) A further examination of effects of cortical stimulation on primate spinothalamic tract cells. *J. Neurophysiol.*, 49: 424–441.

Zamir, N. and Maixner, W. (1986) The relationship between cardiovascular and pain regulatory systems. *Ann. NY Acad. Sci.*, 467: 371–384.

H.L. Fields and J.-M. Besson (Eds.)
Progress in Brain Research, Vol. 77
© 1988 Elsevier Science Publishers B.V. (Biomedical Division)

CHAPTER 4

Peptidergic neurons in the nucleus raphe magnus and the nucleus gigantocellularis: their distributions, interrelationships, and projections to the spinal cord

Robert M. Bowker, Louise C. Abbott and Roger P. Dilts

Department of Veterinary and Comparative Anatomy, Pharmacology, and Physiology, Washington State University, Pullman, WA 99164-6520, USA

Introduction

Our understanding of the anatomy of the neural circuitry underlying the brain stem's control of dorsal horn activity during the presentation of noxious stimuli is incomplete, at least in comparison to the wealth of physiological and pharmacological data on this subject accumulated during the last 10 – 15 years. However, several aspects of the anatomy of raphe-spinal and reticulospinal systems elicit general agreement: (1) both the midline nuclei and the ventrolateral reticular formation of the medulla are important for the descending modulation of noxious inputs to the spinal cord, (2) the main route of this descending inhibition to the spinal cord from these rostral medullary areas is via the dorsolateral funiculus, and (3) perhaps no one single putative neurotransmitter is totally responsible for the descending inhibition to the dorsal horn. Despite agreement on the general outlines of this descending system, several important anatomical questions remain unanswered at this time: (1) which putative neurotransmitters are located in these rostral medullary cell groups, and are thereby potentially involved in these descending control mechanisms? (2) which neurotransmitters localized in these and adjacent nuclei have descending projections to the spinal cord via the dorsolateral funiculus? (3) what

are the chemically defined inputs that may potentially influence, either directly or indirectly, the neurons in the rostral medulla involved in this descending control of sensory transmission? (4) finally, which receptors are present that may potentially mediate the pharmacological actions of these putative neurotransmitters in these nuclei? These questions form the basis of the present report; the answers to them will, hopefully, provide data on the organizational complexity of these nuclei, indicating how they may potentially be involved in descending inhibitory control of nervous activity in the dorsal horn.

To answer these questions several different methodological approaches are employed since each method provides answers to only a small piece of the puzzle. The main technique for identifying the various putative neurotransmitters in the rostral medulla is immunocytochemistry; it provides a very sensitive method for studying the chemical make-up of a nuclear region (Sternberger, 1979). Various antisera, each raised to a different putative neurotransmitter, can localize the chemically identified cell bodies as well as their fibers and terminals within a specific neuropil. Furthermore, when these various antisera are combined with a retrograde cell marker, such as the enzyme horseradish peroxidase (HRP) or a fluorescent dye, the transmitter-defined cell populations

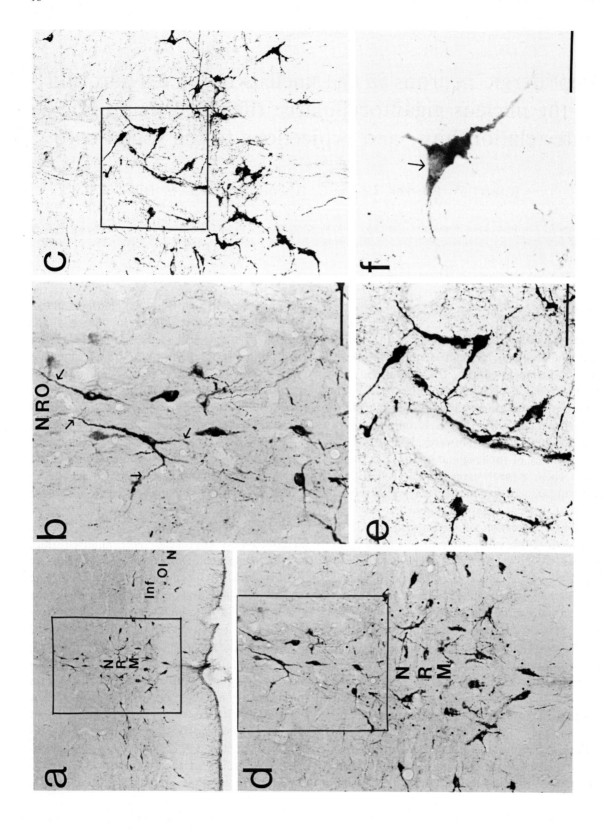

can be defined in terms of their specific origins and locations, their morphological characteristics, and the proportion of each type of chemically defined projection cell in the total efferent projections from that cell group and in the total transmitter-defined population. In addition one can combine two or more immunocytochemical steps on the same tissue section to determine the relationship of two or more chemically defined cell groups, and to chemically identify afferents that influence a particular efferent cell group. This variation of the immunocytochemical method provides an important advantage to understanding the organization of the rostral medulla since the precise cytoarchitectural borders of the various reticular nuclei are difficult to define. The third technique employed in the present studies is quantitative receptor autoradiography (Young and Kuhar, 1979). By this means, the receptors can be visualized and quantitated in specific cell groups and then correlated with different putative neurotransmitters.

Distribution of peptides in the NRM and the NGC

In this presentation several species of peptidergic neurons and their distributions within the nucleus raphe magnus (NRM) and nucleus gigantocellularis (NGC) will be discussed in detail as well as their relationship to the 5HT neurons long known to be present in these same two cell groups. The data on cell bodies represent studies in colchicine pretreated animals. In addition, other peptides and amino acids will be shown to be localized within these nuclei.

Substance P

At the anterior level of the inferior olivary complex, numerous cell bodies having substance P (SP)-like immunoreactivity are located in the nucleus raphe pallidus (NRP) and the more dorsally located NRM, which appears to represent the very caudal part of this nucleus or perhaps a transitional zone between the caudal raphe nuclei and the NRM (Fig. 1, a). These immunoreactive neurons are mainly spindle- or multipolar-shaped with one to several dendritic processes appearing to extend from the cell body whose size ranges from small to medium (10 – 18 μm length + width/2). Extending further dorsally in the most anterior levels of the nucleus raphe obscurus (NRO), several spindle-shaped cells can usually be seen distributed along the midline (arrows in Fig. 1, b). The SP neurons are clustered at the dorsal margins of the inferior olivary lobes and are oriented mainly in a dorsoventral direction with their processes extending dorsally along the raphe and laterally into the NGC (Fig. 1, d). Laterally, in the ventral portions of the NGC (termed the NGC pars alpha by Meessen and Olszewski, 1949), which extend away from the midline immediately dorsal to the inferior olivary complex, few SP-immunoreactive neurons are evident at this caudal level. Only at the lateral extremes of the inferior olive in this reticular nuclear zone are SP cells present. Laterally, SP neurons are restricted to two fairly distinct longitudinal columns along most of the ventral portion of reticular formation: one column is situated in the para-olivary region along the

---

Fig. 1. Photomicrographs showing SP neurons in the rostral medulla from caudal (a) and intermediate (d) levels to more rostral levels (c). (a) Low power view of caudal nucleus raphe magnus (NRM) at the level of the inferior olive nucleus (Inf Ol N). Observe numerous cells in midline with few located laterally dorsal to Inf Ol N. (d) Higher magnifications of the enclosed area in (a) illustrating the morphology of SP cells with oval-shaped cells located mainly ventrally and the spindle-shaped neurons located more dorsally (dotted lines indicate outline of NRM). (b) High power view spindle-shaped cells in nucleus raphe obscurus (NRO) and the processes (arrows) from the enclosed area of (d). (c) Low power view of the NRM at the level of the facial nucleus showing the distribution of SP cells with presence of fewer immunoreactive cells in midline. (e) High magnification of SP cells in (c) at level of the NRM. (f) High magnification of a stained neuron in the NRM having both SP staining in the cytoplasm and 5HT in the nucleus (arrow). Calibration bar, 40 μm.

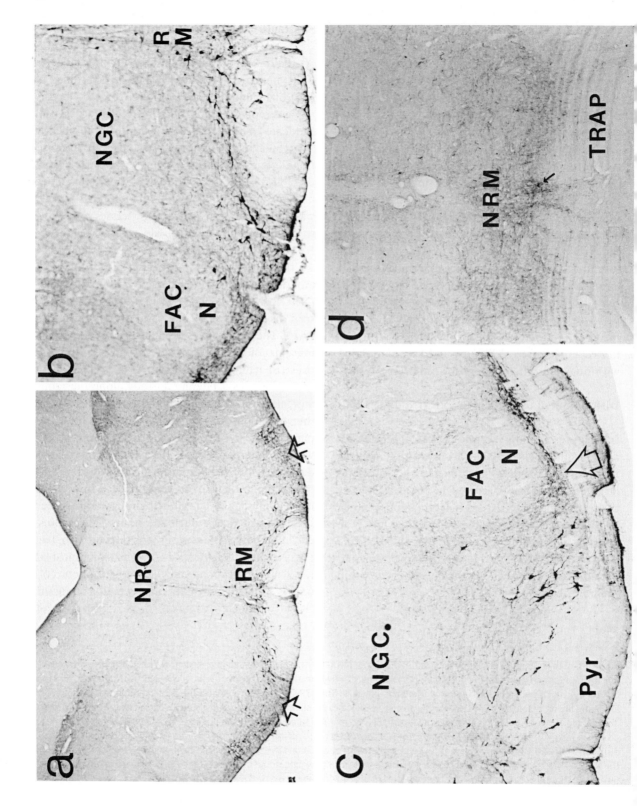

ventral brainstem surface (Fig. 2), while the second population of SP neurons is located further laterally in the lateral reticular nucleus (NRL) and ventral to it (Fig. 2). These more laterally placed SP cells will not be dealt with in great detail in this report. The reader is referred to other studies which analyze in greater detail the functions of these laterally placed SP neurons (Coote and MacLeod, 1974; Henry and Calarescu, 1974; Helke et al., 1982; Pilowsky et al., 1986; Takano et al., 1984).

At a level rostral to the inferior olive, SP-immunoreactive neurons extend from the midline to this lateral para-olivary column of stained neurons along the medullary surface (Fig. 2, a). At this anterior level they appear to form a relatively dense, horizontally oriented sheet of SP-immunoreactive neurons, extending between the NRM and the ventral medullary surface, as well as a dense rostrocaudal plane of SP cells in the ventral NGC between the rostral tip of the inferior olive to the mid-level of the facial nucleus, where the facial motor nerve can be seen to exit from the dorsal aspect of the nucleus. Only a few widely distributed SP neurons can be seen dorsal to this horizontally directed sheet of SP neurons. These SP cells have more multipolar shapes ($18-24\ \mu$m), while the neurons in the ventral NGC have, for the most part, a spindle shape or a tripolar shape with a horizontal orientation (Fig. 2, b). Beginning at the mid-level of the facial nucleus, the relative proportion of SP cells in the NRM decreases in numbers per section. The immunoreactive cells appear to begin to avoid the midline in preference for the laterally placed reticular nuclei, resulting in a fairly substantial collection of SP neurons located laterally in the NGC and immediately ventrally to the facial nucleus and more rostral superior olivary

nucleus (Fig. 2, c). Figs. 2, a, c and d, show the decrease in the relative numbers of SP neurons in the NRM and the NGC at progressively more rostral levels, as well as the gradual apparent displacement of immunoreactive cells to the NGC from the NRM. Thus, between the inferior olivary nucleus and the mid-portion of the facial nucleus lie most of the SP-immunoreactive neurons in the NRM and the ventral parts of the NGC. Rostrally, at the level of the trapezoid body only a few SP cells can be found in the NRM and the ventral parts of the caudal pontine reticular formation – the nucleus pontis caudalis (PoC). While the rostral NRM contains relatively few SP neurons, the NRM at this anterior level does receive a relatively dense innervation of SP-like terminals, some of which make apparent contacts with the cell body profiles of the NRM.

A summary Figure of the localizations of the SP neurons in the NRM and the adjacent NGC is shown in the plotting (Fig. 3, B). On these four coronal sections at representative levels between the rostral level of the inferior olive nucleus and the trapezoid body in the caudal pons, each dot represents a single SP-like neuron seen on the tissue section. SP neurons are usually present, in the normal animal, at these levels; they comprise roughly half of the number of 5HT cells seen in adjacent sections at these same rostrocaudal levels. Beginning at the caudalmost level, SP cells are present within the zone of transition between the NRP and the more rostral NRM, with a few widely distributed cells located more dorsally in the NRO. Another cluster of SP-stained cells is located laterally in the reticular formation near the ventral border of the brain stem. This lateral concentration of SP neurons appears to represent two

Fig. 2. Low power photomicrographs illustrating distribution of the SP cells in the nucleus raphe magnus (NRM) and the nucleus gigantocellularis (NGC) pars alpha. (a) Two clusters of SP neurons can be seen: (1) one group located dorsally to the pyramidal tract which is co-localized with 5HT (Fig. 1, f) and (2) another SP non-5HT cell group located laterally in the medulla ventral to the facial nucleus (lateral to the open arrows). (b) Higher view of SP neurons showing a few SP cells in the nucleus raphe magnus (RM) with more cells in NGC (Fac N, facial nucleus). (c) Rostrally at the mid-facial level photomicrograph showing fewer SP cells medially in raphe magnus and the lateral displacement of the SP cells that do not co-localize with 5HT (lateral to the arrow). (d) Few SP neurons are present at the level of the trapezoid body. The arrow marks the location of the only SP cell on this section.

100

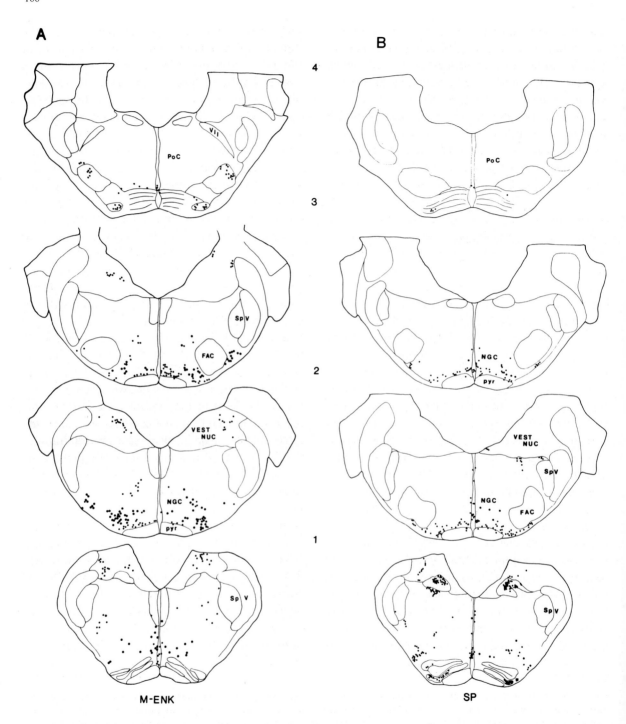

Fig. 3. Plottings showing the distributions of the M-ENK (A) and the SP (B) immunoreactive cells from caudal (1) to more rostral levels (4) of the rostral medulla. Observe that M-ENK cells are concentrated laterally, while SP cells are concentrated ventrally and medially. Sp V, spinal tract of trigeminal nerve; VEST NUC, vestibular nuclei; FAC, facial nucleus; PoC, nucleus reticularis pontis caudalis; VII, 7th nerve; NGC, nucleus gigantocellularis.

populations of neurons which may mediate different functions: those SP cells associated with 5HT neurons are concentrated near the para-olivary area, while the second population of SP cells found along the ventral brain stem appears to be more closely related to other neurotransmitters or neuromodulators other than 5HT. Other locations of SP neurons seen on these same tissue sections include the inferior vestibular nuclei (VEST NUC) and the nucleus of the solitary tract. Most of the SP neurons within the rostral medullary tegmentum appear to be concentrated between the

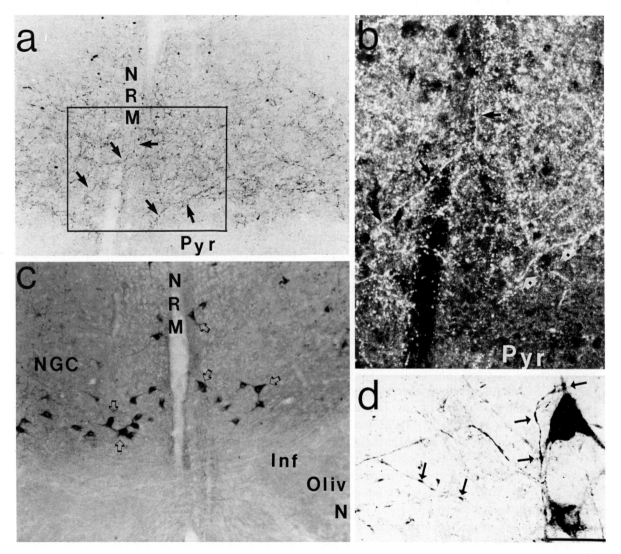

Fig. 4. Photomicrographs illustrating the distribution of SP terminals in the nucleus raphe magnus (NRM) and the ventral nucleus gigantocellularis (NGC) (a and b) and the SOMA cells in these same nuclei of the medulla (c and d). (a) Low power, bright-field view of dense SP-immunoreactive terminals in the NRM and NGC. (b) The approximate enclosed area in (a) is shown under dark-field illumination to illustrate the dense terminal fields in these regions. The arrows mark the same immunoreactive fibers in both photomicrographs. (c) Low power view of SOMA-immunoreactive neurons in the NRM with arrows marking examples of large-size SOMA cells. (d) High power view of SOMA cells and their processes (arrows) in the NRM and the (NGC). Inf Oliv N, inferior olive nucleus; Pyr, pyramidal tract. Calibration bar, 40 μm.

inferior olive and the facial nucleus with few SP cells between the facial nucleus and the more rostral trapezoid body. This skewing of the distributions of the SP neurons in the caudal NRM and adjacent NGC appears to be a common feature of many of the peptidergic neurons to be discussed in this report, in contrast to the more rostral extension of the 5HT population in the NRM which extends to the rostral limits of the trapezoid body.

Immunocytochemistry of brain stem tissue sections for SP terminals can easily be accomplished without the aid of the axonal transport inhibitor colchicine. In this manner, the distributions of the SP terminals can be dissociated from that of the cell bodies. After such a staining procedure in normal animals, the NRM and adjacent NGC have substantial numbers of the SP-like fibers and their terminals (Fig. 4, a and b). Caudally in the NRM, beaded SP fibers can be seen throughout the nucleus as well as projecting laterally into the ventral parts of the NGC as a horizontal band extending from the midline towards the ventrolateral surface of the brain stem. The SP-like immunoreactivity represents a very dense network of stained fibers within the NGC and appears to be much denser than that seen in the midline nucleus. Dorsally in the medullary tegmentum, little SP-like immunoreactivity in fibers was evident. The scant pattern of SP immunoreactivity observed dorsally, as well as ventrally within the pyramidal tract fibers traversing longitudinally through the brain stem, accentuated the SP staining in the ventral NGC and NRM. Such a pattern resulted in the appearance of a horizontal band of SP-like fibers and terminal staining (500 – 800 μm wide) that extended through the ventral NGC and NRM from the lateral-most parts of the reticular nuclei. Further rostrally, this same banding was prominent in the midline and the ventral parts of the nucleus pontis caudalis, but the NRM appeared to have a slightly greater density of terminal fibers in comparison to the more lateral areas. The beaded varicosities of SP-like immunoreactivity appeared to make contacts with cell bodies in the NRM. This observation will, hopefully, become more important to the reader since many of these cell bodies seen in the NRM at this level of the medulla contain 5HT.

Somatostatin

Somatostatin (SOMA) is a 24-amino acid peptide recently discovered in neurons in the medullary tegmentum (Taber-Pierce et al., 1985). These SOMA-like neurons are, for the most part, very striking as they represent many of the largest neurons in the raphe and medullary reticular formation; they are concentrated in two major areas of the medulla. Basically, the SOMA-like cells are present in the anterior half of the medulla beginning in the zone of transition between the rostral parts of the NRP and the NRO and extending through the NRM to the facial nucleus. However, the majority of the neurons stained for SOMA immunoreactivity is concentrated laterally in the NGC and, for the most part, appears to lie dorsal to the areas where the 5HT and SP neurons can be found.

In the midline nuclei at the rostral level of the inferior olivary complex, most of the SOMA-like neurons are located in the ventral parts of the NRO with only an occasional cell present in the NRP. They were usually multipolar, ranging in size from 25 μm to 40 μm with medium- and large-sized neurons predominating (Fig. 4, c and d). Anterior to the inferior olivary complex, progressively fewer SOMA-like cells were seen in the NRM with practically no immunoreactivity present from the mid-facial nucleus to the rostral limits of NRM at the anterior parts of the trapezoid body. In contrast, laterally in the NGC, many SOMA immunoreactive cells can be seen on each section, especially anterior to the inferior olive. Only a few neurons are seen caudally in the ventral reticular formation, the anterior parts of the nucleus reticularis centralis ventralis (NRCV) and the NGC. These few cells appear to form the beginnings of an arch extending from the midline toward the nucleus ambiguus, rather than toward the ventral brain stem surface as do the SP and the 5HT neurons and are located 400 – 800 μm dorsally to the inferior olive (Fig. 5, c). This laterally extending arm of SOMA-like neurons becomes a more discrete entity at the level of the facial nucleus where a band of SOMA-like neurons extends from the midline to a point along the ventral border of the facial nucleus. In addition to this ventral cluster of large-sized SOMA-like neurons, a dorsally located group of SOMA-like neurons was also evident extending from this ventrally situated cluster towards the floor of the IVth ventricle in the nucleus paragigantocellularis dorsalis (NPGD) (Fig. 5, b). These neurons are smaller and spindle shaped in comparison to those SOMA-like neurons clustered

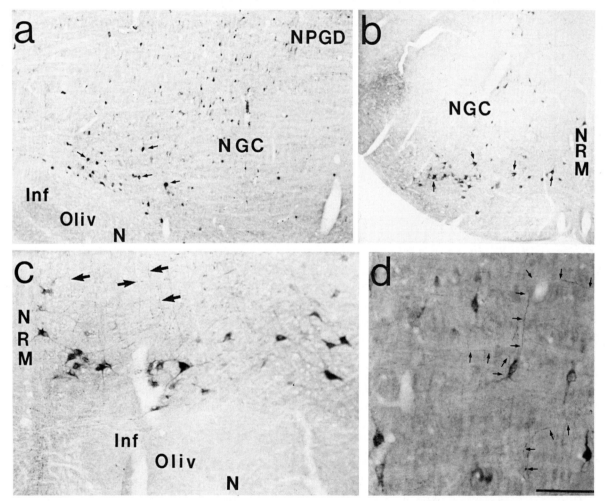

Fig. 5. Photomicrographs of SOMA-immunoreactive neurons illustrating locations and orientations as well as their processes. (a) A parasagittal cut through the rostral medulla showing the inferior olive nucleus (Inf Oliv N) caudally and more rostral the nucleus gigantocellularis (NGC). Arrows mark examples of large-sized SOMA cells. Observe dense concentrations of SOMA cells in the rostral medulla. (b) Coronal section at level anterior to the inferior olive indicating the lateral concentration of SOMA cells in the NGC. Arrows indicate examples of larger sized cells. (c) High power view of SOMA cells showing their processes coursing towards the IVth ventricle (arrows). (d) High magnification of processes from the SOMA cells illustrating their branching and coursing towards the spinal cord and/or the rostral brain stem. Arrows indicate branching of the processes as well as SOMA processes coursing to the spinal cord. NPGD, nucleus paragigantocellularis dorsalis; NRM, nucleus raphe magnus. Calibration bar, 50 μm.

104

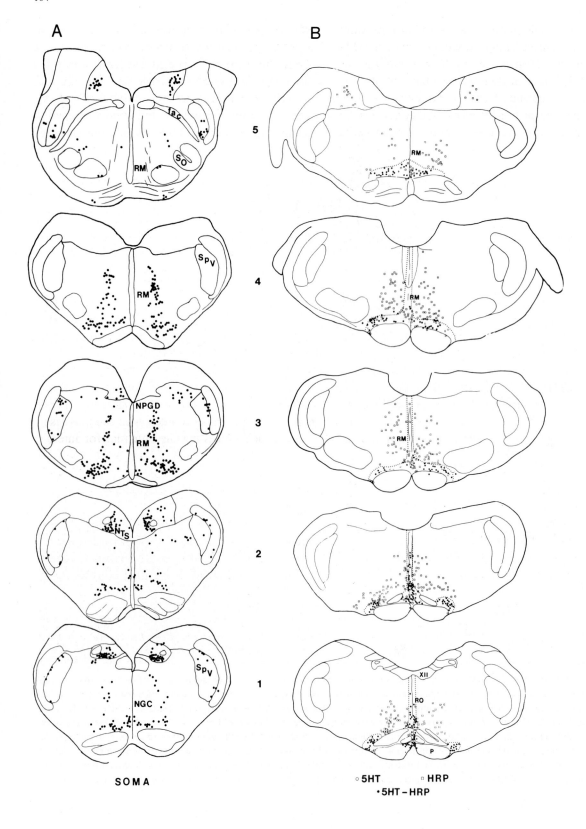

A

B

5

4

3

2

1

SOMA

○ 5HT   □ HRP
• 5HT – HRP

ventrally in the NGC. At the level of the trapezoid body few SOMA-immunoreactive neurons are present.

An interesting aspect of the anatomy of the SOMA-like neurons present in the NGC is that they may be one of the potential candidates for the neurotransmitter(s) or neuromodulator(s) of the classic giant cells, described by the Scheibels nearly three decades ago (Scheibel and Scheibel, 1958). These giant cells located in the rostral medulla and the caudal pons, as seen in thick sections (200 – 1000 μm) stained for Golgi preparations, have dorsal processes from the cell body which extend towards the floor of the IVth ventricle at which point they branch and send processes both towards the spinal cord and the diencephalon. As a result of the widespread anatomical arborization of the same neuron, these cells are believed to integrate the activities of the sensory, motor, and/or autonomic systems of the brain stem with those situated more rostrally in the forebrain as well as those located in the spinal cord. The putative neurotransmitter(s) of these neurons are not known. When the brain stem is cut parasaggitally, one gains a different perspective of a population of these SOMA-identified cells as opposed to the usual coronal section of the brain stem. Due to the technical limitations of immunocytochemistry, however, i.e. short distance of the antiserum penetration, the tissue sections must be cut much thinner than those prepared for Golgi staining. In any event, a parasaggital cut reveals a similar pattern and orientation of the SOMA-like neurons as

that seen in the Golgi stain (Fig. 5, a). These neurons range in size from 27 – 39 μm (length + width/2) and have a dorsal process which appears to course towards the IVth ventricle (Fig. 5, c and d). In addition, they can occasionally be seen to branch (Fig. 5, d) and send a process towards the spinal cord (Fig. 5, d).

The plotting of the SOMA-like neurons present in the NRM and the reticular nuclei of the NGC, NPGD, and the NRCV is shown in Fig. 6, A. Caudally at the transition zone between the NRP and/or the NRO and the NRM, SOMA cells are present mainly in the midline nuclei and the adjacent NGC dorsal to the inferior olive (1). At more anterior levels they can be seen to form a lateral extension into the NGC wherein the SOMA neurons become clustered laterally in the ventral parts of this reticular nucleus (2 – 4). At the rostral-most levels of the NRM and the nucleus pontis caudalis, no SOMA-like cells are present (5).

SOMA terminals are present throughout much of the rostral region of the medullary raphe and adjacent reticular nuclei. The immunoreactive beads appear to make contacts with cell profiles in these nuclei, suggesting the potential for interaction.

Methionine- and leucine-enkephalin

The enkephalins, as represented by the terminal amino acids methionine (M-ENK) and leucine (L-ENK), are also present in these same nuclear regions of the rostral medulla, further com-

---

←

Fig. 6. Plottings showing the distributions of the SOMA neurons (A) and the relationships of the 5HT and descending cells within the rostral medulla (B). (A) The distribution of the SOMA-like neurons are shown on several sections and are located in the midline nuclei with the major component of the staining located in the nucleus gigantocellularis (NGC) of the lateral medulla. (B) The three cell populations of 5HT, spinally projecting 5HT cells (5HT-HRP) and the non-5HT spinally projecting neurons are plotted from the same tissue section and are examples of the distributions used for the quantitative analyses. The open circles show the few 5HT cells that did not appear to contain any retrogradely transported HRP enzyme, while the filled circles show the descending 5HT cells. The open squares indicate the locations of the spinally projecting neurons that did not have any 5HT staining. The dotted lines serve to define the margins from which the quantitative data were obtained and included the raphe nuclei (RP, RO, and the RM) and the pararaphe areas or those areas where 5HT cells are located lateral to the midline. See Table I for the quantitative results. Sp V, spinal tract of trigeminal nerve; RM, nucleus raphe magnus; NPGD, nucleus paragigantocellularis; SO, superior olive nucleus; fac, facial nerve; XII, hypoglossal nucleus; RO, nucleus raphe obscurus.

plicating our understanding of this region and its role in the modulation of somatosensory sensations. However, as will be seen, the enkephalins have several features in their cell body distribution and morphology which distinguish them in their organization from the other peptidergic and aminergic neurons in the rostral medulla, as well as several characteristics that are common to these two classes of chemically identified cells. These differences in the localizations and/or morphologies of M-ENK and L-ENK neurons are useful for subdividing the various neurotransmitter-containing cells into anatomical subsets within the brain stem reticular formation.

Within the transition zone between the NRP, NRO, and the more rostral NRM, M-ENK neurons are present and extend into the adjacent NGC with an average of 15 – 25 neurons per section. Within the NRP, primarily small bipolar cells, 12 – 20 μm (length + width/2), can be seen in a dorsoventral orientation with a few slightly larger globular neurons (18 – 27 μm) being distri-

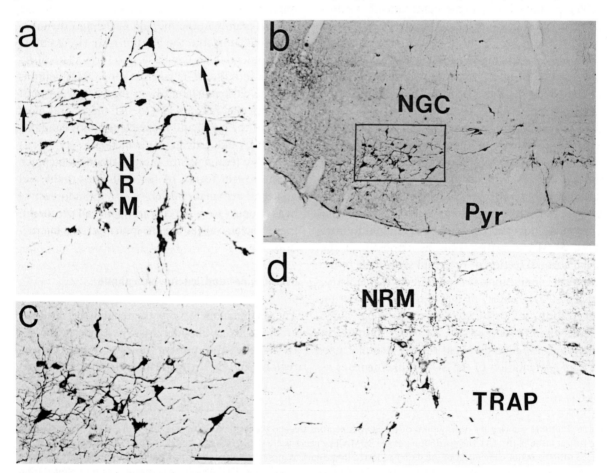

Fig. 7. Photomicrographs show the locations of the neurons having M-ENK immunoreactivity. (a) Low power view of M-ENK cells at the transition zone between the three raphe nuclei at inferior olive level showing the lateral extensions of the M-ENK processes into the adjacent nucleus gigantocellularis (NGC) (arrows). (b) Low power view of the M-ENK in the NGC with lateral and dorsal clustering of these cells. (c) Higher magnification of the M-ENK cells located in the lateral parts of the NGC in (b). Calibration bar, 55 μm. (d) Low power view of M-ENK cell in nucleus raphe magnus (NRM) at the rostral level near trapezoid body illustrating 4 – 10 immunoreactive cells per section. Please compare the greater number of M-ENK cells at this rostral level with the relative lack of immunoreactive cells stained for SP and SOMA.

buted in the dorsal parts of the NRP. At progressively more rostral levels within this transition zone, greater numbers of cells are visible with many larger, horizontally oriented cells and processes extending laterally into the NGC (Fig. 7, a and b). Laterally in the NRL, M-ENK neurons begin to form a cluster with 3 – 6 neurons per section, seen initially at more caudal levels and expanding to a population of 15 – 25 neurons further rostrally. The larger sized neurons (17 – 34 μm) appear to predominate with the NRL cell cluster although medium-sized cells (14 – 24 μm) are evident (Fig. 7, c). Only a few M-ENK neurons can be seen to be distributed dorsally towards the floor of the IVth ventricle. This lack of a major M-ENK-immunoreactive cell population in the dorsal aspects of the NGC and the nucleus paragigantocellularis dorsalis (NPGD) appears to differ from that seen following section staining with the SOMA-like antiserum, indicating a difference in their distribution patterns and in their potential function (see above for the descriptions of the SOMA-like distribution). Between the inferior olive and the facial nucleus in the NGC pars alpha along the dorsal margin of the pyramidal tracts, a few M-ENK neurons are widely distributed in a lateral arc towards the ventrolateral border of the medullary surface (Fig. 3, a). The size of these neurons is mainly small, ranging from 12 – 18 μm in diameter. Dorsal (200 – 300 μm) to this ventral group of M-ENK neurons, the major population of the larger sized (17 – 40 μm) neurons is present and appears to be located in the ventral parts of the NGC rather than in the pars alpha subdivision of the NGC (Fig. 7, c). The M-ENK population within the NGC appears to be concentrated in the caudal half of the rostral medulla between the inferior olivary nucleus and the mid-facial nucleus, rather than rostrally at the level of the trapezoid fibers and its nuclei. However, within the midline isolated M-ENK neurons are present usually as widely scattered entities within this cell group extending to the most anterior border of the NRM (Fig. 7, d).

Fig. 3, A, shows a plotting of the distribution of the M-ENK neurons in the rostral medulla of the rodent. Observe the similarities of the pattern of distribution in the ventral brain stem zones as that of the SOMA-like neurons, while in the dorsal areas few M-ENK appear to be present in contrast to that seen for SOMA-stained cells.

γ-Aminobutyric acid (GABA)

The inhibitory amino acid GABA can also be localized to the midline nuclei and the lateral parts of the brain stem. However, these immunoreactive neurons are not as extensive in their distributions as the above-mentioned peptides, but tend to be clustered into two main regions – the midline nuclei and the para-olivary region – with only an occasional immunoreactive cell being distributed between these two localizations. Few GABA cells are apparent caudally to the inferior olivary nuclei in these regions. In the transition zone of the NRP and the ventral NRO several cells (2 – 5 cells) are present on each section. These GABA neurons appear to be widely distributed in a rostrally extending column in the midline to the trapezoid level in the NRM where there appears to be a tendency to have several more per section than at the more caudal raphe levels (Fig. 8, a). Greater numbers of GABA-like neurons can be located laterally to the para-olivary area or the medial parts of the NRL (Fig. 8, b). These neurons are small to medium-sized, ranging in size from 14 μm to 22 μm and have multipolar shapes (globular and triangular) with several processes extending from the cell body (Fig. 8, b). These GABA-like neurons appear to be localized 400 – 500 μm from the lateral margin of the pyramidal tract, rather than being localized along its border as are the 5HT and a portion of the SP population. This lateral displacement of the GABA neurons is interesting in that some of the GABA-like immunoreactivity can also be co-localized to the 5HT neurons (Belin et al. 1983), suggesting that: (1) the 5HT neurons in this para-olivary group can form several subsets depending upon the species of neurotransmitters co-localized with the 5HT neurons, i.e. SP (and/or TRH) and

5HT and GABA; and (2) these subsets of co-localized transmitter-containing cells appear to be topographically distributed in slightly different regions of NRL and the para-olivary area. A plotting in Fig. 9 shows the relative locations of the GABA-like neurons. Observe that the majority of the cells appears to be situated laterally with fewer located in the midline.

Other peptides: vasoactive intestinal peptide (VIP) and cholecystokinin (CCK)

These two peptides can also be located in cells in these same raphe and reticular nuclei. However, in our experience they are present only as a small population of cells rather than the relatively large population of cells stained for 5HT, SP, M-ENK,

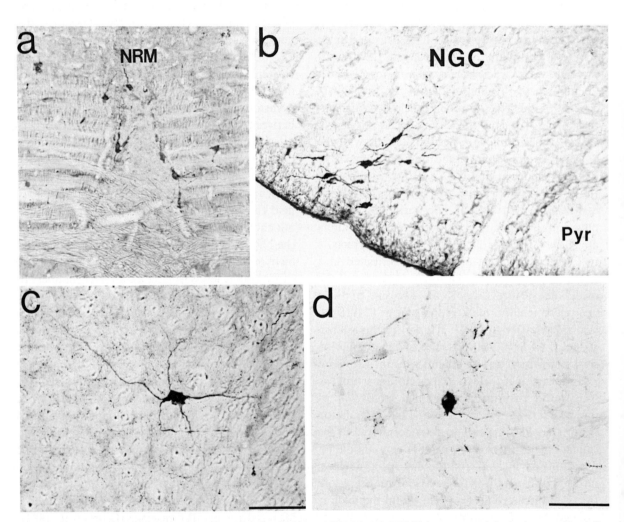

Fig. 8. Photomicrographs showing GABA-like staining (a and b) and VIP (c) and CCK (d) immunoreactivity in the rostral medulla of the nucleus raphe magnus (NRM) and the nucleus gigantocellularis (NGC). (a) GABA cells located in the rostral NRM at the level of the trapezoid body. (b) GABA-stained cells located in the lateral paraolivary area near the ventral brain stem surface. Please observe that the cells are located further laterally than the 5HT and the SP populations of cells. (c) An example of a cell stained for VIP immunoreactivity in the NGC. (d) An example of a CCK-stained cell in the raphe nuclei. Calibration bars, 55 μm.

L-ENK, and SOMA with the same immunocyto-chemical methods. Whether these small populations of VIP and CCK cells represent an underestimation of the total cell groups in these nuclei or the actual relative population, remains to be seen. An underestimation of the population of cells could be explained by the possible differences in the antibody titers and the affinities of the antisera towards the antigens in the tissues sections. In any event, both antigens appear to be located in neurons of these nuclei. Concerning the VIP-like immunoreactive staining, cells are located in the raphe nuclei and usually range from cells of medium size to large-diameter neurons (Fig. 8, c). A few isolated VIP neurons appear to be present in the NGC. The CCK-immunoreactive cells also appeared to be present in the NRM and the NGC, but only as isolated neurons (Fig. 8, d). Only on rare

occasion can one see more than several immunoreactive neurons on a tissue section.

Relation of peptide neurons to 5HT cells in NRM and NGC

As indicated in the introduction, determination of the cytoarchitectural borders of the many reticular nuclei in the medulla can be a very difficult task, especially when one is comparing the locations of the many different peptides in these cell groups. One means of circumventing this problem, while still being able to understand the interrelationships of the many different putative neurotransmitters within the rostral medulla, is to examine several of the transmitters on the same tissue sections by employing two or more different chromagens to identify the neurotransmitter antiseral markers. In

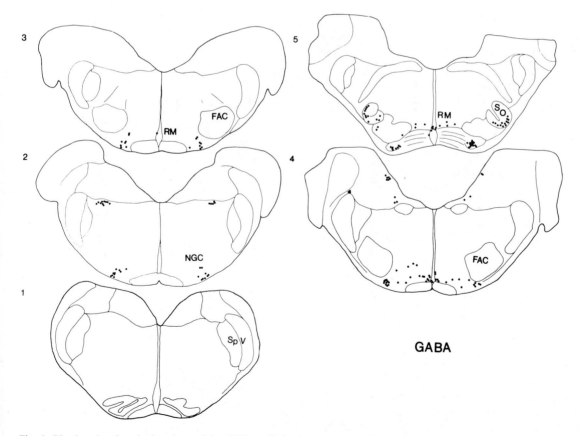

Fig. 9. Plotting showing the locations of the GABA cells in the rostral medulla.

110

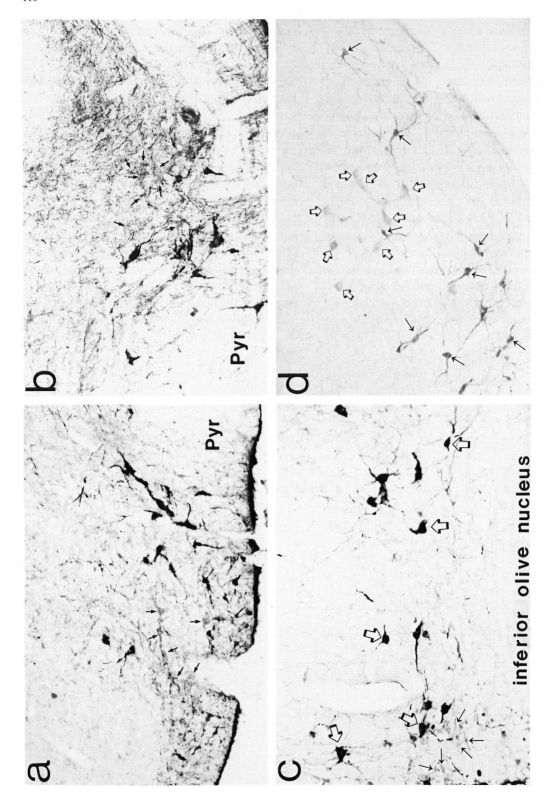

this manner, the relationship of the cell bodies of a specific peptide, such as SP, can be understood in relationship to another neurotransmitter, such as 5HT. In this portion of the presentation, rather than present in great detail the relationships of the various peptides to the 5HT population in different regions of the rostral medulla, we wish only to summarize the data by making several general statements about how these peptidergic and serotonergic neurons may be organized.

Our laboratory has begun to examine the relationships of SP, M-ENK, and SOMA to the locations of the 5HT neurons which are distributed in the same nuclear regions (the reader is referred to several representative works on the distribution and organization of the 5HT neurons in the brain stem: Steinbusch, 1981; Dahlström and Fuxe, 1964, 1965; and Crutcher and Humbertson, 1978). We have thus far determined the following:

(1) At progressively more rostral levels beginning from the anterior part of the inferior olive, the peptides are related in such a manner as to form subpopulations, with the species of neurotransmitter and co-localized neurotransmitter differing in various regions of the reticular nuclei.

(2) Depending upon the animal species, each of the three peptide transmitters (SP, ENK and SOMA), as well as thyrotropin-releasing hormone (TRH) and GABA, is co-localized with 5HT-immunoreactive neurons, but to a variable extent in different regions of these nuclei. SOMA and M-ENK can be shown to be co-localized, but as a subset of the total SOMA and M-ENK population (Bowker, 1987).

(3) In terms of total numbers of cells projecting to the spinal cord from the NRM and the NGC, the 5HT neurons form the major descending projections with the co-localized SP, TRH, and other peptides appearing to form subsets of the descending 5HT system. In the NRM, about one-third of the neurons projecting to the spinal cord do not contain 5HT-like immunoreactivity. Examples of these generalizations will be provided below.

(1) Evidence for neurotransmitter subpopulations

Following immunocytochemical staining for two neurotransmitter markers, two colors − black and brown − can be easily discerned on the same section under the microscope. In those neurons that contain two transmitters in the same neuron, usually both black and the brown colors can be seen, especially since the nucleus is stained brown for 5HT while the cytoplasm can be seen to have both black (peptide) and brown (5HT) colors. Regarding SP and 5HT in the NGC and the medial parts of the NRL, three subpopulations can be seen as a column to the level of the trapezoid body (Fig. 10, a, b, and Fig. 11). Medially, dorsal to the pyramidal tracts, many of the SP neurons appear to be co-localized with 5HT, while dorsolateral to this SP-5HT group lies a population of 5HT-non-SP cells (Fig. 10, a and b). Also, further laterally, ventral to the facial nucleus, one can see a cluster of SP-non-5HT neurons. A plotting in Fig. 11, b, shows the relative distributions of the SP and 5HT-non-SP cells. In a similar fashion SOMA and M-ENK appear to be differentially related to the 5HT neurons in the NRM and the NGC. Caudally the larger-sized SOMA neurons appear to dominate the smaller-sized 5HT cell in the zone of transition between the NRP/NRO and the NRM (Fig. 10, c). Rostrally though, the SOMA cells appear to be concentrated dorsally to the 5HT neurons, while a

---

Fig. 10. Photomicrographs showing the differences in the populations of neurotransmitter markers when viewed on the same tissue section. (a) and (b) Low power views of the para-olivary region showing the relationship of the SP cells (black) and the 5HT-non-SP cells (gray). The SP cells near the pyramidal tract (Pyr) were co-localized with 5HT, while the SP cells ventral to the facial nucleus did not have any 5HT immunoreactivity. The columnar distribution of the SP and the 5HT-non-SP cells persisted rostrally to the level of the trapezoid body in (b). The small arrows indicate the 5HT-non-SP cells. (c) shows the separation of the 5HT cells (gray colored, small arrows) and the laterally located SOMA-stained neurons (open arrows) at caudal levels of the nucleus raphe magnus. (d) Differences in the locations of the 5HT cells (small arrows) and the dorsally located SOMA cells (open arrows) in the nucleus gigantocellularis (NGC) at more rostral levels.

112

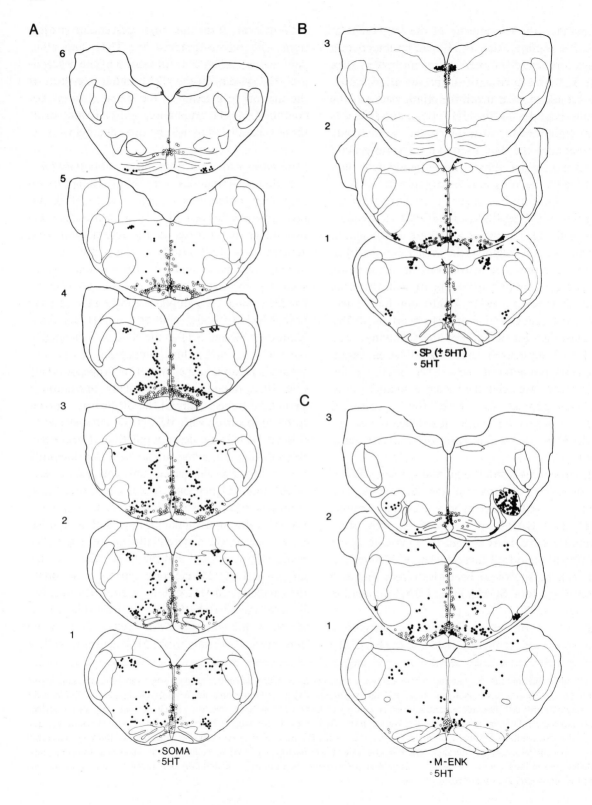

A

6

5

4

3

2

1

• SOMA
○ 5HT

B

3

2

1

• SP (± 5HT)
○ 5HT

C

3

2

1

• M-ENK
○ 5HT

few are intermingled with the 5HT cells (Fig. 10, d and Fig. 11). Several of the latter can be shown to co-exist with the 5HT neurons. A similar relation appears to exist with the M-ENK neurons. These subpopulations of neurotransmitters within these rostral medullary nuclei suggest that the reticular formation does, in fact, have a specific organization according to the species of neurotransmitter and what is or is not co-localized with them (Fig. 11).

(2) Co-localization of peptides with the 5HT neurons

Several groups of scientists have been at the forefront in discovering which putative neurotransmitters are co-localized. Most notably the laboratories of Hökfelt and colleagues (Hökfelt et al., 1978, 1980; Johansson et al., 1981; Hökfelt et al., 1986, and others; Chan-Palay, 1979; Lovick and Hunt, 1983) have shown that many of the SP neurons in the medulla are co-localized with 5HT and/or TRH, while several groups have provided evidence that L-ENK can be co-localized with 5HT neurons (Glazer et al., 1981; Léger et al., 1986). In addition, SOMA and 5HT (unpublished observations), and GABA and 5HT (Belin et al., 1983) can be co-localized, while SOMA and M-ENK have been found to be co-localized in a small population of the SOMA and M-ENK neurons within the rostral medulla (Bowker, 1987). These data provide evidence that the neurotransmitters are segregated into subpopulations depending upon their relationship to the 5HT population as each of these neurotransmitters has a different distribution.

(3) Quantitative reevaluation of descending 5HT projections

Previous work (Bowker et al., 1981b, 1982) had provided evidence in the rat that more than 80% of the neurons that descended to the spinal cord from the distribution of the 5HT neurons in the NRO, NRP, and the NRM, as well as the lateral extensions of the 5HT population, possessed 5HT-like immunoreactivity. The important inference was that the descending SP and TRH neurons from these same cell groups must form a subset of the descending 5HT population if these two peptides are to form a major and significant projection to the spinal cord, since only about 15% of the spinally projecting neurons from these nuclei appeared to be non-5HT containing. No information was provided as to the specific cell groups that contributed to the descending 5HT projections. This finding has been criticized as being an overestimation of the descending projections from the medulla (Johannessen et al., 1984; Skagerberg and Björklund, 1985). As a result of these two studies, we decided to reexamine this question of the descending projections from the 5HT cell group with a special emphasis on the relative contributions of each of the three nuclei. For this presentation only the data from the NRM and the adjacent ventral NGC will be discussed in detail. Two rats received a large injection of HRP enzyme into the lumbar spinal cord and were routinely processed for 5HT immunocytochemistry. Within the NRM from the anterior tip of the inferior olive to the anterior part of the trapezoid, 90% (2 981 5HT-HRP cells out of 3 282 total 5HT neurons) of the

←

Fig. 11. Plotting showing the relationships of the three populations of peptides to the 5HT cell group as seen on the same section. (A) SOMA cells (filled circles) are generally more laterally and dorsally placed than are the 5HT cells (open circles) in the nucleus gigantocellularis (NGC). (B) Plotting showing the SP cells (filled circles) and the 5HT cells (open circles) in the raphe and the NGC. Observe that the SP cells have a near-identical overlap with the 5HT cells ventrally in the medial part of the medulla while laterally a population of SP cells extends beyond the 5HT cell group indicating no co-localization of these two transmitters ventral to facial nucleus. (C) A similar plotting of the M-ENK (filled cells) and the 5HT cells (open circles), with the distribution of the M-ENK cells being mainly lateral and dorsal to the 5HT cell groups. Also observe that M-ENK population of cells distributed further rostrally than either SOMA and SP cell groups.

5HT neurons were seen to project to the lumbar spinal cord. In the ventral parts of the NGC on these same sections nearly 85% (7 014 5HT-HRP cells out of 8 330 total 5HT neurons) of the 5HT cells projected to the lumbar spinal cord. When one examines the 5HT-HRP cells in relationship to the total spinally projecting population within the NRM and the NGC, one obtains an interesting result. In the NRM, only 66% (2 981 5HT-HRP cells out of 4 514 total HRP-filled neurons) of the spinally projecting neurons appeared to contain 5HT immunoreactivity. On the other hand, in the NGC region more than 88% (7 014 5HT-HRP cells out of a total of 7 953 HRP-filled neurons) of the spinally projecting neurons were found to have 5HT staining in the cytoplasm. Overall in the three raphe nuclei, as well as in the NGC, nearly 85% (84.9% − 20 782 5HT-HRP cells out of 24 464 HRP-filled cells) of all the spinally projecting neurons within the 5HT distribution were seen to have 5HT-immunoreactivity. Table I summarizes these results. These results are consistent with our earlier findings (Bowker et al., 1981b). New findings, however, indicating that nearly one-third of

TABLE I

Summary estimation of 5HT-HRP-labelled neurons in relation to 5HT cells (A) and HRP cells (B)

	Rostrocaudal levels:	NRO/NRP	NRM/NGC
A			
$\dfrac{\text{5HT-HRP}}{\text{5HT}}$	raphe:	92.8%	90.8%
	pararaphe:	87.5%	84.2%
B			
$\dfrac{\text{5HT-HRP}}{\text{HRP}}$	raphe:	89.2%	66.0%
	pararaphe:	92.0%	88.2%

Summary − overall estimate:

$\dfrac{\text{5HT-HRP}}{\text{5HT}}$: 88.7% (23 429 5HT cells counted)

$\dfrac{\text{5HT-HRP}}{\text{HRP}}$: 84.9% (24 464 cells projecting to spinal cord counted)

the cells within the NRM that project to the spinal cord have another putative neurotransmitter besides 5HT, raise several interesting questions as to which putative neurotransmitters might be involved in these descending non-5HT projections such as SOMA, M-ENK and L-ENK, as well as potential acetylcholine-containing cells. Furthermore, in the NGC since only about 10 – 15% of the neurons within the ventral NGC (or the NGC pars alpha) appeared to contain another putative neurotransmitter other than 5HT, these data suggest that most of the spinally projecting peptides within the NGC pars alpha must be co-localized with the 5HT neurons and, therefore, form a subset of the descending 5HT system. In view of the differences between the NRM and the NGC projection systems with respect to the percentages of the descending 5HT neurons to the population of spinally projecting neurons, the data indicate further that they should probably be considered as different functional cell populations rather than as a similar system.

Descending projections of peptide cells via the dorsolateral funiculus

With the above presentation of some of the peptidergic neurons in the NRM and their relationships to the 5HT cells, as seen on the same tissue section, the question arises as to which neurotransmitters, specifically the peptides, in these cell groups have descending projections via the dorsolateral funiculus (DLF), and may, as a result, potentially be involved in the modulation of sensory activity in the dorsal horn. Several physiological studies have indicated that the inhibition of dorsal horn neurons, produced by stimulation of the NRM, is greatly reduced or eliminated by the placement of lesions within the DLF (Fields and Basbaum, 1978). Thus, one would surmise that 5HT and peptidergic neurons that might be responsible for at least a portion of this descending inhibition would have their axons located within the DLF. Previous studies, employing the retrograde transport of the HRP enzyme followed by immunocytochemistry, have shown that within the NRM and the adjacent NGC (and NGC pars alpha) cells containing the peptides SP, TRH, and L-ENK have projections as far caudal as the lumbar spinal cord (Bowker et al., 1981a, 1983; Hökfelt et al., 1979). The termination sites of these descending transmitters, particularly in regard to involvement of dorsal horn functions, can be deduced from data in other studies. In studies of anterograde transport of radioactive amino acids or retrograde transport of the HRP in combination with lesions of the various funiculi, the efferent projections from the NRM and the NGC are known to descend to the spinal cord primarily via the DLF (Basbaum et al., 1977; Leichnetz et al., 1978; Martin et al., 1978, 1979, 1982a,b; Goode et al., 1980; Tohyama et al., 1979; Carlton et al., 1983; Watkins et al., 1980). In an attempt to provide evidence that several of these peptides along with the 5HT neurons in these nuclei do potentially have a role in the processing of information of sensory activity in the dorsal horn, the peptides SP, SOMA and M-ENK (L-ENK) can be localized in the dorsolateral and lateral funiculi and traverse the length of the spinal cord via the DLF in several different animal species, including the monkey. These findings provide anatomical support for the idea that they, in all probability, have a role in the descending control of nociception. Fig. 12 illustrates in several photomicrographs that each of the four putative neurotransmitters (SP, M-ENK, SOMA and L-ENK) have immunoreactive fibers in the DLF. The remaining three markers for GABA, CCK, and VIP have not as yet, to the best of our knowledge, been examined on horizontally cut spinal cord sections.

Potential interactions of the peptides and 5HT neurons

In order to visualize chemically coded afferents onto identified NRM/NGC cells, two sequential immunocytochemical reactions need to be performed with two distinct markers. In the present light-microscopic study two markers, M-ENK and SP, will be shown to make contacts upon 5HT cells and that there are differences in relative densities of contacts upon the 5HT neurons in the NRM and the adjacent NGC. One should be aware that the varicosities which appear to make contact with the 5HT neurons are only that − apparent contacts − and may not necessarily form an active synapse with the 5HT cells. On the other hand, to examine a population of 5HT-immunoreactive neurons having chemically identified contacts and to quantify them at the electron microscopic level would be an extremely difficult and time-consuming task.

At the light-microscopic level sections are first processed immunocytochemically for the peptide of either SP, M-ENK or TRH in order that the immunoreactive black punctate profiles can be seen against the amber-colored cell body stained for 5HT. In Fig. 13, a and b illustrate photomicrographs that were immunocytochemically stained first with SP and M-ENK, respectively, followed by 5HT of the cell bodies in the NRM. Both 5HT neurons appear to have immunoreactive profiles against the cell body. Although not appreciated in the photomicrographs due to the inability to obtain all of the possible focal planes of the cell in a single photomicrograph, the relative differences in the apparent contacts on the 5HT neurons in the NRM are shown in camera lucida drawings (Fig. 14, a and b). The M-ENK contacts appear to be denser and more numerous than SP-immunoreactive profiles on the 5HT neurons in the NRM. On the other hand, in the lateral parts of the NGC, no differences could be seen between the densities SP and M-ENK, contacts upon the 5HT neurons since most of the 5HT neurons examined in the para-olivary region and medial to the facial nucleus appeared to receive a very rich innervation of both SP and M-ENK terminals. Thus, these findings would suggest that, at least within the NRM, the 5HT neurons may be under a greater influence of the M-ENK than SP inputs, while laterally the 5HT neurons would appear to be under a similar or equal influence from the SP and M-ENK inputs.

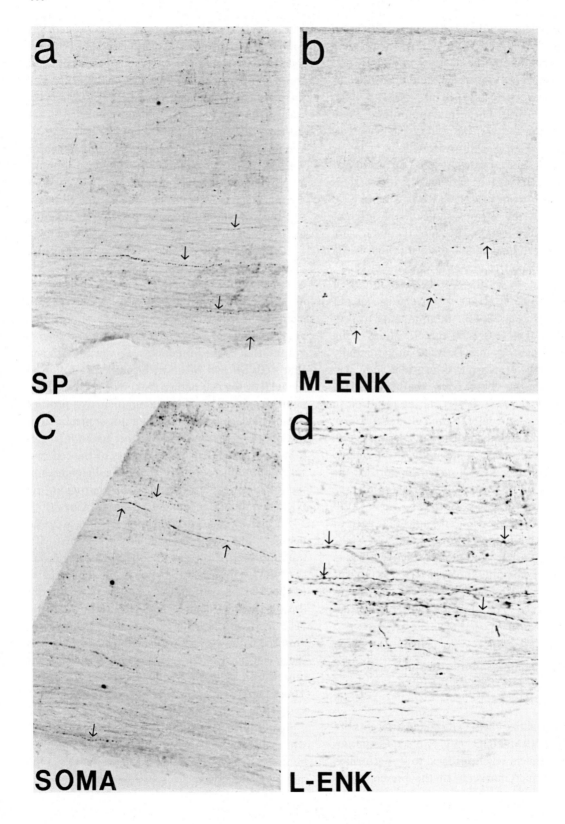

μ receptors in the NRM- and the NGC-quantitative autoradiography

Based on the findings that M-ENK terminals make contacts with the 5HT cells within the NRM and the NGC, one might expect the presence of opioid receptors, for example μ receptors, within these two nuclei. In order to visualize opioid receptors within the NRM and the adjacent nuclei, the ligand D-Ala-Gly-N-MePhe-Gly(ol), which is a specific ligand for the μ receptors, is tagged with a radioactive iodine molecule (^{125}I-DAGO) and then incubated with the brain sections. The radioactive ligand combines with its specific receptors on either the presynaptic terminal and/or the postsynaptic membrane of neural elements within the NRM and NGC prior to exposing them to a photographic film. Such a process enables the experimenter to visualize the receptors in different brain regions. In Fig. 13, c and d illustrate the moderate binding of the opioid receptors in the NRM and denser binding in the dorsal horn of the

spinal nucleus of the trigeminal nerve (Spin V). The latter finding is consistent with most other studies on μ receptors. The surrounding areas of the pyramidal tract and the dorsal medulla and pons have scant binding (see Table II). Table II displays the relative concentrations of the receptors as expressed as $fmol/mm^2/mg$ prot.

Discussion

The present study has provided data that can be summarized into four points for discussion purposes:

(1) The peptidergic neurons and their terminals are differentially distributed within the NRM and the adjacent NGC with respect to each other and to the 5HT neurons, rather than being homogeneously distributed in these cell groups.

(2) Several of these groups of peptidergic neurons include cells that project via the DLF to the spinal cord.

(3) Peptidergic neurons form a subset of the descending 5HT system since the peptides colocalize with 5HT in descending neurons.

(4) One of the potential circuits in the descending control of nociception may include enkephalin afferents onto 5HT and non-5HT neurons. This concept is supported by the demonstration of opiate μ receptors in the NRM and the NGC.

(1) Differential distribution of the peptides in NRM and NGC

The present study has brought together data on the distribution of several different types of peptidergic neurons that can be localized to the rostral medulla, specifically the NRM and the adjacent NGC. The current study shows that their distributions and localizations in these two nuclei are not that dissimilar to the findings of others at least with respect to SP (Hökfelt et al., 1978; Ljungdahl

TABLE II

Quantitative autoradiography determinations ($n = 3$) of ^{125}I-DAGO binding ($fmol/mm^2/mg$ prot) from coronal brain sections

	Brain stem level	
	caudal	rostral
1. Nucleus raphe magnus	1.50 ± 0.39	1.98 ± 0.30
2. Nucleus gigantocellularis	1.51 ± 0.14	1.27 ± 0.11
3. Pyramidal tract	0.24 ± 0.08	0.23 ± 0.04
4. Dorsal tegmentum	0.66 ± 0.05	0.44 ± 0.03
5. Spinal tract and nucleus of V	1.36 ± 0.40	1.31 ± 0.58

Fig. 12. Photomicrographs showing the presence of immunoreactive staining of fibers in the dorsolateral funiculus in the spinal cord for SP (a), M-ENK (b), SOMA (c), and L-ENK (d). The arrows indicate the beaded fibers in these descending axons. All of these transmitters have been shown to have descending projections to the spinal cord from the rostral medulla.

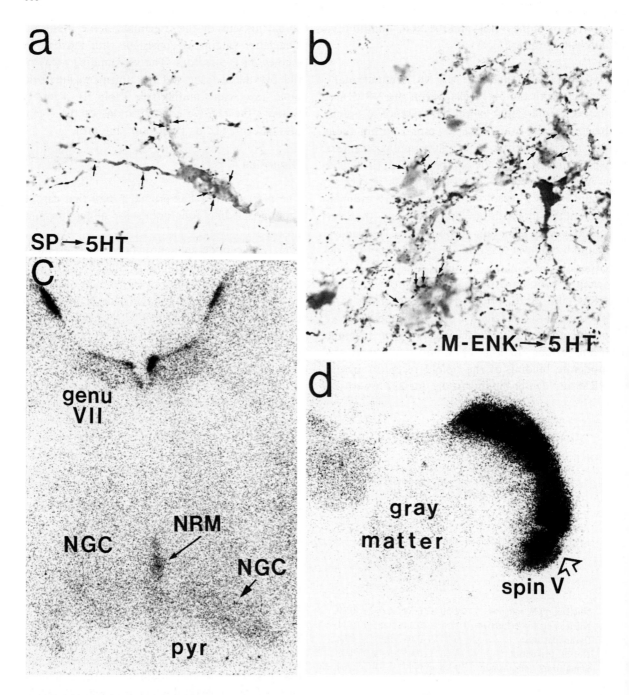

Fig. 13. Photomicrographs showing the apparent contacts of the SP (a) and the M-ENK (b) on the 5HT cells in the nucleus raphe magnus (NRM). Arrows mark the sites of apparent contacts. (c) Moderate μ receptor binding is shown in the NRM and the nucleus gigantocellularis (NGC), as well as dense binding in the spinal trigeminal nucleus (d). Observe the moderate 'button' of receptor binding in rostral NRM with less in ventral NGC. Pyr, pyramidal tract; genu VII, genu of VIIth cranial nerve.

et al., 1978), both M- and L-ENK (Uhl et al., 1979; Hökfelt et al., 1977, 1979; Finley et al., 1981), SOMA (Taber-Pierce et al., 1985), VIP (Jansco et al., 1981), CCK (Kubota et al., 1983; Mantyh and Hunt, 1984) and GABA (Belin et al., 1983), as well as descending TRH cells (Bowker et al., 1983).

There are several other classes of peptide-containing cells within these nuclei that were not presented and include proctolin and galanin, which also coexist with 5HT neurons (Melander et al., 1986). The fact that there are at least 12 – 15 classes of peptide-containing neurons within these

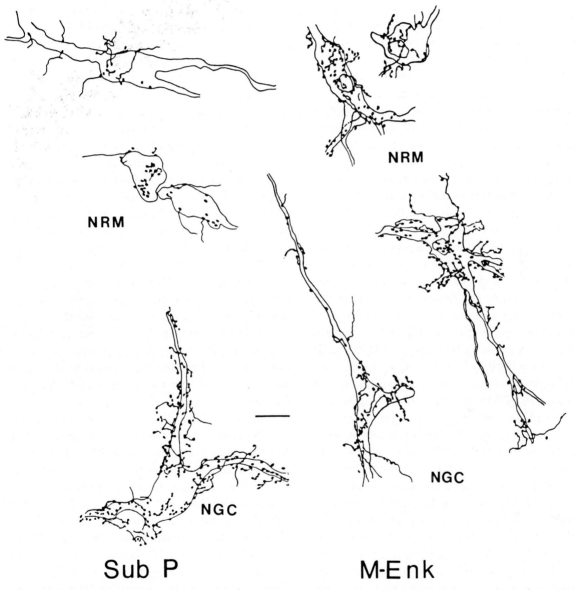

Sub P   M-Enk

Fig. 14. Camera lucida drawings show the SP and M-ENK apparent contacts on 5HT cells in nucleus raphe magnus (NRM) and nucleus gigantocellularis (NGC). Observe the relatively fewer SP contacts on 5HT cells in comparison to the higher density of M-ENK contacts on 5HT cells in NRM. Laterally in NGC on same sections, both peptides had relatively high densities of contacts on 5HT cells. Calibration bar, 25 μm.

two nuclei indicates the complexity and difficulty in understanding the anatomical organization of the rostral medulla in its descending modulation of the spinal cord dorsal horn. Several important aspects of their distributions and localizations within these two nuclei, though, become evident when one analyzes many of these peptides on the same or adjacent tissue sections: these peptides appear to be distributed differentially within these nuclei so as to form subpopulations or clusters of neurons which differ according to the neurotransmitter or transmitters they contain. This differential distribution suggests a specificity to the organization of these cell groups and, hence, a specificity in the functionings of these different groups of neurons. These observations indicate that the reticular formation is very highly organized according to the various neurotransmitters that are found at different medullary levels.

Several examples were used to illustrate the differential distribution of these peptide-containing cells in these nuclei. Three of the peptides that were presented are the SP, SOMA and the M-ENK neurons located in the NRM and the NGC. The SP neurons are mainly distributed in the midline and the ventral NGC, or the pars alpha subdivision, between the anterior parts of the inferior olivary nucleus and the mid-facial nucleus, with few cells present more dorsally in the NGC or rostrally to the mid-facial nucleus and the trapezoid body and nucleus. The SOMA-immunoreactive neurons are present within the NRM, but are larger in size than most of the SP or the 5HT neurons in this nucleus, with the majority of the SOMA cells being located laterally in the NGC. Within the NGC, however, most SOMA neurons are distributed dorsal to the SP and 5HT populations as the SOMA population extends to the floor of the IVth ventricle in the NPGD. Finally, M-ENK neurons are also present in the NRM, but they too tend to be larger in size than the SP and 5HT neurons. The M-ENK population is mainly located in the NGC, with few cells extending dorsally towards the floor of the IVth ventricle, as is the case with the SOMA neurons. Only a few of the M-ENK cells appear to extend rostrally to the trapezoid body level, while no SOMA cells can be found, similar to the rostral extent of the SP neurons. Thus, these three peptides are found in three fairly distinct regions – the SP cells along with the 5HT neurons are located on the midline and in the most ventral part of the NGC, while the SOMA and the M-ENK cells are located more dorsally than either the SP or the 5HT neurons in the NRM and the NGC. Only the 5HT and the M-ENK cells extend as far rostrally in the NRM as the trapezoid body.

The obvious question is: Are there any potential functional implications of this differential distribution of the peptide cells in the rostral medulla? One would expect to see differences in the effects of chemical and perhaps electrical stimulation of the rostral NRM from its most caudal levels as well as differences within the mediolateral direction, since different pools of neurotransmitter-containing cells and potentially their fibers, would be stimulated. To date, few experiments have assessed any differences in the effects of stimulating these various subregions of these nuclei of the NRM and the NGC other than to obtain an effective stimulation site for producing an inhibition in their recording site in the dorsal horn (cf. Willis, 1984). One of the consistent stimulation sites in the NRM for producing spinal cord inhibition is the level immediately caudal to the facial nucleus or at the mid-facial level (Sandkühler and Gebhart, 1984; cf. Willis, 1984). At these medullary levels several peptides are present that may be activated by electrical stimulation. Their relative efficacy may vary since they appear to be present in decreasing relative numbers of neurons at the more anterior levels in the NRM. Those peptide-containing cells that are present, but in dwindling numbers anteriorly, are SP and TRH, while the ENK-, GABA-, and SOMA-containing cells along with the 5HT neurons are present in considerable numbers, suggesting a greater potential to contribute to the descending inhibitory control of the dorsal horn. Few of these peptides are located at the level of the trapezoid body, with the exception of ENK and GABA, suggesting that, at this most rostral level of the NRM, these peptides and/or 5HT may be the most likely candidates involved in the spinal cord inhibition of nociceptive transmission. This type of correlation should probably be performed for each of the putative neuropeptides located in these two nuclei in order to begin determining how they are related to the effective stimulation sites. Such a correlation will, potentially, provide the initial candidates of the medullary circuitry necessary for understanding the functional roles of the NRM and NGC.

(2) Peptidergic neurons with descending projections via the dorsolateral funiculus

Physiological studies have shown that lesions of the DLF abolish or greatly attenuate the effective inhibitory response in the dorsal horn caused by stimulation of the rostral medulla (Fields et al., 1977; cf. Willis, 1984). This indicates the likely course of these descending fibers from the NRM and the NGC which are involved in the antinociceptive effects. In the present study the three peptides, SP, SOMA and ENK, along with 5HT were shown to be present in immunoreactive fibers within the DLF. The origins of these peptides along with the 5HT are from both the NRM and the NGC, both the pars alpha division and the more dorsal NGC (Bowker et al., 1982, 1983). In addition, these peptides are all present within the dorsal horn (Ljungdahl et al., 1978; Hökfelt et al., 1976; Innis et al., 1979).

Anatomical findings of their origins and locations within the DLF, as well as their presence in terminals within the dorsal horn, suggest that these peptides are among the candidates for mediating the descending inhibition from the rostral medulla to the spinal cord. Functionally, SOMA and M-ENK (and L-ENK), and 5HT have been shown to produce an inhibition in the spinal cord, particularly the dorsal horn. ENK, applied iontophoretically, inhibits the activity of dorsal horn cells (Zieglgänsberger and Tulloch, 1979; see, however, Davies and Dray, 1976), similar to the effects of 5HT (Jordan et al., 1978; cf. Willis, 1984). Little information is available about SOMA's ef-

fects in the spinal cord; however in the brain, SOMA nearly always produces an inhibition when it is iontophoresed near recorded neurons, suggesting that this peptide has a generalized inhibitory role in the central nervous system. Together, these findings suggest that these peptides along with 5HT may be likely candidates in the descending inhibitory control of nociceptive activity.

Two important questions to be asked, however, are: To what extent do these descending peptides form a powerful descending inhibitory network from the regions of the NRM and the NGC which are known to produce the antinociceptive effects? Do several or only one of these, and other peptides, form a major (or minor) component in the descending projections from these nuclei to the dorsal horn via the DLF? The answers to these questions should provide an estimate of the relative contribution of these putative neurotransmitters to antinociception originating from these nuclei.

(3) Most descending peptides form a subset of the 5HT system

Several peptides have previously been shown to descend to the spinal cord from the NRM and the adjacent pars alpha subdivision of the NGC; these include SP, TRH, the ENK (Bowker et al., 1983; Hökfelt et al., 1979), CCK (Mantyh and Hunt, 1984) and SOMA (unpublished observations). In a similar fashion, 5HT neurons have been shown by indirect methods (Gilbert et al., 1982; Singer et al., 1979) and by more direct methods (Bowker et al., 1981a and 1983) to originate from these same nuclei as they project to the spinal cord. An important question to ask is: Which of these putative neurotransmitters form the major descending component to the spinal cord, specifically the dorsal horn, from these two nuclei? The quantitative data presented here indicates that from the NRM, the 5HT projections comprise nearly two-thirds of the descending projections, while one-third of the projections appear to be non-5HT containing. On the other hand, only about 15% of the descending projections from the pars alpha subdivision of the NGC are non-5HT containing. While these findings indicate that, quantitatively, the 5HT system forms the major descending projection from the NRM, additional information is inferred regarding the descending peptide-containing cells that have also been shown to coexist with 5HT (Hökfelt et al., 1978; Ljungdahl et al., 1978; Chan-Palay, 1979; Glazer et al., 1981; Belin et al., 1983) and to project to the spinal cord (Bowker et al., 1983). In other words, these descending peptides from the 5HT population in the NRM and the NGC must be a subset of the descending 5HT system if they form a significant descending projection to the spinal cord (Bowker et al., 1983). Thus, the two peptides SP and TRH, which form fairly substantial projections to the spinal cord from the NRM and the NGC (Bowker et al., 1983), appear to be mainly a subset of the descending 5HT system.

What putative neurotransmitter or neurotransmitters make-up the other one-third of the non-5HT neurons from the NRM, or the smaller component (15%) in the pars alpha subdivision in the NGC? The present study and previous works have shown that SOMA (unpublished observations) and ENK (Hökfelt et al., 1979; Bowker et al., 1983) project to the spinal cord from the NRM. To what extent do these two peptides comprise the remainder of the one-third of the descending projections from these nuclei remains to be determined. Within the NGC pars alpha, a few ENK neurons can be seen to project to the spinal cord; but the majority of the descending SOMA and M-ENK are located dorsally to the descending 5HT system in the NGC, rather than within the distribution of 5HT neurons. In all probability there are other peptides that do not co-localize with the 5HT neurons in the NRM but that do project to the spinal cord and thus form a smaller population of the descending non-5HT cells.

Thus, within the rostral medulla, several conclusions can be made regarding the chemical identities of neurons with descending projections and how extensively they form descending pathways to the spinal cord: (1) the peptides SP and TRH (along with GABA and other peptides that are co-localized with 5HT) appear to form a subset of the 5HT system with few non-5HT SP and TRH neurons projecting to the spinal cord from the 5HT population of the rostral medulla; (2) the SOMA and the ENK neurons comprise many of the non-5HT cells that project to the spinal cord from the NRM, while only a very small percentage is situated laterally within the 5HT population of the pars alpha subdivision of the NGC; (3) a population of the SOMA and the ENK neurons projecting to the spinal cord is situated dorsally to the 5HT population in the NGC; (4) other peptides, in all probability, have descending projections from these nuclei to the dorsal horn, but they form a smaller percentage of the projection pathways from the NRM and the ventral NGC, while dorsal to the 5HT system they may comprise a much larger population of descending projections. Future analyses will have to address this possibility.

(4) Potential medullary circuits in the descending control of nociception

While the above discussion focused upon more direct pathways from the rostral medulla to the spinal cord involved in the modulation of dorsal horn activity, an equally important component of the brain's control of these descending pathways is localized within the NRM itself — the chemically identified afferents that may impinge upon the raphe- and reticulospinal projections and the interneurons which are also capable of modulating either the input to these projection neurons or the output from these same cells. Several different neurotransmitter elements are believed to have afferents terminating within these two nuclei, including the peptides SP and TRH and the catecholamines (Hökfelt et al., 1978; Dahlström and Fuxe, 1964). The two peptides presented were employed as examples of a more general hypothesis that definite anatomical differences in the potential peptide-amine interactions may account for at least a portion of the physiological and pharmacological effects observed in the rostral medulla. The anatomical differences were assessed by the relative differences in the immunoreactive profiles which appeared to be making contact with a chemically identified neuron. The two peptides SP and M-ENK make apparent contacts with 5HT neurons in the NRM and the more lateral NGC, but definite differences were evident in the relative densities of these apparent contacts in these two locations. Within the NRM, 5HT neurons appeared to be completely covered with M-ENK immunoreactive profiles, while SP profiles, although present in this nucleus, were relatively sparse. However, on the same tissue section in the NGC, the 5HT cells were completely smothered by both SP- and M-ENK-immunoreactive profiles. Comparison of these two putative neurotransmitters suggests that they may have differential efficacies in activating the 5HT neurons in these two nuclei, suggesting a greater ENK modulatory input to the NRM while the 5HT neurons in the NGC might be more easily affected or under a more rigid control by SP inputs. These implications are only speculation at this point, but the anatomical observations indicate major differences regarding how the various neurotransmitters can effect a cell population. These suggestions will have to await future experiments performed by pharmacologists in order to assess the relative influences of the various peptides onto 5HT cells in the NRM and the NGC. Other questions, such as the distributions of the catecholamines or other peptides, will undoubtedly be of great benefit in unraveling the organization of these two nuclei in the medulla.

With the observation that the ENK-immunoreactive profiles upon 5HT and non-5HT cells are located in the rostral medulla, especially in the NRM, it is perhaps not surprising that opiate receptors are also localized in these two cell groups. This finding is the first, or at least one of the first studies, to document and to quantify the opiate receptors in the NRM. The presence of these μ receptors in the NRM, coupled with the M-ENK-immunoreactive profiles on the 5HT cells, is consistent with the idea that enkephalins act on cells in this region. This hypothesis appears to be sup-ported by fairly extensive pharmacological data implicating the μ receptor in analgesic mechanisms (Fang et al., 1986). Definitive documentation of the localization of the μ receptors on the cell bodies in the NRM is currently being examined. In any event, one avenue to begin documenting the potential circuitry underlying the brainstem's control of nociception is (1) to examine the chemically identified afferents onto descending neurons in these two nuclei and (2) to determine the relative densities of certain receptors in these nuclei that may be mediating the observed effects resulting from administering various drugs. These studies will provide a framework to link pharmacological and physiological studies with anatomical circuitry in order to better understand the descending control of nociception.

Summary

The present study has presented data concerning the identification, distribution and connectivities of several species of peptidergic neurons within the NRM and the NGC. The observation of numerous resident peptides along with 5HT suggests that the anatomical organization of these neurotransmitters within these nuclei is exceedingly complex. Our complete understanding of their organization will, in all probability, encompass years of experimental study to determine whether and how each of these peptides functions in the descending control of nociception. The present study has provided several pieces of the puzzle concerning the anatomical organization of the neurotransmitters in these two nuclei, and is diagramatically shown in Fig. 15. Firstly, the neurotransmitters are not homogeneously distributed throughout these two cell groups. Rather they are segregated into subpopulations, suggesting functional specializations according to the neurotransmitters. Secondly, the major output projection from the NRM and ventral NGC contains 5HT along with one or more colocalized peptides, such as SP and TRH; while a smaller population (approximately one-third) of the descending projections are non-5HT contain-

124

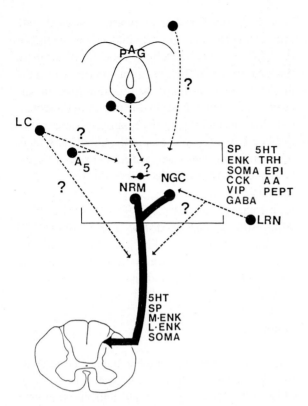

Fig. 15. Diagram showing possible circuitry of peptide cells in nucleus raphe magnus (NRM) and nucleus gigantocellularis (NGC) and their outputs to dorsal horn. Numerous peptides are present in NRM and NGC as either interneurons or projection cells. 5HT, SP, SOMA, M-ENK and L-ENK project to spinal cord in dorsolateral funiculus. Potential inputs are from locus coeruleus (LC), A$_5$, lateral reticular nucleus (LRN), periaqueductal gray (PAG) and higher centers. Many of these inputs to NRM and NGC are not known. SP, substance P; ENK, enkephalin; SOMA, somatostatin, CCK, cholecystokinin; VIP, vasoactive intestinal peptide; GABA, γ-aminobutyric acid; 5HT, serotonin; TRH, thyrotropin-releasing hormone; EPI, epinephrine; AA, various amino acids; pept, other peptides.

neurons are perhaps equally complex, as inputs to the NRM/NGC are believed to originate from many brain areas, including the locus coeruleus, the A$_5$ cell group and the periaqueductal gray (PAG) area, as well as the lateral reticular nucleus (LRN) and higher brain centers. While the neurotransmitter identities of several of these inputs are known, including the catecholamines, ENK and neurotensin, many inputs to these cell groups are not yet identified. Future work designed to unravel the anatomical complexities of these nuclei in order to better understand the circuitry involved in the descending control of nociception must focus not only upon a small number of these neurotransmitter elements within the NRM/NGC region, but must analyze all potential transmitter interactions in terms of their coded afferents and efferent projections, the intrinsic neurons and the receptor organization. Only then can these two critical links in the rostral medulla in the descending control of nociception be understood.

Acknowledgements

The authors would like to acknowledge the excellent technical assistance of B. Gideon, L. Roth, K. Hook and T. Boles and the typing and editorial assistance of C. Smith, J. Ho and C. Sosna.

References

Basbaum, A.I., Marley, N.J.E., O'Keefe, J. and Clanton, C.H. (1977) Reversal of morphine and stimulus-produced analgesia by subtotal spinal cord lesions. *Pain*, 3: 43 – 56.

Belin, M.F., Nanopoulos, D., Didier, M., Aguera, M., Steinbusch, H., Verhofstad, A., Maitre, M. and Pujol, J.-F. (1983) Immunohistochemical evidence for the presence of gamma-aminobutyric acid and serotonin in one nerve cell. A study on the raphe nuclei of rat using antibodies to glutamate decarboxylase and serotonin. *Brain Res.*, 275: 329 – 339.

Bowker, R.M. (1987) Evidence for the colocalization of somatostatin- and methionine-enkephalin-like immunoreactivities in raphe and gigantocellularis nuclei. *Neurosci. Lett.*, 81: 75 – 81.

Bowker, R.M., Steinbusch, H. and Coulter, J.D. (1981a)

ing. These other non-5HT projections from the NRM/NGC do contain SOMA, ENK and probably other peptides not as yet identified. Some neurotransmitter candidates that are potentially involved in nociceptive control, have been shown to be present in axons that descend via the DLF to innervate the dorsal horn. They include 5HT, SP, M-ENK and L-ENK and SOMA. The chemically coded inputs to these peptidergic and 5HT-containing

Serotonergic and peptidergic projections to the spinal cord demonstrated by a combined retrograde HRP histochemical and immunocytochemical staining method. *Brain Res.*, 211: 412 – 417.

Bowker, R.M., Westlund, K.N. and Coulter, J.D. (1981b) Origins of serotonergic projections to the spinal cord in rat: an immunocytochemical-retrograde transport study. *Brain Res.*, 226: 187 – 199.

Bowker, R.M., Westlund, K.N. and Coulter, J.D. (1982) Organization of descending serotonergic projections to the spinal cord. In H.G.J.M. Kuypers and G.F. Martin (Eds.), *Descending Pathways to the Spinal Cord, Progress in Brain Research, Vol. 57*, Elsevier, Amsterdam, pp. 239 – 265.

Bowker, R.M., Westlund, K.N., Sullivan, M.C., Wilbur, J.F. and Coulter, J.D. (1983) Descending serotonergic, peptidergic and cholinergic pathways from the raphe nuclei: a multiple transmitter complex. *Brain Res.*, 288: 33 – 48.

Carlton, S.M., Leichnetz, G.R., Young, E.G. and Mayer, D.J. (1983) Supramedullary afferents of the nucleus raphe magnus in the rat: a study using the transcannula HRP gel and autoradiographic techniques. *J. Comp. Neurol.*, 214: 43 – 58.

Chan-Palay, V. (1979) Combined immunocytochemistry and autoradiography after in vivo injections of monoclonal antibody to substance P and ^{3}H-serotonin: co-existence of two putative transmitters in single raphe cells and fiber plexuses. *Anat. Embryol.*, 156: 241 – 254.

Coote, J.H. and MacLeod, V.H. (1974) The influence of bulbospinal monoaminergic pathways on sympathetic nerve activity. *J. Physiol. (Lond.)*, 241: 453 – 475.

Crutcher, K.A. and Humbertson, A.O. (1978) The organization of monoamine neurons within the brainstem of the North American opossum *(Didelphis virginiana)*. *J. Comp. Neurol.*, 179: 195 – 222.

Crutcher, K.A., Humbertson, A.O. and Martin, G.F. (1978) The origin of brainstem-spinal pathways in the North American opossum *(Didelphis virginiana)*. Studies using the horseradish peroxidase method. *J. Comp. Neurol.*, 179: 169 – 194.

Dahlström, A. and Fuxe, K. (1964) Evidence for the existence of monoamine-containing neurons in the central nervous system. I. Demonstration of monoamines in the cell bodies of brain stem neurons. *Acta Physiol. Scand.*, 62, Suppl. 232: 1 – 55.

Dahlström, A. and Fuxe, K. (1965) Evidence of the existence of monoamine-containing neurons in the central nervous system. II. Experimentally induced changes in the intraneuronal amine levels of the bulbospinal neuron systems. *Acta Physiol. Scand.*, 64, Suppl. 247: 1 – 36.

Davies, J. and Dray, A. (1976) Effects of enkephalin and morphine on Renshaw cells in feline spinal cord. *Nature*, 262: 603 – 604.

Fang, F.G., Fields, H.L. and Lee, N.M. (1986) Action at the μ receptor is sufficient to explain the supraspinal analgesic effect of opiates. *J. Pharmacol. Exp. Ther.*, 238: 1039 – 1044.

Fields, H.L. and Basbaum, A.I. (1978) Brainstem control of spinal pain – transmission neurons. *Annu. Rev. Physiol.*, 40: 217 – 248.

Fields, H.L., Basbaum, A.I. and Clanton, C.T. (1977) Nucleus raphe magnus inhibition of spinal cord dorsal horn neurons. *Brain Res.*, 126(3): 441 – 453.

Finley, J.C.W., Maderdrut, J.L. and Petrusz, P. (1981) The immunocytochemical localization of enkephalin in the central nervous system of the rat. *J. Comp. Neurol.*, 198: 541 – 565.

Gilbert, R.F.T., Emson, P.C., Hunt, S.P., Bennett, G.W., Marsden, C.A., Sandberg, B.E.B., Steinbusch, H.W.M. and Verhofstad, A.A.J. (1982) The effects of monoamine neurotoxins on peptides in the rat spinal cord. *Neuroscience*, 7: 69 – 87.

Glazer, E.J., Steinbusch, H., Verhofstad, A. and Basbaum, A.I. (1981) Serotonin neurons in nucleus raphe dorsalis and paragigantocellularis of the cat contain enkephalin. *J. Physiol. (Paris)*, 77: 241 – 245.

Goode, G.E., Humbertson, A.O. and Martin, G.F. (1980) Projections from the brain stem reticular formation to laminae I and II of the spinal cord: studies using light and electron microscopic techniques in the North American opossum. *Brain Res.*, 189: 327 – 342.

Helke, C.J., Neill, J.J., Marsari, V.J. and Loewy, A.D. (1982) Substance P neurons project from the ventral medulla to the intermediolateral cell column and ventral horn in the rat. *Brain Res.*, 243: 147 – 152.

Henry, J.L. and Calarescu, F.R. (1974) Excitatory and inhibitory inputs from medullary nuclei projecting to spinal cardioacceleratory neurons in the cat. *Exp. Brain Res.*, 20: 485 – 504.

Hökfelt, T., Elde, R., Johansson, O., Luft, R., Nilsson, G. and Arimura, A. (1976) Immunohistochemical evidence for separate populations of somatostatin-containing and substance P-containing primary afferent neurons in the rat. *Neuroscience*, 1: 131 – 136.

Hökfelt, T., Elde, R., Johansson, O., Terenius, L. and Stein, L. (1977) The distribution of enkephalin-immunoreactive cell bodies in the rat central nervous system. *Neurosci. Lett.*, 5: 25 – 31.

Hökfelt, T., Ljungdahl, A., Steinbusch, H., Verhofstad, A., Nilsson, G., Brodin, E., Pernow, B. and Goldstein, M. (1978) Immunohistochemical evidence of substance P-like immunoreactivity in some 5-hydroxytryptamine-containing neurons in the rat central nervous system. *Neuroscience*, 3: 517 – 538.

Hökfelt, T., Terenius, L., Kuypers, H.G.J.M. and Dann, O. (1979) Evidence for enkephalin immunoreactive neurons in the medulla oblongata projecting to the spinal cord. *Neurosci. Lett.*, 14: 55 – 60.

126

Hökfelt, T., Johansson, O., Ljungdahl, J.M. and Schultzberg, M. (1980) Peptidergic neurons. *Nature*, 284: 515–521.

Hökfelt, T., Fried, G., Hansen, S., Holets, V., Lundberg, J.M. and Skirbol, L. (1986) Neurons with multiple messengers – distribution and possible functional significance. In J.M. van Ree and S. Matthysse (Eds.) *Psychiatric Disorders: Neurotransmitters and Neuropeptides, Progress in Brain Research, Vol. 65*, Elsevier, Amsterdam, pp. 115–137.

Hunt, S.P. and Lovick, T.A. (1982) The distribution of serotonin metenkephalin and B-lipotropin-like immunoreactivity in neuronal perikarya of the cat brainstem. *Neurosci. Lett.*, 30: 139–145.

Innis, R.B., Correa, F.M.A., Uhl, G.R., Schneider, B. and Snyder, S.H. (1979) Cholecystokinin octapeptide-like immunoreactivity: Histochemical localization in rat brain. *Proc. Natl. Acad. Sci. USA*, 76: 521–525.

Jansco, G., Hökfelt, T., Lundberg, J.M., Kuraly, E., Halasz, N., Nilsson, G., Terenius, L., Rehfeld, J., Steinbusch, H., Verhofstad, A., Elde, R., Said, S. and Brown, M. (1981) Immunohistochemical studies on the effect of capsaicin on spinal and medullary peptides and monoamine neurons using antisera to Substance P, gastrin/CCK, somatostatin, VIP, enkephalin, neurotensin and 5-hydroxytryptamine. *J. Neurocytol.*, 10: 963–980.

Johannessen, J.N., Watkins, L.R. and Mayer, D.J. (1984) Non-serotonergic origins of the dorsolateral funiculus in the rat ventral medulla. *J. Neurosci.*, 4: 757–766.

Johansson, O., Hökfelt, T., Pernow, B., Jeffcoate, S.L., White, N., Steinbusch, H.W.M., Verhofstad, A.A.J., Emson, P.C. and Spindel, E. (1981) Immunohistochemical support for three putative transmitters in one neuron: coexistence of 5-hydroxytryptamine, substance P- and thyrotropin releasing hormone-like immunoreactivity in medullarly neurons projecting to the spinal cord. *Neuroscience*, 6: 1857–1881.

Jordan, L.M., Kenshalo, D.R., Jr., Martin, R.F., Haber, L.H. and Willis, W.D. (1978) Depression of primate spinothalamic tract neurons by iontophoretic application of 5-hydroxytryptamine. *Pain*, 5: 135–142.

Kubota, Y., Inagaki, S., Shiosaka, S., Chol, S.J., Tateishi, K., Hashimura, E., Hamaoka, T. and Tohyama, M. (1983) The distribution of cholecystokinin octapeptide-like structures in the lower brainstem of the rat: An immunohistochemical analysis. *Neuroscience*, 9: 587–604.

Léger, L., Charnay, Y., Dubois, P.M. and Jouvet, M. (1986) Distribution of enkephalin-immunoreactive cell bodies in relation to serotonin-containing neurons in the raphe nuclei of the cat: immunohistochemical evidence for the coexistence of enkephalins and serotonin in certain cells. *Brain Res.*, 362: 63–73.

Leichnetz, G.R., Watkins, L., Griffin, G., Murfin, R. and Mayer, D.J. (1978) The projection from nucleus raphe magnus and other brainstem nuclei to spinal cord in the rat: a study using the HRP blue-reaction. *Neurosci. Lett.*, 8: 118–124.

Ljungdahl, S., Hökfelt, T. and Nilsson, G. (1978) Distribution of substance P-like immunoreactivity in the rat. I. Cell bodies and nerve terminals. *Neuroscience*, 3: 861–943.

Lovick, T.A. and Hunt, S.P. (1983) Substance P – immunoreactive and serotonin-containing neurones in the ventral brainstem of the cat. *Neurosci. Lett.*, 36: 223–228.

Mantyh, P.W. and Hunt, S.P. (1984) Evidence for cholecystokinin-like immunoreactive neurons in the rat medulla oblongata which project to the spinal cord. *Brain Res.*, 291: 49–54.

Martin, G.F., Humbertson, A.O., Laxson, C. and Panneton, W.M. (1979) Evidence for direct bulbospinal projections to laminae IX, X and the intermediolateral cell column. Studies using axonal transport techniques in the North American opossum. *Brain Res.*, 170: 165–171.

Martin, G.F., Cabana, T., DiTirro, F.J., Ho, R.H. and Humbertson, A.D. (1982a) Reticular and raphe projections to the spinal cord of the North American opossum. Evidence for connectional heterogeneity. In H.G.J.M. Kuypers and G.F. Martin (Eds.), *Descending Pathways to the Spinal Cord, Progress in Brain Research, Vol. 57*, Elsevier, Amsterdam, pp. 131–144.

Martin, G.F., Cabana, T., DiTirro, F.J., Ho, R.H. and Humbertson, A.O. (1982b) Raphespinal projections in the North American opossum: evidence for connectional heterogeneity. *J. Comp. Neurol.*, 208: 67–84.

Martin, R.F., Jordan, L.M. and Willis, W.D. (1978) Differential projections of cat medullary raphe neurons demonstrated by retrograde labeling following spinal cord lesions. *J. Comp. Neurol.*, 182: 77–78.

Meessen, H. and Olszewski, J. (1949) *A Cytoarchitectonic Atlas of the Rhombencephalon of the Rabbit*, Karger, Basel.

Melander, T., Hökfelt, T., Rökaeus, A., Cuello, A.C., Oertel, W.H., Verhofstad, A. and Goldstein, M. (1986) Coexistence of galanin-like immunoreactivity with catecholamines, 5-hydroxytryptamine, GABA and neuropeptides in the rat CNS. *J. Neurosci.*, 6: 3640–3654.

Pilowsky, P.M., Kapoor, V., Minson, J.B., West, M.J. and Chalmers, J.P. (1986) Spinal cord serotonin release and raised blood pressure after brainstem kainic acid injection. *Brain Res.*, 366: 354–357.

Sandkühler, J. and Gebhart, G.F. (1984) Relative contributions of the nucleus raphe magnus and adjacent medullary reticular formation to the inhibition by stimulation in the periaqueductal gray of a spinal nociceptive reflex in the pentobarbital-anesthetized rat. *Brain Res.*, 305: 77–87.

Scheibel, M.E. and Scheibel, A.B. (1958) Structural substrates for integrative patterns in the brain stem reticular cove. In H. Jasper et al. (Eds.), *Reticular Formation of the Brain*, Little, Brown and Co., Boston, pp. 31–55.

Singer, E., Sperk, G., Placheta, P. and Leeman, S.E. (1979)

Reduction of substance P levels in the ventral cervical spinal cord of the rat after intracisternal 5,7-dihydroxytryptamine injection. *Brain Res.*, 174: 362 – 365.

Skagerberg, G. and Björklund, A. (1985) Topographic principles of serotonergic and non-serotonergic brainstem neurons in the rat. *Neuroscience*, 15: 445 – 480.

Steinbusch, H.W.M. (1981) Distribution of serotonin-immunoreactivity in the central nervous system of the rat cell bodies and terminals. *Neuroscience*, 6: 557 – 618.

Sternberger, L.A. (1979) The unlabeled antibody peroxidase-antiperoxidase (PAP) method. In L. Sternberger (Ed.), *Immunocytochemistry*, Wiley, New York, pp. 104 – 169.

Taber-Pierce, E., Lichtenstein, E. and Feldman, S.C. (1985) The somatostatin systems of the guinea-pig brainstem. *Neuroscience*, 15: 215 – 235.

Takano, Y., Martin, J.E., Leeman, S.E. and Loewy, A.D. (1984) Substance P immunoreactivity released from rat spinal cord after kainic acid excitation of the ventral medulla oblongata: a correlation with increases in blood pressure. *Brain Res.*, 291: 168 – 172.

Tohyama, M., Sakai, K., Touret, M., Slavert, O. and Jouvet, M. (1979) Spinal projections from the lower brain stem in the cat as demonstrated by the horseradish peroxidase technique. II. Projections from the dorsolateral pontine tegmentum and raphe nuclei. *Brain Res.*, 176: 215 – 231.

Uhl, G.R., Goodman, R.R., Kuhar, M.J., Childers, S.R. and Snyder, S.H. (1979) Immunohistochemical mapping of enkephalin containing cell bodies, fibers and nerve terminals in the brainstem of rat. *Brain Res.*, 166: 79 – 94.

Watkins, L.R., Griffin, G., Leichnetz, G.R. and Mayer, D.J. (1980) The somatotopic organization of the nucleus raphe magnus and surrounding brainstem structures as revealed by HRP slow-release gels. *Brain Res.*, 181: 1 – 15.

Willis, W.D. (1984) The raphe-spinal system. In C.D. Barnes (Ed.), *Brainstem Control of Spinal Cord Function*, Academic Press, New York, pp. 141 – 214.

Young, W.S. III and Kuhar, M.J. (1979) A new method for receptor autoradiography: [^{3}H] opioid receptors in rat brain. *Brain Res.*, 179: 255 – 270.

Zieglgänsberger, W. and Tulloch, I.F. (1979) The effects of methionine- and leucine-enkephalin on spinal neurones of the cat. *Brain Res.*, 167: 53 – 64.

H.L. Fields and J.-M. Besson (Eds.)
Progress in Brain Research, Vol. 77
© 1988 Elsevier Science Publishers B.V. (Biomedical Division)

CHAPTER 5

Spinal dorsal horn circuitry involved in the brain stem control of nociception

M.A. Ruda

Neurobiology and Anesthesiology Branch, National Institute of Dental Research, National Institutes of Health, Bethesda, MD 20892, USA

Introduction

Higher centers of the neuraxis which contribute afferents to the spinal cord include the cerebral cortex, hypothalamus and several nuclear groups in the brain stem. In the previous chapter of this volume, Bowker has reviewed some of the putative biogenic amine and peptide neurotransmitters that have been found in brain stem neurons that project to the spinal cord. These include the monoamines serotonin (5HT), noradrenaline and dopamine (Dahlström and Fuxe, 1964, 1965; Björklund and Skagerberg, 1979; Hökfelt et al., 1979a; Glazer and Ross, 1980; Westlund and Coulter, 1980; Westlund et al., 1981, 1982; Stevens et al., 1982; Skagerberg et al., 1982); the peptides substance P (SP), enkephalin (ENK), thyrotropin-releasing hormone (TRH) and cholecystokinin (CCK) which originate from the brain stem (Hökfelt et al., 1979b; Johansson et al., 1981; Helke et al., 1982; Bowker et al., 1982; Mantyh and Hunt, 1984); and the hypothalamic peptides vasopressin, oxytocin and their respective neurophysins (Millan et al., 1984; Lang et al., 1983; Swanson and McKellar, 1979; Gibson et al., 1981). Analysis of the function of these descending projections is rendered more difficult by the co-localization of one or more peptides with a monoamine in the dorsal horn terminals of single axons that originate from brain stem nuclei.

Descending afferent inputs from the brain stem may interact with several different neural elements in the dorsal horn. These include projection neurons which relay information from the spinal cord to higher centers of the neuraxis; local circuit neurons which either have an axonal arbor in the spinal cord or vesicle-containing dendrites presynaptic to other dorsal horn elements; and the terminals of primary afferent neurons. Multiple label studies have been extremely useful in identifying potential interactions between descending afferents and other dorsal horn components. Retrograde labeling or intracellular staining of dorsal horn neurons, when combined with immunocytochemistry, provides information on the neurochemicals in afferents to identified neurons or the neurochemicals they themselves contain. The double immunofluorescence method provides information on the colocalization of neurochemicals within single neurons or axon terminals. The combination of electrophysiological methods with these anatomical ones provides further information about the potential functional aspects of the system.

The role of several neurochemicals in brain stem projections to dorsal horn sensory systems has been examined (for review see Basbaum and Fields, 1978, 1984; Dubner and Bennett, 1983). However, anatomical studies have focused on the role of 5HT and co-localized peptides. This paper

130

will review the contribution of 5HT axons to dorsal horn circuitry. Most studies employ the immunocytochemical method. It should be noted that immunocytochemistry does not unequivocally identify the substance that is labeled (Petrusz et al., 1976, 1977). Immunocytochemical labeling should therefore be referred to as 'like immunoreactive' (LI).

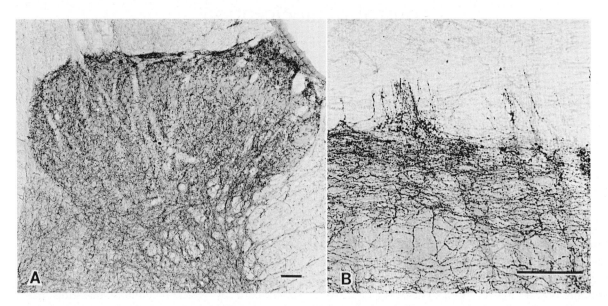

Fig. 1. Light-microscopic demonstration of 5HT-LI axons in cat lumbar spinal cord. In transverse section (A), a dense plexus of dark, PAP-labeled axons can be observed in all laminae of the dorsal horn. In sagittal section, the 5HT-LI axons in the superficial dorsal horn laminae display a predominant rostrocaudal orientation (B). Scale bar represents 100 μm. (From Ruda et al., 1982).

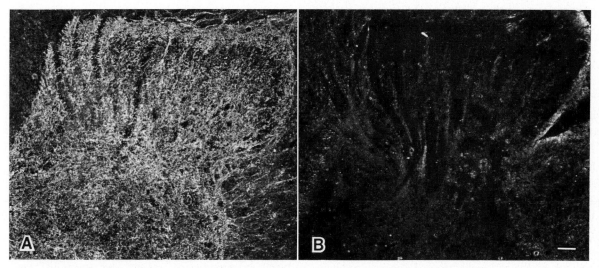

Fig. 2. Dark-field light micrographs of 5HT-LI axons in the cervical (A) and lumbar (B) enlargements of the same cat, 8 weeks following transection of the thoracic spinal cord. The sections illustrate the dense 5HT-LI immunoreactive plexus of fibers above the transection site (A), while below the transection (B) no 5HT-LI immunoreactive fibers are visible. Magnification × 50. Scale bar represents 100 μm.

Morphology of serotonin axons in the dorsal horn

5HT-LI axons have been observed in all laminae of the dorsal horn (Fig. 1, A) in the rat, cat, dog and monkey (Steinbusch, 1981; Ruda et al., 1982; Kojima et al., 1982, 1983; LaMotte and De Lanerolle, 1983; Light et al., 1983; Maxwell et al., 1983). In the superficial dorsal horn, the 5HT-LI axons display a predominant rostrocaudal orientation (Fig. 1, B). Essentially all the 5HT-LI axons in the spinal cord originate from supraspinal sites. In the cat, spinal transection at the thoracic level results in a loss of all 5HT labeling at lumbar levels (Fig. 2; Ruda et al., 1986). In the rat and monkey, a few 5HT-LI cell bodies have been identified, especially around the central canal (LaMotte et al., 1982; Newton et al., 1986). Their potential contribution to dorsal horn circuitry is unclear. 5HT-LI axons have been shown to travel in the dorsolateral funiculus (Fig. 3; Kojima et al., 1983; Hylden et al., 1985; Basbaum et al., 1987), an area of descending axons which likely terminate in the dorsal

horn. They include both unmyelinated and small myelinated axons (Basbaum et al., 1987).

The ultrastructural features of 5HT-LI axons have been described by several investigators (Maxwell et al., 1983b; Ruda et al., 1982; Light et al., 1983; LaMotte and De Lanerolle, 1983). Axon terminals immunoreactive for 5HT are typically dome-shaped and contain a mixture of small oval agranular vesicles and a few dense core vesicles (Fig. 4). Most synaptic specializations are symmetrical. They are found mainly on small caliber dendritic shafts and occasionally on spines and cell bodies. At the EM level, there is little morphological evidence for 5HT-LI varicosities presynaptic to other axons.

5-HT innervation of dorsal horn neurons

The relationship between retrogradely labeled thalamic projection neurons and 5HT-LI containing axonal varicosities has been investigated in the monkey using previously described methodology (Ruda and Coffield, 1983; Ruda et al., 1984). Due to the technical limitations of retrograde labeling,

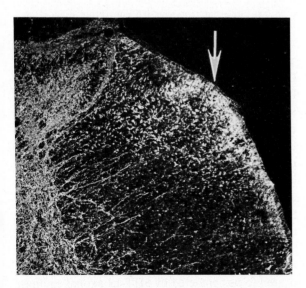

Fig. 3. Dark-field photomicrograph of PAP-labeled 5HT-LI axons in the dorso-lateral funiculus of cat lumbar spinal cord. In the transverse plane, the 5HT-LI axons display a wedgeshaped focus directly under the surface of the spinal cord. Magnification × 33. (From Hylden et al., 1985).

TABLE I

Number of thalamic projection neurons contacted by 5HT immunoreactive axonal endings

	Cervical enlargement	Lumbar enlargement
Lamina I cells 2 – 10 contacts	44 (73%)	34 (89%)
Lamina I cells no contacts	16 (27%)	4 (11%)
Lamina V cells 2 – 10 contacts	19 (50%)	30 (49%)
Lamina V cells > 10 contacts	4 (11%)	9 (15%)
Lamina V cells no contacts	15 (39%)	22 (36%)

Number in parentheses indicates percentage of total number of cells in each lamina.

132

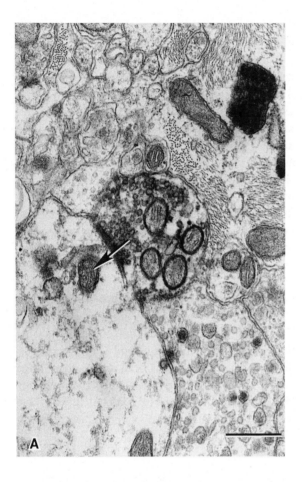

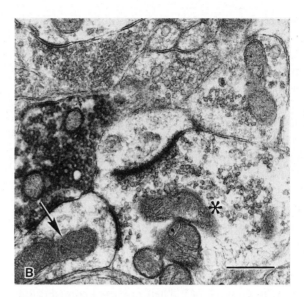

Fig. 4. Ultrastructure of 5HT-LI axonal endings in laminae I and II of the cat lumbar spinal cord. The endings typically contain oval agranular vesicles and form symmetrical synaptic contacts on dendritic shafts (A). 5HT-LI varicosities which synapse on dendritic spines (B) are less frequent. In B, the spine-head receiving a synapse (arrow) from a 5HT-LI varicosity is also postsynaptic to an unlabeled central ending (*). Magnification × 36 000. Scale bar represents 0.5 μm. (From Ruda et al., 1982.)

only the cell body and proximal dendrites could be identified and examined for the presence of 5HT contacts. Light microscopic observation revealed that the 5HT-LI varicosities contacted the cell body and proximal dendrites of thalamic projection neurons (Fig. 5). Most contacts were located on the dendrites rather than the cell body. In lamina I, bipolar and multipolar projection neurons (10–25 μm cell body short diameter) received a variable number of contacts. In lamina V, the larger multipolar neurons (25–35 μm cell body short diameter) typically received more contacts than the small bipolar projection neurons.

The number of thalamic projection neurons contacted by 5HT-LI axonal endings in the cervical and lumbar enlargements was quite high (Table I).

Cells with contacts were slightly more common in lamina I than in lamina V. Regardless of laminar location, the projection neurons with proximal contacts represented approximately two-thirds of the retrogradely labeled neurons in the lamina. The number of neurons with 5HT-LI contacts in the lumbar enlargement was slightly higher than in the cervical enlargement. The number of contacts on the cell body and proximal dendrites typically ranged from two to ten (Table I).

Ultrastructural analysis of thalamic projection neurons, which at the light microscopic level appeared to be contacted by 5HT-LI axonal endings, identified a synaptic relationship between the two elements. The labeled projection neurons were identified by the presence of electron dense HRP granules while the 5HT-LI varicosities contained the distinctive PAP reaction product (Figs. 6 and 7). The 5HT-LI axonal endings contacting the projection neurons ranged in length from 0.8–2.5 µm. They contained oval agranular vesicles and a few dense core vesicles. A symmetrical synaptic specialization was typically found; slightly asymmetrical synapses were infrequently observed. The thalamic projection neurons which received synaptic contacts from 5HT-LI axonal varicosities often received synapses from numerous other endings containing unidentified neurochemicals (Fig. 7).

These observations of 5HT innervation of thalamic projection neurons have been confirmed and extended in studies of physiologically identified lamina I neurons (Hoffert et al., 1983; Miletic et al., 1984) and lamina I projection neurons with terminals in either the thalamus or mesencephalon (Hylden et al., 1986). The intracellular HRP technique used in these studies has the advantage of labeling the complete dendritic arbor of the neuron, allowing a more complete determination of the contact distribution on the neuron. Both nociceptive-specific and wide-dynamic-range neurons terminating in either the thalamus or mesencephalon received a variable number of 5HT-LI contacts on their somata and

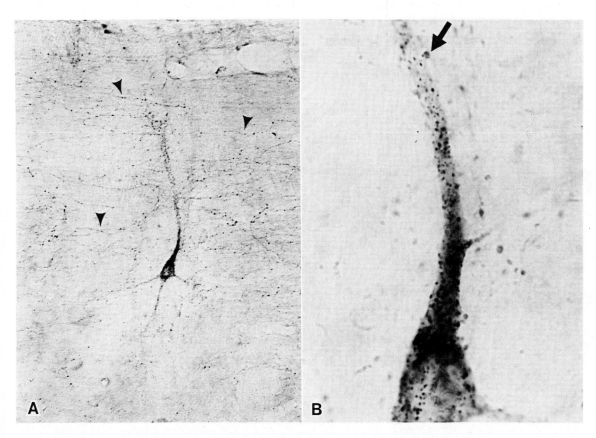

Fig. 5. (A) Light-micrograph of a retrogradely labeled lamina V thalamic projection neuron in a sagittal section of monkey lumbar spinal cord, immunocytochemically stained for 5HT. The projection neuron has a large dorsally directed dendrite and three ventrally directed dendrites visible. Numerous strands of 5HT-LI varicosities course through the section (arrowheads). Magnification × 220. (B) At higher magnification, a 5HT-LI varicosity (arrow) contacts the dendrite of the labeled neuron. The axonal varicosities are typically larger in size than the retrograde HRP granules and are marked by a brown chromogen as opposed to a black chromogen in the labeled cell. Magnification × 1300.

134

dendrites. The contacts were preferentially located on the dendritic shafts rather than spines. Several 5HT-LI varicosities on a single strand often contacted the identified neuron. The density of 5HT innervation was independent of the physiological

innervation was independent of the physiological characteristics of the neuron and the location of its axon terminal.

An additional population of dorsal horn long distance projection neurons, dorsal column postsynaptic (DCPS) neurons, have been shown to receive contacts from 5HT-LI varicosities (Nishikawa et al., 1983). Following retrograde HRP labeling of the DCPS neurons, most DCPS neurons were observed at the light-microscopic level to be contacted on their somata and proximal dendrites by 5HT-LI varicosities. At the EM level, the labeled varicosities were observed to form symmetrical synapses on the retrogradely labeled DCPS neurons. Since the DCPS population of neurons is known to contain almost equal numbers of nociceptive and non-nociceptive neurons (Lu et al., 1983), the frequency of 5HT contacts on DCPS neurons suggests that 5HT modulates the output of both classes of neurons.

In addition to 5HT contacts on dorsal horn neurons which are part of long distance projection

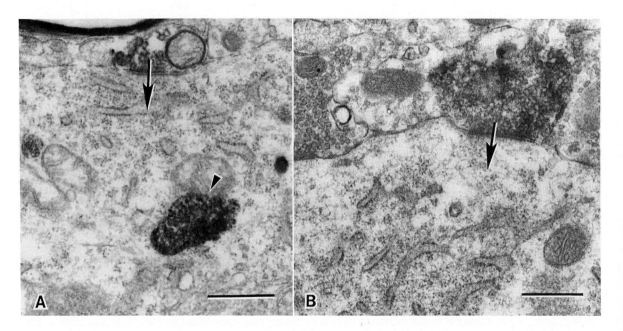

Fig. 6. 5HT-LI varicosities contacting thalamic projection neurons typically formed a symmetrical type of synaptic specialization (arrows). They contained a mixture of oval agranular and a few dense core vesicles (not illustrated). Retrograde HRP reaction product is visible in (A) (arrowhead). The morphological features of 5HT-LI varicosities were similar in lamina I (A) and lamina V (B). Magnification in (A) × 39 000; in (B) × 36 000. Scale bar represents 0.5 μm.

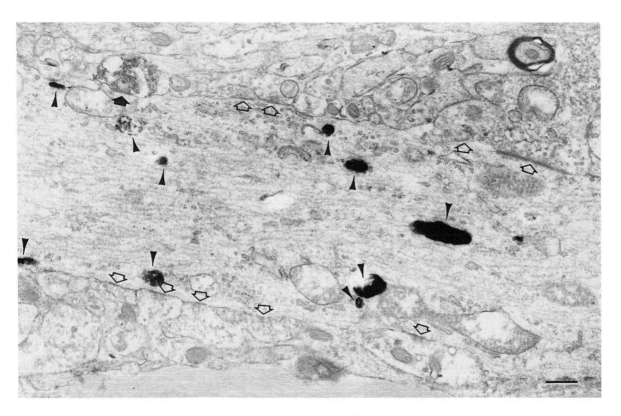

Fig. 7. A 5HT-LI varicosity (filled arrow) contacts a dentritic shaft in lamina I of monkey cervical enlargement. The dendrite is from the proximal portion of a thalamic projection neuron, labeled with retrogradely transported HRP (arrowheads). Numerous unlabeled vesicle-containing profiles (open arrows) also contact the dendrite. Magnification × 21 330. Scale bar represents 0.5 μm.

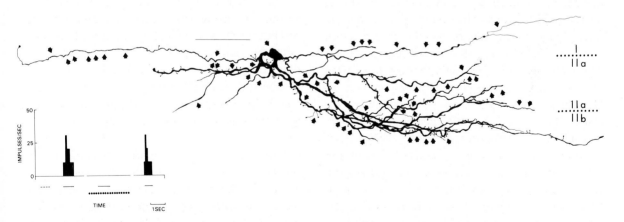

Fig. 8. An intracellular HRP-filled nociceptive-specific stalked cell is illustrated using the camera lucida technique. Tissue sections containing the neuron were stained for 5HT immunoreactivity. The location of 5HT-LI contacts on the neuron are indicated with arrows. Although many dendritic spines are found on the neuron, all 5HT-LI contacts occurred on dendritic shafts. Lamina borders are indicated by dotted lines at right. The response of the neuron to peripheral stimulation (innocuous touch, dashed lines; noxious pinch, solid lines) is indicated at the left. NRM stimulation (dots) abolished the neuron's response to noxious pinch. Scale bar represents 50 μm. (From Miletic et al., 1984.)

pathways, 5HT input to local circuit neurons has also been investigated. Using the intracellular HRP method combined with immunocytochemistry (Fig. 8), stalked cells, a morphologically separable subpopulation of local circuit neurons in lamina II, were observed to be contacted by numerous 5HT-LI varicosities (average of 63) (Hoffert et al., 1983; Miletic et al., 1984). Islet cells, a distinct morphological cell type in lamina II, were found to receive few contacts (average of 25 and 8). The observation of potential 5HT innervation could be correlated with the effects of nucleus raphe magnus (NRM) stimulation. The responses of stalked cells to noxious stimulation were suppressed during NRM stimulation (Fig. 8) while no effect was observed on the responses of islet cells (Miletic et al., 1984).

A subpopulation of enkephalin immunoreactive (ENK-LI) neurons in the superficial dorsal horn have also been shown to receive contacts from axonal varicosities which take up [^{3}H]5HT (Glazer and Basbaum, 1984). It is likely that most of these ENK-LI neurons are local circuit neurons rather than long-distance projection neurons (Basbaum, 1982; Nahin, 1987, 1988; Nahin and Micevych, 1986). The observation of 5HT input onto enkephalin neurons provides an anatomical substrate for descending monoaminergic modulation of dorsal horn opioid neurons. The opioid neurons may in turn modulate the output of dorsal horn projection neurons (Ruda et al., 1984). Although some excitatory effects of 5HT iontophoresis have been observed in the dorsal horn, the predominant effect appears to be inhibitory (Willcockson et al., 1984a; Randic and Yu, 1976; Belcher et al., 1978; Headley et al., 1978; Jordan et al., 1979). ENK iontophoresis likewise produces inhibition (Zieglgansberger and Tulloch, 1979; Willcockson et al., 1984b). The observation of 5HT input to ENK neurons suggests that activation of a descending 5HT pathway would result in inhibition of some ENK neurons. This effect may be tonically present. Recent evidence suggests this possibility. *In situ* hybridization histochemistry demonstrates an increase in enkephalin mRNA following spinal cord transection. Immunocytochemical analysis of ENK immunoreactivity also suggests an elevation following transection (Ruda, unpublished observations).

Colocalization of neurochemicals in descending axons

The identification of several different peptides colocalized with 5HT in the brain stem raphe nuclei, raises the possibility that some of these neurons contribute afferents to the dorsal horn. 5HT neurons have been shown to co-localize SP, ENK, CCK and TRH (Johansson et al., 1981; Hökfelt et al., 1978; Lovick and Hunt, 1983; Glazer et al., 1981; Hunt and Lovick, 1982; Mantyh and Hunt, 1984). Experiments employing the 5HT neurotoxins 5,6- or 5,7-dihydroxytryptamine demonstrate a loss of 5HT, SP, and TRH in the spinal cord as assayed by radioimmunoassay and immunocytochemistry (Hökfelt et al., 1978; Björklund et al., 1979; Singer et al., 1979; Johansson et al., 1981; Gilbert et al., 1982). In the ventral horn, almost all of the SP and all of the TRH immunoreactivity disappeared following neurotoxin treatment. In the dorsal horn, an approximate 25% decrease in SP immunoreactivity was detected. Since the neurotoxin is likely to be specific for axons containing 5HT and a peptide rather than those containing a peptide alone, these data provide evidence for co-localized axons descending to the spinal cord. These studies clearly demonstrate the presence of co-localized 5HT-LI/SP-LI axons in the ventral horn; however, their potential role in dorsal horn circuitry is less defined.

Using a double immunofluorescence staining protocol with species-specific antisera, a direct demonstration of co-localized 5HT and peptide in individual spinal cord axon terminals has been made. Colocalization of 5HT and SP has been examined in the spinal cord of the rat (Wessendorf and Elde, 1987) and cat (Tashiro and Ruda, 1988). In both species, the vast majority of axons containing the co-localized neurochemicals were found in the ventral horn, most often associated with the motoneuronal cell groups. In the dorsal horn, the density of co-localized axons varied in the different dorsal horn laminae. Few were found in laminae I and II. In laminae V and VI they were observed more often than in the superficial layers, but still represented only a small percentage of the populations of either 5HT-LI or SP-LI axons (Fig. 9).

The infrequency of co-localized 5HT-LI/SP-LI axons in the dorsal horn provides some insight into the brain stem origin of 5HT neurons involved in dorsal horn circuitry. Co-localization of 5HT-LI/SP-LI is found in neurons throughout the nuclei raphe magnus, pallidus and obscurus (Hökfelt et al., 1978) but is most common in the more caudal part of the brain stem complex (Ruda et al., 1986). The brain stem neurons co-localizing 5HT-LI/SP-LI are unlikely candidates to play a major role in dorsal horn function, since axons co-localizing 5HT-LI/SP-LI are found infrequently in the dorsal horn. They are more likely at the spinal level to be involved in ventral horn function. Since the neurons which co-localized 5HT-LI/SP-LI and those which do not are intermingled in the raphe nuclei, the observations on the differential laminar distribution in the spinal cord may provide a

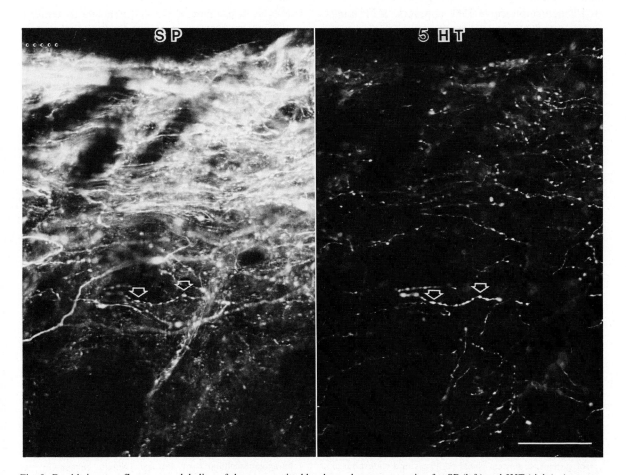

Fig. 9. Double immunofluorescence labeling of the same sagittal lumbar enlargement section for SP (left) and 5HT (right). An example of a 5HT-LI/SP-LI axon is indicated by arrows. The lamina I dorsal column border (dots) is marked for orientation. Scale bar represents 50 μm. (From Tashiro and Ruda, 1988).

method for differentiating neurons more likely to be involved in sensory than in motor function at spinal levels.

Conclusions

In summary, descending 5HT modulation of dorsal horn neuronal activity exhibits a predominantly postsynaptic mechanism which occurs at a variety of sites. 5HT contacts are found on several different populations of long distance projection neurons as well as interneurons (Table II). There is no strong morphological support for 5HT presynaptic effects on primary afferent axons. Since spinomesencephalic, spinothalamic and DCPS neurons receive 5HT contacts, 5HT innervation of projection pathways appears to be a common feature of monoaminergic modulation of dorsal horn neural circuits. The different classes of projection neurons receiving 5HT inputs suggest that 5HT plays a role in modulating output systems having a diversity of function.

Acknowledgements

I would like to acknowledge my colleagues at the Neurobiology and Anesthesiology Branch of the National Institute of Dental Research whose work over the past several years has formed the basis for this review. I would also like to thank Ms. J.J. Johannes for her help in preparing this manuscript.

References

Basbaum, A.I. (1982) Anatomical substrates for the descending control of nociception. In B. Sjölund and A. Björklund (Eds.), *Brain Stem Control of Spinal Mechanisms*, Elsevier, Amsterdam, pp. 119–133.

Basbaum, A.I. and Fields, H.L. (1978) Endogenous pain control mechanisms: review and hypothesis. *Ann. Neurol.*, 4: 451–462.

Basbaum, A.I. and Fields, H.L. (1984) Endogenous pain control systems: brainstem spinal pathways and endorphin circuitry. *Annu. Rev. Neurosci.*, 7: 309–338.

Basbaum, A.I., Zahs, K., Lord, B.A.P. and Lakos, S. (1987) The fibre caliber of 5-HT immunoreactive axons in the dor-

solateral funiculus of the rat and cat. *Somatosensory Res.,* 5: 177–185.

Belcher, G., Ryall, R.W. and Schaffner, R. (1978) The differential effects of 5-hydroxytryptamine, noradrenaline and raphe stimulation on nociceptive and non-nociceptive dorsal horn interneurones in the cat. *Brain Res.*, 151: 307–321.

Björklund, A. and Skagerberg, G. (1979) Evidence for a major spinal cord projection from the diencephalic A11 dopamine cell group in the rat using transmitter-specific fluorescent retrograde tracing. *Brain Res.*, 117: 170–175.

Björklund, A.J., Emson, P.C., Gilbert, R.F.T. and Skagerberg, G. (1979) Further evidence for the possible coexistence of 5-hydroxytryptamine and substance P in medullary raphe neurons of rat brain. *Br. J. Pharmacol.*, 66: 112–113.

Bowker, R.M., Westlund, K.N., Sullivan, M.C., Wilber, J.F. and Coulter, J.D. (1982) Transmitters of the raphe-spinal complex: immunocytochemical studies. *Peptides*, 3: 291–298.

Dahlström, A. and Fuxe, K. (1964) Evidence for the existence of monoamine-containing neurons in the central nervous system. I. Demonstration of monoamines in the cell bodies of brain stem neurons. *Acta Physiol. Scand.*, 62, Suppl. 232: 1–55.

Dahlström, A. and Fuxe, K. (1965) Evidence for the existence of monoamine-containing neurons in the central nervous system. II. Experimentally induced changes in the intraneuronal amine levels of bulbospinal neuron systems. *Acta Physiol. Scand.*, 64, Suppl. 247: 7–36.

Dubner, R. and Bennett, G.J. (1983) Spinal and trigeminal mechanisms of nociception. *Annu. Rev. Neurosci.*, 6: 381–418.

Gibson, S.J., Polak, J.M., Bloom, S.R. and Wall, P.D. (1981) The distribution of nine peptides in rat spinal cord with special emphasis on the substantia gelatinosa and on the area around the central canal (lamina X). *J. Comp. Neurol.*, 201: 65–79.

Gilbert, R.F.T., Emson, P.C., Hunt, S.P., Bennett, G.W., Marsden, C.A., Sandberg, B.E.B., Steinbusch, H.W.M. and Verhofstad, A.A.J. (1982) The effects of monoamine neurotoxins on peptides in the rat spinal cord. *Neuroscience*, 7: 69–87.

Glazer, E.J. and Basbaum, A.I. (1984) Axons which take up [^{3}H]serotonin are presynaptic to enkephalin immunoreactive neurons in cat dorsal horn. *Brain Res.*, 298: 386–391.

Glazer, E.J. and Ross, L.L. (1980) Localization of noradrenergic terminals in sympathetic preganglionic nuclei of the rat: demonstration by immunocytochemical localization of dopamine-β-hydroxylase. *Brain Res.*, 185: 39–49.

Glazer, E.J., Steinbusch, H., Verhofstad, A. and Basbaum, A.I. (1981) Serotonin neurons in nucleus raphe dorsalis and paragigantocellularis of the cat contain enkephalin. *J. Physiol. (Paris)* 77: 241–245.

Headley, P.M., Duggan, A.W. and Griersmith, B.T. (1978) Selective reduction by noradrenaline and 5-hydroxytryptamine of nociceptive responses of cat dorsal horn neurones. *Brain Res.*, 145: 185–189.

Helke, C.J., Neil, J.L., Massari, V.J. and Loewy, A.D. (1982) Substance P neurons project from the ventral medulla to the intermediolateral cell column and ventral horn in the rat. *Brain Res.*, 243: 147–152.

Hoffert, M.J., Miletic, V., Ruda, M.A. and Dubner, R. (1983) Immunocytochemical identification of serotonin axonal contacts on characterized neurons in laminae I and II of the cat dorsal horn. *Brain Res.*, 267: 361–364.

Hökfelt, T., Ljungdahl, A., Terenius, L., Elde, R. and Nilsson, G. (1977) Immunohistochemical analysis of peptide pathways possibly related to pain and analgesia: enkephalin and substance P. *Proc. Natl. Acad. Sci. USA*, 74: 3081–3085.

Hökfelt, T., Ljungdahl, A., Steinbusch, H., Verhofstad, A.N., Nilsson, G., Brodin, E., Pernow, B. and Goldstein, M. (1978) Immunohistochemical evidence of substance P-like immunoreactivity in some 5-hydroxytryptamine containing neurons in the rat central nervous system. *Neuroscience*, 3: 517–538.

Hökfelt, T., Phillipson, O. and Goldstein, M. (1979a) Evidence for a dopaminergic pathway in the rat descending from the A11 cell group to the spinal cord. *Acta Physiol. Scand.*, 107: 393–395.

Hökfelt, T., Terenius, L., Kuypers, H.G.J.M. and Dann, O. (1979b) Evidence for enkephalin immunoreactive neurons in the medulla oblongata projecting to the spinal cord. *Neurosci. Lett.* 14: 55–60.

Hunt, S.P. and Lovick, T.A. (1982) The distribution of serotonin, metenkephalin and β-lipotropin-like immunoreactivity in neuronal perikarya of the cat brain stem. *Neurosci. Lett.*, 30: 139–145.

Hunt, S.P., Kelly, J.S., Emson, P.C., Kimmel, J.R., Miller, R.J. and Wu, J.-Y. (1981) An immunohistochemical study of neuronal populations containing neuropeptides or gamma-aminobutyrate within the superficial layers of the rat dorsal horn. *Neuroscience*, 6: 1883–1898.

Hylden, J.L.K., Ruda, M.A., Hayashi, H. and Dubner, R. (1985) Descending serotonergic fibers in the dorsolateral and ventral funiculi of cat spinal cord. *Neurosci. Lett.*, 62: 299–304.

Hylden, J.L.K., Hayashi, H., Ruda, M.A. and Dubner, R. (1986) Serotonin innervation of physiologically identified lamina I projection neurons. *Brain Res.*, 370: 401–404.

Johansson, O., Hökfelt, T., Pernow, B., Jeffcoate, S.L., White, N., Steinbusch, H.W.M., Verhofstad, A.A.J., Emson, P.C. and Spindel, E. (1981) Immunohistochemical support for three putative transmitters in one neuron: coexistence of 5-hydroxytryptamine, substance P- and thyrotropin releasing hormone-like immunoreactivity medullary neurons projecting to the spinal cord. *Neuroscience*, 6: 1857–1881.

Jordan, L.M., Kenshalo, Jr., D.R., Martin, R.F., Haber, L.H. and Willis, W.D. (1979) Two populations of spinothalamic

tract neurons with opposite responses to 5-hydroxytryptamine. *Brain Res.*, 164: 342–346.

Kanazawa, I., Sutoo, D., Oshima, I. and Saito, S. (1979) Effect of transection on choline acetyltransferase, thyrotropin releasing hormone and substance P in the cat cervical spinal cord. *Neurosci. Lett.*, 13: 325–330.

Kojima, M., Takeuchi, Y., Goto, M. and Sano, Y. (1982) Immunohistochemical study on the distribution of serotonin fibers in the spinal cord of the dog. *Cell Tiss. Res.*, 226: 477–491.

Kojima, M., Takeuchi, Y., Goto, M. and Sano, Y. (1983) Immunohistochemical localization of serotonin fibers and terminals in the spinal cord of the monkey *(Macca fuscata)*. *Cell Tiss. Res.*, 229: 23–36.

LaMotte, C.C. and DeLanerolle, N.C. (1983) Ultrastructure of chemically defined neuron systems in the dorsal horn of the monkey. III. Serotonin immunoreactivity. *Brain Res.*, 274: 65–77.

LaMotte, C.C., Johns, D.R. and DeLanerolle, N.C. (1982) Immunohistochemical evidence of indolamine neurons in monkey spinal cord. *J. Comp. Neurol.*, 206: 359–370.

Lang, R.E., Heil, J., Ganten, D., Hermann, K., Rascher, W. and Unger, Th. (1983) Effects of lesions in the paraventricular nucleus of the hypothalamus on vasopressin and oxytocin contents in brainstem and spinal cord of rat. *Brain Res.*, 260: 326–329.

Light, A.R., Kavookjian, A.M. and Petrusz, P. (1983) The ultrastructure and synaptic connections of serotonin-immunoreactive terminals in spinal laminae I and II. *Somatosens. Res.*, 1: 33–50.

Lovick, T.A. and Hunt, S.P. (1983) Substance P-immunoreactive and serotonin-containing neurones in the ventral brainstem of the cat. *Neurosci. Lett.*, 36: 223–228.

Lu, G.-W., Bennett, G.J., Nishikawa, N., Hoffert, M.J. and Dubner, R. (1983) Extra- and intracellular recordings from dorsal column postsynaptic spinomedullary neurons in the cat. *Exp. Neurol.*, 82: 456–477.

Mantyh, P.W. and Hunt, S.P. (1984) Evidence for cholecystokinin-like immunoreactive neurons in the rat medulla oblongata which project to the spinal cord. *Brain Res.*, 291: 49–54.

Maxwell, D.J., Leranth, C. and Verhofstad, A.A.J. (1983) Fine structure of serotonin-containing axons in the marginal zone of the rat spinal cord. *Brain Res.*, 266: 253–259.

Miletic, V., Hoffert, M.J., Ruda, M.A., Dubner, R. and Shigenaga, Y. (1984) Serotonergic axonal contacts on identified cat spinal dorsal horn neurons and their correlation with nucleus raphe magnus stimulation. *J. Comp. Neurol.*, 228: 129–141.

Millan, M.J., Millan, M.H., Czlonkowski, A. and Herz, A. (1984) Vasopressin and oxytocin in the rat spinal cord: distribution and origins in comparison to (Met)enkephalin, dynorphin and related opioids and their irresponsiveness to stimuli modulating neurohypophyseal secretion. *Neuro-*

140

science, 13: 179 – 188.

Nahin, R.L. (1987) Immunocytochemical identification of long ascending peptidergic neurons contributing to the spinoreticular tract in the rat. *Neuroscience*, 23: 859 – 896.

Nahin, R.L. (1988) Immunocytochemical identification of long ascending peptidergic lumbar spinal neurons terminating in either the medial or lateral thalamus in the rat. *Brain Res.*, 443: 345 – 349.

Nahin, R.L. and Micevych, P.E. (1986) A long ascending pathway of enkephalin-like immunoreactive spinoreticular neurons in the rat. *Neurosci. Lett.*, 65: 271 – 276.

Newton, B.N., Maley, B.E. and Hamill, R.W. (1986) Immunohistochemical demonstration of serotonin neurons in autonomic regions of the rat spinal cord. *Brain Res.*, 376: 155 – 163.

Nishikawa, N., Bennett, G.J., Ruda, M.A., Lu, G.-W. and Dubner, R. (1983) Immunocytochemical evidence for a serotonergic innervation of dorsal column postsynaptic neurons in cat and monkey. *Neuroscience*, 10: 1333 – 1340.

Petrusz, P., Sar, M., Ordronneau, P. and DiMeo, P. (1976) Specificity in immunocytochemical staining. *J. Histochem. Cytochem.* 24: 1110 – 1115.

Petrusz, P., Sar, M., Ordronneau, P. and DiMeo, P. (1977) Reply to the letter of Swaab et al. Can specificity ever be proved in immunocytochemical staining? *J. Histochem. Cytochem.*, 25: 390 – 391.

Randic, M., and Yu, H.H. (1976) Effects of 5-hydroxytryptamine and bradykinin on cat dorsal horn neurones activated by noxious stimuli. *Brain Res.*, 111: 197 – 203.

Ruda, M.A. and Coffield, J. (1983) Light and ultrastructural immunocytochemical localization of serotonin synapses on primate spinothalamic tract neurons. *Soc. Neurosci. Abstr.*, 9: 1.

Ruda, M.A., Coffield, J. and Steinbusch, H.W.M. (1982) Immunocytochemical analysis of serotonergic axons in laminae I and II of the lumbar spinal cord of the cat. *J. Neurosci.*, 2: 1660 – 1671.

Ruda, M.A., Coffield, J. and Dubner, R. (1984) Demonstration of postsynaptic opioid modulation of thalamic projection neurons by the combined techniques of retrograde horseradish peroxidase and enkephalin immunocytochemistry. *J. Neurosci.*, 4: 2117 – 2132.

Ruda, M.A., Bennett, G.J. and Dubner, R. (1986) Neurochemistry and neural circuitry in the dorsal horn. In P.C. Emson, M. Rossor and M. Tohyama (Eds.), *Peptides and Neurological Disease, Progress in Brain Research, Vol. 66*, Elsevier Science Publishers, Amsterdam, pp. 216 – 268.

Singer, E., Sperk, G., Placheta, P. and Leeman, S.E. (1979) Reduction of substance P levels in the ventral cervical spinal cord of the rat after cisternal 5,7-dihydroxytryptamine injec-

tion. *Brain Res.*, 174: 362 – 365.

Skagerberg, G., Björklund, A., Lindvall, O. and Schmidt, R.H. (1982) Origin and termination of the diencephalospinal dopamine system in the rat. *Brain Res. Bull.*, 9: 237 – 244.

Steinbusch, H.W.M. (1981) Distribution of serotonin immunoreactivity in the central nervous system of the rat — cell bodies and terminals. *Neuroscience*, 6: 557 – 618.

Stevens, R.T., Hodge, Jr., C.J. and Apkarian, A.V. (1982) Kölliker-Fuse nucleus: the principal source of pontine catecholaminergic cells projecting to the lumbar spinal cord of cat. *Brain Res.*, 239: 589 – 594.

Swanson, L.W. and McKellar, S. (1979) The distribution of oxytocin and neurophysin stained fibers in the spinal cord of the rat and monkey. *J. Comp. Neurol.*, 188: 87 – 106.

Tashiro, T. and Ruda, M.A. (1988) Immunocytochemical identification of axons containing coexistent serotonin and substance P in the cat lumbar spinal cord. *Peptides,* 9: 383 – 391.

Wessendorf, M.W. and Elde, R.P. (1987) The coexistence of serotonin- and substance P-like immunoreactivity in the spinal cord of the rat as shown by immunofluorescent double-labeling. *J. Neurosci.*, 7: 2352 – 2363.

Westlund, K.N. and Coulter, J.D. (1980) Descending projections of the locus coeruleus and subcoeruleus/medial parabrachial nuclei in monkey: axonal transport studies and dopamine-β-hydroxylase immunocytochemistry. *Brain Res. Rev.*, 2: 235 – 264.

Westlund, K.N., Bowker, R.M., Ziegler, M.G. and Coulter, J.D. (1981) Origins of spinal noradrenergic pathways demonstrated by retrograde transport of antibody to dopamine-β-hydroxylase. *Neurosci. Lett.*, 25: 243 – 249.

Westlund, K.N., Bowker, R.M., Ziegler, M.G. and Coulter, J.D. (1982) Descending noradrenergic projections and their spinal terminations. In H.G.J.M. Kuypers and G.F. Martin (Eds.), *Descending Pathways to the Spinal Cord, Progress in Brain Research, Vol. 57*, Elsevier, Amsterdam, pp. 219 – 238.

Willcockson, W.S., Chung, J.M., Hori, Y., Lee, K.H. and Willis, W.D. (1984a) Effects of iontophoretically released amino acids and amines on primate spinothalamic tract cells. *J. Neurosci.*, 4: 732 – 740.

Willcockson, W.S., Chung, J.M., Hori, Y., Lee, K.H. and Willis, W.D. (1984b) Effects of iontophoretically released peptides on primate spinothalamic tract cells. *J. Neurosci.*, 4: 741 – 750.

Zieglgangsberger, W. and Tulloch, I.F. (1979) The effects of methionine- and leucine-enkephalin on spinal neurones of the cat. *Brain Res.*, 167: 53 – 64.

H.L. Fields and J.-M. Besson (Eds.)
Progress in Brain Research, Vol. 77
© 1988 Elsevier Science Publishers B.V. (Biomedical Division)

CHAPTER 6

Stimulation-produced analgesia in animals: behavioural investigations

Jean-Louis Oliveras and Jean-Marie Besson

INSERM, U. 161, Unité de Recherches de Neurophysiologie Pharmacologique, 2 rue d'Alésia, 75014 Paris, France

Introduction

Since the initial observations of Reynolds (1969), showing that rats could support severe painful interventions such as laparotomies during and after periaqueductal gray matter (PAG) electrical stimulation, this type of 'stimulation-produced analgesia' (SPA) has been extensively studied using numerous behavioural, anatomical, electrophysiological, biochemical and neuropharmacological techniques in various species such as cat, rat and monkey (see reviews in: Liebeskind et al., 1976; Mayer and Price, 1976; Basbaum and Fields, 1978, 1984; Mayer, 1979; Besson et al., 1981, 1982).

Despite the fact that SPA has been reported from various regions such as the locus coeruleus (Segal and Sandberg, 1977), the habenula (Benabid and Mahieux, 1984; Cohen and Melzack, 1986), the lateral hypothalamus (Carr and Loons, 1982), the nucleus tractus solitarius (Lohof et al., 1987), the septal preoptic area (Schmidek et al., 1971), the pontine parabrachial region (Desalles et al., 1985), the ventral tegmental area (Moreau et al., 1984) and the prefrontal cortex (Hardy, 1985), the most extensive studies have been performed at the level of the mesencephalic PAG and the more caudal medullary region including the nucleus raphe magnus (NRM) and its immediate vicinity. Anatomical and electrophysiological studies have also shown that SPA obtained from the PAG and raphe systems is at least in part sustained by the so-called 'descending control systems' which can exert a powerful modulatory effect upon nociceptive transmission at the spinal and trigeminal levels (see Willis, this volume).

Although there is a general agreement that PAG and medullary raphe stimulation produces SPA in animals, and sufficient data to support the reality of such a system in the brain, the use of this type of stimulation in patients suffering from chronic pain is controversial (Meyerson, this volume), after the initial rush of enthusiasm of the different neurosurgical teams involved in this approach (Adams, 1976; Gybels et al., 1976; Hosobuchi et al., 1977, 1979; Richardson and Akil, 1977a,b).

This paper is essentially an overview of current knowledge of the behavioural aspects of SPA in animals and considers some of the pitfalls arising from brain stem electrical stimulation which could partly explain some controversies between different neurosurgical groups.

SPA induced by PAG stimulation

In rat and cat, many studies have shown that moderate electrical stimulation of PAG can produce antinociceptive effects as judged behaviourally (i.e., disappearance of reflex and gross behavioural reactions to painful stimuli). However, in these species, and in monkey and humans, the reliability of 'analgesia' and the exact localization of the stimulating targets are still a subject of

142

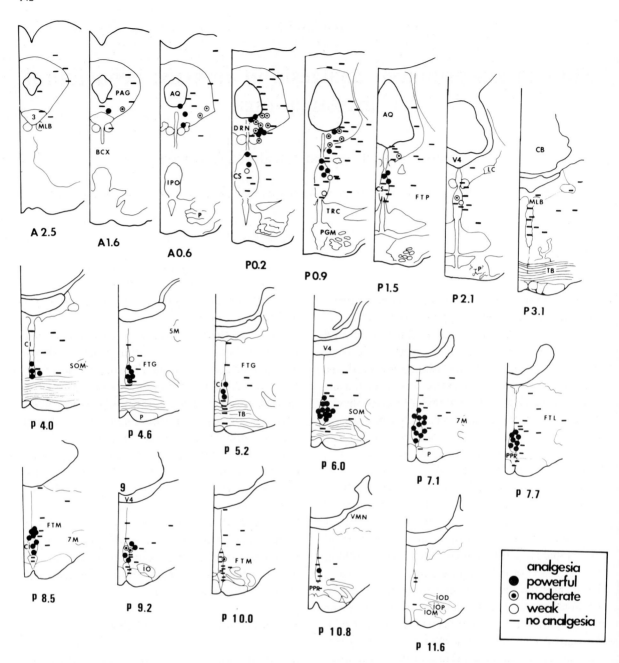

Fig. 1. Localization of stimulation-produced analgesia (SPA) efficacious sites throughout the mesencephalon and the medulla in the awake, freely moving cat. The most powerful analgesic effects were triggered by stimulation of nuclei raphe dorsalis (DRN), centralis superior (CS) and centralis inferior (CI, nucleus raphe magnus). Abbreviations refer to the stereotactic atlas of Berman.

much discussion. We will consider below the data obtained in cat and rat.

SPA from PAG stimulation in the cat

In parallel with many studies at the PAG level in the rat (see below), we performed from 1972 to 1978, in the cat, a very extensive mapping which included more than 300 stimulation sites spread over the brain stem, from the mesencephalon (fourth nucleus) to the medulla (inferior olive) (Fig. 1). This initial mapping was based on gauging the gross behavioural reactions in response to strong pinches applied to various body regions from the head to the tail (Guilbaud et al., 1972; Liebeskind et al., 1973; Oliveras et al., 1974a, 1979). Any moderate (up to 100 μA) central electrical stimulation which attenuated or suppressed all the reactions to pinch (e.g. vocalization, withdrawal, biting, flight, etc.) with no other observable behavioural modification due to the central stimulation itself was considered to be antinociceptive. Fig. 1 illustrates that, at the mesencephalic level in the cat, the analgesic sites were restricted to the ventral PAG. Indeed, stimulation of dorsal and dorsolateral PAG did not trigger analgesia but, by contrast, induced aversive reactions such as escape or coordinated attacks which indicate intense emotional disturbances. In the mesencephalic reticular formation adjacent to the PAG, no analgesia was obtained, and central stimulation occasionally triggered emotional effects but mainly motor disturbances. A closer examination of effective sites in the cat ventral PAG reveals that the main target for SPA is, in fact, the dorsal raphe nucleus (DRN). Indeed, at this level, we found powerful analgesia (total suppression of nocifensive manifestations during central stimulation) and, sometimes, moderate analgesia (nocifensive reactions strongly attenuated but still present during central stimulation). It is noteworthy that sites which triggered moderate analgesia were also found outside the DRN, in the ventrolateral aspect of the PAG.

Subsequently, we performed other tests such as tooth pulp electrical stimulation which allowed the quantification of cat SPA and the assessment of the potency of SPA on the trigeminal system (Oliveras et al., 1974b, 1977, 1979). In Fig. 2, the effects of central stimulation on the tooth pulp induced jaw-opening reflex (JOR, the analog of a nociceptive spinal reflex) is shown. We observed that DRN stimulation provoked robust increases of the JOR threshold (5 to 10 times). As with the pinch test, no effects upon the tooth pulp induced JOR were triggered during the stimulation of dorsolateral PAG, whereas strong emotional reactions did appear.

In summary in the cat, the combination of the pinch test and tooth pulp stimulation data clearly establish the reliability of SPA elicited from the ventral and ventrolateral PAG, since at this level, central stimulation strongly attenuates nociceptive reflexes and more integrated forms of nocifensive behaviour with no other disturbances. These pioneering data were confirmed in the same species using other tests such as subcutaneous formalin (Dubuisson and Melzack, 1977) and shuttle-box avoidance coupled with radial nerve electrical stimulation (Gebhart and Toleikis, 1978).

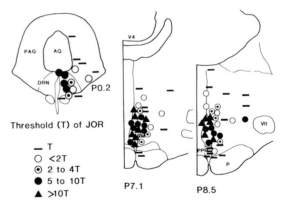

Fig. 2. Effects of periaqueductal gray (PAG) and nucleus raphe magnus (NRM) central stimulations upon the threshold of the jaw-opening reflex (JOR) in the freely moving cat. Robust increases of the JOR threshold (5 to 10 times reference threshold, T) were obtained during stimulation of DRN and NRM. Note that at NRM level massive threshold increases were frequently observed (more than 10 times, 100 or 200, even) as compared to DRN. Abbreviations refer to Fig. 1.

SPA from PAG stimulation in the rat

In the rat, SPA from the PAG has been extensively studied and there are important interspecies differences from the cat. The numerous studies performed in the rat from 1969 to 1982 (Reynolds, 1969; Mayer et al., 1971; Akil and Mayer, 1972; Mayer and Liebeskind, 1974; Akil and Liebeskind, 1975; Basbaum et al., 1976; Giesler et al., 1976; Morrow and Casey, 1976; Pert and Walter, 1976; Soper, 1976; Yaksh et al., 1976a; Lewis and Gebhart, 1977a,b; Yeung et al., 1977; Rhodes and Liebeskind, 1978; Dennis et al., 1980; Cannon et al., 1982) clearly indicate that analgesic effects can be induced by stimulation of areas throughout the PAG. In addition, with the exception of the study of Basbaum et al. (1976), few ineffective stimulation sites have been described; in this latter study, ineffective areas were generally found in the dorsal and lateral PAG. As already mentioned in the cat, we found that stimulation of the dorsal and lateral parts of the PAG produced behavioural effects, notably aversive reactions. These dramatic behavioural responses have not been clearly described in the rat by the main groups studying SPA. These discrepancies between cat and rat seem surprising (see Kiser et al., 1978), since it is well known that stimulation of the dorsal PAG, in the rat, can also trigger behavioural effects which have been used as a model of aversive reactions (Olds and Olds, 1962; Kiser et al., 1978; Schmitt and Karli, 1980).

In our opinion the more extensive analgesic zone in the rat compared to the cat could be due to the fact that several of these studies have used restrained animals, a condition which could mask the marked side effects induced by stimulation of the dorsal PAG. In order to check this hypothesis, we have reexamined the effects of SPA in the rat with two major objectives (Fardin et al., 1984a): (a) to define, as accurately as possible, the effective analgesic zones based on an extensive number of sites of stimulation, and (b) to consider, in freely moving animals, the possible side effects of central stimulation. Analgesia was evaluated (during central stimulation) by measuring the change of the vocalization threshold induced by electrical tail shocks or by considering the reaction of the animal to pinch.

The most striking result of our study, carried out on 129 freely moving rats, was that in order to obtain antinociceptive effects from all parts of the PAG as has been previously described in the rat, it is necessary to apply intensities of central stimulation which also trigger other marked behavioral responses (Fig. 3, II). Except for two studies these concomitant behavioral reactions have not been reported by previous investigators (Pert and Walter, 1976; Yeung et al., 1977).

Using intensities of PAG stimulation which did not induce such side effects (Fig. 3, I) very few effective analgesic sites were found (21/129 sites of which 14/83 were strictly located in the ventral PAG). In this condition, it was possible to define two 'pure analgesic regions', both located in the ventral PAG: one centered on the dorsomedial part of the DRN and the other one situated in the ventrolateral PAG. No change of nociceptive threshold was observed when stimulating the dorsal and dorsolateral parts of the PAG or adjacent structures. In fact, in some rats, an increase in pain reactivity was noted.

When the intensity of central stimulation (applied to the various parts of the PAG) was increased, some stereotyped 'behavioural responses' occurred depending on the location of the stimulation site: motor effects (gnawing, rotation or tremor) in the ventral PAG and aversive effects (flight, jumping and, on accasions, distress vocalizations) in the dorsal, dorsolateral PAG and in the ventral region just surrounding the cerebral aqueduct. Under these conditions, analgesia was obtained from practically the entire PAG, the vocalization threshold being increased dramatically on occasions.

It must be emphasized that antinociceptive effects associated with other obvious behavioural manifestations (aversive ones) were also obtained from sites located outside the PAG (colliculi and tectum adjacent to the dorsal and dorsolateral PAG).

Although the stereotyped behavioural reactions

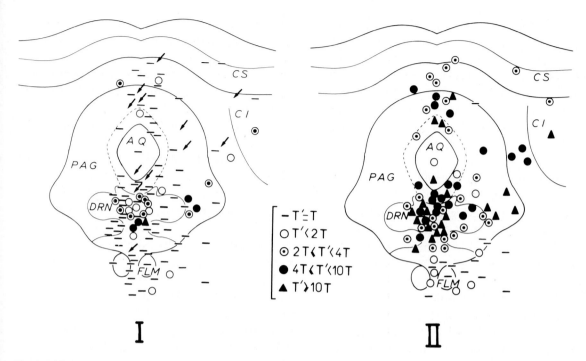

Fig. 3. Differential effects of PAG stimulation on the vocalization threshold induced by electrical tail shocks according to the absence (I) or to the presence (II) of additional noticeable behavioural reactions in the freely moving rat (T′, vocalization threshold before central stimulation; T′, vocalization threshold during central stimulation). Without any behavioural manifestations due to the central stimulation itself, very few analgesic sites were found, which were almost exclusively located to the DRN (ventromedial part) and a more lateral zone.

have generally not been described by previous investigators studying SPA in the rat, our observations agree with much of the data previously reported in the literature. It is well established that stimulation of dorsal and dorsolateral parts of the PAG and the adjacent dorsal midbrain tectum induces behavioral reactions which include intensive 'emotional effects' in the rat (Olds and Olds, 1962; Valenstein, 1965; Gardner and Malmo, 1969; Wolfe et al., 1971; Schmitt et al., 1974; Kiser and Lebovitz, 1975; Waldbillig, 1975), the cat (Spiegel et al., 1954; Hunsperger, 1956, 1959; Wada et al., 1970; Oliveras et al., 1974a) and the monkey (Delgado, 1955; Jürgens, 1976). The first investigations of the effects of stimulation of the mesencephalic and diencephalic central gray noted the 'unpleasant' nature of the induced effects (Magoun et al., 1937; Kelly et al., 1946). In man, feelings of anxiety, distress, panic and even pain have been

described during stimulation of these regions (Nashold et al., 1969; Nashold et al., 1974; Cosyns and Gybels, 1979). In animals, these behavioural reactions which have been described as 'fear-like' or 'pain-like', reactions are rather similar to those induced by a peripheral noxious stimulation: avoidance and flight, vocalization, attack or rage reactions, neurovegetative reactions such as pupillary dilatation, piloerection and alterations of cardiac and respiratory frequencies have all been described. Nocifensive reactions have also been observed during stimulation of the PAG (Hunsperger, 1956; Oliveras et al., 1974a) and the colliculi (Spiegel et al., 1954).

Within the ventral part of the PAG as well as in the subjacent mesencephalic reticular formation, the behavioural reactions were generally gnawing and automatic motor effects which did not seem to be aversive. Gnawing has been elicited in the rat either by electrical stimulation of the DRN (Schmitt et al., 1974) or by stimulation of the hypothalamus (Waldbillig, 1975; Roberts, 1980) which projects to the PAG (Wolf and Sutin, 1966; Saper et al., 1979; Mantyh, 1982; and see Holstege, this volume). Moreover, gnawing can also be induced by microinjection of the GABA agonist, muscimol, within the DRN (Przewlocka et al., 1979).

The rotation of the animal, which is rarely described in the cat (Oliveras et al., 1974a) has been noted in the rat during stimulation of the ventrolateral part of the PAG (Kiser et al., 1978) and after unilateral electrolytic or chemical destruction of the DRN (Jacobs et al., 1977; Giambalvo and Snodgrass, 1978; Nicolaou et al., 1979; Blackburn et al., 1980). As the DRN projects to the substantia nigra and striatum (Conrad et al., 1974; Azmitia and Segal, 1979; Dray et al. 1978; Van de Kar and Lorens, 1979; Van der Kooy and Hattori, 1980; Steinbush et al., 1981) some authors have proposed that serotoninergic neurons of the DRN influence the nigrostriatal pathways.

The existence and the importance of these additional behavioural effects which were elicited in association with SPA, call into question the physiological significance of the analgesia triggered by stimulation of all areas of the PAG. Indeed, it is not clear whether these concomitant behavioural manifestations should be considered to be side effects which are independent of SPA. In other words, when the central stimulation simultaneously produces complex marked behavioural reactions, part of the analgesia may result either from an inability of the animal to respond due to a block of motor function as in the case of rotation or tremor, or from stress phenomena which may result from stimulation of aversive regions. This problem is particularly obvious using stimulation sites from which we were able to induce, in the same animals, an increase in pain reactivity during stimulation subthreshold for analgesia and, with stimulation that caused aversive reactions, an 'analgesia' which could have been secondary to stress. Although increases in

pain reactivity from PAG stimulation have, in general, not been reported, our observations are in good agreement with those of Schmidek et al. (1971) who occasionally found, in awake monkeys, decreases in the vocalization threshold during the stimulation of the PAG.

However, we cannot exclude that the differential effects that we observed from the PAG result from the activation of independent neural substrates which could be, in some cases, activated concomitantly by the electrical stimulation. On the basis of this hypothesis, it should be possible to separate the antinociceptive effect from the other behavioural reactions by suitable pharmacological means. Nevertheless, our study indicates that analgesia can be elicited from areas which are not restricted to the PAG but which include other structures such as the colliculi, the intercollicular commissure as well as the tectum immediately adjacent to the lateral PAG. Indeed, in these areas, analgesia could be elicited in some animals by low levels of current intensities and, thus, cannot be a result of current spread to the PAG.

Our results, demonstrating the major role of the ventral PAG in SPA in the rat, are in good agreement with our previous observations in the cat. In contrast, they disagree with some data in the rat reported in the literature, and raise the problem of the possible involvement of 'stress-produced analgesia' and motor disturbances in the appearance of most of the analgesic effects elicited by lateral or dorsolateral PAG stimulation. Consequently, we have extended our investigations (Fardin et al., 1984b) in order to analyse whether the analgesic effects present different characteristics when induced from various PAG areas. For this purpose we studied the degree of both analgesic effects and behavioural reactions as a function of the current intensity of the central stimulation.

Within the ventral PAG the changes in vocalization threshold as a function of the central stimulation intensities illustrate that graded increases in stimulation intensity induce a progressive rise in vocalization threshold. On average, the increase in vocalization threshold appears before the induction of any behavioural reaction when the stimulation sites are located in the dorsomedial subdivision of the dorsal raphe nucleus and in the ventrolateral zone lying under the mesencephalic nucleus of the trigeminal nerve. These results corroborate the existence of analgesic regions distinct from any obvious side effects as previously described. At higher current intensities, we noted an enlargement of effective analgesic areas within the ventral PAG, but the analgesia was always associated with motor effects (mainly rotation). However, several observations strongly suggest that these motor reactions do not interfere with the antinociceptive effects. For example, there was no relationship between the strength of the analgesic effects and the motor disturbances. Furthermore, stimulation of the most ventral part of the PAG or adjacent mesencephalic reticular formation could induce considerable motor effects without any modification in vocalization threshold. In fact, on the basis of the limited extent of the different areas into which we subdivide the ventral PAG, this extension of analgesic areas could result, at least in part, from a spread of current to the pure analgesic zones.

Within the dorsal and dorsolateral PAG as well as in the ventral region just surrounding the aqueduct, analgesia appeared suddenly, was generally less pronounced and was always accompanied by strong aversive reactions. These latter characteristics were also obtained from stimulation of regions located outside the PAG (colliculi, intercollicular commissure and tectum adjacent to the dorsolateral PAG).

Our behavioural observations are reminiscent of pharmacological data which illustrate the heterogeneity of the PAG, especially with regard to its ventral and dorsal areas: (a) although antinociceptive effects have been observed during morphine microinjections within various PAG areas (see Yaksh and Rudy, 1978, for review), Sharpe et al. (1974), in the rat, have shown that small doses of morphine (3 μg) were effective only when they were injected in the ventral part of the PAG; similar results have been obtained by Yaksh et al. (1976b).

Interestingly, using higher doses (10 – 50 μg), morphine became effective at sites over the whole PAG but the analgesia was accompanied by pronounced behavioural modifications such as 'episodes of violent uncoordinated motor activity accompanied occasionally with vocalization, ipsilateral circling behaviour and hyperreactivity as a response to a variety of stimuli' (see also the results of Jacquet and Lajtha (1973, 1974)); (b) Cannon et al. (1982) using the tail flick test, showed that the morphine antagonist, naloxone, was effective in reducing analgesia induced by stimulation of the ventral but not the dorsal PAG; (c) Akil and Mayer (1972) and Akil and Liebeskind (1975) have observed that analgesia triggered by stimulation of the ventral PAG was markedly reduced after administration of a serotonin synthesis inhibitor, p-chlorophenylalanine (p-CPA). These authors did not note any alteration in the analgesic effects induced from stimulation sites within the dorsal or lateral PAG.

The PAG dorso-ventral dichotomy was also observed when considering self-stimulation phenomena: (a) the rat never exhibits self-stimulation behaviour with an electrode placed within the dorsal and dorsolateral PAG; in fact, the animal will terminate electrical stimulation of these regions (Olds and Olds, 1962; Valenstein, 1965; Gardner and Malmo, 1969; Schmitt et al., 1974, 1977); (b) in contrast, self-stimulation phenomena have been reported in the ventral part of the PAG (Liebman et al.. 1970; Schmitt et al., 1974, 1977). According to these latter authors, these effects were more pronounced the nearer the electrode was to the dorsomedial part of the dorsal raphe nucleus. However, other investigators have not found a systematic relation between effective sites for SPA and self-stimulation (Mayer and Liebeskind, 1974; Soper, 1976). This issue should be re-examined on the basis of the location of the pure analgesic regions we have described.

Finally, regarding the possible role of the behavioural reactions in the production of analgesia, the present study leads us to conclude that analgesia induced by ventral PAG stimulation is due to the activation of a neural substrate distinct from that producing motor effects. By contrast, the different characteristics of analgesia from dorsal PAG areas, taken together with the inability to produce rises in vocalization threshold without aversive reactions, further question the 'authenticity' and the nature of the analgesia elicited from aversive regions. Indeed, several hypotheses could be proposed to explain the simultaneous appearance of both analgesic effects and aversive reactions: (a) there may be a simple concomitance of analgesia and aversion. In this case, one must presume that the electrical stimulation activates two independent systems. One can speculate that the aversion results, for example, from the activation of structures such as the medial thalamus or the hypothalamus which receive projections from the PAG (Chi, 1970; Hamilton, 1973; Smith and Flynn, 1980; Comans and Snow, 1981) and which are believed to play an important role in the emotional component of pain; (b) the analgesia might be a consequence of the aversion. In this case, one can suppose that the violent aversive reactions that we have observed are a form of 'central pain' triggered by the stimulation of these regions. On this assumption, the analgesia induced by threshold or suprathreshold stimulation of these PAG regions could result from a situation in which pain of peripheral origin (electrical stimulation of the tail) is negligible by comparison to that of central origin.

Another possibility is that these analgesic effects are similar to those triggered by certain stressful conditions (Akil et al., 1976; Amir and Amit, 1978; Chance et al., 1978; Hayes et al., 1978; Bodnar et al., 1980; Lewis et al., 1980). Indeed, we have already mentioned that the stimulation of these regions induces emotional phenomena and intensive neurovegatative reactions in animals (Kelly et al., 1946; Delgado, 1955; Hunsperger, 1959; Skultety, 1959; Gardner and Malmo, 1969; Duggan and Morton, 1983) as well as in humans (Nashold et al., 1969; Nashold et al., 1974; Cosyns and Gybels, 1979). These effects outlast the duration of the stimulation since we have often noticed

that the rat remained static with gasping respiration following stimulation. The existence and the persistence of these behavioural modifications could explain the marked analgesic post-effects obtained by stimulation of these regions.

Clinical considerations

The various side effects of PAG stimulation that we have reported are particularly important since deep brain stimulation is used for the treatment of severe chronic pain in humans. Our study indicates that, in two different species, rat and cat, there is a good correspondence of the various behavioural reactions induced by stimulation of the PAG, especially as to the location of aversive and analgesic areas. The limited extent of the pure analgesic zones and the presence, in their immediate vicinity, of aversive areas (which also exist in humans in these regions (Nashold et al., 1974; Cosyns and Gybels, 1979)) complicate this form of treatment and may partly explain some of the contradictory clinical results using stimulation of the PAG (see Meyerson, this volume). However, great care must be taken in the comparison of results obtained in rat and cat with those described in man since, in man, the stimulation is applied in order to relieve chronic pain of pathological origin and is generally ineffective against acute pain. Moreover, in man, the exact location of the stimulating electrodes is not known with precision. Effective sites have been reported within either the PAG or more rostral periventricular structures.

It, therefore, seems essential to precisely locate the analgesic zones in periventricular and periaqueductal regions in a species more closely related to humans. It is surprising that no systematic mapping has been performed as yet in the monkey. Indeed both analgesic effects (Goodman et al., 1976; Hayes et al., 1979) and aversive reactions (Schmidek and Fohanno, 1971; Oleson et al., 1980) have been reported in the primate, but the results as a whole are contradictory and include only very few stimulation sites. At the present time surgeons must be guided by previous work in human subjects.

SPA from ventromedial medulla (VMM)

As shown for PAG stimulation, the location of the effective stimulation sites in or close to the DRN, suggests the involvement of serotoninergic mechanisms in stimulation-produced analgesia. This hypothesis is supported by the fact that, in the rat, injection of a serotonin synthesis inhibitor, p-chlorophenylalanine (p-CPA), blocks the analgesic effect of stimulation from electrode sites in the ventral part of the periaqueductal grey matter (Akil and Mayer, 1972). For these reasons we have investigated in the cat the effects elicited by the stimulation of pontine and medullary raphe nuclei rich in serotonin-containing neurons.

SPA from NRM in the cat

The exploration of more posterior areas of the mesencephalon and medulla confirmed the importance of the raphe nuclei in analgesia (Redjemi et al., 1974; Oliveras et al., 1975, 1977, 1978a, 1979). In these pioneering studies we showed that stimulation of the central superior raphe nucleus (CS) triggered analgesic effects like those from the DRN (Fig. 1). Indeed, electrical stimulation of the dorsal part of CS induced powerful analgesia as judged by the pinch test, and greatly modified, by 5 to 10 times, the JOR threshold during central stimulation. But, for the majority of stimulating sites located at pontine and medullary levels, the most reliable structure for SPA in the cat was definitely the NRM. Taking into account that stimulation of certain regions of the reticular formation including the nucleus reticularis gigantocellularis did not provoke analgesia but rather strong motor disturbances, all the stimulating sites within NRM produced a very powerful analgesia as revealed by the pinch test. During NRM stimulation reactions to pinch disappeared but the animals remained quiet and alert. They were able to move and to respond to other kinds of sensory stimuli such as visual,

auditory and tactile. In addition, NRM stimulation triggered dramatic elevations of the JOR threshold of between 5 and 10 times, but for a large number of stimulation sites, the threshold was elevated by more than 10 times, in some cases even 100- and 200-fold.

In Fig. 2, the comparison of data from DRN and NRM does give a good idea of the differences between both nuclei the strength of central stimulation gauged with the JOR. Either with the pinch test or JOR, no analgesic effects were obtained by stimulating the more posterior raphe nuclei such as pallidus and obscurus (Figs. 1 and 2).

The importance of NRM in SPA in the cat was further tested using post-stimulation effects as an index of central stimulation effectiveness. We clearly demonstrated that after prolonged NRM stimulation (several min), huge post-effects were observed. The JOR threshold was still elevated for almost 1 h after the termination of central stimulation (Oliveras et al., 1977). We observed the same kind of effect at the DRN level, but is was not so pronounced.

Finally, still using the tooth pulp electrical stimulation as the quantifiable stimulus to measure the strength of analgesia, we found that, in the cat, NRM stimulation blocks the most integrated nocifensive manifestations induced by strong tooth pulp stimulation. Indeed, the four different reactions (JOR, head hyperextension, head rotations and scratching) provoked by increasing tooth pulp electrical stimulation intensity were highly modified during central stimulation. NRM stimulation was able to totally suppress all the reactions; and the highest intensities of tooth pulp stimulation only triggered reflexes such as JOR and head hyperextension.

Using a neurophysiological approach in freely moving cats we demonstrated that the effects of central stimulation were not due to motor blockade (Fig. 4). In this approach, realized in six animals we showed that NRM stimulation totally suppressed the JOR of peripheral tooth pulp origin, but not of central trigeminal origin (obtained by direct trigeminal stimulation at the level of the trigeminal subnucleus oralis). Taking into account that only one interneuron is interposed between tooth pulp primary afferents and trigeminal motoneurons in the JOR (Sumino, 1971), this data indicates that NRM-induced JOR suppression is not occurring at the motoneuronal level, but rather at interneuronal and/or primary afferent sites. Without jumping from reflexes to sensation, it is, however, reasonable to think that more integrated nocifensive reactions are inhibited by a similar mechanism, i.e. not at the motoneuronal level.

SPA from NRM and adjacent structures in the rat

SPA induced by NRM stimulation in the rat was initially reported by Proudfit and Anderson (1975) and subsequently confirmed by other groups using various nociceptive tests (Akaike et al., 1978; Oliveras et al., 1978b, Satoh et al., 1980; Zorman et al., 1981; Hammond and Yaksh, 1984; Barbaro et al., 1985). In contrast with the cat, however, it appears that SPA can be elicited not only by midline structures (i.e., NRM) but also by a region extending over the pyramidal tract which corresponds to the nucleus reticularis paragigantocellularis (NRPG) (see Basbaum and Fields, 1984). A few studies have reported that electrical stimulation of the ventral part of the nucleus reticularis gigantocellularis is potentially able to produce antinociceptive effects (Satoh et al., 1980; Zorman et al., 1981). Since the majority of the above-mentioned studies utilized simple reflexes such as the tail flick, for gauging SPA, we performed a study in which the integrated vocaliza-

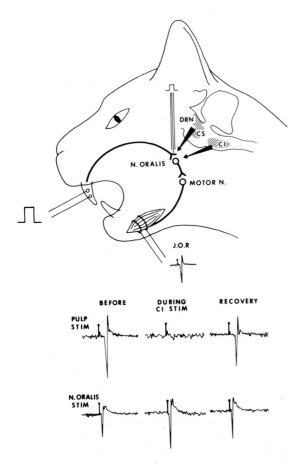

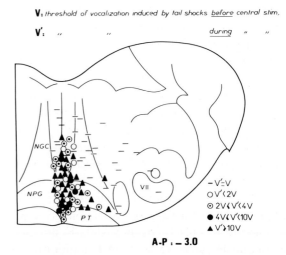

Fig. 5. Modifications of the vocalization threshold (T) induced by tail shocks, by stimulation (T') of NRM and adjacent structures in the freely moving rat. For a great number of stimulation sites located either in the NRM or in the nucleus reticularis paragigantocellularis (NPG), central stimulation elevates the vocalization threshold in huge proportions (more than 10 times during central stimulation).

Fig. 4. Effects of central stimulation (NRM) upon the JOR evoked by tooth pulp and spinal trigeminal nucleus (oralis subdivision) stimulations in the freely moving cat. The upper part shows the disynaptic organization of the JOR. Stimulation of the CI (NRM) totally blocks the JOR of tooth-pulp origin but slightly facilitates the JOR of trigeminal origin.

tion reflex was used as the nociceptive index (Oliveras et al., 1978b). It clearly appears (Fig. 5) that stimulation of NRM and NRPG elevates the vocalization threshold induced by electrical tail shocks to a remarkable extent; for example: 5- to 10-fold, and very often more than 10-fold. By comparison, 3 mg/kg of i.v. morphine induces a 4-fold threshold increase (Oliveras et al., 1978b). The robustness of NRM-NRPG stimulations was confirmed with the pinch test in some studies (Oliveras et al., 1978b; Satoh et al., 1980; Hammond and Yaksh, 1984). Like in the cat, NRM and NRPG stimulations were more effective for SPA than for NDR stimulation (compare Figs. 3 and 5). Additionally, NRM and NRPG do not appear to trigger side effects when analgesia is present. However, in agreement with another study (Akaike et al., 1978), high central stimulation intensities provoked motor disturbances and aversive effects. In contrast, stimulation of the nuclei raphe pallidus and obscurus had no effect, while motor disturbances (rotation) were generally observed when stimulating the nucleus reticularis gigantocellularis.

Finally, in the rat, the localization of medullary analgesic sites to NRM and NRPG suggests, like in the cat, serotoninergic mechanisms involved in SPA at this level; indeed, these two nuclei overlap the serotoninergic B3 cellular group initially described by Dahlström and Fuxe (1964).

Concluding remarks

More than 15 years of investigation in freely moving animals have clearly established the important role of the PAG and NRM-NRPG areas in stimulation-produced analgesia. As extensively reviewed in this paper, the effects induced by PAG stimulation are extraordinarily complex and, in fact, in both rat and cat the stimulation sites from which 'pure antinociception' is reported have a limited extent. Consequently one could presume that these zones are difficult to locate in humans.

At pontomedullary levels powerful analgesia was obtained by stimulation of the NRM-NRPG area. On the basis of quantitative studies, using the JOR tests in the cat and the vocalization threshold in the rat, we have been able to demonstrate unambiguously that electrical activation of this area gives rise to stronger analgesic effects than the PAG.

The powerful inhibitory effects produced by brain stem stimulation on spinal or trigeminal reflexes evoked by noxious stimulation could be partly mediated by the activation of descending inhibition exerted on spinal and trigeminal dorsal horn neurons thought to participate in the central transmission of the painful messages. Initially reported in the cat (Guilbaud et al., 1972; Liebeskind et al., 1973; Oliveras et al., 1974a), strong depressive effects can be induced by PAG stimulation on the activities of neurons of the spinal cord. In some of these experiments, we had previously checked that some sites of stimulation produced strong analgesia in freely moving animals. All subsequent studies have confirmed that PAG and NRM stimulation inhibits, to a marked extent, the responses of dorsal horn neurons to natural (pinch, heat) nociceptive stimuli and electrical stimuli, activating C fibers (see Refs. in Besson and Chaouch, 1987).

A major difficulty in correlating electrophysiological and behavioural data arises from the fact that the inhibition of dorsal horn neuronal activities can be obtained from sites, particularly the adjacent mesencephalic and bulbar reticular structures, where stimulation does not induce analgesia in freely moving animals. Inhibition of dorsal horn neurons can be elicited from more different brain stem areas than can 'pure' analgesic effects. To approach this problem under suitable conditions, it would be necessary to develop experiments in awake, freely moving animals where the evaluation of the analgesic effects and the recording of dorsal horn neurons could be carried out simultaneously.

In spite of these difficulties, the involvement of descending control systems in stimulation-produced analgesia is strongly suggested by experiments (Basbaum et al., 1977) that showed that analgesia induced by stimulation of the medioventral PAG is almost totally suppressed by lesions of the dorsolateral funiculus (DLF) which contains numerous fibers originating from the NRM. However, even though a section of the dorsolateral funiculus reduces the analgesia, one cannot exclude that the stimulation modulates the transmission and integration of nociceptive messages at the supraspinal levels. On the other hand, the functional importance of the DLF in respect of nociception and pain leads to a brief consideration of the nature of the fibers in this tract (see Refs. in Besson and Chaouch, 1987). In addition to propriospinal fibers, this tract contains ascending fibers, among which are spinocervical tract fibers. Dorsal horn neurons send mesencephalic and thalamic projections in this quadrant of the cord. In addition, descending fibers passing in this pathway have various origins such as the ventromedial medulla, locus coeruleus, paralemniscal reticular formation, mesencephalic central gray, red nucleus, hypothalamic paraventricular nucleus, etc. The multiple origins of fibers comprising the DLF stress the need for care in interpreting the results of behavioural studies based on lesions of this tract.

Since direct spinal projections from the PAG are not particularly dense, it has been proposed that PAG analgesic effects could be relayed by the NRM which does massively project to the dorsal horn (see Holstege this volume and Basbaum and Fields, 1984). In fact, there is extensive anatomical and electrophysiological evidence for a direct link between PAG and NRM. Interestingly, in the rat, NRM lesions reduce the analgesia obtained by stimulation of the ventral PAG (Prieto et al., 1983) but do not affect that produced from dorsal regions where the stimulation is often aversive. Even though the existence of connections between the PAG and NRM has been clearly established, involvement of other relays in the antinociceptive effects from the PAG cannot be excluded. For example, the PAG also projects onto bulbopontine reticular formation, areas of which, i.e. the nucleus reticularis gigantocellularis, are at the origin of bulbospinal pathways. It, therefore,

seems necessary to reconsider in detail the relative roles of these different components (the various zones of the PAG-bulbopontine nuclei-spinal cord areas) in the analgesia obtained from the mesencephalon.

Together, the NRM and its adjacent lateral zone corresponding to the nucleus reticularis gigantocellularis pars alpha and to the nucleus paragigantocellularis have been looked upon as a functional entity under the term rostral ventromedial medulla (RVM) (Basbaum et al., 1978; Basbaum and Fields, 1984). This opinion is justified by at least four lines of evidence: (1) behaviourally their stimulation induces a pure analgesia; (2) all give rise to descending axons to the spinal cord via the DLF; (3) they also receive projections from the PAG; (4) all contain 5-hydroxytryptamine (5HT) neurons.

In conclusion, the RVM from which the strongest antinociceptive effects were induced and which massively projects to the spinal cord, seems to form a relay or final common pathway for SPA, since the effects of PAG stimulation are partly exerted via this zone. In addition, the RVM receives afferents from various structures, including the cerebral cortex, the hypothalamus, the caudate nucleus, the nucleus cuneiformis, the bulbopontine reticular formation, and the locus coeruleus (see Refs. in Besson et al., 1982; Carlton et al., 1983; and Holstege, this volume). This is well illustrated throughout this volume by the complexity of the pharmacological aspects of descending control systems and the multiple afferents onto the RVM, which give rise to the problem of the role of individual systems and the circumstances of their activation.

Acknowledgements

We are grateful to Dr. A.H. Dickenson for help with the English and to M. Hoch and M. Cayla for typing the manuscript. This work was supported by l'Institut National de la Santé et de la Recherche Médicale (INSERM).

References

Adams, J.E. (1976) Naloxone reversal of analgesia produced by brain stimulation in the human. *Pain*, 2: 161 – 166.

Akaike, A., Shibata, T., Satoh, H. and Tagaki, H. (1978) Analgesia induced by microinjection of morphine into, and electrical stimulation of, the nucleus reticularis paragigantocellularis of rat medulla oblongata. *Neuropharmacology*, 17: 775 – 778.

Akil, H. and Liebeskind, J.C. (1975) Monoaminergic mechanisms of stimulation-produced analgesia. *Brain Res.*, 94: 279 – 296.

Akil, H. and Mayer, D.J. (1972) Antagonism of stimulation-produced analgesia by p-CPA, a serotonin synthesis inhibitor. *Brain Res.*, 44: 692 – 697.

Akil, H., Madden, J., Patrick, R.L. and Barchas, J.D. (1976) Stress-induced increase in endogenous opiate peptides: concurrent analgesia and its partial reversal by naloxone. In H.W. Kosterlitz (Ed.), *Opiate and Endogenous Opioid Peptides*, Elsevier Biomedical Press, Amsterdam, pp. 63 – 70.

Amir, S. and Amitz, Z. (1978) Endogenous opioid ligands may mediate stress-induced changes in the affective properties of pain related behavior in rats. *Life Sci.*, 23: 1143 – 1152.

Azmitia, E.C. and Segal, M. (1979) An autoradiographic analysis of the different ascending projections of the dorsal and median raphe nuclei in the rat. *J. Comp. Neurol.*, 179: 641 – 668.

Barbaro N.M., Hammond, D.L. and Fields, H.L. (1985) Effects of administered methysergide and yohimbine on microstimulation-produced antinociception in the rat. *Brain Res.*, 343: 220 – 223.

Basbaum, A.I. and Fields, H.L. (1978) Endogenous pain control mechanisms: review and hypothesis. *Ann. Neurol.*, 4: 451 – 462.

Badbaum, A.I. and Fields, H.L. (1984) Endogenous pain control systems, brainstem spinal pathways and endorphin circuitry. *Annu. Rev. Neurosci.*, 7: 309 – 338.

Basbaum, A.I., Marley, N.J.E. and O'Keefe, J. (1976) Spinal cord pathways involved in the production of analgesia by brain stimulation. In J.J. Bonica and D. Albe-Fessard (Eds.), *Advances in Pain Research and Therapy, Vol. 1*, Raven Press, New York, pp. 511 – 515.

Basbaum, A.I., Marley, N.J.E., O'Keefe, J. and Clanton, C.H. (1977) Reversal of morphine and stimulation produced analgesia by subtotal spinal cord lesion. *Pain*, 3: 43 – 56.

Benabid, A.L. and Mahieux, G. (1984) Electrical stimulation of the rat habenular complex induces a naloxone reversible analgesia. *Soc. Neurosci. Abst.*, 10: 102.

Besson, J.M. and Chaouch, A. (1987) Peripheral and spinal mechanisms of nociception. *Physiol. Rev.*, 67: 67 – 186.

Besson, J.M., Oliveras, J.L., Chaouch, A. and Rivot, J.P. (1981) Role of raphe nuclei in stimulation producing analgesia. In B. Haber, S. Gabay, M.R. Issirorides and S.G.A. Alivisatos (Eds), *Serotonin-neurochemistry and Function, Advances in Experimental Biology and Medicine, Vol. 133*, Plenum Press, New York, pp. 153 – 176.

Besson, J.M., Guilbaud, G., Abdelmoumene, M. and Chaouch, A. (1982) Physiologie de la nociception. *J. Physiol. (Paris)*, 78: 7 – 107.

Blackburn, T.P., Forster, G.A., Heapy, C.G.and Kemp, J.O. (1980) Unilateral 5,7-dihydroxytryptamine lesions of the dorsal raphe nucleus (DRN) and rat rotational behaviour. *Eur. J. Pharmacol.*, 67: 427 – 438.

Bodnar, R.J., Kelly, D.D. Brutus, M. and Glusman, M. (1980) Stress-induced analgesia: neural and hormonal determinants. *Neurosci. Biobehav. Rev.*, 4: 87 – 100.

Cannon, J.T., Prieto, G.J. and Liebeskind, J.C. (1982) Evidence for opioid and non-opioid forms of stimulation-produced analgesia in the rat. *Brain Res.*, 243: 315 – 321.

Carlton, S.M., Leichnetz, G.R., Young, E.G. and Mayer, D.J. (1983) Supramedullary afferents of the nucleus raphe magnus in the rat: a study using the transcannula HRP gel and autoradiographic techniques. *J. Comp. Neurol.*, 214: 43 – 58.

Carr, K.D. and Loons, E.E. (1982) Rats self-administer nonrewarding brain stimulation to ameliorate aversion. *Science*, 215: 1516 – 1517.

Chance, W.T., White, A.C., Krynock, G.M. and Rosecrans, J.A. (1978) Conditional fear-induced antinociception and decreased binding of (^{3}H)N-leuenkephalin to rat brain. *Brain Res.*, 151: 371 – 374.

Chi, C.C. (1970) An experimental silver study of the ascending projections of the central gray substance and adjacent tegmentum in the rat with observations in the cat. *J. Comp. Neurol.*, 139: 259 – 272.

Cohen, S.R. and Melzack, R. (1986) Habenular stimulation produces analgesia in the formalin test. *Neurosci. Lett.*, 70: 165 – 169.

Comans, P.E. and Snow, P.J. (1981) Ascending projections to nucleus parafascicularis of the cat. *Brain Res.*, 230: 337 – 341.

Conrad, L.C., Leonard, C.M. and Pfaff, D.W. (1974) Connections of the median and dorsal raphe nucleus in the rat: an autoradiographic and degeneration study. *J. Comp. Neurol.*, 156: 179 – 206.

Cosyns, P. and Gybels, J. (1979) Electrical central gray stimulation for pain in man. In J.J. Bonica, D. Albe-Fessard and J.C. Liebeskind (Eds.), *Advances in Pain Research and Therapy, Vol. 3*, Raven Press, New York, pp. 511 – 514.

Dahlström, A. and Fuxe, K. (1964) Evidence for the existence of monoamine-containing neurons in the central nervous system. I. Demonstration of monoamines in the cell bodies of brainstem neurons. *Acta Physiol. Scand.*, 62, Suppl. 232: 1 – 55.

Delgado, J.M.R. (1955) Cerebral structures involved in transmission and elaboration of noxious stimulation. *J. Neurophysiol.*, 18: 267 – 275.

154

Dennis, S.G., Choiniere, M. and Melzack, R. (1980) Stimulation-produced analgesia in rats: assessment by two pain tests and correlation with self-stimulation. *Exp. Neurol.*, 68: 295 – 309.

Desalles, A.F., Katayama, Y., Becker, M.P. and Hayes, R.L. (1985) Pain suppression induced by electrical stimulation of the pontine parabrachial region. *J. Neurosurg.*, 62: 397 – 407.

Dray, A., Davies, J., Oakley, N.R., Tongroach, D. and Vellucci, S. (1978) The dorsal and medial raphe projections to the substantia nigra in the rat: electrophysiological, biochemical and behavioural observations. *Brain Res.*, 151: 431 – 442.

Dubuisson, D. and Melzack, R. (1977) Analgesic brain stimulation in the cat: effects of intraventricular serotonin, norepinephrine and dopamine. *Exp. Neurol.*, 57: 1059 – 1066.

Duggan, A.W. and Morton, C.R. (1983) Periaqueductal grey stimulation: an association between selective inhibition of dorsal horn neurons and changes in peripheral circulation. *Pain*, 15: 237 – 248.

Fardin, V., Oliveras, J.L. and Besson, J.M. (1984a) A reinvestigation of the analgesic effects induced by stimulation of the periaqueductal gray matter in the rat. I. The production of behavioral side effects together with analgesia. *Brain Res.*, 306: 105 – 123.

Fardin, V., Oliveras, J.L. and Besson, J.M. (1984b) A reinvestigation of the analgesic effects induced by stimulation of the periaqueductal gray matter in the rat. II. Differential characteristics of the analgesia induced by ventral and dorsal PAG stimulation. *Brain Res.*, 306: 125 – 139.

Gardner, L. and Malmo, R.B. (1969) Effects of low-level septal stimulation on escape: significance for limbic-midbrain interactions in pain. *J. Comp. Physiol. Psychol.*, 68: 65 – 73.

Gebhart, G.F. and Toleikis, J.R. (1978) An evaluation of stimulation produced analgesia in the cat. *Exp. Neurol.*, 62: 570 – 579.

Giambalvo, C.T. and Snodgrass, S.R. (1978) Biochemical and behavioural effects of serotonin neurotoxins on the nigrostriatal dopamine system: comparison of injection sites. *Brain Res.*, 152: 555 – 566.

Giesler, G.J. and Liebeskind, J.C. (1976) Inhibition of visceral pain by electrical stimulation of the periaqueductal gray matter. *Pain*, 2: 43 – 48.

Goodman, S.J. and Holocombe, V. (1976) Selective and prolonged analgesia in monkey resulting from brain stimulation. In J.J. Bonica and D. Albe-Fessard (Eds.), *Advances in Pain Research and Therapy, Vol. 1*, Raven Press, New York, pp. 495 – 502.

Guilbaud, G., Besson, J.M., Liebeskind, J.C. and Oliveras, J.L. (1972) Analgésie induite par stimulation de la substance grise périaqueducale chez le chat: données comportementales et modifications de l'activité des interneurones de la corne dorsale de la moelle. *C.R. Hebd. Seances Acad. Sci. Ser. D. Sci. Nat.*, 275: 1055 – 1057.

Gybels, J., Van Hees, J. and Peluso, F. (1976) Modulation of experimentally produced pain in man, by electrical stimulation of some cortical, thalamic and basal ganglia structures. In J.J. Bonica and D. Albe-Fessard (Eds.), *Advances in Pain Research and Therapy, Vol. 1*, Raven Press. New York, pp. 475 – 478.

Hamilton, B.L. (1973) Projections of the nuclei of the periaqueductal gray matter in the cat. *J. Comp. Neurol.*, 152: 45 – 48.

Hammond, D. and Yaksh, I. (1984) Antagonism of stimulation-produced antinociception by intrathecal administration of methysergide or phentolamine. *Brain Res.*, 298: 329 – 337.

Hardy, S.G. (1985) Analgesia elicited by prefrontal stimulation. *Brain Res.*, 339: 281 – 284.

Hayes, R.L., Bennett, G.L., Newlon, P.G. and Mayer, D.J. (1978) Behavioral and physiological studies of non-narcotic analgesia in the rat elicited by certain environmental stimuli. *Brain Res.*, 155: 69 – 90.

Hayes, R.L., Price, D.D., Ruda, M. and Dubner, R. (1979) Suppression of nociceptive responses in the primate by electrical stimulation of the brain or morphine administration: behavioral and electrophysiological comparisons. *Brain Res.*, 167: 417 – 421.

Hosobuchi, Y., Adams, J.E. and Linchitz, R. (1977) Pain relief by electrical stimulation of the central gray matter in humans and its reversal by naloxone. *Science*, 197: 183 – 186.

Hosobuchi, Y., Rossier, J., Bloom, F.E. and Guillemin, R. (1979) Stimulation of human periaqueductal gray for pain relief increases immunoreactive β-endorphin in ventricular fluid. *Science*, 203: 279 – 281.

Hunsperger, R.W. (1956) Role of substantia grisea centralis mesencephali in electrically-induced rage reactions. In J. Ariens Kappers (Ed.), *Progress in Neurobiology*, Elsevier, New York, pp. 289 – 292.

Hunsperger, R.W. (1959) Les représentations centrales des réactions affectives dans le cerveau antérieur et dans le tronc cérébral. *Neurochirurgie*, 2: 207 – 233.

Jacobs, B.L., Simon, S.M., Ruimy, D.D. and Trulson, M.E. (1977) A quantitative rotational model for studying serotoninergic function in the rat. *Brain Res.*, 124: 271 – 281.

Jacquet, Y.F. and Lajtha, A. (1973) Morphine action at central nervous system sites in rat: analgesia or hyperalgesia depending on site and dose. *Science*, 182: 490 – 492.

Jacquet, Y.F. and Lajtha, A. (1974) Paradoxical effects after microinjection of morphine in the periaqueductal gray matter in the rat. *Science*, 185: 1055 – 1057.

Jürgens, V. (1976) Reinforcing concomitants of electrically elicited vocalizations. *Exp. Brain Res.*, 26: 203 – 214.

Kelly, A.H., Beaton, L.E. and Magoun, H.W. (1946) A midbrain mechanism for facio-vocal activity. *J. Neurophysiol.*, 1: 181 – 189.

Kiser, R.S. and Lebovitz, R.M. (1975) Monoaminergic mechanisms in aversive brain stimulation. *Physiol. Rev.*, 15: 47 – 53.

Kiser, R.S., Lebovitz, R.M. and German, D.C. (1978) Anatomic and pharmacologic differences between two types of aversive midbrain stimulation. *Brain Res.*, 155: 331–342.

Lewis, V.A. and Gebhart, G.F. (1977a) Morphine-induced and stimulation-produced analgesias at coincident periaqueductal central gray loci: evaluation of analgesic congruence, tolerance and cross-tolerance. *Exp. Neurol.*, 57: 934–955.

Lewis, V.A. and Gebhart, G.F. (1977b) Evaluation of the periaqueductal central gray (PAG) as a morphine specific locus of action and examination of morphine-induced and stimulation-produced analgesia at coincident PAG loci. *Brain Res.*, 124: 283–303.

Lewis, J.W., Cannon, J.T. and Liebeskind, J.C. (1980) Opioid and non opioid mechanisms of stress analgesia. *Science*, 208: 623–625.

Liebeskind, J.C., Guilbaud, G., Besson, J.M. and Oliveras, J.L. (1973) Analgesia from electrical stimulation of the periaqueductal gray matter in the cat: behavioral observations and inhibitory effects on spinal cord interneurons. *Brain Res.*, 50: 441–446.

Liebeskind, J.C., Giesler, G.J. Jr. and Urca, G. (1976) Evidence pertaining to an endogenous mechanism of pain inhibition in the central nervous system. In I. Zotterman (Ed.), *Sensory Functions of the Skin in Primates*, Pergamon Press, Oxford, pp. 561–573.

Liebman, J.M., Mayer, D.J. and Liebeskind, J.C. (1970) Mesencephalic central gray lesions and fear-motivated behavior in rats. *Brain Res.*, 23: 353–370.

Lohof, A.M., Morgan, M.M., John, J.H. and Liebeskind, J.C. (1987) Stimulation produced analgesia from the nucleus tractus solitarius in the rat: spinal pharmacology. *Pain*, Suppl. 4: S287.

Magoun, H.W., Atlas, D., Ingersoll, E.H. and Ranson, S.W. (1937) Associated facial, vocal and respiratory components of emotional expression: an experimental study. *J. Neurol. Psychopathol.*, 17: 241–255.

Mantyh, P.W. (1982) The ascending input to the midbrain periaqueductal gray in the primate. *J. Comp. Neurol.*, 211: 50–64.

Mayer, D.J. (1979) Endogenous analgesia systems: neural and behavioral mechanisms. In J.J. Bonica, J.C. Liebeskind and D. Albe-Fessard (Eds.), *Advances in Pain Research and Therapy, Vol. 3*, Raven Press, New York, pp. 385–410.

Mayer, D.J. and Liebeskind, J.C. (1974) Pain relief by focal electrical stimulation of the brain: an anatomical and behavioral analysis. *Brain Res.*, 68: 73–93.

Mayer, D.J. and Price, D.D. (1976) Central nervous system mechanisms of analgesia. *Pain*, 2: 379–404.

Mayer, D.J., Wolfle, T.L., Akil, H., Carder, B. and Liebeskind, J.C. (1971) Analgesia from electrical stimulation in the brain stem of the rat. *Science*, 174: 1351–1354.

Moreau, J.L., Cohen, E. and Lieblich, I. (1984) Ventral tegmental analgesia in two strains of rats: effects of amphetamine, naloxone and parachlorophenylalanine. *Brain Res.*, 300: 1–8.

Morrow, T.J. and Casey, K.L. (1976) Analgesia produced by mesencephalic stimulation: effect on bulboreticular neurons.

In J.J. Bonica and D. Albe-Fessard (Eds.), *Advances in Pain Research and Therapy, Vol. 1*, Raven Press, New York, pp. 503–510.

Nashold, B.S. Jr., Wilson, W.P. and Slaughter, D.G. (1969) Sensations evoked by stimulation in the midbrain of man. *J. Neurosurg.*, 30: 14–24.

Nashold, B.S., Jr., Wilson, W.P. and Slaughter, D.G. (1974) The midbrain on pain. In J.J. Bonica (Ed.), *Advances in Neurology, Vol. 4*, Raven Press, New York, pp. 157–166.

Nicolaou, N.H., Garcia-Munoz, M., Arbuthnott, G.W. and Eccleston, D. (1979) Interactions between serotoninergic and dopaminergic systems in rat brain demonstrated by small unilateral lesions of the raphe nuclei. *Eur. J. Pharmacol.*, 57: 295–305.

Olds, M.E. and Olds, J. (1962) Approach escape interaction in rat brain. *Annu. J. Physiol.*, 203: 803–810.

Oleson, T.D., Kirkpatrick, D.B. and Goodman, S.J. (1980) Elevation of pain threshold to tooth shock by brain stimulation in primates. *Brain Res.*, 194: 79–95.

Oliveras, J.L., Besson, J.M., Guilbaud, G. and Liebeskind, J.C. (1974a) Behavioral and electrophysiological evidence of pain inhibition from midbrain stimulation in the cat. *Exp. Brain Res.*, 20: 32–44.

Oliveras, J.L., Woda, A., Guilbaud, G. and Besson, J.M. (1974b) Inhibition of the jaw opening reflex by electrical stimulation of the periaqueductal gray matter in the awake, unrestrained cat. *Brain Res.*, 72: 328–331.

Oliveras, J.L., Redjemi, F., Guilbaud, G. and Besson, J.M. (1975) Analgesia induced by electrical stimulation of the inferior centralis nucleus of the raphe in the cat. *Pain*, 1: 139–145.

Oliveras, J.L., Guilbaud, G. and Besson, J.M. (1977) The use of tooth pulp stimulation to evaluate the analgesia induced by stimulation of raphé nuclei in the cat. In D.J. Anderson and B. Matthews (Eds.), *Pain in the Trigeminal Region*, Elsevier, Amsterdam, pp. 319–330.

Oliveras, J.L., Hosobuchi, Y., Guilbaud, G. and Besson, J.M. (1978a) Analgesic electrical stimulation of the feline nucleus raphe magnus: development of tolerance and its reversal by 5-HTP. *Brain Res.*, 146: 404–409.

Oliveras., J.L., Hosobuchi, Y., Bruxelle, J., Passot, C. and Besson, J.M. (1978b) Analgesic effects induced by electrical stimulation of the nucleus raphe magnus in the rat: interaction with morphine analgesia. *Abstracts 7th International Congress of Pharmacology (Paris), Vol. 1*, p. 119.

Oliveras, J.L., Guilbaud, G. and Besson, J.M. (1979) A map of serotoninergic structures involved in stimulation producing analgesia in unrestrained freely moving cats. *Brain Res.*, 164: 317–322.

Pert, A. and Walter, M. (1976) Comparison between naloxone reversal of morphine and electrical stimulation-induced analgesia in the rat mesencephalon. *Life Sci.*, 19: 1023–1032.

Prieto, G.J., Cannon, J.T. and Liebeskind, J.C. (1983) N. Raphe magnus lesions disrupt stimulation-produced anal-

156

gesia from ventral but not dorsal midbrain areas in the rat. *Brain Res.*, 261: 53–57.

Proudfit, H.K. and Anderson, E.G. (1975) Morphine analgesia: blockade by raphe magnus lesions. *Brain Res.*, 98: 612–618.

Przewlocka, B., Stala, L. and Scheel-Kruger, J. (1979) Evidence that GABA in the nucleus dorsalis raphe induces stimulation of locomotor activity and eating behavior. *Life Sci.*, 25: 937–846.

Redjemi, F., Oliveras, J.L., Guilbaud, G. and Besson, J.M. (1974) Analgésie induite par la stimulation du noyau central inférieur du raphé chez le cat. *C.R. Hebd. Séances Acad. Sci. Ser. D. Sci. Nat.*, 279: 1105–1107.

Reynolds, D.V. (1969) Surgery in the rat during electrical analgesia induced by focal brain stimulation. *Science*, 164: 444–445.

Rhodes, D.L. and Liebeskind, J.C. (1978) Analgesia from rostral brainstem stimulation in the rat. *Brain Res.*, 143: 521–532.

Richardson, D.E. and Akil, H. (1977a) Pain reduction by electrical brain stimulation in man. I. Acute administration in periaqueductal and periventricular sites. *J. Neurosurg.*, 47: 178–183.

Richardson, D.E. and Akil, H. (1977b) Pain reduction by electrical brain stimulation in man. Part II: chronic self-administration in the periventricular gray matter. *J. Neurosurg.*, 47: 184–194.

Roberts, W.W. (1980) [^{14}C]Deoxyglucose mapping of first-order projections activated by stimulation of lateral hypothalamic sites eliciting gnawing, eating and drinking in rats. *J. Comp. Neurol.*, 194: 617–638.

Saper, C.B., Swanson, L.W. and Cowan, R.J. (1979) An autoradiographic study of the efferent connections of the lateral hypothalamic area in the rat. *J. Comp. Neurol.*, 183: 689–706.

Satoh, M., Akaike, A., Nakazawa, T. and Takagi, H. (1980) Evidence for involvement of separate mechanisms in the production of analgesia by electrical stimulation of the nucleus reticularis paragigantocellularis and nucleus raphe magnus in the rat. *Brain Res.*, 194: 525–529.

Schmideck, H.H., Fohanno, D., Ervin, F.R. and Sweet, W.H. (1971) Pain threshold alterations by brain stimulation in the monkey. *J. Neurosurg.*, 35: 715–722.

Schmitt, P. and Karli, P. (1980) Escape induced by combined stimulation in medial hypothalamus and central gray. *Physiol. Behav.*, 24: 111–121.

Schmitt, P., Echancher, F. and Karli, P. (1974) Etude des systèmes de renforcement négatif et de renforcement positif au niveau de la substance grise centrale chez le rat. *Physiol. Behav.*, 12: 271–279.

Schmitt, P., Abou-Hamed, H. and Karli, P. (1977) Effets aversifs et appétitifs induits par stimulation mésencéphalique et hypothalamique. *Brain Res.*, 130: 521–530.

Segal, M. and Sandberg, D. (1977) Analgesia produced by elec-

trical stimulation of catecholamine nuclei in the rat brain. *Brain Res.*, 123: 369–372.

Sharpe, L.G., Garnett, J.E. and Cicero, T.J. (1974) Analgesia and hypersensivity produced by intracranial microinjections of morphine into the periaqueductal gray matter of the rat. *Behav. Biol.*, 11: 303–313.

Skultety, F.M. (1959) Relation of periaqueductal gray matter to stomach and bladder motility. *Neurology*, 9: 190–197.

Smith, D.A. and Flynn, J.P. (1980) Afferent projections to affective attack sites in cat hypothalamus. *Brain Res.*, 194: 41–51.

Soper, W.Y. (1976) Effects of analgesic midbrain stimulation on reflex withdrawal and thermal escape in the rat. *J. Comp. Physiol. Psychol.*, 90: 91–101.

Spiegel, E.A., Kletzkin, M. and Szekely, E.G. (1954) Pain reactions upon stimulation of the tectum mesencephali, *J. Neuropathol. Exp. Neurol.*, 13: 212–220.

Steinbusch, H.W.M., Nieuwenhuys, R., Verhofstad, A.A.J. and Van der Koyd, D. (1981) The nucleus raphe dorsalis of the rat and its projection upon the caudoputamen. A combined architectonic, immunohistochemical and retrograde transport study. *J. Physiol. (Paris)*, 77: 157–174.

Sumino, R. (1971) Central nervous pathways involved in the jaw-opening reflex in the cat. In R. Dubner and Y. Kawamura (Eds.), *Oral-facial Sensory and Motor Mechanisms*, Appleton-Century-Crofts, New York, pp. 315–331.

Swajkoski, A.R., Mayer, D.J. and Johnson, J.H. (1981) Blockade by nalextrone of analgesia produced by stimulation of the dorsal raphe nucleus. *Pharmacol. Biochem. Behav.*, 15: 419–423.

Valenstein, E.S. (1965) Independence of approach and escape reactions to electrical stimulation of the brain. *J. Comp. Physiol. Behav. Psychol.*, 60: 120–130.

Van de Kar, L.D. and Lorens, S.A. (1979) Differential serotoninergic innervation of individual hypothalamic nuclei and other forebrain regions by the dorsal and median midbrain raphe nuclei. *Brain Res.*, 162: 45–54.

Van der Kooy, D. and Hattori, T. (1980) Dorsal raphe cells with collateral projections to the caudate-putamen and substantia nigra: a fluorescent retrograde double labeling study in the rat. *Brain Res.*, 186: 1–7.

Wada, J.A., Matsuda, M., Jung, E. and Hamm, A.E. (1970) Mesencephalically induced escape behavior and avoidance performance. *Exp. Neurol.*, 29: 215–220.

Waldbillig, R.J. (1975) Attack, eating, drinking and gnawing elicited by electrical stimulation of rat mesencephalon and pons. *J. Comp. Physiol. Psychol.*, 89: 200–212.

Willis, W.D. (1982) Control of nociceptive transmission in the spinal cord. In *Progress in Sensory Physiology, Vol. 3*, Springer-Verlag, Berlin, p. 159.

Wolf, G. and Sutin, J. (1966) Fiber degeneration after lateral hypothalamic lesions in the rat. *J. Comp. Neurol.*, 127: 137–156.

Wolfe, T.L., Mayer, D.J., Carder, B. and Liebeskind, J.C.

(1971) Motivational effects of electrical stimulation in dorsal tegmentum of the rat. *Physiol. Behav.*, 7: 569 – 574.

Yaksh, T.L. and Rudy, T.A. (1978) Narcotics, analgetics: CNS sites and mechanisms of action as revealed by intracerebral injection techniques. *Pain*, 4: 299 – 359.

Yaksh, T.L., Yeung, J.C. and Rudy, T.A. (1976a) An inability to antagonize with naloxone the elevated nociceptive thresholds resulting from electrical stimulation of the mesencephalic central gray. *Life Sci.*, 18: 1193 – 1198.

Yaksh, T.L., Yeung, J.C. and Rudy, T.A. (1976b) Systematic examination in the rat of brain sites sensitive to the direct application of morphine: observation of differential effects within the periaqueductal gray. *Brain Res.*, 114: 83 – 103.

Yeung, J.C., Yaksh, T.L. and Rudy, T.A. (1977) Concurrent mapping of brain sites for sensitivity of the direct application of morphine and focal electrical stimulation in the production of antinociception in the rat. *Pain*, 4: 23 – 40.

Zorman, G., Hental, I.D., Adams, J.E. and Fields, H.W. (1981) Naloxone-reversible analgesia produced by microstimulation in the rat medulla. *Brain Res.*, 219: 137 – 148.

H.L. Fields and J.-M. Besson (Eds.)
Progress in Brain Research, Vol. 77
© 1988 Elsevier Science Publishers B.V. (Biomedical Division)

CHAPTER 7

Stimulation-produced antinociception

Jonathan O. Dostrovsky

Department of Physiology, Faculty of Medicine, University of Toronto, Toronto, Ontario, M5S 1A8 Canada

The previous paper by Oliveras and Besson on stimulation-produced analgesia or antinociception (SPA) has presented detailed evidence for the involvement of the periaqueductal gray matter (PAG) and the nucleus raphe magnus (NRM) in SPA. They discussed in particular the findings of their recent studies (Fardin et al., 1984a,b) which have helped to resolve many of the seemingly inconsistent results of previous studies on SPA induced from the PAG, and clearly implicated this structure in SPA.

Although the most extensive studies of SPA have concerned the roles of the PAG and NRM, these are by no means the only structures which have been implicated in descending antinociceptive mechanisms. The previous paper has only very briefly mentioned the possible involvement of other structures in SPA. In order to provide a more complete description of the current state of knowledge regarding the possible mechanisms and sites involved in SPA, this short paper will briefly introduce the possible roles of other structures within the central nervous system in SPA*. This paper is not intended to be a comprehensive review of this large research field, and only a few recent studies will be specifically cited. The reader is

referred to other papers in this book and to the following reviews for further details on the actual studies alluded to here (Willis, 1982; Hammond, 1986; Gebhart, 1986; Besson and Chaouch, 1987).

The antinociception induced by PAG or NRM stimulation is believed to result primarily if not exclusively by an inhibitory action on nociceptive neurons in the spinal cord or trigeminal brain stem nuclear complex, as has been described in the previous paper and in other papers in this volume. It would seem that the converse should also be true: that stimulation at any supraspinal site which inhibits nociceptive neurons should also induce antinociception. However, if this were true then there should be many sites capable of inducing SPA, since in recent years many investigators have reported the inhibition of the responses of spinal or trigeminal nociceptive neurons by stimulation at numerous sites within the CNS (see Table I). Although not all of these sites have been investigated to determine their possible effectiveness in eliciting antinociception, it is obvious that not all of these sites are SPA sites. How can we explain the failure of a site which inhibits nociceptive neurons to elicit antinociception? The following are some possible reasons:

(1) Stimulation at the site may produce aversive and/or motor effects in the unanesthetized animal which may be too powerful to allow testing whether antinociception is also present (in the anesthetized animal aversive effects might not be discernible, especially in those experiments in which the animals are paralyzed). The previous

---

* Although the term stimulation-produced antinociception could refer to very diverse sites and mechanisms such as transcutaneous nerve stimulation, in this paper we will use the term in the more usual and restricted sense to include only CNS stimulation sites at supraspinal levels.

paper very clearly demonstrated how at some sites within the PAG the stimulus elicited aversive and/or motor effects in addition to antinociception. It is likely that at some other sites the aversive or motor effects are so much more powerful that it would be impossible to test for antinociception.

(2) The presence of the anesthetic may alter the normal balance and function of the various pathways in such a way that the inhibition observed in the anaesthetized animal may be very weak or even absent in the unanesthetized animal.

(3) The inhibition produced may be too short and habituate markedly with repeated stimulation so that it would not be possible to maintain a pro-

TABLE I

Structures giving rise to stimulation-induced inhibition of nociceptive neurons in the dorsal horn

'PAIN INHIBITORY SYSTEM'
Periaqueductal/periventricular gray
Nucleus raphe magnus
Nucleus reticularis paragigantocellularis
Nucleus reticularis magnocellularis

SOMATOSENSORY SYSTEM
Dorsal column nuclei
Ventrobasal thalamus
Somatosensory cortex
Trigeminal nucleus

MOTOR SYSTEM
Lateral reticular nucleus
Nucleus reticularis gigantocellularis
Red nucleus
Vestibular nucleus
Substantia nigra
Caudate
Motor cortex

OTHER
Anterior pretectal nucleus
Medial preoptic area
Septum
Medial diencephalon
Lateral hypothalamus
Locus coeruleus

longed depression of nociceptive neurons with a long maintained train of stimuli. In the electrophysiological studies the inhibitory effects seen even with stimulation in the PAG and NRM are generally of short duration, much shorter than the duration of antinociception observed in the unanesthetized animal (however, this is apparently not the case for anterior pretectal stimulation (APT, Rees and Roberts, 1987)). It is not clear why this is so, and the possibility remains that the inhibition usually studied in the anesthetized animal is not the same as that giving rise to SPA in the unanesthetized animal (see (4) below). Part of this problem may be due simply to the common use of short trains in the electrophysiological studies and lower frequency prolonged trains in the behavioral studies. It is possible that some of the inhibitory effects summate with prolonged trains but others not and/or some may be shortened in the presence of anesthesia and others short in both states. Thus, it is possible that the occurrence of short duration inhibition to a short high frequency train in the anesthetized animal may be a poor predictor of the effectiveness of that inhibitory system in the unanesthetized animal and when prolonged low frequency trains are used.

(4) It is usually assumed that the inhibition of the responses of dorsal horn neurons as a result of stimulation in the PAG or NRM is at least partly, if not totally, responsible for the antinociception observed in the unanesthetized animal. Although this is a very reasonable assumption, there are discrepancies between the electrophysiological findings in anesthetized animals and the behavioral findings. In particular, non-nociceptive neurons in the spinal cord, lateral cervical nucleus and dorsal column nuclei, can frequently be inhibited from the same stimulation sites, and at similar or lower intensities compared to nociceptive neurons (e.g. see Fig. 1, and Dostrovsky, 1980, 1984; Gray and Dostrovsky, 1983, 1985). Furthermore, nociceptive neurons can frequently be inhibited at lower current intensities from sites lateral to the sites in the PAG and NRM (Figs. 1 and 2, A). These findings can be obtained even in experiments where

pairs of electrodes are placed such that one electrode is in the PAG or NRM and the other lateral to it in nucleus cuneiformis (CU) or nucleus reticularis magnocellularis or gigantocellularis. The same neuron can thus be tested from both sites. The fact that the stimulation thresholds (to induce inhibition) at the lateral sites are frequently lower than at the more medial sites (e.g. see Fig. 2, B, for example, of CU in comparison with PAG) implies that the inhibition is unlikely to have resulted from current spread to the PAG and/or NRM. And yet the behavioral studies indicate that the thresholds for inducing analgesia are lower for the more medial sites. Even when one maps out the relative effectiveness of stimulation sites in inhibiting the jaw-opening reflex in the anesthetized cat, one finds that the lateral sites are generally more effective (Dostrovsky et al., 1982). Additionally, stimulation of the red nucleus has been found to be more effective in inhibiting the responses of spinal dorsal horn neurons on the

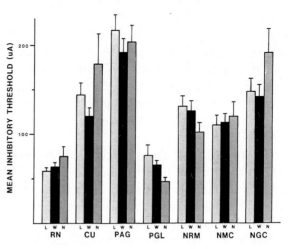

Fig. 1. Bar graphs showing the average current thresholds for inhibiting low threshold mechanoreceptive (L), wide dynamic range (W), and nociceptive-specific (N) neurons in the cat lumbar spinal cord dorsal horn by stimulation in red nucleus (RN), nucleus cuneiformis (CU), PAG, nucleus paragigantocellularis lateralis (PGL), NRM, nucleus reticularis magnocellularis (NMC), and nucleus reticularis gigantocellularis (NGC). (From Gray and Dostrovsky, unpublished data.)

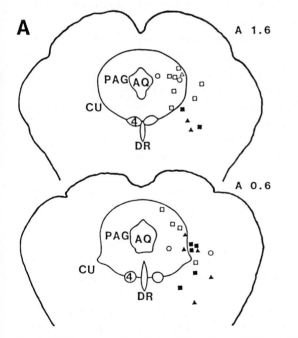

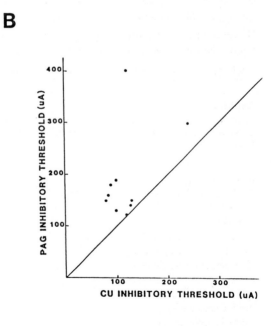

Fig. 2. (A) Reconstruction of stimulation sites in PAG and CU. The shape of each symbol indicates the average current threshold needed to inhibit nociceptive cells in cat lumbar spinal cord dorsal horn in that particular experiment. Insert gives the range of values for each symbol in microamperes. Abbreviations: DR, dorsal raphe; Aq, cerebral aqueduct; 4, trochlear nucleus. (B) Plot comparing the relative effect of stimulating in the PAG and CU. Each point represents the thresholds for inhibiting the same nociceptive cell from the two sites. Points above the $y = x$ (45°) line signify that the threshold stimulation current for inhibiting the neurons was lower in CU than in PAG. (From Gray and Dostrovsky, unpublished data).

basis of current intensities, than PAG or NRM (Fig. 1, Gray and Dostrovsky, 1984). There is no satisfactory explanation for these discrepancies, and they indicate that one has to be careful in predicting efficacy of a site for SPA on the basis of the efficacy of that site in inhibiting dorsal horn neuronal responses or reflexes in the anesthetized animal.

(5) Stimulation-produced antinociception may result only if a specific population of spinal cord neurons is inhibited. It is even possible that some neurons may be excited. Stimulation at most sites inhibits low threshold mechanoreceptive neurons as well as nociceptive neurons, but the relative effectiveness of different sites in inhibiting the different classes of neurons differs. Stimulation in APT has been reported to inhibit only wide dynamic range neurons (convergent) and not low threshold mechanoreceptive- or nociceptive-specific neurons (Rees and Roberts, 1987). Stimulation of the dorsolateral funiculus, which contains most of the descending axons terminating in the dorsal horn, has been shown to excite some lamina I and II neurons. Stimulation in nucleus reticularis gigantocellularis has been shown to excite some nociceptive neurons deep in the cord. Since at present we do not know with certainty the roles of the different classes of neurons in the spinal cord and trigeminal brain stem complex in nociception and modulation of nociception, it is difficult to predict which neurons must be inhibited in order to elicit antinociception.

Nevertheless quite a large number of structures have been suggested as sites from which SPA may be elicited and many of these are listed in Table II. Are all these sites components of descending modulatory systems? Does stimulation at these sites really produce antinociception, and are they potentially useful as sites for the treatment of chronic pain in humans? Does the brain really possess such a large number of distinct parallel modulatory systems? It is difficult to provide clear answers to these questions at the present time. The following factors need to be considered:

(1) The behavioral tests employed in many of the studies consist of a determination of the effects of stimulation on a spinal reflex, usually the tail flick reflex. Inhibition of a nociceptive reflex is not necessarily equivalent to antinociception and even less so to analgesia, which strictly speaking only be evaluated in man. The effects of stimulation of many of these other sites have not been tested extensively on a variety of behavioral tests for antinociception.

(2) The antinociception elicited at some sites may not reflect different parallel control systems but rather effects mediated by relay in PAG and/or NRM. Not much is known concerning those pathways and structures which can activate the PAG/NRM system, and it is reasonable to expect that stimulation at some more rostral sites may activate this system. Nevertheless, we know from experiments that have employed lesions to pathways or nuclei, that there are multiple descending pathways capable of controlling nociceptive information and giving rise to antinociception.

(3) In humans, deep brain stimulation is usually reported to alleviate chronic pain but not to significantly affect pain thresholds and acute experimental pain. Moreover, the effects frequently

TABLE II

Sites from which stimulation-produced antinociception has been reported

Prefrontal cortex
Septal-preoptic area
Caudate
Habenula
Ventrobasal complex (in man)
Dorsomedial hypothalamus
Ventromedial hypothalamus
Anterior pretectal nucleus
Periventricular gray (in man)
Periaqueductal gray
Nucleus raphe magnus
Nucleus paragigantocellularis
Cerebellum
Lateral reticular nucleus
Dorsal column nuclei

last for long periods of time. Thus, the effects studied in animals are quite different from those obtained in man and may thus represent different mechanisms.

(4) Recent studies have tended to pay more attention to aversive and motor effects of stimulation at SPA sites. It appears from these recent studies (e.g. Fardin et al., 1984a,b; Prado and Roberts, 1985) that at most sites, despite denials in the earlier literature, antinociception does not occur without concomitant aversive and/or motor effects. In the study of Prado and Roberts many sites in the CNS were assessed for antinociceptive and aversive effects. The only site in their study that yielded analgesia without any detectable aversive effects was the anterior pretectal nucleus. Even the SPA resulting from the PAG was reported to be accompanied by aversive effects, although, according to the findings of Fardin et al., this would have been due to inability to selectively stimulate the 'pure' analgesic zone within the PAG.

The fact that SPA is usually accompanied by other effects could simply be a reflection of the non-selective nature of electrical stimulation. At most sites, it is impossible to selectively activate the neurons involved in descending controls, either because the effective site is too small, its boundaries are very ragged, or it is a heterogeneous region, and the other neural elements within or surrounding induce motor and/or aversive effects when activated. This is the case for the ventral PAG, as has been clearly demonstrated by Fardin et al. (1985).

Another possibility is that the neurons that give rise to descending inhibition and, thus, antinociception, have axon collaterals which activate other neural structures to give rise to aversive or motor effects.

A third possibility is that the stimulation activates a system which gives rise to aversive reactions and that the aversive 'centers' activate an antinociceptive system as well as typical aversive responses. There have been many recent studies that have clearly shown the existence of multiple stress-induced antinociceptive systems activated by a variety of stressors, although not all stress situations apparently activate these antinociception systems. It is likely that centrally induced aversive stimulation is stressful.

One potential problem with some of these studies is determining from the stimulus-induced behavior of the animal that the stimulation is indeed aversive or stress-inducing. For example, the stimulus by being unexpected and unphysiological may provoke an alerting response, exploration, or even escape, without it really being unpleasant. In human patients undergoing stereotactic surgery we frequently stimulate in the thalamus. These stimuli in almost all cases induce paraesthesiae which are definitely not aversive or painful and, in fact, when referred to the region of the chronic pain, may alleviate the pain. If this stimulus is unexpectedly turned on, the patient will frequently make an orienting response (movement), and may even vocalize in surprise. This type of behavior in an experimental animal could be mistaken for an aversive response. It is interesting that stimulation in the medial lemniscus, which in man produces this type of paraesthetic sensation, has been reported in the rat to produce an aversive reaction. Thus, the fact that stimulation at a given site in an animal has been identified as aversive does not necessarily mean that stimulation at such a site in man would be aversive and of no use, therefore, as a potential site for SPA.

A number of studies have shown that stimulation of structures, usually associated with the motor system, can produce inhibition of nociceptive neurons. These findings suggest the possibility that during execution of movements (perhaps only certain types) nociceptive reflexes and possibly also nociception may be depressed. If this is the case, then the fact, that at some SPA sites movements are also evoked, may not be due to current spread to a component of the motor system in addition to activation of a separate descending modulatory system, but rather that the stimulus is activating only the motor system which in turn directly or indirectly also activates a descending antinociception system.

In summary, since the initial discoveries of SPA induced from the PAG region, our knowledge of the mechanisms and details concerning these controls has increased tremendously. However, as this short paper has pointed out, these new findings have revealed an amazingly complex system of descending pathways which appear capable of depressing nociception and which, apart from the PAG/NRM pathway, are still poorly understood. More studies are required before we can clearly determine the roles and interrelationships of the various sites implicated in SPA and their usefulness in the clinical treatment of pain conditions.

References

Besson, J.-M. and Chaouch, A. (1987) Peripheral and spinal mechanisms of nociception. *Physiol. Rev.*, 67: 67 – 186.

Dostrovsky, J.O. (1980) Raphe and periaqueductal gray induced suppression of non-nociceptive neuronal responses in the dorsal column nuclei and trigeminal sub-nucleus caudalis. *Brain Res.*, 200: 184 – 189.

Dostrovsky, J.O. (1984) Brainstem influences on transmission of somatosensory information in the spinocervicothalamic pathway. *Brain Res.*, 292: 229 – 238.

Dostrovsky, J.O., Hu, J.W., Sessle, B.J. and Sumino, R. (1982) Stimulation sites in periaqueductal gray, nucleus raphe magnus and adjacent regions effective in suppressing oral-facial reflexes. *Brain Res.*, 252: 287 – 297.

Fardin, V., Oliveras, J.-L. and Besson J.-M. (1984a) A reinvestigation of the analgesic effects induced by stimulation of the periaqueductal gray matter in the rat. I. The production of behavioral side effects together with analgesia. *Brain Res.*, 306: 105 – 123.

Fardin, V., Oliveras, J.-L. and Besson J.-M. (1984b) A reinvestigation of the analgesic effects induced by stimulation of the periaqueductal gray matter in the rat. II. Differential characteristics of the analgesia induced by ventral and dorsal PAG stimulation. *Brain Res.*, 306: 125 – 139.

Gebhart, G.F. (1986) Modulatory effects of descending systems on spinal dorsal horn neurons. In T.L. Yaksh (Ed.), *Spinal Afferent Processing*, Plenum, New York, pp. 390 – 416.

Gray, B.G. and Dostrovsky, J.O. (1983) Descending inhibitory influences from periaqueductal gray, nucleus raphe magnus and adjacent reticular formation. I. Effects on lumbar spinal cord nociceptive and nonnociceptive neurons. *J. Neurophysiol.*, 49: 932 – 947.

Gray, B.G. and Dostrovsky, J.O. (1984) Red nucleus modulation of somatosensory responses of cat spinal cord dorsal horn neurons. *Brain Res.*, 311: 171 – 175.

Gray, B.G. and Dostrovsky, J.O. (1985) Inhibition of feline spinal cord dorsal horn neurons following electrical stimulation of nucleus paragigantocellularis lateralis. A comparison with nucleus raphe magnus. *Brain Res.*, 348: 261 – 273.

Hammond, D.L. (1986) Control systems for nociceptive afferent processing: the descending inhibitory pathways. In T.L. Yaksh (Ed.), *Spinal Afferent Processing*, Plenum, New York, pp. 363 – 390.

Prado, W.A. and Roberts, M.H.T. (1985) An assesement of the antinociceptive and aversive effects of stimulating identified sites in the rat brain. *Brain Res.*, 340: 219 – 228.

Rees, H. and Roberts, M.H.T. (1987) Anterior pretectal stimulation alters the responses of spinal dorsal horn neurones to cutaneous stimulation in the rat. *J. Physiol. (Lond.)*, 385: 415 – 436.

Willis, W.D. (1982) Control of nociceptive transmission in the spinal cord. *Progress in Sensory Physiology, Vol. 3*, Springer-Verlag, Berlin.

H.L. Fields and J.-M. Besson (Eds.)
Progress in Brain Research, Vol. 77
© 1988 Elsevier Science Publishers B.V. (Biomedical Division)

CHAPTER 8

Studies of PAG/PVG stimulation for pain relief in humans

Nicholas M. Barbaro

Department of Neurological Surgery, 787-M, UCSF, San Francisco, CA 94143, USA

Introduction

Neurosurgeons interested in the treatment of patients with chronic pain had been using electrical stimulation of the brain for a number of years before the PAG was found to be an effective analgesia-producing site in animals. As early as the mid 1950's, electrodes were implanted in the septal region and the supraoptic nuclei (Heath, 1954; Pool et al., 1956). Mazars and his colleagues (1973) began stimulating the sensory thalamus to treat patients with various forms of 'deafferentation pain' in the 1960's. The first report of thalamic stimulation in the United States was by Adams and Hosobuchi in 1973. Thus, when the initial report by Reynolds (1969), that PAG electrical stimulation produced a profound analgesia without other obvious neurological effects, was confirmed by others (Mayer et al., 1971; Akil et al., 1976), neurosurgeons were eager to utilize this new target in the treatment of patients with chronic pain. By 1977, two independent groups reported promising results in the treatment of intractable chronic pain with electrical stimulation of the human PAG. Although there has been some criticism of the rapidity with which seemingly preliminary animal data were applied to human treatment, it must be pointed out that the technology for human stereotaxic brain stimulation had been developing for nearly 20 years, and that the PAG and PVG were seen simply as new targets for an established

technique rather than as a completely new form of treatment. In addition, the knowledge that stimulation of the human PAG produced analgesia placed great impetus on animal research in this area.

Technique of PAG stimulation

Electrodes are implanted using standard stereotaxic techniques which vary somewhat among centers. I prefer the Leksell stereotaxic frame (Leksell Stereotaxic System, AB Elekta Instruments, Stockholm, Sweden) but several other available stereotaxic systems are adequate. Although some neurosurgeons have begun to use CT- or MRI-guided stereotaxic systems, I use a positive-contrast ventriculogram as the basis for stereotaxic location of targets. This is because the entire procedure can be carried out in the operating room and because the ventriculogram gives a precise outline of the aqueduct. The new contrast agent iohexol (Omnipaque, Winthrop-Breon Laboratories, New York, NY, USA) has reduced the morbidity (nausea, seizures) of this procedure significantly (Shaw and Potts, 1985). A stereotaxic atlas is not needed since the aqueduct is the only landmark necessary for implantation.

The PAG target is 3 mm from the midline at the most rostral and ventral portion of the aqueduct. Platinum 4-contact electrodes are implanted with the most distal contact at the target. Fig. 1 shows

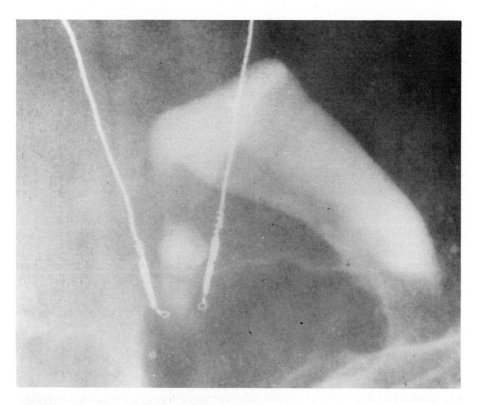

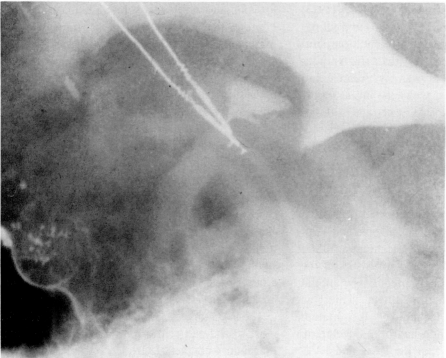

Fig. 1. Intraoperative ventriculogram showing the relationship of the ventricular system and the electrodes. (A) Anteroposterior view showing bilateral PAG electrodes in relationship to the third ventricle. (B) Lateral view showing electrode tips at the ventral edge of the aqueduct, just beneath the anterior commissure.

a ventriculogram with bilateral PAG electrodes in place. Electrodes are implanted under local anesthesia so that intraoperative stimulation can be employed to assess electrode location. Electrical stimulation of the ventral PAG is often associated with subjective sensations, such as a feeling of warmth, which are poorly localized but frequently are in midline regions such as the neck, chest or abdomen. Electrodes placed dorsal and lateral to the appropriate region may produce feelings of fear or aversion or well-localized sensory paresthesias.

A major difference between stimulation of human PAG and techniques used in animal studies is that it is not possible to determine whether or not a particular electrode is effective in relieving pain during the initial implantation procedure in human subjects. This is one reason for the bilateral implantation of PAG electrodes in a single patient. There has not been an increased morbidity associated with bilateral implantation (Hosobuchi, 1986), and the need for an additional stereotaxic procedure in a given patient is reduced.

Although the electrode employed has four contacts, the early hardware used to provide permanent stimulation utilized only a single pair of electrodes. Thus, a trial stimulation period was necessary to determine which pair of electrodes was most effective in relieving the patient's pain. This trial stimulation period lasted from a few days to a few weeks during which the electrode was connected by wires through the skin to a temporary stimulation system. Unfortunately, some patients who had excellent pain relief developed infections because the wires created a direct passage through the skin. Technological advances now permit early implantation of the entire electrode array and subsequent electronic selection of electrode combinations. This obviates the need for transcutaneous wires, thus reducing the chance of infection. In fact, although the number of cases using this new technique is small, I have not had an electrode infection with the newer hardware.

The intracranial electrode is attached to a receiver which is placed in a subcutaneous pocket, usually in the pectoral region (Fig. 2). This in-

volves tunnelling a wire from the scalp to the subcutaneous pocket. This procedure is performed under general anesthesia, usually 1 or 2 days following electrode implantation. Patients can

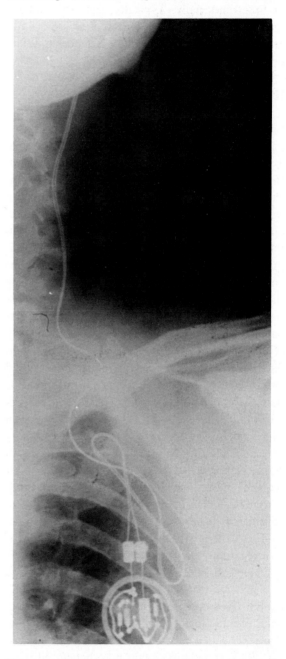

Fig. 2. Radiograph showing subcutaneous receiver in the anterior chest region and wire passing in lateral neck to reach electrode at cranial site (not seen).

then activate their electrode using a battery-operated external transmitter with an antenna placed directly over the receiver. The PAG electrode is usually activated for 15 min at a maximum of four times daily. Typically, the visual analog scale and the need for oral narcotics are used to evaluate the efficacy of a given electrode combination.

Human PAG stimulation and opiates

Early studies indicated that SPA could be at least partially blocked by systemically-administered naloxone (Mayer and Hayes, 1975; Akil et al., 1976). In addition, cross-tolerance between systemically-administered opiates and PAG stimulation was shown. Taken with the observation that naloxone reversed the pain relief associated with human PAG stimulation, these findings indicated that there was an opiate link with this form of analgesia. Further confirmation was obtained by showing that levels of β-endorphin were significantly increased in the cerebrospinal fluid of patients following PAG electrical stimulation (Akil et al., 1978; Hosobuchi et al., 1979). These findings formed the basis for the morphine test used to evaluate patients with severe chronic pain as potential candidates for PAG stimulation (Hosobuchi, 1982). In this test, patients were given successive doses of intravenous morphine (usually to a maximum of 30 mg) and evaluated for pain relief. Naloxone was then used to reverse the effects of morphine. Patients who reported naloxone-reversible pain relief with morphine were considered to be good candidates for PAG electrodes. Although this test provided useful information regarding the degree of opiate responsiveness in a given patient, no study has ever demonstrated that patients who do not respond to systemically administered opiates are responsive to PAG electrical stimulation. In fact, it is not known how many patients who were excluded from treatment with PAG stimulation might have benefitted from such treatment.

Recent studies have raised doubts regarding the opioid link in PAG electrical stimulation. Some animal studies have not replicated the earlier findings that analgesia produced by electrical stimulation in the PAG is reversed by naloxone (Yaksh et al., 1976 (Fig. 3); Gebhart and Toleikis, 1978). Furthermore, recent data from Young et al. (1987) indicate that pain relief from PVG stimulation in humans is not reversed by naloxone, and that there is no cross-tolerance between systemic opiates and PAG stimulation. Recent attempts to replicate the rise in β-endorphin levels in cerebrospinal fluid have suggested that this is an artifact of the contrast agents used for ventriculography during the procedure (Dionne et al., 1984 (Fig. 4); Fessler et al., 1984). Furthermore, many patients have been treated with a combination of PAG and thalamic electrodes in order to alleviate both 'nociceptive' and 'central' forms of pain (see Meyerson's Chapter). This approach, while clinically useful,

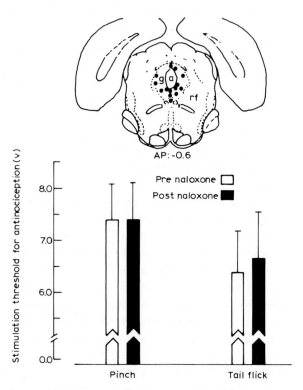

Fig. 3. Inability of naloxone to raise the stimulation threshold for antinociception at a variety of sites in the PAG of the rat. (From Yaksh et al., 1976; reprinted with permission.)

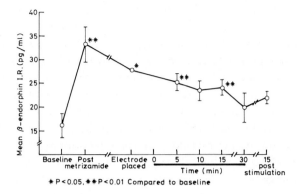

* P<0.05, ** P<0.01 Compared to baseline

Fig. 4. Relationship between β-endorphin levels in human cerebrospinal fluid and various aspects of the PAG electrode implantation procedure. The rise in β-endorphin level is correlated with the injection of contrast material into the ventricle rather than with electrical stimulation. (From Dionne et al., 1984; reprinted with permission.)

has actually confounded the question of whether different types of pain are responsive to stimulation at different sites and whether opiate responsiveness is important in predicting success with PAG stimulation.

Efforts to reconcile differences in the data described above have centered on electrode location as one major difference between studies. Opioid and non-opioid forms of SPA have been postulated as arising from ventral and dorsal PAG, respectively (Cannon et al., 1982). Young et al. placed their electrodes in periventricular gray rather than PAG. However, Richardson and Akil (1977a) reported naloxone reversal of electrical stimulation of PVG in their initial studies. Given the inability to accurately determine electrode location in human subjects, it is not possible to say whether differences in electrode location are a sufficient explanation for apparent differences in opiate effects. As reviewed extensively elsewhere in this volume, there is considerable evidence that the PAG is involved in opioid analgesia, and that opioid mechanisms are involved in the function of the PAG. At present it is unclear whether pain relief from electrical stimulation of the human PAG involves an opioid mechanism or if the

response to opiates is predictive of the effectiveness of PAG stimulation in a given patient.

Long-term results of PAG stimulation

In spite of these difficulties, we now have long-term follow-up on a fairly large number of patients treated at several centers. A recent compilation of these data by Levy et al. (1987) shows that there is an overall success rate of 49% using PAG or PVG stimulation for a variety of painful conditions (Table I). The success rate approaches 60% if so-called deafferentation pain states are excluded. This is in agreement with recent data from Hosobuchi (1986) and from Young et al. (1985). Furthermore, Hosobuchi has shown that his success rate has improved yearly as the indications for brain stimulation have been better defined.

There are several problems with existing studies on the use of PAG stimulation for pain relief in humans. The criteria for judging success differ significantly among centers. For example, Young et al. (1985) used the patient's subjective report of pain relief as well as the patient's ability to taper narcotic analgesics. Others have defined success according to whether the patient continued to use electrical stimulation in long-term follow-up

TABLE I

Results of PAG/PVG stimulation for nociceptive pain[a]

Author	Year	Patients	Long-term success	Percentage
Adams	1987	52	18	35
Hosobuchi	1986	65	50	77
Plotkin	1982	44	35	80
Ray	1980	19	14	74
Mazars	1979	17	0	0
Meyerson	1979	74	41	55
Richardson	1977	20	14	70
Total		291	172	59

[a] Adapted from Levy et al., 1987.

(Levy, Lamb and Adams, 1987). Although subjective reports of pain relief are useful clinical measures of treatment success, a variety of other, more objective indicators such as functional activity scales and ability to return to work would be useful. Furthermore, no study has provided a statistical comparison of pain levels following stimulation of different electrode combinations on a given electrode array. Such data would not only establish the efficacy of this form of treatment, but would also help to pinpoint more effective stimulation targets.

What can be said is that many patients with medically refractory pain report definite relief from the use of PAG or PVG stimulation. Efforts to improve the success rate with this procedure will depend on the application of information obtained from animal experiments on descending control of pain transmission. One example of this is the use of L-tryptophan in patients with PAG electrodes in order to enhance the availability of serotonin at brain stem levels. Hosobuchi et al. (1980) have stated that tolerance to the effects of PAG stimulation and cross-tolerance between systemically administered opiates can be reduced by the oral administration of L-tryptophan. However, these data were not compared with a placebo nor were the examiners blinded as to the use of this agent. The use of tricyclic antidepressants may also provide similar benefit, but sufficient data are not available to anwer this question.

Human vs. animal PAG stimulation

The transition from animal studies to human treatment is a difficult one. There are numerous differences between the phenomenon of SPA in animals and the analgesia experienced by patients using PAG electrodes. SPA has an immediate onset and nearly immediate termination when studied using nociceptive reflexes such as the tail flick. Patients may or may not notice an immediate relief of pain when stimulating the PAG, and the analgesia lasts several hours. Although some animal studies have looked at post-stimulation analgesia (see Oliveras' Chapter), the type of painful stimuli used to study SPA are frequently brief, cutaneous, and very reproducible. The type of patients treated by PAG electrodes have pain that is chronic and arises from deep tissues. Furthermore, electrode location can be precisely determined in animal studies by using electrolytic lesions and examining histological preparations. Not only can human electrode placement not be determined with the same precision as in animal studies, but the relatively large electrodes and high current levels used make precise definition of the region stimulated impossible. In fact, the method used to set stimulation levels is to increase the stimulus current until there are subjective effects such as involuntary eye movements and then reduce the current to just below the threshold for these effects. Occasionally, patients report feelings of fear when certain electrodes are activated. These are generally somewhat dorsal and lateral to sites which produce pain relief and may correspond with areas in animal studies which produce vocalization or escape behavior (see Oliveras' Chapter).

Although precise histological localization is not feasible in patients, magnetic resonance imaging has recently enhanced the evaluation of electrode location in a limited number of patients. An example of one such study is shown in Fig. 5. Of interest in this patient is the finding that the distal pair of electrodes, which appears to be along the ventrolateral PAG, produced excellent relief of severe low-back pain and produced a sensation of cold in the mid-chest and abdomen. The more proximal pair of electrodes (more dorsal and lateral) produced the same feeling of cold but provided no pain relief. Thus, although temperature paresthesias are useful in localizing electrodes at the time of implantation, they are not, in themselves, predictive of electrode efficacy. The use of MRI is likely to provide useful information regarding target localization, which hopefully will improve the success rate for this procedure.

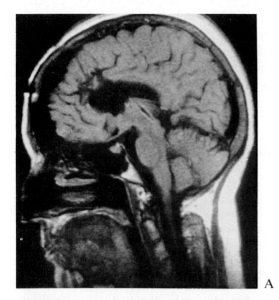

A

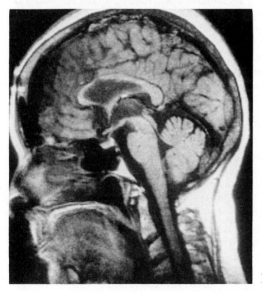

B

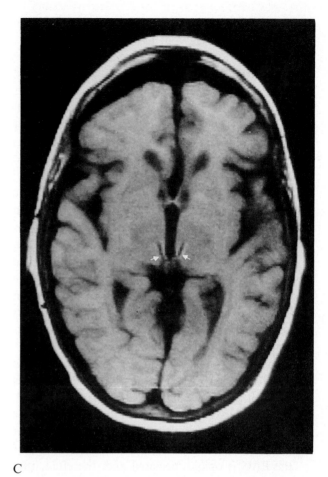

C

Fig. 5. Magnetic resonance image (MRI) showing bilateral PAG electrodes. (A) Sagittal image 3 mm lateral to midline shows one electrode in dorsal midbrain. Lesions in the medial frontal lobe are from a cingulumotomy performed at another institution in an effort to treat this patient's pain. (B) Mid-line sagittal MRI shows the aqueduct of Sylvius. By comparing electrode location in (A) with aqueduct location in (B) an estimate of the exact electrode location can be made. (C) Axial MRI through the third ventricle at the level of the posterior commissure showing two electrodes (white arrows) near the PAG. Next lower image showed the aqueduct but was below the level of the electrodes. Bilateral cingulumotomy lesions can also be seen.

Conclusions

The above considerations indicate that further study is necessary to evaluate the use of PAG electrical stimulation in humans suffering from severe chronic pain. Such studies must take into account the quality and location of pain, the responsiveness to opiates and other analgesic agents, psychological variables and electrode location.

Questions which remain to be answered include whether analgesia can be proven to result from PAG stimulation in these patients, the precise indications for the use of PAG stimulation, which electrode sites are most effective in relieving pain and whether there is any clear relationship between the opiate responsiveness of a painful condition and the effectiveness of PAG stimulation.

Summary

Although electrical stimulation of human peri-aqueductal gray (PAG) has been employed for more than 15 years, a number of questions remains unanswered. These include the types of pain problems which are best treated using this modality, the optimal site for stimulation and whether the analgesia produced by stimulation of this region involves an opioid link. The latter two questions are more difficult to answer in human studies than in animal experiments. Furthermore, because the analgesic effects seen in animals are of immediate onset and are often short-lived while those in humans have a slower onset and last longer, it is not clear that all information gained in animal experiments applies to human analgesia studies.

Initial reports stated that PAG stimulation was best for 'nociceptive' as opposed to 'central' pains and that patients with pains relieved by systemically administered opiates were good candidates for this procedure. This fits well with the concept that the analgesia produced by electrical stimulation of the PAG is opioid mediated and, therefore, that only pains responsive to opiates would respond to PAG stimulation. Subsequent studies have not confirmed these findings, and surgeons who implant PAG electrodes do not use morphine responsiveness as an absolute criterion for patient selection. This and the increasing use of both thalamic and PAG electrodes in the same patient for the same pain problem have made the patient selection process seem even more empirical.

In spite of these difficulties, electrical stimulation of the PAG continues to be used for treatment of patients with severe, medically-refractory pain problems. A review of the existing literature suggests that long-term success can be obtained in 50 – 60% of patients. However, the criteria by which success is determined differ significantly among studies. Well-designed prospective studies are essential for a better understanding of analgesic mechanisms in humans and to improve success rates for this procedure. In order to better study this modality, strict attention must be given to the type and location of the pain, its response to opiates and other centrally acting analgesics, psychological variables and to electrode location.

References

Adams, J.E. (1976) Naloxone reversal of analgesia produced by brain stimulation in the human. *Pain*, 2: 161 – 166.

Adams, J.E., Hosobuchi, Y. and Fields, H.L. (1974) Stimulation of internal capsule for relief of chronic pain. *J. Neurosurg.*, 41: 740 – 744.

Akil, H., Mayer, D.J. and Liebeskind, J.C. (1976) Antagonism of stimulation-produced analgesia by naloxone, a narcotic antagonist. *Science*, 191: 961 – 962.

Akil, H., Richardson, D.E., Hughes, J. and Barchas, J.D. (1978) Enkephalin-like material elevated in ventricular cerebrospinal fluid of pain patients after analgetic focal stimulation. *Science*, 201: 463 – 465.

Cannon, J.T., Prieto, G.J. and Liebeskind, J.C. (1982) Evidence for opioid and non-opioid forms of stimulation-produced analgesia in the rat. *Brain Res.*, 243: 315 – 321.

Dieckmann, G. and Witzmann, A. (1982) Initial and long-term results of deep brain stimulation for chronic intractable pain. *Appl. Neurophysiol.*, 45: 167 – 172.

Dionne, R.A., Mueller, G.P., Young, R.F., Greenberg, R.P., Hargreaves, K.M., Gracely, R. and Dubner, R. (1984) Contrast medium causes the apparent increase in β-endorphin levels in human cerebrospinal fluid following brain stimulation. *Pain*, 20: 313 – 321.

Fessler, R.G., Brown, F.D., Rachlin, J.R. and Mullan, S. (1984) Elevated beta-endorphin in cerebrospinal fluid after electrical brain stimulation: artifact of contrast infusion? *Science*, 224: 1017 – 1019.

Gebhart, G.F. and Toleikis, J.R. (1978) An evaluation of stimulation-produced analgesia in the cat. *Exp. Neurol.*, 62: 570 – 579.

Heath, R.G. (1954) *Studies in Schizophrenia*, Harvard University Press, Cambridge.

Hosobuchi, Y. (1978) Tryptophan reversal of tolerance to analgesia induced by central grey stimulation. *Lancet*, 2: 47.

Hosobuchi, Y. (1983) Combined electrical stimulation of the periaqueductal gray matter and sensory thalamus. *Appl. Neurophysiol.*, 46: 112 – 115.

Hosobuchi, Y. (1986) Subcortical electrical stimulation for control of intractable pain in humans. *J. Neurosurg.*, 64: 543 – 553.

Hosobuchi, Y., Adams, J.E. and Rutkin, B. (1973) Chronic thalamic stimulation for the control of facial anaesthesia dolorosa. *Arch. Neurol.*, 29: 158 – 161.

Hosobuchi, Y., Adams, J.E. and Linchitz, R. (1977) Pain relief by electrical stimulation of the central gray matter in humans and its reversal by naloxone. *Science*, 197: 183 – 186.

Hosobuchi, Y., Rossier, J., Bloom, F.E. and Guillemin, R. (1979) Stimulation of human periaqueductal gray for pain relief increases immunoreactive beta-endorphin in ventricular fluid. *Science*, 203: 279 – 281.

Hosobuchi, Y., Lamb, S. and Bascom, D. (1980) Tryptophan loading may reverse tolerance to opiate analgesics in humans: a preliminary report. *Pain*, 9: 161 – 169.

Levy, R., Lamb, S. and Adams, J. (1987) Long-term success for deep brain stimulation for chronic pain: standardized outcomes in 965 reported cases. *Pain*, Suppl. 4: S9.

Levy, R., Lamb, S. and Adams, J. (1987) Treatment of chronic pain by deep brain stimulation: long-term follow-up and review of the literature. *Neurosurgery*, 21: 885 – 893.

Mayer, D.J. and Hayes, R.L. (1975) Stimulation-produced analgesia: development of tolerance and cross-tolerance to morphine. *Science*, 188: 941 – 943.

Mayer, D.J., Wolfle, T.L., Akil, H., Carder, B. and Liebeskind, J.C. (1971) Analgesia from electrical stimulation of the brain stem of the rat. *Science*, 174: 1351 – 1354.

Mazars, G.J., Merienne, L. and Cioloca, C. (1973) Stimulations thalamiques intermittentes antalgiques. Note préliminaire. *Rev. Neurol.*, 128: 273 – 279.

Mazars, G.J., Merienne, L. and Cioloca, C. (1979) Comparative study of electrical stimulation of posterior thalamic nuclei, periaqueductal gray and other midline mesencephalic structures in man. In J.J. Bonica (Ed.), *Advances in Pain Research and Therapy, Vol. 3*, Raven Press, New York, pp. 541 – 546.

Plotkin, R. (1982) Results in 60 cases of deep brain stimulation for chronic intractable pain. *Appl. Neurophysiol.*, 45: 173 – 178.

Pool, J.L., Clark, W.K. and Hudson, P. (1956) *Hypothalamic-hypophysical Interrelationships*, C.C. Thomas, Springfield, IL.

Ray, C.D. and Burton, C.V. (1980) Deep brain stimulation for severe, chronic pain. *Acta Neurochir.*, 30 (Suppl.): 289 – 293.

Reynolds, D.V. (1969) Surgery in the rat during electrical analgesia induced by focal brain stimulation. *Science*, 164: 444 – 445.

Richardson, D.E. and Akil, H. (1977a) Pain reduction by electrical brain stimulation in man. I. Acute administration of periaqueductal and periventricular sites. II. Chronic self-administration in the periventricular gray matter. *J. Neurosurg.*, 47: 184 – 194.

Richardson, D.E. and Akil, H. (1977b) Long-term results of periventricular gray self-stimulation. *Neurosurgery*, 1: 199 – 202.

Shaw, D.D. and Potts, D.G. (1985) Toxicology of iohexol. *Invest. Radiol.*, Suppl., 20: S10 – S13.

Yaksh, T.L., Yeung, J.C. and Rudy, T.A. (1976) An inability to antagonize with naloxone the elevated nociceptive thresholds resulting from electrical stimulation of the mesencephalic central gray. *Life Sci.*, 18: 1193 – 1198.

Young, R.F. and Chambi, V.I. (1987) Pain relief by electrical stimulation of the periaqueductal and periventricular gray matter: evidence for a non-opioid mechanism. *J. Neurosurg.*, 66: 364 – 371.

Young, R.F., Kroening, R., Fulton, W., Feldman, R.A. and Chambi, I. (1985) Electrical stimulation of the brain in treatment of chronic pain. *J. Neurosurg.*, 62: 389 – 396.

H.L. Fields and J.-M. Besson (Eds.)
Progress in Brain Research, Vol. 77
© 1988 Elsevier Science Publishers B.V. (Biomedical Division)

CHAPTER 9

Problems and controversies in PVG and sensory thalamic stimulation as treatment for pain

Björn A. Meyerson

Department of Neurosurgery, Karolinska Hospital, S-104 01 Stockholm, Sweden

Introduction

In the late seventies a number of clinical studies provided evidence that intracerebral stimulation (ICS) * was a reliable method for dealing with pain otherwise resistant to conventional treatment (reviews, see Hosobuchi, 1980; Gybels, 1983; Meyerson, 1983, 1985; Turnbull, 1984). Intracerebral stimulation, as well as other forms of electric stimulation for pain, appeared to be particularly attractive in view of the fact that theoretically it offered the possibility of manipulating endogenous pain-controlling mechanisms. However, many of the ensuing studies failed to confirm the first, optimistic reports (e.g. Dieckmann and Witzmann, 1982). Recently, three major studies with long-term follow-ups have been published (Young et al., 1985; Hosobuchi, 1986; Siegfried, 1986). The number of successful cases in these series is comparatively high and the authors maintain that ICS is a valuable tool in pain treatment. However, they base their conclusions on different grounds. Thus, as will be further discussed below, there are discordant opinions on the preferred stimulation target, incidence of tolerance and possible counter-measures, biochemical mechanisms involved, etc. An inquiry to a number of established neurosurgeons with long experience in

pain treatment has shown that several of them have ceased to practice ICS because they only rarely find a good indication for the procedure, that the outcome is unpredictable and that they have failed to obtain satisfactory results, particularly by midbrain stimulation.

The fact that ICS presently is practised in only a few centers gives the impression that the development of the method has come to a standstill and that no major progress leading to improved efficacy and reliability has been made lately. It appears that it has not yet been possible to exploit novel experimental data on the functioning of endogenous pain controls in the further development of ICS. For example, the recently discovered intricate interplay between spinal serotonergic and noradrenergic mechanisms involved in the descending control of nociception (e.g. Archer et al., 1986; reviews, see Fitzgerald, 1986; Hammond, 1986) has so far not led to systematic trials to enhance the efficacy of midbrain stimulation by the use of a supplementary pharmacological therapy.

ICS has evolved along two lines, corresponding to the two major target regions for stimulation: the sensory thalamic nuclei (VPM/VPL) and the periaqueductal-periventricular grey region (PAG/PVG). Conceivably, stimulation in these two regions may influence pain by the activation of different mechanisms and/or systems. There is evidence that stimulation in the sensory thalamus

---

* Often referred to as deep brain stimulation (DBS).

(STh) is selectively effective for neuropathic (deafferentation) pain whereas PAG/PVG stimulation (in the following referred to as PVG) appears to affect only nociceptive pain. This conceptualisation of two fundamentally different forms of somatic pain has only recently been recognized. In clinical pain literature, 'pain' is still often referred to as an entity specified in terms of underlying disease, location and intensity. The distinction of nociceptive vs. neuropathic pain has important clinical implications as they respond differently to various treatment modalities. The most salient distinguishing feature is that exogenous opioids as well as peripherally acting analgesics are effective in a typical dose-response fashion only for the nociceptive type of pain. In contrast, neuropathic pain is generally resistant to common analgesics (cf. Arnér and Meyerson, 1988). As will be dealt with further on, there is evidence that the distinction between these two forms of pain is crucial for defining the indications for ICS and the choice of stimulation target. In this context, it should be recalled that research related to supraspinal control has principally focused on the nociceptive type of pain. Therefore, it can be questioned whether, for example, studies on effects of stimulation in the sensory thalamic nuclei on nociceptive spinal neurons are indeed relevant for the clinical application of stimulation in this same target region (e.g. Dickenson, 1983; Gerhart et al., 1983). Vice versa, it is likewise unclear whether data derived from experiments with upper midbrain stimulation in an animal model of neuropathic-deafferentation pain (e.g. autotomy behaviour) are applicable to therapeutic stimulation in the corresponding region.

Background

The history of the development of PVG stimulation is too well known to need recapitulation. However, it is of interest to note that in 1971 Schmideck et al., in experiments in monkeys, stimulated the PAG and the centromedian-parafascicular complex without any consistent effects on pain thresholds. Actually, the first observation in man that stimulation in the PVG region could suppress pain was made in 1973 by Richardson and Akil during the course of stereotactic operations (thalamotomy) (see Richardson and Akil, 1977). The pioneers in the further development of PVG stimulation for clinical use have been Hosobuchi and Adams (e.g. Hosobuchi et al., 1977; Hosobuchi, 1986).

Although North-American neurosurgeons are generally given credit for having introduced sensory thalamic stimulation, this approach to pain treatment was used in the late sixties by Mazars in Paris. That was some years before the introduction of the gate-control theory, and Mazars had based his trials with thalamic stimulation on the classical theory advanced by Head and Holmes in 1911 (for ref., see Mazars et al., 1976). Unfortunately, these early studies were not published until 1973 and it is only recently that Mazars' pioneering work has been recognized outside France (Mazars et al., 1973, 1974). A series of some hundred patients, suffering from various types of neuropathic pain treated with sensory thalamic stimulation and with a surprisingly high rate of success was published later (Mazars et al., 1979).

It is reasonable to assume that the rationale for trying stimulation in the sensory thalamus, as well as in the sensory limb of the internal capsule, as introduced in 1973 by Hosobuchi et al. (1973, 1974), was the favourable experience previously made with stimulation applied to the skin, peripheral nerves and spinal cord. Supraspinal lemniscal stimulation would be the logical way of dealing with painful conditions in which there are insufficient primary afferent neurons available as 'substrate' for stimulation, for example in cases with complete spinal cord lesions, avulsion of the brachial plexus, facial anaesthesia dolorosa, etc.

Clinical results and indications

Cooperative studies have been performed both in the US and in Europe and they account for results reported from the major centers. The North-

American study comprised 339 patients treated by seven different neurosurgeons until 1982 (Groth et al., 1982). About 75% of the patients experienced sufficient pain control by temporary test stimulation to warrant permanent electrode implantation. About 75% of these patients maintained satisfactory control of pain but the mean follow-up lasted only about 17 months. In the European cooperative study from 1979 some 180 patients subjected to sensory thalamic stimulation for neuropathic pain were reported and about 60% had experienced useful pain reduction (Lazorthes, 1979). The outcome of treating such pain with PVG stimulation was relatively poor except when applied for 'low back pain' which was successfully treated in about 2/3 of the patients.

PVG-stimulation

One of the reasons why PVG stimulation has provided variable results, and has fallen into disrepute among some neurosurgeons, may be that it has been almost exclusively applied for 'low back pain'. For obvious reasons, this term, as well as 'failed back surgery', does not connotate a true clinical entity but rather a heterogenous syndrome which may include pain due to arachnoiditis, spinal root lesions, diseased intervertebral discs, facet joint arthrosis, secondary muscular spasm and inflammation, etc. The pains produced by these conditions may be both nociceptive and neuropathic, and a single patient may have both types of pain simultaneously. Unless the pain in such cases is thoroughly analysed in order to assess the type of pain which dominates, indiscriminate use of either stimulation target may produce inconsistent results. In this context it should be noted that the same line of reasoning applies for spinal cord stimulation when considered for the same type of pain (cf. Winkelmüller, 1981). As elegantly demonstrated by Hosobuchi (1986), the rational way of dealing with 'low back pain' comprising both nociceptive and neuropathic pain components, is to implant electrodes in both stimulation targets (see also Young et al., 1985). This ap-

proach appears to have been very rewarding in that about 70% of patients with this condition have enjoyed satisfactory long-term pain relief. A few other studies (Plotkin, 1982; Richardson, 1982a) have also claimed a high proportion of successful cases of 'low back pain', although implantation was done in PVG only.

As previously mentioned, several neurosurgeons have failed to demonstrate the usefulness of PVG stimulation. However, a thorough search in the literature reveals that, apart from the studies cited above, other neurosurgeons have not tried such stimulation with the indication of 'low back pain'. Instead, the negative reports with the use of PVG stimulation are mostly based on experiences with pain conditions which appear to have been predominantly neuropathic (e.g. Gybels and Cosyns, 1976; Amano et al., 1982). On the whole, the only other major indication for which PVG stimulation has been tried is cancer pain. In a group of 18 patients nine were reported to have had a satisfactory pain relief (Meyerson, 1983), and this proportion of successful cases compares well with what has been reported by others (e.g. Lazorthes, 1979; Groth et al., 1982). With the development of spinal − and intraventricular − administration of opioids, pain due to malignancy has become a rare indication for PVG stimulation. It should be emphasized that a neuropathic type of pain is often present as result of neoplastic invasion of nervous tissue, and this form of cancer pain still constitutes a major therapeutic problem, as it appears to be largely resistant to opioids also, when administred spinally (Arnér and Arnér, 1985). As already mentioned, such pain appears to be resistant to PVG stimulation; a few other indications for PVG stimulation have been reported (e.g. pancreatitis, osteoporosis) but the number of cases is too small to permit an evaluation.

Considering the favourable outcome reported by some with PVG stimulation for pain in the low back, it is surprising that similar conditions causing pain in the cervical region have not become an indication. One may also ask why the remarkably positive North-American studies on the efficacy of

PVG stimulation for 'low back pain' have apparently not appealed to neurosurgeons outside the US. It might be that the important psychosocial problems, which often play a major role in complicating pain management in these patients, render advanced somatic treatment unsuitable. Perhaps, there is also a feeling that intracerebral stimulation is an almost experimental method which is hardly justifiable for a 'trivial' condition such as chronic pain in the low back. No doubt, there are also methodological problems involved, and frustrating, previous experiences with PVG stimulation – conceivably applied on wrong indications – may have deterred many neurosurgeons from continuing the use of this stimulation target.

In the early reports on ICS there were accounts of occasional cases diagnosed as having neuropathic pain who nevertheless benefitted from PVG stimulation. Thus, for example Richardson and Akil (1977), reported five patients out of 11 with definite diagnoses of neuropathic pain who had excellent pain control, but the length of follow-up was not given. It should also be noted that in the above-mentioned North-American cooperative study there were some patients with central pain, 'facial pain', and pain due to spinal cord injury who had good pain relief with PVG stimulation. Similar results were documented in the European cooperative study from 1979, where about a fourth of the patients with neuropathic pains enjoyed relief. However, the period of follow-up in the latter study was comparatively short. It should be mentioned that in a recent study Young et al. (1985) reported that a few patients, among them one with facial postherpetic neuralgia, unexpectedly experienced almost complete pain relief from PVG stimulation whereas STh stimulation provided only partial alleviation. However, these occasional reports are at variance with several other studies supplying evidence that PVG stimulation is ineffective for neuropathic pain (Boëthius et al., 1976; Hosobuchi, 1980, 1986; Siegfried, 1983; Meyerson, 1983; Tsubokawa et al., 1985). The latter studies are thus in agreement with the assump-

tion that PVG stimulation operates via morphine-like mechanisms and exclusively influences pain which responds to opioids to which neuropathic pain as a rule is resistant.

It might be that PVG stimulation is effective only for pain which also responds to exogenous opioids. This would, however, not necessarily exclude the possibility that PVG stimulation may also operate via the activation of non-endorphinergic systems. This being the case, one would expect that some morphine-resistant pains would respond to PVG stimulation, but the problem becomes difficult to overcome since, unfortunately, no drugs which mimic a non-endorphinergic, endogenous pain control have been identified, for example, for neuropathic pain. That would perhaps help to solve the problem of why some rare cases of neuropathic pain might in fact respond to PVG stimulation.

Sensory thalamic stimulation

In contrast to PVG stimulation, stimulation in the specific sensory thalamic nuclei apparently has become a more commonly employed form of treatment. Some of the same neuropathic pain conditions for which STh stimulation has been applied may also respond to spinal cord stimulation, and in clinical practice this form of stimulation is often tried before ICS is considered. Typical examples are lumbosacral rhizopathy and peripheral neuralgias. However, in the literature there is no direct comparison of the effectivness of ICS with spinal stimulation. Some neuropathic pain conditions are characterized by deafferentation, phantom limb pain being the most conspicuous example. In a few of these cases, spinal stimulation-induced paraesthesiae can not be evoked in the painful region, suggesting an extensive transganglionic degeneration of dorsal column fibers. For these cases, as well as for pain which may be classified as central (pain in paraplegia, plexus avulsion, pain due to brain stem or thalamic lesions), stimulation has to be applied at a supraspinal relay station of the lemniscal system, i.e. in the sensory thalamus.

The largest recent series of patients with neuropathic pain subjected to thalamic stimulation is that reported by Siegfried (1986). In this study, comprising 103 patients with a mean follow-up of 32 months, 80 initially enjoyed significant pain relief as measured by a visual analogue scale. After the first 4 months, there was a slight tendency of the pain to increase but it still remained substantially reduced as compared to the pretreatment level. The majority of the patients had pain located in the face. In an earlier report no less than 10 out of 13 patients with follow-ups between 5 and 32 months suffering from postherpetic facial pain enjoyed satisfactory pain relief (Demierre and Siegfried, 1983). Tsubokawa et al. (1984) have reported good results, in 14 out of 23 patients, also in pain associated with malignancy but where the pain apparently was largely neuropathic in nature. Somewhat less favourable outcome with STh stimulation applied to various forms of neuropathic pain has recently been recorded by Hosobuchi (1986): 25 out of 55 patients obtained satisfactory relief.

It is of particular interest that Young et al. (1985) recently reported that only two patients out of six obtained partial relief, and none of his cases enjoyed complete control of their pain. A review of the literature with regard to the outcome of specific pain diagnoses reveals that, in general, 'thalamic pain' (many cases subjected to stimulation in the sensory limb of the internal capsule) and peripheral nerve injury appear to be good indications (e.g. Lazorthes, 1979; Groth et al., 1982; references, see Meyerson, in press). Also postcordotomy dysaesthesia often responds favourably (Hosobuchi, 1986).

Sensory thalamic stimulation has also been applied for lumbosacral rhizopathy and, as mentioned above, Hosobuchi has in such patients (referred to as 'low back pain') employed dual stimulation in both targets which resulted in an exceptionally high rate of success. Thus, of 49 patients treated with ICS for this diagnosis, 39 were deemed to be successful and no less than 19 had two electrodes implanted. Also Turnbull et al. (1980) applied STh stimulation for 'low back pain' and found 12 out of 14 patients to be effectively relieved. However, these excellent results do not concur with those of several others and, for example Young et al. (1984) conclude that, in their experience, stimulation in the sensory thalamus is rarely useful.

From the above it is obvious that the results of ICS are highly variable in different clinical reports and that there are discordant views on its usefulnes and reliability as well as on the indications. This applies to both stimulation targets. In particular, the importance and nature of opioid mechanisms in PVG stimulation has been subject to debate (cf. Barbaro, this volume; see also Young et al., 1987). In the following, some crucial technical and methodological problems which may account for part of the variability of the clinical results of ICS, will be addressed.

Electrode design and stimulation parameters

In the vast majority of patients commercial 4-pole electrodes have been utilized, the stimulating poles being 1 mm in length and 2 mm apart (Medtronic DBS electrode). There are no data suggesting that the interpolar distance and the surface of the stimulating pole are of importance for the efficacy of stimulation, although Mazars (1976) has claimed that the interpolar distance should be 4 mm and the surface area of the stimulating pole 4 mm^2. It has been estimated that a current of $0.5 - 1$ mA, which is usually employed in ICS, does not effectively spread more than 1.5 mm outside the electrode (Comte, 1982; see also Ranck, 1975). That a comparatively small volume of nervous tissue around the electrode is activated is further substantiated by the fact that when a 4-pole array is employed, the coupling of the poles is generally of decisive importance for the effect. This applies to stimulation in both targets. It should also be noted that stimulation is always applied with an intensity just above (STh) or below (PVG) the threshold for evoking subjective sensations.

With PVG stimulation it has become routine (cf. Young et al., 1985) to employ the stimulator with some restriction, applying stimulation not more than twice or three times daily and with a stimulus frequency typically kept at 30 Hz. The background for this stimulation regime has been the idea that a certain restriction in the use of the stimulator would diminish the risk of developing tolerance. However, there are no data supporting this assumption.

With stimulation in the sensory thalamus, patients are left to employ the stimulator as much as they like. As with spinal cord stimulation there are no observations suggesting that 'over-stimulation' is likely to 'fatigue' the system. It has been reported that in STh ramp-stimulation, which means that during a period of 10 – 30 s the stimulus intensity slowly increases to a pre-set level and then abruptly shuts off, is more effective than a continuous mode of stimulation (Hosobuchi, 1986). This finding, however, has not been confirmed by other investigators (e.g. Siegfried, 1985).

With PVG stimulation satisfactory control of pain may be obtained with two or three daily stimulation periods lasting 15 – 30 min. Reports on the time course of pain suppression with STh stimulation are markedly discordant. Thus, both Young et al. (1985) and Hosobuchi (1986) maintain that the effect of such stimulation is generally short-lasting and only partial, requiring the patients to use their stimulator almost continuously. At variance with these studies, Siegfried (1986) in a large series of patients subjected to this treatment, has found that the average daily stimulation time was about 50 min. It should be noted in this context that Mazars et al. (1976), in the early reports, claimed that several of their patients could obtain complete abolition of pain with stimulation only two or three times weekly, and in a few patients we have obtained the same remarkably long-lasting effects with short periods of stimulation (unpublished).

Characteristics of target regions

PVG

There are in the literature numerous observations indicating that the region in the medial diencephalic-mesencephalic junction zone, from where stimulation-produced pain relief can be obtained, is very small indeed. In spite of general agreement on the stereotactic coordinates which define the stimulation target, the precision of the electrode placement is exceedingly critical (Hosobuchi et al., 1977; Meyerson et al., 1979). Even though most stereotactic systems theoretically provide a high degree of accuracy, a slight deviation of the insertion device used for electrode implantation can occur and may then result in a displacement of a few millimeters. In particular, the mediolateral extension of the susceptible region is very limited indeed, perhaps not more than 2 – 3 mm. This is illustrated by one of our patients in whom two electrodes were implanted, one located 2 mm laterally to the other but with the same X and Y coordinates. Only the most medial electrode proved to be effective. In another patient two parallel electrodes were placed in the same sagittal plane, one 2 mm in front of the other. With this arrangement pain relief could be produced by stimulating via either of the electrodes (Fig. 1). On the basis of this and similar observations (cf. Adams, 1976), it is possible to delineate the approximate extension of the critical region for stimulation.

However, more conclusive information can be derived from correlative neuroanatomical and clinical studies based on autopsy material. There are in the literature only three such studies of patients having had electrodes in the PVG/PAG region. Three cases were reported by Hosobuchi et al. (1977), who commented on the specificity of the location of the effective stimulation pole. Gybels et al. (1980) and Boivie and Meyerson (1982) have reported on two groups of patients each including five cases. If the results with regard to stimulation site and clinical effects are compared, it appears that an electrode trajectory in the PVG, 2–3 mm in front of the center of the posterior commissure, is more effective than one where the electrode is aimed towards the commissure and passes through the parafascicular and centromedian nuclei. In the Boivie-Meyerson study the relationship between an

effective stimulation site and the parafascicular nucleus was discussed, and it was concluded that only the most medial portion of this nucleus, or rather the transitional zone to the so-called endymal nucleus (Strenge et al., 1981) constitutes the effective region (Fig. 2).

Akil and Richardson (1977), in their first trials with intraoperative stimulation, assumed that the parafascicular nucleus was particularly effective, but it should be realized that it is difficult on the basis of stereotactic radiographs to tell the exact anatomical location of a stimulating probe. Besides, the medial border of the parafascicular nucleus is anatomically not well defined. Corroborative information based on reported and observed responses to intraoperative stimulation is often difficult to interpret and seems to be of limited predictive value. Such responses have been described in detail by Amano et al. (1982), and claimed to be useful for anatomical identification of the stimulated region. Several autonomic and psychological effects of periaqueductal stimulation were monitored but their presence or absence was not correlated with pain relief. Stimulation of the PVG region often gives rise to a pleasant, though short-lasting sensation of warmth felt in the abdomen, but this sensation does not necessarily imply that pain relief can be achieved. It has also been claimed that stimulation-produced ocular oscillation indicates a proper placement of the electrode, but in our experience this is not reliable. It is reasonable to assume that the variable results reported with PVG stimulation are partly due to the extreme precision required when implanting electrodes in this target region. It is evident that there is still a great need for improving the anatomical and functional precision and accuracy of electrode placement in the ideal PVG stimulation target. As pointed out by Gybels (1983), it might be possible to activate this same pain-controlling system by stimulating more rostral portions of the endorphinergic system (cf. Richardson, 1982) or to find other target sites from where it could be indirectly activated.

It has recently been reported in a large series of

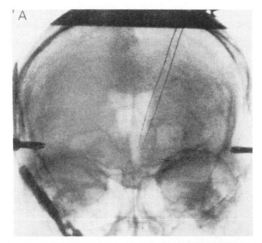

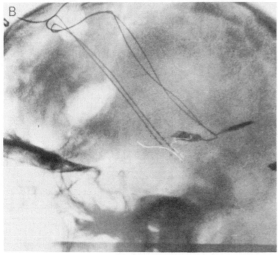

Fig. 1. Stereotactic radiographs showing electrodes implanted in the PVG region in two patients with cancer pain. In (A) the two electrodes were separated in the mediolateral dimension only, about 2 mm apart. Only the medial electrode was effective. In (B) two electrodes were implanted, one 2 mm anterior to the other. Stimulation via either of the electrodes provided pain relief.

182

patients subjected to long-term PVG stimulation, that electrodes were initially implanted for trial stimulation on both sides of the aqueduct (Hosobuchi, 1986). It was found that virtually all patients obtained better pain relief with stimulation in the left PVG than in the right. There are in the literature no reports confirming this interesting observation. It should be recalled that PVG stimulation produces bilateral effects and that there are no data suggesting a somatotopic organization in this region.

Sensory thalamic nucleus

In man, this nucleus is comparatively large, measuring about 10 mm in the mediolateral dimension and 8 mm antero-posteriorly. Thanks to the pioneering studies by Tasker, summarized in a most useful stereotactic atlas (Emmers and Tasker, 1975), detailed data are available on the somatotopic organization of this nucleus. It is well known that the larger, medial part (VPM) represents the face and the hand, and the smaller,

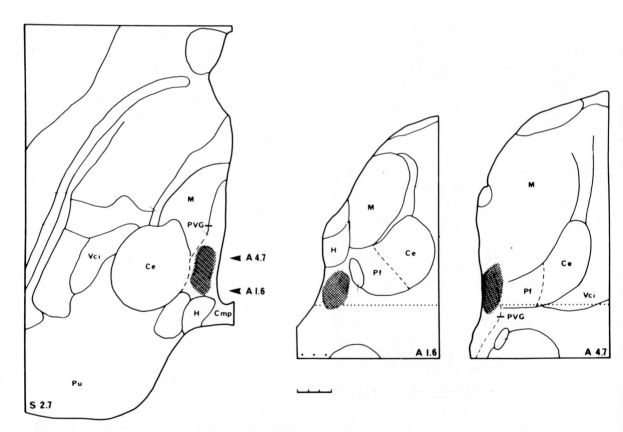

Fig. 2. The approximate extent of the region from which pain relief can be obtained by electric stimulation (hatched area), as based on autopsy data. Slightly modified drawings of horizontal plane S 2.7 (left) and frontal planes A 1.6 and A 4.7 from Van Buren and Borke's stereotactic atlas of the human thalamus. Millimeter scale below plane A 1.6.Cma-Cmp level indicated by dotted line in planes A 1.6 and A 4.7. Ce, nucleus centromedianus thalami; Cmp, commissura posterior; H, nucleus habenularis; M, nucleus medialis; Pf, nucleus parafascicularis; PGV, periventricular grey region; Vci, nucleus ventralis caudalis internus. (From Boivie and Meyerson, 1982; reproduced by permission, Elsevier Biomedical Press.)

lateral one contains projection from the leg. In practice, it is very difficult to find the location in the nucleus from where stimulation-induced paraesthesiae may be evoked in the head, the neck, the back and the trunk. Apparently, these are masked by sensations simultaneously evoked from the more extensive face and hand portions. Another problem of practical importance is that in some cases of long-standing peripheral deafferentation it may be very difficult, or impossible, to find the projection site corresponding to the affected limb, for example in paraplegia or phantom limb (unpublished observations; Tasker, personal communication). It might be that functional changes, similar to those observed in experimental animals (Albe-Fessard and Lombard, 1980; Gautron and Guilbaud, 1982; Morpurgo et al. 1983), have occurred as a result of distorted afferent input.

As with spinal cord stimulation, it is generally accepted that the presence of paraesthesiae in the painful region in response to thalamic stimulation at low intensity, is a prerequisite for obtaining pain relief. Therefore, the placement of the electrode can sometimes be very critical as illustrated by one of our cases. That patient suffered from causalgia-like pain in the ulnar region of the arm and hand. During trial stimulation it was eventually discovered that the patient felt the stimulation-induced paraesthesiae in the radial part of the arm only. Somatosensory responses evoked from the ulnar nerve were of comparatively low amplitude. As shown in Fig. 3, the responses obtained with this electrode site (A) had the highest amplitude when stimulation was applied to the lip, whereas no response would be recorded with stimulation of the tibial nerve. In a study where evoked potentials were used to map the somatotopy of the sensory nucleus, the region corresponding to the projection from the radial fingers is located only 2 mm medially from that representing the ulnar ones (Giorgi et al., 1980). On the basis of these data we changed the location of the electrode to a location 2 mm more laterally, and from this new position more prominent responses could be obtained by

stimulation of the ulnar nerve. At this electrode site (Fig. 3, B), responses to lip stimulation displayed a reduced amplitude and it was now also possible to obtain responses to tibial stimulation. Stimulation in this new target provided satisfactory pain relief. This particular case further illustrates that at low-intensity stimulation the functional spread of current apparently does not exceed about 1 mm.

It is possible to evoke paraesthesiae by stimulation both in the sensory nucleus itself and in the junction zone between the nucleus and the lemniscus, where the threshold for producing paraesthesiae is generally lower. It has been claimed by Mazars et al. (1974) that the intensity of stimulation should be kept just sub-threshold to

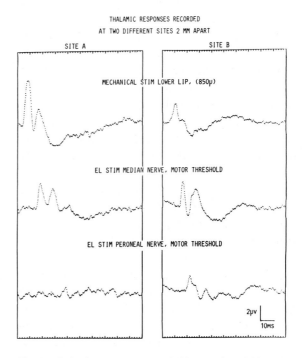

Fig. 3. Thalamic responses recorded in a patient subjected to ICS for causalgic pain in the ulnar region. Stimulation in site A produced paraesthesiae confined to the radial portion of the arm. The electrode was repositioned 2 mm more laterally, site B, from where paraesthesiae could be produced also in the ulnar region. Note the difference in relative amplitude of the responses recorded at the two sites (Hallström and Meyerson, in preparation).

paraesthesiae and that instead a sensation of warmth is preferable. In some of our patients who have enjoyed exceptionally long-lasting and effective poststimulatory suppression of pain, such sensations of pleasant feelings of warmth dominated, and paraesthesiae could only be evoked with comparatively high stimulus intensity. These observations are in accordance with the view maintained by Mazars. However, it is not yet known whether the presence of 'thermal paraesthesiae' is a favourable sign in STh stimulation (cf. Namba et al., 1985).

Problems in the clinical application of ICS

Tolerance

The development of tolerance is considered to be one of the major problems with stimulation in either of the two targets. With stimulation in PVG a failing effect with time has been claimed to be equivalent to tolerance to exogenous opioids, as substantiated by the finding that cross-tolerance to morphine can generally be demonstrated. This would imply that stimulation-produced analgesia in man is solely the result of activation of mechanisms associated with opioid substances. For reasons discussed above this assumption has been questioned, and it should also be emphasized that tolerance to PVG stimulation is not a regular phenomenon, since there are patients who have maintained the positive effect of stimulation for many years.

Different strategies have been tried to counteract the development of tolerance. The most interesting approach has been the use of oral L-tryptophan with the intent to enhance the synthesis of serotonin, which in experimental animals may reverse tolerance to PVG stimulation (reviews, see Rivot et al., 1984; Hammond, 1986). The effectiveness of L-tryptohan has been reported in two studies only, but it should be recalled that PVG stimulation is presently practised in very few centers (Hosobuchi et al., 1980, 1986; Tsubokawa, personal communication). Another way of trying

to enhance serotonergic mechanisms in PVG stimulation is to utilize drugs which interfere with the re-uptake of serotonin. However, these drugs generally have composite effects as they also act on both noradrenergic and cholinergic systems. There are as yet no controlled studies proving the reinforcement of PVG stimulation by use of such drugs.

The reported incidence of failures to maintain the effect of STh stimulation varies in different studies. As the physiological mechanism to the pain relief obtained with such stimulation is virtually unknown, it is difficult to speculate on the possible reasons why tolerance – or fatigue or habituation – may occur. It has been claimed (Tsubokawa et al., 1984; Hosobuchi, 1986) that a regular medication with L-dopa may improve the efficacy of STh stimulation and even reverse 'habituation'. However, these observations remain to be confirmed.

Criteria for patient-target selection

Based on the assumption that PVG and STh are selectively efficacious for nociceptive and neuropathic pain, respectively, and that these two forms of pain can be differentiated by their responsiveness to opioids, the so-called morphine test has become a principal element in the selection of patients and targets (Plotkin, 1982; Young, 1985; Hosobuchi, 1986). Morphine is administered i.v. in incremental doses, randomly interspersed with placebo injections, and the pain is assessed using a visual analogue scale (VAS). Reported pain relief is interpreted as a sign of the pain being of nociceptive origin whereas a lack of response suggests that the pain is neuropathic. Although the responsiveness to opioids is useful in differentiating nociceptive and neuropathic pain, there are certain difficulties inherent in the interpretation of morphine tests in general and in particular, when designed as outlined above. Thus, in practice it is often difficult to separate a true analgesic effect from the sedation which inevitably accompanies morphine in high doses. Besides, many of the patients considered for ICS are regular users of opioids (cf. Young et al., 1986) and they may be capable of recognizing the secondary effects of an active drug versus placebo. Moreover, they are often tolerant and/or dependent. Therefore, it is desirable for patients to be free of narcotic analgesics for some time before subjected to the test. Instead of using morphine in incremental doses, we have found it useful to administer a standard dose (10 – 15 mg) given double-blind randomly interspersed with placebo injections (Arnér and Meyerson, 1988). Whatever design of test is employed, a potential problem to overcome is that some chronic pain conditions, and in particular those referred to as 'low back pain', may include a mixture of various nociceptive and neuropathic pain components. In addition, pain classified as psychogenic or idiopathic may be unresponsive to narcotic analgesics (Arnér and Meyerson, 1988).

It has been reported (Tasker et al., 1980; Plotkin, 1982) that barbiturates i.v. can be used to alleviate neuropathic pain and can thus be employed as a test to differentiate such pain from nociceptive pain. However, this possibility has not been systematically explored and sedation could make the interpretation difficult.

The relevance and reliability of the morphine test can only be accepted if, in fact, PVG stimulation-induced pain relief occurs only as a result of endorphinergic activation. This notion has been challenged on the basis that the elevation of endorphins in CSF associated with stimulation may be unrelated to the pain-relieving effect (Amano et al., 1980). Moreover, as discussed elsewhere in this volume (see Chapter by Barbaro) naloxone reversal of relief following PVG stimulation is not a regular finding (Meyerson, 1983). However, it should be recalled that the effects of this drug, particularly when used in the very high doses required to induce reversal, are exceedingly complex (review, see Millan, 1986). An experimental finding which may be of particular relevance in this context is that, in rats, stimulation in the dorsal part of PAG brings into operation an antinociceptive

system which is not influenced by naloxone, whereas stimulation applied in the ventral part of the same region is naloxone-sensitive (Liebeskind et al., 1982). Similar results are reported by Hosobuchi in this volume.

When discussing the possible physiological mechanisms of pain relief resulting from stimulation regardless of whether applied in PVG or in STh, reference to data derived from experimental work should be done with utmost care. It should be recalled that little experimental work has been performed on subhuman primates and there are likely to be significant species differences. More important is the often neglected fact that stimulation-produced analgesia in animals signifies a reduction of responsiveness to acute, noxious stimuli whereas in patients no appreciable augmentation of thresholds or of tolerance to painful stimuli has yet been demonstrated – in contrast, chronic pain can be abolished. It is indeed a challenge to find an explanation to these seemingly contradictory phenomena.

Possible ways of exploring the biochemical background to ICS

One of the striking differences between stimulation-produced analgesia in animals and pain relief with ICS in man is the time course. In animals, it is rarely possible to produce effects that last more than a few minutes whereas the poststimulatory suppression of chronic pain in man may persist for many hours, in exceptional cases even for days. This intriguing feature of ICS may represent changes in the neurohumoral milieu at the site of stimulation or occurring as a result of activation of pathways projecting to remote regions. Deepened understanding of the nature of these changes can promote the further development of ICS. In principal, two different approaches to the study of the biochemical background to ICS in man are available: (1) measurements of different transmitter substances, or their metabolites, in lumbar or ventricular CSF, or even locally at the stimulation site by micro-dialyses (in preparation) in order to assess changes induced by stimulation, (2) administration of drugs, systemically or intrathecally, which may have transmitter antagonistic of agonistic properties with regard to the effect of stimulation.

There are several problems involved in designing and performing studies concerned with analyses of CSF. It is likely that the release of endogenous substances associated with ICS is more directly influencing the composition of ventricular than of lumbar CSF, and long-term implantation of a ventricular catheter for research purposes only is ethically questionable. A trivial but real problem is the selection of relevant substances for analysis. Apart from the commonly studied transmitter/modulator substances (endorphins, enkephalins, monoamines, substance P, etc.), there are a multiplicity of substances which in animal experiments have been shown to be directly related to pain and anti-nociception (review, see Aronoff and Sweet, 1985), though it is questionable whether this information is relevant to chronic pain (discussion, see Millan, 1986).

In view of solid experimental evidence for the participation in stimulation-produced analgesia of both supraspinal and spinal serotonergic and noradrenergic pathways and mechanisms, it is surprising that so few attempts have been made to assess the possible involvement of monoamines in ICS. Over the years we have collected lumbar CSF, before and subsequent to both PVG and STh stimulation, as well as spinal cord stimulation, and performed analyses of monoamine metabolites as well as substance P, somatostatin, cholecystokinin (CCK), VIP and neurotensin (Meyerson et al., 1986). No consistent changes as a result of either form of stimulation could be found in any of these measurements with the exception of substance P. In view of the postulated transmitter function of substance P at the first spinal relay of nociception, one would expect a high concentration of this substance in lumbar CSF obtained from patients in severe pain prior to stimulation. That was not the case. Unexpectedly, stimulation caused an augmentation of the substance P content which,

however, seemed to occur also in a few patients who did not enjoy pain relief. Therefore, it is conceivable that changes of the substance P concentration induced by stimulation were unrelated to pain and pain relief. These findings illustrate the difficulties involved in trying to relate a release, or consumption, of transmitters/modulators assumed to be associated with pain-relieving stimulation.

The practicality of using agonistic and antagonistic drugs which may influence the effect of ICS is limited by the fact that there are relatively few such drugs available for human use. Besides, they are often not sufficiently receptor-selective to permit definite conclusions. As already mentioned, L-tryptophan and L-dopa have been employed as putative agonists in order to restore the efficacy of PVG and STh stimulation, respectively. It might be that a systematic study of the effects of serotonin and dopamine, as well as noradrenaline and acetylcholine blockers would supply corroborative evidence of the involvement of these transmitters in ICS. Such studies could perhaps help to bridge some of the gaps in our understanding of the biochemical background to ICS in man.

Acknowledgements

Part of the data presented in this article have been supported by grants from Karolinska institutets fonder and Märta Hedborgs fond.

References

Adams, J.E. (1976) Naloxone reversal of analgesia produced by brain stimulation in the human. *Pain*, 2: 161–166.

Albe-Fessard, D.G. and Lombard, M.C. (1980) Animal models for chronic pain. In H.W. Kosterlitz and L.Y. Terenius (Eds.), *Pain and Society*, Verlag Chemie GmbH, Weinheim, pp. 299–310.

Amano, K., Tanikawa, T., Kawamura, H., Iseki, H., Notani, M., Kawabatake, H., Shiwaku, T., Suda, T., Demura, H. and Kitamura, K. (1982) Endorphins and pain relief. Further observations on electrical stimulation of the lateral part of the periaqueductal gray matter during rostal mesencephalic reticulotomy for pain relief. *Appl. Neurophysiol.*, 45: 123–135.

Archer, T., Jonsson, G., Minor, B.G. and Post, C. (1986) Noradrenergic-serotonergic interactions and nociception in the rat. *Eur. J. Pharmacol.*, 120: 295–307.

Arnér, S. and Arnér, B. (1985) Differential effect of epidural morphine in the treatment of cancer-related pain. *Acta Anaesthesiol. Scand.*, 29: 332–336.

Arnér, S. and Meyerson, B.A. (1988) Lack of analgesic effect of opioids on neuropathic and idiopathic forms of pain. *Pain*, 33: 11–23.

Aronoff, G. and Sweet, W.H. (1985) The future of pain management. In G. Aronoff (Ed.), *Evaluation and Treatment of Chronic Pain*. Urban and Schwarzenberg, New York, pp. 640–658.

Boëthius, J., Lindblom, U., Meyerson, B.A. and Widén, L. (1976) Effects of multifocal brain stimulation on pain and somatosensory functions. In Y. Zotterman (Ed.), *Sensory Functions of the Skin in Primates*, Pergamon Press, Oxford, New York, pp. 531–548.

Boivie, J. and Meyerson, B.A. (1982) A correlative anatomical and clinical study of pain suppression by deep brain stimulation. *Pain*, 13: 113–126.

Comte, P. (1982) Monopolar versus bipolar stimulation. *Appl. Neurophysiol.*, 45: 156–159.

Demierre B. and Siegfried, J. (1983) Traitement neurochirurgical de la névralgie postherpétiforme. *Méd. et Hyg.* (Genève), 1519: 1960–1966.

Dickenson, A. (1983) The inhibitory effects of thalamic stimulation on the spinal transmission of nociceptive information in the rat. *Pain*, 17: 213–224.

Dieckmann, G. and Witzmann, A. (1982) Initial and long-term results of deep brain stimulation for chronic intractable pain. *Appl. Neurophysiol.*, 45: 167–172.

Emmers, R. and Tasker, R.R. (1975) *The Human Somesthetic Thalamus*. Raven Press, New York, 111 pp.

Fitzgerald, M. (1986) Monoamines and descending control of nociception. TINS, 9: 51–52.

Gautron, M. and Guilbaud, G. (1982) Somatic response of ventrobasal thalamic neurons in polyarthritic rats. *Brain Res.*, 237: 459–471.

Gerhart, K.D., Yezierski, R.P., Fang, Z.R. and Willis, W.D. (1983) Inhibition of primate spinothalamic tract neurons by stimulation in the ventral posterior lateral (VPL) thalamic nucleus: possible mechanisms. *J. Neurophysiol.*, 49: 406–423.

Giorgi, G., Kelly, P.J., Eaton, D.C., Guiot, G. and Derome, P. (1980) A study of the tridimensional distribution of somatosensory evoked responses in human thalamus to aid the placement of stimulating electrodes for treatment of pain. *Acta Neurochir.*, Suppl. 30, 279–287.

Groth, K., Adams, J., Richardson, D., Hosobuchi, Y., Ray, C., Turnbull, I. and Long, D. (1982) Deep brain stimulation for chronic intractable pain. Medtronic Inc., Minneapolis.

Gybels, J. (1983) Analgesic brain stimulation in chronic pain in man and rat. In T. Yokota, and R. Dubner (Eds.), *Current Topics in Pain Research and Therapy* (ICS), Excerpta Medica, Amsterdam, pp. 137–144.

Gybels, J. and Cosyns, P. (1976) Modulation of clinical and experimental pain in man by electrical stimulation of the thalamic periventricular gray. In Y. Zotterman (Ed.), *Sensory Functions of the Skin in Primates*, Pergamon Press, Oxford, pp. 521–530.

Gybels, J., Dom, R. and Cosyns, P.C. (1980) Electrical stimulation of the central gray for pain relief in human: autopsy data. *Acta Neurochir.*, Suppl. 30: 259–268.

Hammond, D.L. (1986) Control systems for nociceptive afferent processing: the descending inhibitory pathways. In T.L. Yaksh (Ed.), *Spinal Afferent Processing*, Plenum Publ. Co., New York, pp. 363–380.

Hosobuchi, Y. (1980) The current status of analgesic brain stimulation. *Acta Neurochir.*, Suppl. 30: 219–227.

Hosobuchi, Y. (1986) Subcortical electrical stimulation for control of intractable pain in humans. *J. Neurosurg.*, 64: 543–553.

Hosobuchi, Y., Adams, J.E. and Rutkin, B. (1973) Chronic thalamic stimulation for the control of facial anesthesia dolorosa. *Arch. Neurol.*, 29: 158–161.

Hosobuchi, Y., Adams, J.E. and Fields, H.L. (1974) Chronic thalamic and internal capsular stimulation for the control of facial anesthesia dolorosa and dysesthesia of thalamic syndrome. *Adv. Neurol.*, 4: 783–787.

Hosobuchi, Y., Adams, J.E. and Linchitz, R. (1977) Pain relief by electrical stimulation of the central gray matter in humans and its reversal by naloxone. *Science*, 197: 183–186.

Hosobuchi, Y., Rossier, J. and Bloom, F.E. (1980) Oral loading with L-tryptophan may augment the simultaneous release of ACTH and β-endorphin that accompanies periaqueductal stimulation in humans. In E. Costa and M. Trabucchi (Eds.), *Neural Peptides and Neuronal Communication*, Raven Press, New York, pp. 563–569.

Lazorthes, Y. (1979) European study on deep brain stimulation. Resumé of the 3rd European Workshop on Electrical Neurostimulation. Medtronic Inc., Paris (In mimeo).

Liebeskind, J.C., Cannon, J.T., Prieto, G.J. and Lee, A. (1982) Evidence for opioid and non-opioid forms of stimulation-produced analgesia in the rat. *Brain Res.*, 243: 315–321.

Mazars, G., Mérienne, L. and Cioloca, C. (1973) Stimulations thalamiques intermittentes analgiques. Note préliminaire. *Rev. Neurol.* (Paris), 128: 273–279.

Mazars, G., Mérienne, L. and Cioloca, C. (1974) Traitement de certains types de douleurs par des stimulateurs thalamiques implantables. *Neuro-chir.* (Paris), 20: 117–124.

Mazars, G., Mérienne, L. and Cioloca, C. (1976) Etat actuel de la chirurgie de la douleur. *Neuro-chir.* (Paris), Suppl. 1, 22, 164 pp.

Mazars, G.J., Mérienne, L. and Cioloca, C. (1979) Comparative study of electrical stimulation of posterior thalamic nuclei, periaqueductal gray, and other midline mesencephalic structures in man. In J.J. Bonica, J.C. Liebeskind and D.G. Albe-Fessard (Eds.)., *Advances in Pain Research and Therapy, Vol. 3*, Raven Press. New York, pp. 541–546.

Meyerson, B.A. (1983) Electrostimulation procedures: effects, presumed rationale, and possible mechanisms. In J.J. Bonica, U. Lindblom and A. Iggo (Eds.), *Advances in Pain Research and Therapy, Vol. 5*, Raven Press, New York, pp. 495–534.

Meyerson, B.A. (1989) Intracerebral stimulation. In J.J. Bonica (Ed.), *Management of Pain in Clinical Practice*, Lea and Febiger, Philadelphia, Chapter 72: D, in press.

Meyerson, B.A., Boëthius, J. and Carlsson, A.M. (1979) Alleviation of malignant pain by electrical stimulation in the periventricular-periaqueductal region: pain relief as related to stimulation sites. In J.J. Bonica, J. Liebeskind and D.G. Albe-Fessard (Eds.), *Advances in Pain Research and Therapy, Vol. 3*, Raven Press, New York, pp. 525–533.

Meyerson, B.A., Brodin, E. and Linderoth, B. (1985) Possible neurohumoral mechanisms in CNS stimulation for pain suppression. *Appl. Neurophysiol.*, 48: 175–180.

Millan, M.J. (1986) Multiple opioid systems and pain. *Pain*, 27: 303–347.

Morpurgo, C.V., Gavazzi, G., Pollin, B., Amsallem, B. and Lombard, M.C. (1983) Changes of somatic organization in thalamic ventrobasal nucleus of chronic awake cats associated with persistent nociceptive stimulation. In J.J. Boica, U. Lindblom and A. Iggo (Eds.), *Advances in Pain Research and Therapy, Vol. 5*, Raven Press, New York, 5: 179–183.

Namba, S., Wani, T., Shimizu, Y., Fujiwara, N., Namba, Y., Nakamua, S. and Nishimoto, A. (1985) Sensory and motor responses to deep brain stimulation. *J. Neurosurg.*, 63: 224–234.

Ranck, Jr., J.B. (1975) Which elements are excited in electrical stimulation of mammalian central nervous system: a review. *Brain Res.*, 98: 417–440.

Richardson, D.E. (1982a) Long-term follow-up of deep brain stimulation for relief of chronic pain in the human. In M. Brock (Ed.), *Modern Neurosurgery*, Springer Verlag, Berlin-Heidelberg, pp. 449–453.

Richardson, D.E. (1982b) Analgesia produced by stimulation of various sites in the human β-endorphin system. *Appl. Neurophysiol.*, 45: 116–122.

Richardson, D.E. and Akil, H. (1977) Pain reduction by electrical brain stimulation in man. *J. Neurosurg.*, 47: 178–183.

Rivot, J.P., Weil-Fugazza, J., Godefroy, F., Bineau-Thurotte, M., Ory-Lavollée, L. and Besson, J.-M. (1984) Involvement of serotonin in both morphine and stimulation-produced analgesia: electrochemical and biochemical approaches. In L. Kruger and J.C. Liebeskind (Eds.), *Advances in Pain Research and Therapy, Vol. 6*, Raven Press, New York, pp. 135–150.

Schmidek, H.H., Fohanno, D., Ervin, F.R. and Sweet, W.

(1971) Pain threshold alterations by brain stimulation in the monkey. *J. Neurosurg.*, 35: 715–722.

Siegfried, J. (1983) Long term results of electrical stimulation in the treatment of pain by means of implanted electrodes (epidural spinal cord and deep brain stimulation). In R. Rizzi and M. Visentin (Eds.), *Pain Therapy*, Elsevier Biomedical Press, Amsterdam, pp. 463–475.

Siegfried, J. (1985) Long-term results of intermittent stimulation of the sensory thalamic nuclei and 67 cases of deafferentation pain. In Y. Lazorthes and A.R.M. Upton (Eds.), *Neurostimulation, an Overview*, Futura Publ. Co. Inc., New York, pp. 129–140.

Siegfried, J. and H. Van Loveren (1986) Thalamic stimulation: effects on deafferentation pain and movement disorders. In M. Samii (Ed.), *Surgery in and around the Brain Stem and the Third Ventricle*. Springer-Verlag, Berlin-Heidelberg. pp. 540–546.

Strenge, H., Braak, E., Braak, H. and Muhtaroglu, U. (1981) On the nucleus endymalis of the human thalamus. *J. Hirnforsch.*, 22: 243–252.

Tasker, R.R., Organ, L.W. and Hawrylyshyn, P. (1980) Deafferentation and causalgia. In J.J. Bonica (Ed.), *Pain*, Raven Press, New York, pp. 305–329.

Tsubokawa, T., Yamamoto, T., Katayama, Y., Hirayama, T. and Shibuya, H. (1984) Thalamic relay nucleus stimulation for relief of intractable pain. Clinical results and β-endorphin immunoreactivity in the cerebrospinal fluid. *Pain*, 18: 115–126.

Tsubokawa, T., Katayama, Y., Yamamoto, T. and Hirayama, T. (1985) Deafferentation pain and stimulation of the thalamic sensory relay nucleus: clinical and experimental study. *Appl. Neurophysiol.*, 48: 166–171.

Turnbull, I.M. (1984) Brain stimulation. In P.D. Wall and R. Mezack (Eds.), *Textbook of Pain*, Churchill Livingstone, Edinburgh, pp. 706–714.

Turnbull, I.M., Shulman, R. and Woodhurst, B. (1980) Thalamic stimulation for neuropathic pain. *J. Neurosurg.*, 52: 486–493.

Winkelmüller, W. (1981) Experience with the control of low back pain by the dorsal column stimulation (DCS) system and by the peridural electrode system (PISCES). In Y. Hosobuchi and T. Corbin (Eds.), *Indications for Spinal Cord Stimulation*, Excerpta Medica, Amsterdam, pp. 34–40.

Young, R.F. and Chambi, I. (1987) Pain relief by electrical stimulation of the periaqueductal and periventricular gray matter. *J. Neurosurg.*, 66: 364–371.

Young, R.F., Feldman, R.A., Kroening, R., Fulton, W. and Morris, J. (1984) Electrical stimulation of the brain in the treatment of chronic pain in man. In L. Kruger and J.C. Liebeskind (Eds.), *Advances in Pain Research and Therapy, Vol. 6*, Raven Press, New York, pp. 289–303.

Young, R.F., Kroening, R., Fulton, W., Feldman, R.A. and Chambi, I. (1985) Electrical stimulation of the brain in treatment of chronic pain. *J. Neurosurg.*, 62: 389–396.

H.L. Fields and J.-M. Besson (Eds.)
Progress in Brain Research, Vol. 77
© 1988 Elsevier Science Publishers B.V. (Biomedical Division)

CHAPTER 10

Current issues regarding subcortical electrical stimulation for pain control in humans

Yoshio Hosobuchi

Section of Functional and Stereotactic Surgery, Department of Neurological Surgery, School of Medicine, University of California, San Francisco, San Francisco, CA, USA

Introduction

Electrical stimulation of specific sites in the human brain has been used to provide relief or suppression of pain since 1960, when Heath and Mickle (1960) reported suppression of pain in patients by stimulation of the septal area. Others subsequently used therapeutic stimulation of subcortical areas, such as the median forebrain bundle (Balagura and Ralph, 1973) and caudate nucleus (Erwin et al., 1966), but for more than a decade little attention was paid to these sporadic clinical efforts.

In 1973, Mazars and colleagues (1973) and our group at the University of California, San Francisco (Hosobuchi et al., 1973) reported independently that electrical stimulation from electrodes permanently implanted in the region of the sensory thalamus satisfactorily alleviated deafferentation pain, a syndrome caused by damage to the peripheral or central nervous system that generally respond poorly to opiate analgesic agents (Hosobuchi, 1982). These findings led to the commercial manufacture of a stimulation system consisting of an implantable electrode made of an inert metal which is connected to a radiofrequency-coupled transcutaneous stimulator. On the basis of studies by Reynolds (1969) and others showing the behavioral antinociceptive effect of stimulation of the periaqueductal gray region of the brain in animals, this system was assessed to determine the thera-

peutic efficacy of stimulation of the comparable area of the human brain. The encouraging preliminary results were reported in 1977 by our group (Hosobuchi et al., 1977) and by Richardson and Akil (1977). Since that time, further clinical studies have established the safety of the technique and a general consensus that stimulation of the somatosensory area of the thalamus (STh) is effective in the control of deafferentation or neuropathic pain syndromes (Hosobuchi, 1980; Siegfried, 1985) that may be refractory to conventional opiate medication, and stimulation of the periaqueductal gray matter (PAG) is effective for pain syndromes that respond to opiates (Hosobuchi, 1980, 1982).

Despite large clinical series of patients undergoing subcortical stimulation for pain control that have recently been reported (Hosobuchi, 1986; Meyerson, 1979; Plotkin, 1982, Siegfried, 1985; Young et al., 1985), there seems to be considerable disagreement regarding the precise targets for stimulation, stimulation parameters, actual effect on sensory perception beyond clinical pain relief, and, finally, the possible mechanism for the pain suppression achieved by stimulation of these subcortical structures. Although a general consensus is lacking on these questions, I will discuss these issues based on my 17 years of experience in the area of stimulation-produced analgesia (SPA) in humans.

The target for stimulation

Sensory thalamus

The effect of stimulation of the subcortical STh in relieving deafferentation pain in humans was discovered empirically (Hosobuchi et al., 1973; Mazars et al., 1973). No histologic verification of the precise sites of electrode implantation has been made in patients who have had an electrode placed in this region. Computer-aided tomography (CAT) scans have defined the general location of the effective site to be in the posterior ventral lateral region of the thalamus, and have excluded the previously held notion that the posterior limb of the internal capsule also may be an effective target site (Hosobuchi, 1986).

It required the introduction of magnetic resonance (MR) imaging to precisely define the target in the thalamus. Our recent MR analysis of 17 patients with implanted thalamic electrodes (9 unilateral, 8 bilateral) showed that, in patients who experienced therapeutic efficacy, the contact point of the electrodes was situated just at the most ventral portion of the sensory thalamic nuclei, as the medial lemniscus enters the thalamus (Fig. 1). Because electrical stimulation at any point in this region will produce similar paresthesias in the body, the precise anatomic site of the electrode cannot be localized with certainty on the basis of the quality of paresthesia reported by the patient alone (Hosobuchi, 1986; Tasker et al., 1983).

A few studies performed recently in animals and humans have also suggested that stimulation of the ventral area of the sensory thalamus, where maximum peripheral sensory evoked responses can be recorded, provides the most effective control of deafferentation pain (Nishimoto et al., 1984; Yingling and Hosobuchi, 1984). Thus, what initially was thought to be a relatively wide target area in which electrical stimulation would produce therapeutic efficacy may actually be a considerably smaller area. This would explain the marked variations in clinical results that have been reported (Hosobuchi, 1986; Plotkin, 1982; Siegfried, 1985;

Young et al., 1985). We have not used somatosensory evoked response recordings routinely to delineate the target point for the implantation of thalamic electrodes because it is often difficult to elicit sensory evoked responses from a deafferented portion of the body.

Electrical impedance measurement does provide useful guidance during electrode placement. When measurements show a change from the electrical

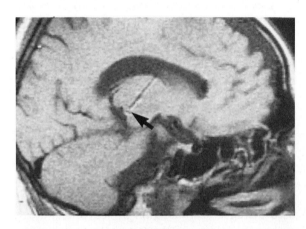

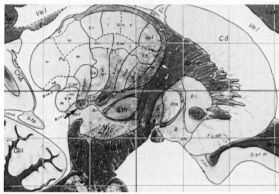

Fig. 1. (Top) Sagittal magnetic resonance image of a patient with a left sensory thalamic electrode. The patient had right postcordotomy dysesthesia which was relieved by the thalamic stimulation. The electrode is seen as a dark line in the thalamus. The most inferior contact point of the electrode is placed just above the medial lemniscus. The sagittal section is 15 mm from the midline of the brain. A T_2-weighted image was selected to present a clear image of the electrode. Note the location of the medial lemniscus on the T_2-weighted image (arrow). (Bottom) A comparable sagittal section of human brain at 14.5 mm from midline according to the Schaltenbrand and Bailey Atlas (1959). The arrow indicates the location of the medial lemniscus.

impedance in the gray matter (450 Ω) to that in white matter (600 Ω) using a Radionics® stimulation probe with a 3-mm exposed tip, one generally can be assured that the electrode tip is entering the medial lemniscus. Such electrical impedance measurements, providing neurophysiologic definition of the electrode implantation site, accompanied by confirmation on postoperative MR images, may further improve success rates in the control of difficult deafferentation pain by thalamic stimulation.

Periaqueductal gray and periventricular gray (PVG) region

In contrast to the lack of histologic verification of electrode placement in patients with thalamic stimulation, there are at least four reports documenting autopsy findings on patients who have had electrodes implanted in the PAG-PVG region (Baskin et al., 1986; Boivie and Meyerson, 1982; Gybels et al., 1980; Hosobuchi et al., 1977). Among those, the patients who had experienced definite therapeutic efficacy had the electrode placed in the ventral portion of the PAG and PVG. Those who had had limited or no effect appeared to have their electrode(s) located outside or more lateral to this narrow band of gray matter surrounding the CSF passage.

These findings raise a serious technical question about whether stereotactic surgery can be performed with sufficient accuracy to place a rather sizeable electrode in such a small area in humans — but this technical challenge may be answered in the viable clinical results reported (Hosobuchi, 1986; Meyerson, 1979; Plotkin, 1982; Young et al., 1985). In fact, in animals there may be significant differences in the analgesia produced by ventral as opposed to dorsal PAG stimulation. The SPA obtained with ventral PAG stimulation is reversed by naloxone (Besson, 1980; Mayer, 1979), whereas dorsal PAG stimulation-produced analgesia is not (Cannon et al., 1982; Fardin et al., 1984).

In 1975, Dr. Jay Law told me of one of his patients who was dying of a cancer producing severe abdominal pain. This pain was controlled successfully by PAG stimulation but, to be free of pain, the patient had to self-stimulate continuously. This was somewhat different from our experience with similar types of pain problems, as our patients used intermittent stimulation. The relief this patient obtained by stimulation was not reversed by naloxone. A CAT scan showed the electrode tip to be located in the dorsal PAG at the level of the superior colliculus.

This observation differed significantly from my observations up to that time (Hosobuchi et al., 1977). Over the past 9 years, therefore, I have assessed the analgesic effect of dorsal PAG stimulation in my patients undergoing mesencephalic reticulotomy for relief of the pain of head and neck cancer (Hosobuchi, 1987). In these patients, SPA was obtained by stimulation of the area described by Dr. Law. SPA from this region did require continuous stimulation, and occasionally was accompanied by an unpleasant sensation, such as fear. The pain relief obtained was not reversed by naloxone nor was it accompanied by alterations in the endorphin level in ventricular cerebral spinal fluid (Hosobuchi, 1987).

These findings also implied a possibility of heterogeneity of the analgesic system existing at the PAG level in humans. Until research can clearly define the site of electrode placement in this region by either autopsy studies or at least by MR images, arguments regarding whether or not PAG stimulation in humans relates to the stimulation of an opioid descending pain-inhibitory system, and whether or not the stimulation of PAG is accompanied by a release of endorphins, is entirely superfluous.

Summary

The empirical evidence supports the efficacy of deep brain stimulation in the management of chronic pain. Although the implantation of electrodes and chronic stimulation of the subcortical area in humans are not entirely without risk or complications, the technique provides safe, satisfactory control of pain for patients who have severe and intractable pain that is difficult or impossible to manage by medical means. Despite large, recently compiled clinical series of subcortical stimulation for pain control, there seems to be considerable disagreement regarding precise targets for stimulation, stimulation parameters, actual effect on sensory perception beyond clinical pain relief, and, finally, a possible mechanism of the pain suppression achieved by the stimulation of subcortical structures in humans. The primary reason for confusion in these areas is focused in one main area: that is, the failure to provide either radiologic or histologic documentation of the stimulation site. Recently introduced magnetic resonance imaging techniques may rapidly resolve such problems.

References

Balagura, S. and Ralph, T. (1973) The analgesic effect of electrical stimulation of the diencephalon and the mesencephalon. *Brain Res.,* 60: 369 – 379.

Baskin, D., Mehler, W.R., Hosobuchi, Y., Richardson, D.E., Adams, J.E. and Flitter, M.A. (1986) Autopsy analysis of the safety, efficacy and cartography of electrical stimulation of the central gray in humans. *Brain Res.,* 371: 231 – 236.

Besson, J.-M.R. (1980) Supraspinal modulation of the segmental transmission of pain. In H.W. Kosterlitz and L.Y. Terrenius (Eds.), *Pain and Society,* Verlag Chemie, Weinheim, pp. 161 – 182.

Boivie, J. and Meyerson, B.A. (1982) A correlative anatomical and clinical study of pain suppression by deep brain stimulation. *Pain,* 13: 113 – 126.

Cannon, J.T., Prieto, G.J. and Liebeskind, J.C. (1982) Evidence for opioid and non-opioid forms of stimulation produced analgesia in rat. *Brain Res.,* 243: 315 – 321.

Erwin, F.R., Brown, C.E. and Mark, V.H. (1966) Striatal influence on facial pain. *Confin. Neurol.,* 27: 75 – 90.

Fardin, V., Oliveras, J.L. and Besson, J.M. (1984) A reinvestigation of the analgesic effects induced by stimulation of the periaqueductal gray matter in cats. *Brain Res.,* 306: 105 – 123.

Gybels, J., Dom, R. and Cosyns, P.C. (1980) Electrical stimulation of the central gray for pain relief in humans: autopsy data. *Acta Neurochir.* Suppl., 30: 259 – 268.

Heath, R.G. and Mickle, W.A. (1960) Evaluation of seven years experience with depth electrode studies in human patients. In E.R. Ramey and D.S. O'Doherty (Eds.), *Electrical Studies on the Unanesthetized Brain,* Hoeber Inc., New York, pp. 214 – 247.

Hosobuchi, Y. (1980) The current status of analgesic brain stimulation. *Acta Neurochir.* Suppl., 30: 219 – 227.

Hosobuchi, Y. (1982) Analgesia induced by brain stimulation with chronically implanted electrodes. In H.H. Schmidek and W.H. Sweet (Eds.), *Operative Neurological Techniques, Vol. 2,* Grune and Stratton, New York, pp. 981 – 991.

Hosobuchi, Y. (1986) Subcortical electrical stimulation for control of intractable pain in humans. *J. Neurosurg.,* 64: 543 – 553.

Hosobuchi, Y. (1987) Dorsal periaqueductal gray-matter stimulation in humans. *Pace,* 10: 213 – 216.

Hosobuchi, Y., Adams, J.E. and Rutkin, B. (1973) Chronic thalamic stimulation for the control of facial anesthesia dolorosa. *Arch. Neurol.,* 29: 158 – 161.

Hosobuchi, Y., Adams, J.E. and Linchitz, R. (1977) Pain relief by electrical stimulation of the central gray matter in humans and its reveral by naloxone. *Science,* 197: 183 – 186.

Mayer, D.J. (1979) Endogenous analgesia systems: neural and behavioral mechanisms. In J.J. Bonica, J.C. Liebeskind and D.G. Albe-Fessard (Eds.), *Advances in Pain Research and Therapy, Vol. 3,* Raven Press, New York, pp. 385 – 410.

Mazars, G.J., Merienne, L. and Ciolocca, C. (1973) Stimulations thalamiques intermittentes antalgiques. Note préliminaire. *Rev. Neurol.,* 128: 273 – 279.

Meyerson, B.A. (1979) Stimulation electrique du systeme nerveux central pour le soulagement des douleurs chroniques. In D.G. Albe-Fessard and J. Gybels (Eds.), *La Douleur,* 42° Congres Français Médical, Masson, Paris, pp. 71 – 89.

Nishimoto, A., Namba, S., Nakao, Y., et al. (1984) Inhibition of nociceptive neurons by internal capsule stimulation. *Appl. Neurophysiol.,* 47: 117 – 127, 1984.

Plotkin, R. (1982) Results in 60 cases of deep brain stimulation for chronic intractable pain. *Appl. Neurophysiol.,* 45: 173 – 178.

Reynolds, D.V. (1969) Surgery in the rat during electrical analgesia induced by focal brain stimulation. *Science,* 164: 444 – 445.

Richardson, D.E. and Akil, H. (1977) Pain reduction by electrical brain stimulation in man. 2. Chronic self-administration in the periventricular gray matter. *J. Neurosurg.,* 47: 184 – 194.

Siegfried, J. (1985) Long-term results of intermittent stimulation of the sensory thalamic nuclei in 67 cases of deafferentation pain. In Y. Lazorthes and A.R.M. Upton (Eds.), *Neurostimulation: an Overview,* Futura Publishing Co., Mt. Kisco, New York, pp. 129 – 143.

Tasker, R.R., Tsuda, T. and Hawrylyshyor, P. (1983) Clinical neurophysiological investigation of deafferentation pain. *Adv. Pain Res. Ther.,* 5: 713 – 738.

Yingling, C.D. and Hosobuchi, Y. (1984) A subcortical correlate of P300 in man. *Electroencephalogr. Clin. Neurophysiol.,* 59: 72 – 76.

Young, R.F., Kroening, R., Fulton, W., Feldman, R.A., Chambi, I. (1985) Electrical stimulation of the brain in treatment of chronic pain. *J. Neurosurg.,* 62: 389 – 396.

H.L. Fields and J.-M. Besson (Eds.)
Progress in Brain Research, Vol. 77
© 1988 Elsevier Science Publishers B.V. (Biomedical Division)

CHAPTER 11

Tonic descending inhibition and spinal nociceptive transmission

A.W. Duggan and C.R. Morton

Department of Pharmacology, John Curtin School of Medical Research, Australian National University, Canberra ACT, Australia

Introduction

A commonly used preparation in neurophysiological and neuropharmacological experiments on the spinal cord and nociception is an anaesthetized cat, subjected to extensive surgery, and with the spinal cord transected at the thoracolumbar junction. Such a preparation is lively with neurons responding vigorously to appropriate noxious stimuli. But much of this liveliness is artifactual and stems from the severance of spinal neurons from the brain.

The consequences of spinal transection have been studied for over 100 years beginning with the description of spinal shock by Hall (1843) and considerably developed by the subsequent studies of Sherrington (1906). Spinal shock refers to the total suppression of reflexes in spinal segments distal to the site of section, and is most prolonged in primates. Following a period of reflex suppression, flexor reflexes recover relatively rapidly and typically become hyperactive. Extensor reflexes may never adequately recover. While early explanations of the results of spinal transection emphasized withdrawal of tonic supraspinal facilitation, in 1926 Fulton suggested that suppression of monosynaptic extensor reflexes from spinal transection resulted from withdrawal of tonic supraspinal inhibition of antagonistic multisynaptic flexor withdrawal reflexes. The latter were

known to inhibit extensor reflexes. This view was supported by Liddell et al. (1932) who found that sectioning the dorsolateral and ventral funiculi of the spinal cord increased flexor reflexes in the cat.

Tonic supraspinal inhibition of flexor reflexes has been extensively studied by Lundberg and his colleagues (Holmqvist and Lundberg, 1961; Engberg et al., 1968; Lundberg, 1982). In *intact* animals, the flexor reflex is best elicited by a noxious cutaneous stimulus (Sherrington, 1906). Lundberg has defined a further group of primary afferents in the cat, which includes group II and III muscle afferents, joint afferents and both high and low threshold cutaneous afferents as the 'flexor reflex afferents' (FRA) and which may elicit flexor reflexes in *spinal* preparations. Transmission of impulses in these afferents to motoneurons, to ascending fibres and to the spinal interneurons responsible for generating dorsal root potentials, was shown to be under powerful tonic supraspinal control in intact animals.

More recent studies have emphasized that the excitation of many neurons of the dorsal horn by peripheral noxious stimuli is tonically inhibited from the brain, both in decerebrate, and in barbiturate or chloralose anaesthetized animals. Such inhibition is readily demonstrated by comparing the activities of these neurons in the presence and absence of reversible block of spinal conduction produced by localized cooling of the spinal cord cephalic to the neurons under study. Fig. 1 illustrates typical apparatus and the increases in neuronal firing produced by cold block of the spinal cord. With decerebrate cats, Wall (1967) found that cold block at the thoracolumbar junction expanded the peripheral receptive fields and increased the excitabilities of lumbar neurons of laminae IV, V, and VI. Subsequent studies have noted, however, that the tonic descending inhibition of lamina V or spinocervical tract neurons in decerebrate cats is exerted predominantly on excitation by noxious stimuli or by impulses evoked electrically in unmyelinated fibres, with little effect on non-nociceptive responses (Brown, 1971; Besson et al., 1975).

Investigations with anaesthetized cats have produced similar results. With multireceptive dorsal horn neurons in barbiturate or chloralose anaesthetized cats, cold block at the thoracolumbar junction has increased responses to noxious cutaneous heat and to impulses in unmyelinated primary afferents together with spontaneous firing, but non-nociceptive responses have been little or not affected (Handwerker et al., 1975; Duggan et al., 1977, 1981; Soja and Sinclair, 1980, 1983a,b; Morton et al., 1983, 1984; Dickhaus et

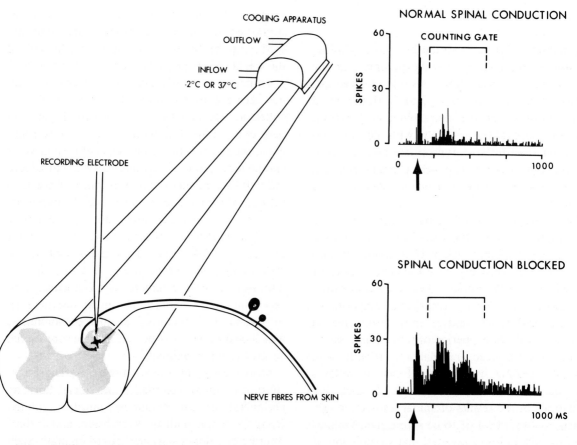

Fig. 1. Enhanced firing of a lumbar dorsal horn neuron following spinal cold block at the thoracolumbar junction. Typical cooling apparatus is shown on the left. The peristimulus histograms illustrate summed cell firing in response to 16 stimuli (marked by an arrow) to the ipsilateral tibial nerve at an intensity adequate to excite both myelinated and unmyelinated afferent fibres. The counting gate above each record indicates the period following each stimulus in which action potentials evoked by impulses in unmyelinated afferents were totalled and an analogue of each count plotted continuously as a gated C response (see Fig. 2).

al., 1985). Cervero et al. (1976) similarly found tonic descending inhibition on nociceptive-specific neurons of lamina I in chloralose anaesthetized cats, but such inhibition could not be detected on neurons of the substantia gelatinosa (Cervero et al., 1979).

Tonic descending inhibition also occurs in other species. In anaesthetized rats, this inhibition was found on the excitation of dorsal horn neurons by noxious cutaneous thermal stimuli (Necker and Hellon, 1978). In anaesthetized monkeys, the responses of spinothalamic tract neurons to impulses in Aδ sural primary afferents were found to be tonically inhibited (Willis et al., 1977). A recent report has also described tonic descending inhibition of nociceptive reflexes in a non-mammalian vertebrate preparation, the decerebrate stingray (Livingston and Leonard, 1985).

Several important questions need to be addressed when considering tonic descending inhibition and nociception. The first is whether this control is present in conscious animals or is it an artifact of the experimental preparation? Secondly, is tonic decending inhibition primarily concerned with nociception, and thus can influence the perception of pain, or is its real function to control spinal withdrawal reflexes to a number of peripheral stimuli? Are there multiple descending controls inhibiting spinal transmission of nociceptive information or is there predominantly one? The source of the inhibition needs to be considered, as well as the mechanisms of the inhibition in the spinal cord and the neurotransmitters involved. In the account which follows the inhibition will be referred to as 'tonic descending inhibition', with no implication that this is necessarily a homogeneous entity in terms of cells of origin, transmitters released or neurons affected.

Tonic descending inhibition and conscious animals

Several studies have described hyperalgesia following spinal or supraspinal lesions, suggesting that a tonically active supraspinal system, for suppressing the perception of noxious stimuli, is indeed operative in conscious animals.

In rats, nociception is often measured by determining the tail flick latency in response to a noxious thermal stimulus to the tail surface. Acute spinalization at the thoracic level has produced either a marked decrease in this latency (Grossmann et al., 1973; Woolf et al., 1980) or a more vigorous tail flick response (Irwin et al., 1951). Inactivation of supraspinal regions has also shortened the latency of this nociceptive reflex (discussed later in this chapter). In monkeys, lesions of the dorsolateral column, have decreased the latency, and increased the force of escape, from a noxious electrical stimulus to the ipsilateral hindlimb, although thresholds were not altered (Vierck et al., 1971). Cats observed for up to 9 months following lumbar intrathecal administration of alumina cream were found to be hyperalgesic (Kennard, 1950). Lesions of the dorsal cervical cord have also enhanced responsiveness to noxious mechanical stimulation in cats (Melzack et al., 1958). Importantly in awake, drug-free cats, spinal dorsal horn neurons showed little spontaneous activity, suggesting the presence of tonic inhibition (Collins, 1984, 1987). Furthermore, almost all neurons sampled in this preparation responded only to low-threshold mechanical stimuli, raising the possibility that some were multireceptive cells with tonic inhibition of their nociceptive excitation. Collectively this evidence supports the presence of tonic descending inhibition in conscious animals.

The sources of tonic descending inhibition

In determining the supraspinal source or sources of tonic descending inhibition, one approach has been to observe such inhibition before and after inactivation of various supraspinal regions. Such experiments have examined many areas but particularly those where electrical stimulation produces descending inhibition of spinal neurons and behavioural analgesia, such as the mesencephalic periaqueductal grey matter (PAG) and the medullary nucleus raphe magnus (NRM).

In rats, the NRM has been proposed as a source of tonic inhibition since inactivation of this region, either irreversibly by lesions (Proudfit and Anderson, 1975), or reversibly by microinjection of local anaesthetic (Proudfit, 1980), decreased tail flick latency (but see Prieto et al., 1983). Lesions of the adjacent nuclei gigantocellularis and paragigantocellularis failed to alter nociceptive (tail flick and hot plate tests) thresholds (Mohrland et al., 1982). Electrolytic lesions and local anaesthetic inactivate both cell bodies and fibres of passage and, therefore, these studies do not exclude the participation of higher centres in tonic inhibition. Thus, a decreased tail flick latency in rats has also been produced by lesions (Rhodes, 1979) or microinjection of local anaesthetic (Carlsson and Jurna, 1987) in the PAG, and by lesions in the caudal medial thalamus (Rhodes, 1979) or medial hypothalamus (Vidal and Jacob, 1980).

In the decerebrate cat, medial and paramedial lesions of the caudal medulla have reduced tonic inhibition of the flexor withdrawal reflex. Holmqvist and Lundberg (1961) made midline medullary lesions 3 mm in width and found reduced tonic inhibition of transmission of impulses in cutaneous and high threshold muscle and joint afferents. Wolstencroft and West (1982) found that electrolytic lesions of the NRM, nucleus raphe pallidus and adjacent reticular formation reduced inhibition of flexor withdrawal to noxious pinch.

In anaesthetized cats, the present evidence suggests that such midline brain regions do not contribute significantly to tonic descending inhibition. Extensive lesions of the PAG neither reduced this tonic inhibition in anaesthetized cats (Hall et al., 1982), nor enhanced sensitivity to noxious stimulation in behavioural tests on awake cats (Melzack et al., 1958; Kelly and Glusman, 1968). Destruction of many supraspinal regions, such as the dorsal raphe nucleus, various medullary raphe nuclei, the locus coeruleus, and the medullary nuclei gigantocellularis and magnocellularis, did not alter tonic descending inhibition of dorsal horn neurons in anaesthetized cats (Hall et al., 1981, 1982). This tonic inhibition was reduced by bilateral lesions in the ventrolateral medulla, in the region of the lateral reticular nuclei (Hall et al., 1982; Morton et al., 1983, 1984). Selective reversible inactivation of

neuronal cell bodies can be achieved by microinjection of an inhibitory amino acid analogue such as piperidine-4-sulphonate. By this technique, the region exerting tonic inhibition in the anaesthetized cat was subsequently localized more precisely in the ventrolateral medulla, just ventral to the facial nuclei (Foong and Duggan, 1986). Fig. 2 illustrates such an experiment and shows that a shift of 0.5 mm was sufficient to differentiate active and inactive injection sites.

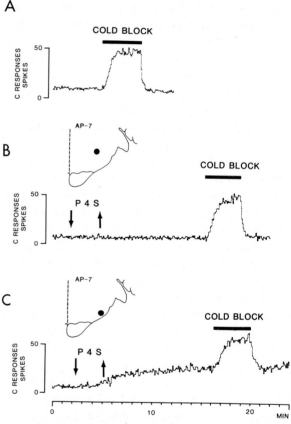

Fig. 2. Reduction of tonic descending inhibition by microinjections of piperidine-4-sulphonate (P4S) in the ventrolateral medulla. The records plot the gated C responses (see Fig. 1) of a lamina V neuron in response to electrical stimulation of the ipsilateral tibial nerve. (A) Gated C-responses were increased by cold block of the thoracolumbar junction. (B) Microinjection of 0.5 μl of a 5 mM solution of P4S at the site indicated by a filled circle had no effect on cell firing. (C) Microinjection of P4S at the indicated site increased gated C responses, and the decreased change produced by cold block indicates that this was due to a decrease in tonic descending inhibition.

It is possible that anaesthesia reduces the contribution of medial and paramedial medullary neurons to tonic inhibition. It also appears that the experiments on decerebrate preparations did not explore, sufficiently, the effects of lesions of lateral reticular areas. Thus it is possible that, in conscious cats, both of these areas contribute to tonic inhibition in the spinal cord.

The spinal mechanisms of tonic inhibition

The possible mechanisms of a supraspinal control on spinal events are several (Lundberg, 1982; Duggan, 1985). If the descending fibres are directly inhibitory, then the inhibition could occur presynaptically, to reduce transmitter release from the central terminals of primary afferents, or could produce postsynaptic inhibition of spinal interneurons. Alternatively, the descending fibres could excite inhibitory interneurons of the spinal cord which could act either pre- or postsynaptically on the relevant structures. These possible mechanisms of tonic descending inhibition are illustrated in Fig. 3.

If tonic descending inhibition is exerted presynaptically, then all spinal neurons ultimately excited by impulses in the relevant primary afferent fibres should be inhibited. In the experiments of Holmqvist and Lundberg (1961), however, there was evidence that this was not always true. Thus, transmission in impulses from tendon afferents to motoneurons was subject to tonic supraspinal con-

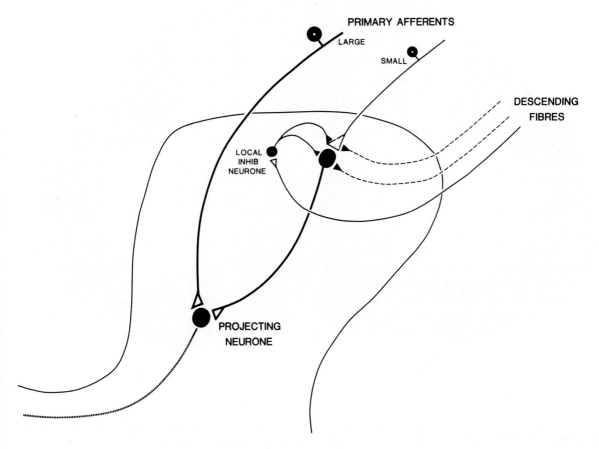

Fig. 3. Mechanisms of tonic descending inhibition in the dorsal horn. Excitatory synapses are unfilled, inhibitory synapses are filled. Descending fibres: broken lines, inhibitory; unbroken line, excitatory.

198

trol, whereas that to interneurons generating dorsal root potentials was not. In addition, lesions reducing tonic inhibition of transmission of FRA impulses to interneurons inhibiting extensor motoneurons had no effect on transmission from the same fibres to flexor motoneurons.

There is now considerable evidence that substance P (SP) is released centrally by impulses in peripheral nociceptors. Release of SP has been shown by perfusion of the surface of the spinal cord (Yaksh et al., 1980), by push-pull cannulae in the dorsal horn (Kuraishi et al., 1985), and in the substantia gelatinosa by the antibody microprobe technique (Duggan and Hendry, 1986; Duggan et al., 1987). This latter device is a microelectrode coated with antibodies to a neuropeptide which, if

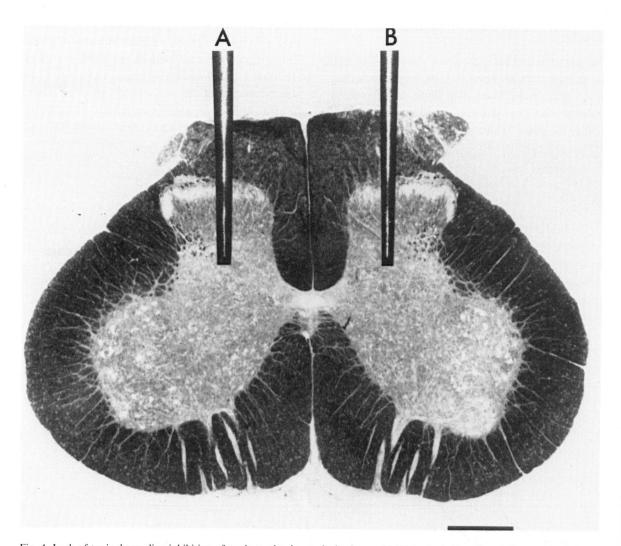

Fig. 4. Lack of tonic descending inhibition of noxious stimulus-evoked release of irSP in the substantia gelatinosa. Photographic enlargements of autoradiographs of microprobes bearing immobilized antibodies to SP have been superimposed on a spinal cord section. Both microprobes were 30 min in the lower lumbar spinal cord while noxious mechanical stimulation (calibrated clamps) was applied to the digital pads of the ipsilateral hind limb. (A) With normal spinal conduction; (B) spinal conduction blocked by cooling at the thoracolumbar junction. Note the reduced binding of ^{125}I-SP centered on the substantia gelatinosa, indicating prior binding of endogenous irSP released by the noxious stimulus. Calibration bar, 1 mm.

released, will bind to the microprobe. Release is detected on autoradiographs as zones of inhibition of binding of a radiolabelled form of the neuro-peptide, in which microprobes are subsequently incubated. The antibody microprobe has shown that noxious cutaneous stimuli to the skin produce release of immunoreactive SP (irSP) in the substantia gelatinosa of the spinal cord, and in the overlying pia mater. Cold block or transection of the spinal cord at the thoracolumbar junction failed to alter such release. Fig. 4 illustrates autoradiographic images of microprobes showing release of irSP in the substantia gelatinosa, in response to peripheral noxious stimuli. There is no difference in release with normal spinal conduction (A) and with cold block of spinal conduction (B).

Fig. 5 contains computer-compiled mean image density scans of antibody microprobes, and the noxious stimulus-evoked release of irSP in the substantia gelatinosa is shown to be unchanged by spinal transection. These experiments provide direct evidence to support the proposal of Lundberg (1982) that tonic inhibition is exerted on interneurons of the spinal cord. One study, using push-pull cannulae (Kuraishi et al., 1985), reported that spinal transection does increase noxious stimulus-evoked SP release. The amounts of SP released by noxious stimuli before and after transection were 136 fmol/min ± 37, SEM, and 265 ± 139, respectively. The large variance in the evoked release of SP after spinal transection casts doubt on the validity of this finding.

A failure to observe tonic descending control of noxious stimulus-evoked release of SP argues against a termination of descending fibres on the central terminals of nociceptors and also against an activation, by descending fibres, of local inhibitory interneurons acting presynaptically to inhibit transmitter release from the central terminals of nociceptors. This conclusion is supported by pharmacological evidence (discussed later in this chapter), and by the anatomical finding that axo-axonic synapses, the structural bases of presynaptic inhibition, are very rare in the upper dorsal horn. Both in the rat (Zhu et al., 1981) and cat

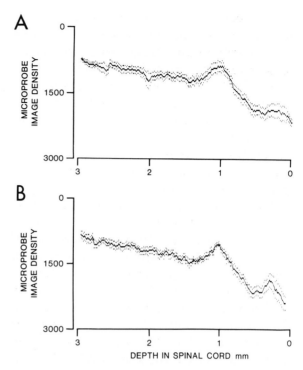

Fig. 5. Averaged image density scans of antibody microprobes for SP with normal spinal conduction (A: $n = 21$), and with the spinal cord transected (B: $n = 16$). The images of microprobes were scanned with a video camera. A computer digitized the mean optical density in squares, 16 × 16 μm, to a grey scale value of 0 to 255. A transverse integration (in 16-μm steps) was then performed across the image of each probe and these integrals plotted with respect to depth in the spinal cord. (A) and (B) plot the mean image densities (SEM) of microprobes inserted into the lower lumbar dorsal horn of cats with the ipsilateral hind paw immersed in water at 52°C for 30 min. In both there is a zone of decreased binding of ^{125}I-SP in the substantia gelatinosa. This represents release of irSP. There is a lesser release of irSP at the cord surface. There is no significant difference in the release of irSP in the presence (B) and absence (A) of tonic descending inhibition.

(Duncan and Morales, 1978) less than 1% of synapses in the substantia gelatinosa were found to be axo-axonic. In the substantia gelatinosa of the cat, boutons either containing (Light et al., 1983) or taking up 5HT (Ruda and Gobel, 1980) made no axo-axonic contacts. Studies of the distribution of enkephalins in the upper dorsal horn have not favoured a release of these compounds at axo-axonic synapses (Hunt et al., 1980).

Collectively, these findings make it very unlikely that there is a significant tonic supraspinal control of transmitter release from the spinal terminations of peripheral nociceptors.

If tonic descending inhibition is exerted postsynaptically on spinal interneurons, an important consideration is the location of the neurons in the spinal cord primarily (monosynaptically), affected by impulses in the relevant descending fibres. This is particularly important if this inhibition is to be studied adequately by iontophoretic methods.

Engberg et al. (1968) recorded intracellularly from dorsal horn neurons while stimulating at brain stem sites tonically inhibiting transmission of FRA impulses. They observed very few potential changes in the cells studied but frequent reductions in the potentials evoked by FRA impulses. It was suggested that the primary inhibition was exerted on, or near, first order interneurons. Intracellular recordings have shown that electrical stimulation in the region of the NRM and PAG of the cat hyperpolarizes a proportion of spinothalamic tract neurons (Giesler et al., 1981) and nociceptive-specific and multireceptive neurons of laminae I and II (Light et al., 1986). It is difficult to relate these studies directly to tonic descending inhibition.

Although these studies on the mechanisms of tonic inhibition do not permit definitive conclusions, it is probable that this control is exerted postsynaptically on neurons of the superficial dorsal horn. If these neurons are located near the sites of nociceptive afferents in the substantia gelatinosa, it is perhaps surprising that one study of this area found that the neurons examined were not subject to tonic supraspinal inhibition (Cervero et al., 1979).

Pharmacology of tonic supraspinal inhibition of nociception

To be sure that a drug modifies tonic descending inhibition, it is necessary to measure this inhibition directly. Few experiments have done this. Since there is evidence that spinal monoamines are wholly of supraspinal origin (Carlson et al., 1964), changes in the baseline of a spinal nociceptive reflex, following caudal intrathecal administration of antagonists of catecholamines, can reasonably be attributed to effects on tonically active processes of supraspinal origin. The same cannot be said for compounds contained within intrinsic neurons of the spinal cord, since effects on spinal reflexes following drug application could equally be due to effects on the actions of compounds released from spinal neurons, as well as on transmitter release from descending fibres.

Amino acids

Bicuculline and strychnine have been examined for effects on tonic inhibition since they reduce inhibition by γ-aminobutyric acid (Curtis et al., 1970) and glycine (Curtis et al., 1968), respectively. Neither compound reduced tonic inhibition of the excitation of laminae IV and V neurons of the cat by peripheral noxious stimuli (Duggan et al., 1981a). These drugs were given intravenously, near the bodies of the neurons studied and more dorsally, up to and including the substantia gelatinosa, and in amounts adequate to reduce a segmental inhibition.

Monoamines

An important distinction needs to be made between results obtained in the rat and the cat. In the rat there is considerable evidence for the involvement of monoamines in tonic inhibition but in the cat such evidence is sparse.

Receptors for 5HT are now divided into three subtypes (Bradley et al., 1986). Pharmacological studies on tonic inhibition have used antagonist drugs with high affinity for $5HT_1$ receptors (methysergide) and $5HT_2$ receptors (methysergide, cinanserin, ketanserin) but not compounds binding to $5HT_3$ receptors (cocaine, MDL 72222).

In the rat, intrathecal administration of methysergide produced hyperactive responses to peripheral noxious stimuli, suggesting that a tonic inhibition had been reduced (Proudfit and Hammond, 1981). Berge (1982) found that spinal transection shortened tail flick latency and that systemic administration of metergoline, mianserin or methiothepin produced a similar change. These drugs were without effect on the latency of the response in spinally transected animals. Systemic cinanserin and methysergide enhanced the excitation of dorsal horn neurons of the halothane anaesthetized rat by impulses in unmyelinated primary afferents (Rivot et al., 1987). Collectively, these observations support a tonic release of 5HT in the spinal cord, acting to suppress spinal nociceptive transmission in the rat.

Results in the cat have been less convincing. Intravenous methysergide and bromolysergic acid diethylamide reduced tonic inhibition of transmission of impulses in FRA to inhibitory interneurons of the decerebrate cat (Engberg et al., 1968). In the anaesthetized cat, intravenous methysergide did reduce tonic inhibition of the excitation of dorsal horn neurons by impulses in unmyelinated primary afferents, but this reduction was accompanied by a powerful depression of such excitation at the spinal level (Griersmith et al., 1981). Both in this, and in a subsequent study (Foong et al., 1985), it was considered that a supraspinal depressant action of methysergide could not be excluded as a cause of the reduction in supraspinal inhibition. Such an explanation can also apply to the results of Engberg et al. (1968) cited above. Iontophoretic methysergide, administered near spinal neurons (Foong et al., 1985) or more dorsally in the substantia gelatinosa (Griersmith et al., 1981), had no effect on the excitation of dorsal horn neurons of the anaesthetized cat by peripheral noxious stimuli.

The illustrations of Carstens et al. (1981) show that doses of methysergide, reducing inhibition from PAG stimulation of the excitation of dorsal horn neurons of the anaesthetized cat by noxious heating of the skin, did not alter the uninhibited responses, suggesting a lack of effect on tonic inhibition. Prior treatment with fluoxetine (a 5HT-uptake blocker), or parachlorophenylalanine (a depleter of 5HT), did not alter tonic descending inhibition in anaesthetized cats (Soja and Sinclair, 1980). In anaesthetized monkeys, the noxious stimulus-evoked firing of spinothalamic neurons was not altered by doses of methysergide and cinanserin reducing inhibition of the responses from PAG stimulation (Yezierski et al., 1982).

As suggested previously, the medullary raphe contribution to tonic descending inhibition may be reduced in anaesthetized animals. The failure to modify this inhibition with 5HT antagonists may indicate that the ventrolateral medullary component, which accounts for nearly all of tonic inhibition in anaesthetized animals, does not involve release of 5HT in the spinal cord. In conscious or decerebrate preparations it appears probable that this inhibition is, in part, dependent on 5HT release.

In the rat, depletion of spinal noradrenaline by administration of 6-hydroxydopamine produced hyperresponsiveness to noxious thermal stimuli, suggesting a reduction in a tonic inhibition of spinal nociception (Howe and Yaksh, 1982). It would be expected that intrathecal administration of antagonists of noradrenaline would also produce hyperalgesia. This has been observed with the relatively non-selective compound phentolamine (Proudfit and Hammond, 1981), but more readily with the partially selective $\alpha 2$ adrenoceptor antagonist yohimbine (Sagen and Proudfit, 1984).

In the cat there is little evidence that tonic descending inhibition involves spinal release of noradrenaline. In studies on transmission of impulses in the FRA, systemic administration of precursors of noradrenaline inhibited such transmission in spinal cats (Anden et al., 1966). It was not shown, however, that antagonists of noradrenaline reduced tonic inhibition in the intact animal. Two studies (Jurna and Grossmann, 1976; Soja and Sinclair, 1983b) depleted cats of noradrenaline by reserpine administration, but found no reduction of tonic descending inhibition. Indeed in the work of Soja and Sinclair (1983b), this inhibition was increased by reserpine treatment. Zhao and Duggan (unpublished observations) found that intravenous idazoxan, a selective $\alpha2$ adrenoceptor antagonist, had no effect on tonic inhibition of spinal nociceptive transmission in the anaesthetized cat.

Carlton et al. (1987) have proposed that adrenaline may be important in tonic descending inhibition. Both in the monkey (Carlton et al., 1987) and rat (Ross et al., 1984), spinally projecting adrenaline synthesizing neurons have been found in the ventrolateral medulla in an area approximating to that shown to be the major source of tonic descending inhibition in the anaesthetized cat (Foong and Duggan, 1986). The spinal projection of these neurons is mainly to the intermediolateral cell column of the thoracic spinal cord (Ross et al., 1984), but Carlton et al. (1987) observed additional projections to laminae I and V of the spinal cord at all levels. This interesting finding has not been investigated pharmacologically as a mechanism of tonic descending inhibition.

Opioid peptides

Because opioid peptides are contained within intrinsic neurons of the spinal cord (Hökfelt et al., 1977; Hunt et al., 1980; Bennett et al., 1982), changes in the amplitude and latency of spinal reflexes to peripheral noxious stimuli produced by opioid antagonists cannot necessarily be related to changes in supraspinal controls. They could equally result from changes in tonic inhibition intrinsic to the spinal cord. Intrathecal naloxone has produced hyperalgesia in conscious rats (Dickenson et al., 1981), and increased the amplitude of ascending spinal volleys in response to electrical stimulation of unmyelinated primary afferents in decerebrate rats (Bernatsky et al., 1983). There is, however, abundant evidence that systemic naloxone increases events in spinal animals including spinal reflexes (Goldfarb and Hu, 1976; Bell and Martin, 1977; Morton et al., 1982; Catley et al., 1983; Duggan et al., 1984), the firing of neurons to peripheral stimuli (Henry, 1979; Rivot et al., 1979; Sinclair et al., 1980), and the amplitude of ascend-

ing volleys produced by peripheral nerve stimulation (Duggan et al., 1985).

Tonic descending inhibition has been measured in anaesthetized cats for effects by systemic naloxone. Although intravenous naloxone increased the excitation of neurons of laminae IV and V by noxious heating of the skin (Duggan et al., 1977), and ascending volleys in the spinal anterolateral funiculus from electrical stimulation of unmyelinated primary afferents of the contralateral tibial nerve (Duggan, 1985), the cold block method showed that this was due to a spinal action and not to a decrease in tonic descending inhibition.

Collectively, these pharmacological studies have been largely unsuccessful in attempting to implicate neurotransmitters in tonic descending inhibition. Mention needs to be made, however, of two pharmacological procedures that have reduced tonic descending inhibition. Analgesic doses of morphine reduced tonic descending inhibition in the decerebrate (Jurna and Grossmann, 1976) and barbiturate anaesthetized cat (Duggan et al., 1981b). It is this reduction of tonic inhibition which results in the modest effects of systemic morphine on the firing of spinal neurons in the intact cat, when compared with its powerful depressant action in the spinal animal. Administration of capsaicin to neonatal rats produced a reduction in the frequency with which tonic descending inhibition was observed on spinal neurons of the same animals when adult (Cervero and Plenderleith, 1985). It was suggested that the reduction of tonic inhibition was responsible for the normal nociceptive responses of these animals despite their severe reductions in numbers of unmyelinated primary afferent fibres.

The significance of tonic inhibition

To a lower organism, flexor reflexes can be a significant component of normal behavioural responses, since they serve to withdraw from potential or actual sources of obstruction and/or injury. With the development of more complex behaviour, however, flexor reflexes become a potential hindrance to the execution of skilled motor performance. Sherrington (1906) termed nociceptive flexor reflexes 'prepotent' since they dominate, and consequently displace, all other types of reflex competing for a common pathway (Fulton, 1938). Hence it appears appropriate that, in the alert state, flexor reflexes should be inhibited. If nociceptive afferents are the most powerful in eliciting flexor reflexes, it is not surprising that actual injury can interrupt motor performance, since the preservation of flexor reflexes to damaging stimuli is of obvious importance to an animal. In life-threatening situations, however, it can be appropriate to suppress all flexor reflexes, including those to nociceptive impulses, so that an organized motor response to enable defensive or escape behaviour can occur. Thus, stress-induced analgesia can be regarded as an extreme form of tonic inhibition of flexor reflexes.

Viewed in this way, tonic descending inhibition can be regarded as a control directed at peripheral inputs which can potentially interrupt voluntary movement. As such, it is possible to reconcile the earlier work which emphasized control of transmission of impulses in non-noxious cutaneous and high threshold muscle and joint afferents (FRA) (Lundberg, 1982), with the later emphasis on inhibition of nociceptive transmission.

Placing the emphasis on motor events, however, raises the question: Does this control result in diminished perception of pain? This question cannot be answered definitively, but the scheme suggested below does favour alterations in pain perception by changes in the level of tonic descending inhibition.

It has been shown that monosynaptic transmission of impulses in low threshold cutaneous afferents is not subject to tonic supraspinal control, whereas polysynaptic transmission of the same impulses is (Holmqvist et al., 1961). One interpretation of this finding is that fast transmission of the non-noxious mechanoreceptive information, needed for perception of touch, is not subject to tonic inhibition but that the spinal connections of this information, which can evoke flexor reflexes, is

under such control. Fig. 3 depicts monosynaptic excitation of a projecting neuron as free of supraspinal inhibition. This hypothesis predicts that information transmitted through the dorsal column nuclei is not subject to tonic inhibition. There is no evidence for monosynaptic transmission of nociceptive to supraspinal areas. It may exist for the faster Aδ afferents which arborize mainly in lamina I (Light and Perl, 1979), and may make monosynaptic contacts with spinothalamic tract neurons of this area. Unmyelinated primary afferents, however, mainly terminate in lamina II, and neurons of this area do not project to supraspinal areas (Cervero and Iggo, 1981). It is probable, therefore, that supraspinal transmission of impulses in unmyelinated nociceptors is polysynaptic and subject to tonic supraspinal inhibition. It is important to emphasize that impulses in unmyelinated nociceptors do result in pain perception (Torebjörk, 1985). If this hypothesis is correct, it follows that alterations in tonic inhibition result in alterations in the perception of pain.

Experiments in cats and monkeys have shown that inhibition of the spinal transmission of nociceptive information induced by electrical stimulation in supraspinal regions, is associated with hypoalgesia or analgesia (Oliveras et al., 1974; Hayes et al., 1979). In anaesthetized cats, such spinal inhibition from stimulation in the PAG is interrupted by lesions in the ventrolateral medulla which abolish tonic inhibition (Morton et al., 1984). Such findings suggest not only that these stimulation-produced descending controls and tonic descending inhibition share common pathways, but that the degree of tonic inhibition is indeed relevant to the perception of pain in conscious animals.

This hypothesis on the functional significance of tonic descending inhibition is consistent with findings linking inhibition of nociception to the visceral alerting response. The latter is a cardiovascular response to brain stimulation, consisting of increased cardiac output, increased blood flow to skeletal muscle, but reduced cutaneous and splanchnic perfusion (Abrahams et al., 1960; Hilton et al., 1983). The areas evoking this response include the hypothalamus, PAG, and the ventrolateral medulla (Abrahams et al., 1960; McDougall et al., 1985; Lovick and Hilton, 1985), all regions which produce analgesia when electrically stimulated (Oliveras et al., 1974; Richardson and Akil, 1977; Gebhart and Ossipov, 1986). Importantly, it was shown in the anaesthetized cat that the visceral alerting response was associated with inhibition of spinal nociceptive responses from stimulation in the PAG (Duggan and Morton, 1983) and the hypothalamus (Morton and Duggan, 1986).

The visceral alerting response has been proposed as an essential component of cardiovascular control in the conscious state (Hilton, 1982). With the findings of Collins (1984, 1987) that tonic descending inhibition is powerfully present in conscious cats, it is not unrealistic to associate this inhibition with alertness and to propose that one function is to suppress flexor reflexes, and thus to permit conscious motor performance. That is not to say that tonic inhibition is a single entity in terms of cells of origin, spinal neurons affected, and mechanisms of inhibition. Neurochemically it may turn out to be very diverse.

References

Abrahams, V.C., Hilton, S.M. and Zbrozyna, A. (1960) Active muscle vasodilatation produced by stimulation of the brain stem: its significance in the defence reaction. *J. Physiol. (Lond.),* 154: 491 – 513.

Andén, N.E., Jukes, M.G.M., Lundberg, A. and Vyklicky, L. (1966) The effect of DOPA on the spinal cord. I. Influence on transmission from primary afferents. *Acta Physiol. Scand.,* 67: 373 – 386.

Bell, J.A. and Martin, W.R. (1977) The effects of the narcotic antagonists naloxone, naltrexone and nalorphine on spinal cord C-fibre reflexes evoked by electrical stimulation or radiant heat. *Eur. J. Pharmacol.,* 42: 147 – 154.

Bennett, G.J., Ruda, M.A., Gobel, S. and Dubner, R. (1982) Enkephalin immunoreactive stalked cells and lamina IIb islet cells in cat substantia gelatinosa. *Brain Res.,* 240: 162 – 166.

Berge, O.-G. (1982) Effects of 5-HT receptor agonists and antagonists on a reflex response to radiant heat in normal and spinally transected rats. *Pain,* 13: 253 – 266.

Bernatzky, G., Doi, T. and Jurna, I. (1983) Effects of in-

trathecally administered pentobarbital and naloxone on the activity evoked in ascending axons of the rat spinal cord by stimulation of afferent A and C fibres. Further evidence for a tonic endorphinergic inhibition in nociception. *Naun. Schmiedeberg's Arch. Pharmacol.,* 323: 211 – 216.

Besson, J.M., Guilbaud, G. and Le Bars, D. (1975) Descending inhibitory influences exerted by the brain stem upon the activities of dorsal horn lamina V cells induced by intra-arterial injection of bradykinin into the limbs. *J. Physiol.,* 248: 725 – 739.

Bradley, P.B., Engel, G., Fenwick, W., Fozard, J.R., Humphrey, P.A., Middlemiss, D.N., Nylecharane, E.J., Richardson, B.P. and Saxena, P.R. (1986) Proposals for the classification and nomenclature of functional receptors for 5-hydroxytryptamine. *Neuropharmacology,* 25: 564 – 576.

Brown, A.G. (1971) Effects of descending impulses on transmission through the spinocervical tract. *J. Physiol.,* 219: 103 – 125.

Carlsson, A.B., Falch, B., Fuxe, K. and Hillarp, N.A. (1964) Cellular localization of neuroamines in the spinal cord. *Acta Physiol. Scand.,* 60: 112 – 119.

Carlsson, L.-H. and Jurna, I. (1987) The role of descending inhibition in the anti-nociceptive effects of the pyrazolone derivatives, metamizol (dipyrone) and aminophenazone ('Pyramidon'). *Naun.-Schmiedeberg's Arch. Pharmacol.,* 335: 154 – 159.

Carlton, S.M., Honda, C.N., Denoroy, L. and Willis, W.D. Jr. (1987) Descending phenylethanolamine-*N*-methyltransferase projections to the monkey spinal cord: an immunohistochemical double labeling study. *Neurosci. Lett.,* 76: 133 – 139.

Carstens, E., Fraunhofer, M. and Zimmermann, M. (1981) Serotonergic mediation of descending inhibition from midbrain periaqueductal gray, but not reticular formation, of spinal nociceptive transmission in the cat. *Pain,* 10: 149 – 167.

Catley, D.M., Clarke, R.W. and Pascoe, J.E. (1983) Naloxone enhancement of spinal reflexes in the rabbit. *J. Physiol.,* 339: 61 – 73.

Cervero, F. and Iggo, A. (1981) The substantia gelatinosa of the spinal cord: a critical review. *Brain,* 103: 717 – 772.

Cervero, F. and Plenderleith, M.B. (1985) C-fibre excitation and tonic descending inhibition of dorsal horn neurones in adult rats treated at birth with capsaicin. *J. Physiol.,* 365: 223 – 238.

Cervero, F., Iggo, A. and Ogawa, H. (1976) Nociceptor-driven dorsal horn neurones in the lumbar spinal cord of the cat. *Pain,* 2: 5 – 24.

Cervero, F., Molony, V. and Iggo, A. (1979) Supraspinal linkage of substantia gelatinosa neurones: effects of descending impulses. *Brain Res.,* 175: 351 – 355.

Collins, J.G. (1984) Neuronal activity recorded from the spinal dorsal horn of physiologically intact awake drug free restrained cats: a preliminary report. *Brain Res.,* 322: 301 – 304.

Collins, J.G. (1987) Inhibition of spontaneous activity of spinal dorsal horn neurons in the intact cat is naloxone-insensitive. *Brain Res.*, 401: 95–102.

Curtis, D.R., Hosli, L., Johnston, G.A.R. and Johnston, I.H. (1968) The hyperpolarization of spinal motoneurones by glycine and related amino acids. *Exp. Brain Res.*, 5: 235–258.

Curtis, D.R., Duggan, A.W., Felix, D. and Johnston, G.A.R. (1970) GABA, bicuculline and central inhibition. *Nature,* 226: 1222–1224.

Dickenson, A.H., Le Bars, D. and Besson, J.M. (1981) Endogenous opiates and nociception: a possible functional role in both pain inhibition and detection as revealed by intrathecal naloxone. *Neuroscience Lett.*, 24: 161–164.

Dickhaus, H., Pauser, G. and Zimmermann, N. (1985) Tonic descending inhibition affects intensity coding of nociceptive responses of spinal dorsal horn neurones. *Pain*, 23: 145–158.

Duggan, A.W. (1985) Pharmacology of descending control systems. *Phil. Trans. Roy. Soc. Lond. B*, 308: 375–391.

Duggan, A.W. and Hendry, I.A. (1986) Laminar localization of the sites of release of immunoreactive substance P in the dorsal horn with antibody coated microelectrodes. *Neurosci. Lett.*, 68: 134–140.

Duggan, A.W. and Morton, C.R. (1983) Periaqueductal grey stimulation: an association between selective inhibition of dorsal horn neurones and changes in peripheral circulation. *Pain*, 15: 237–248.

Duggan, A.W., Hall, J.G., Headley, P.M. and Griersmith, B.T. (1977) The effect of naloxone on the excitation of dorsal horn neurones of the cat by noxious and non-noxious cutaneous stimuli. *Brain Res.*, 138: 185–189.

Duggan, A.W., Griersmith, B.T. and Johnson, S.M. (1981a) Supraspinal inhibition of the excitation of dorsal horn neurones by impulses in unmyelinated primary afferents: lack of effect by strychnine and bicuculline. *Brain Res.*, 210: 231–241.

Duggan, A.W., Griersmith, B.T. and North, R.A. (1981b) Morphine and supraspinal inhibition of neurones: evidence that morphine decreases tonic descending inhibition in the anaesthetized cat. *Br. J. Pharmacol.*, 69: 461–466.

Duggan, A.W., Morton, C.R., Johnson, S.M. and Zhao, Z.Q. (1984) Opioid antagonists and spinal reflexes in the anaesthetized cat. *Brain Res.*, 297: 33–40.

Duggan, A.W., Hall, J.G., Foong, F.W. and Zhao, Z.Q. (1985) A differential effect of naloxone on transmission of impulses in primary afferents to ventral roots and ascending spinal tracts. *Brain Res.*, 344: 316–321.

Duggan, A.W., Morton, C.R., Zhao, Z.Q. and Hendry, I.A. (1987) Noxious heating of the skin releases immunoreactive substance P in the substantia gelatinosa of the cat: a study with antibody microprobes. *Brain Res.*, 403: 345–349.

Duncan, D. and Morales, R. (1978) Relative numbers of several types of synaptic connections in the substantia gelatinosa of the cat spinal cord. *J. Comp. Neurol.*, 182: 601–610.

Engberg, I., Lundberg, A. and Ryall, R.W. (1968) Is the tonic decerebrate inhibition of reflex paths mediated by monoaminergic pathways? *Acta Physiol. Scand.*, 72: 123–133.

Foong, F.W. and Duggan, A.W. (1986) Brain stem areas tonically inhibiting dorsal horn neurones: studies with microinjection of the GABA analogue piperidine-4-sulphonic acid. *Pain*, 27: 361–371.

Foong, F.W., Terman, G. and Duggan, A.W. (1985) Methysergide and spinal inhibition from electrical stimulation in the periaqueductal grey. *Eur. J. Pharmacol.*, 116: 239–248.

Fulton, J.F. (1926) *Muscular Contraction and the Reflex Control of Movement,* Williams and Wilkins, Baltimore.

Fulton, J.F. (1938) *Physiology of the Nervous System,* Oxford University Press, New York.

Gebhart, G.F. and Ossipov, M. (1986) Characterization of inhibition of the spinal nociceptive tail flick reflex in the rat from the medullary lateral reticular nucleus. *J. Neurosci.*, 6: 701–713.

Giesler, G.J., Gerhart, K.D., Yezierski, R.P., Wilcox, T.K. and Willis, W.D. (1981) Postsynaptic inhibition of primate spinothalamic neurons by stimulation in nucleus raphe magnus. *Brain Res.*, 204: 184–188.

Goldfarb, J. and Hu, J.W. (1976) Enhancement of reflexes by naloxone in spinal cats. *Neuropharmacology*, 15: 785–792.

Griersmith, B.T., Duggan, A.W. and North, R.A. (1981) Methysergide and supraspinal inhibition of the transmission of nociceptive information in the anaesthetized cat. *Brain Res.*, 204: 147–158.

Grossmann, W., Jurna, I., Nell, T. and Theres, C. (1973) The dependence of the anti-nociceptive effect of morphine and other analgesic agents on spinal motor activity after central monoamine depletion. *Eur. J. Pharmacol.*, 24: 67–77.

Hall, J.G., Duggan, A.W., Johnson, S.M. and Morton, C.R. (1981) Medullary raphe lesions do not reduce descending inhibition of dorsal horn neurones of the cat. *Neurosci. Lett.*, 25: 25–29.

Hall, J.G., Duggan, A.W., Morton, C.R. and Johnson, S.M. (1982) The location of brainstem neurones tonically inhibiting dorsal horn neurones of the cat. *Brain Res.*, 244: 215–222.

Hall, M. (1843) *New Memoir on the Nervous System.* H. Ballière, London.

Handwerker, H.O., Iggo, A. and Zimmermann, M. (1975) Segmental and supraspinal actions on dorsal horn neurones responding to noxious and non-noxious skin stimuli. *Pain*, 1, 147–165.

Hayes, R.L., Price, D.D., Ruda, M. and Dubner, R. (1979) Suppression of nociceptive responses in the primate by electrical stimulation of the brain or morphine administration:

behavioural and electrophysiological comparisons. *Brain Res.*, 167: 417–421.

Henry, J.L. (1979) Naloxone excites nociceptive units in the lumbar dorsal horn of the spinal cat. *Neuroscience*, 4: 1485–1491.

Hilton, S.M. (1982) The defence-arousal system and its relevance for circulatory and respiratory control. *J. Exp. Biol.*, 100: 159–174.

Hilton, S.M., Marshall, J.M. and Timms, R.J. (1983) Ventral medullary relay neurones in the pathway from the defence areas of the cat and their effect on blood pressure. *J. Physiol.*, 345: 149–166.

Hökfelt, T., Ljungdahl, A., Terenius, L., Elde, R. and Nilsson, G. (1977) Immunohistochemical analysis of peptide pathways possibly related to pain and analgesia: enkephalin and substance P. *Proc. Natl. Acad. Sci. USA*, 74: 3081–3085.

Holmqvist, B. and Lundberg, A. (1961) Differential supraspinal control of synaptic actions evoked by volleys in the flexion reflex afferents in alpha motoneurones. *Acta Physiol. Scand.*, 54: Suppl. 186, 1–61.

Howe, J.R. and Yaksh, T.L. (1982) Changes in sensitivity to intrathecal norephinephrine and serotonin after 6-hydroxydopamine (60HDA), 5,6 dihydroxytryptamine (5,6 DHT) or repeated monoamine administration. *J. Pharmacol. Exp. Ther.*, 220: 311–321.

Hunt, S.P., Kelly, J.S. and Emson, P.C. (1980) The electron microscopic localization of methionine-enkephalin within the superficial layers (I and II) of the spinal cord. *Neuroscience*, 5: 1871–1890.

Irwin, S., Houde, R.W., Bennett, D.R., Hendershot, L.C. and Seevers, M.H. (1951) The effects of morphine, methadone and meperidine on some reflex responses of spinal animals to nociceptive stimulation. *J. Pharmacol. Exp. Ther.*, 101: 132–143.

Jurna, I. and Grossmann, W. (1976) The effect of morphine on the activity evoked in ventrolateral tract axons of the cat spinal cord. *Exp. Brain Res.*, 24: 473–484.

Kelly, D.D. and Glusman, M. (1968) Aversive thresholds following midbrain lesions. *J. Comp. Physiol. Psychol.*, 66: 25–34.

Kennard, M.A. (1950) Chronic focal hyper-irritability of sensory nervous system in cats. *J. Neurophysiol.*, 13: 215–222.

Kuraishi, Y., Hirota, N., Sato, Y., Kaneto, S., Satoh, M. and Takagi, H. (1985) Noradrenergic inhibition of the release of substance P from the primary afferents in the rabbit spinal dorsal horn. *Brain Res.*, 359: 177–182.

Liddell, E.G.T., Matthes, K., Oldberg, E. and Ruch, T.C. (1932) Reflex release of flexor muscles by spinal section. *Brain*, 55: 239–246.

Light, A.R. and Perl, E.R. (1979) Re-examination of the dorsal root projection to the spinal dorsal horn including observations on the differential termination of coarse and fine fibres.

J. Comp. Neurol., 186: 117–132.

Light, A.R., Kavookjian, A.M. and Petrusz, P. (1983) The ultrastructure and synaptic connections of serotonin-immuno reactive terminals in spinal laminae I and II. *Somatosensory Res.*, 1: 33–50.

Light, A.R., Casale, E.J. and Menetrey, D.M. (1986) The effects of focal stimulation in nucleus raphe magnus and periaqueductal gray on intracellularly recorded neurons in spinal laminae I and II. *J. Neurophysiol.*, 56: 555–571.

Livingston, C.A. and Leonard, R.B. (1985) Tonic descending inhibition in the stingray's spinal cord. *Brain Res.*, 358: 339–342.

Lovick, T.A. and Hilton, S.M. (1985) Vasodilator and vasoconstrictor neurones of the ventrolateral medulla in the cat. *Brain Res.*, 331: 353–357.

Lundberg, A. (1982) Inhibitory control from the brain stem of transmission from primary afferents to motoneurons, primary afferent terminals and ascending pathways. In B. Sjölund and A. Björklund (Eds.), *Brain Stem Control of Spinal Mechanisms*, Elsevier Biomedical Press, Amsterdam, pp. 179–224.

McDougall, A., Dampney, R. and Bandlen, R. (1985) Cardiovascular components of the defence reaction evoked by excitation of neuronal cell bodies in the midbrain periaqueductal grey of the cat. *Neurosci. Lett.*, 60: 69–75.

Melzack, R., Stotler, W.A. and Livingston, W.K. (1958) Effects of discrete brainstem lesions in cats on perception of noxious stimulation. *J. Neurophysiol.*, 21: 353–367.

Mohrland, J.S., McManus, D.Q. and Gebhart, G.F. (1982) Lesions in nucleus reticularis gigantocellularis: effect on the antinociception produced by microinjection of morphine and focal electrical stimulation in the periaqueductal gray. *Brain Res.*, 231: 143–152.

Morton, C.R. and Duggan, A.W. (1986) Inhibition of spinal nociceptive transmission accompanies cardiovascular changes from stimulation in diencephalic 'defence' regions of cats. *Behav. Brain Res.*, 21: 183–188.

Morton, C.R., Zhao, Z.Q. and Duggan, A.W. (1982) A function of opioid peptides in the spinal cord of the cat: intracellular studies of motoneurones during naloxone administration. *Neuropeptides*, 3: 83–91.

Morton, C.R., Johnson, S.M. and Duggan, A.W. (1983) Lateral reticular regions and the descending control of dorsal horn neurones of the cat: selective inhibition by electrical stimulation. *Brain Res.*, 275: 13–21.

Morton, C.R., Duggan, A.W. and Zhao, Z.Q. (1984) The effects of lesions of medullary midline and lateral reticular areas on inhibition in the dorsal horn produced by periaqueductal gray stimulation in the cat. *Brain Res.*, 301: 121–130.

Necker, R. and Hellon, R.F. (1978) Noxious thermal input from the rat tail: modulation by descending inhibitory influences. *Pain*, 4: 231–242.

Oliveras, J.L., Besson, J.M., Guilbaud, G. and Liebeskind, J.C. (1974) Behavioural and electrophysiological evidence of pain inhibition from midbrain stimulation in the cat. *Exp. Brain Res.,* 20: 32–44.

Prieto, G.J., Cannon, J.T. and Liebeskind, J.C. (1983) N. raphe magnus lesions disrupt stimulation-produced analgesia from ventral but not dorsal midbrain areas in the rat. *Brain Res.,* 261: 53–57.

Proudfit, H.K. (1980) Reversible inactivation of raphe magnus neurons: effects on nociceptive threshold and morphine-induced analgesia. *Brain Res.,* 201: 459–464.

Proudfit, H.K. and Anderson, E.G. (1975) Morphine analgesia: blockade by raphe magnus lesions. *Brain Res.,* 98: 612–618.

Proudfit, H.K. and Hammond, D.L. (1981) Alterations in nociceptive thresholds and morphine-induced analgesia produced by intrathecally administered amine antagonists. *Brain Res.,* 218: 393–399.

Rhodes, D.L. (1979) Periventricular system lesions and stimulation-produced analgesia. *Pain,* 7: 51–63.

Richardson, D.E. and Akil, H. (1977) Pain reduction by electrical brain stimulation in man. *J. Neurosurg.,* 47: 178–194.

Rivot, J.P., Chaouch, A. and Besson, J.M. (1979) The effect of naloxone on the C-fiber response of dorsal horn neurons and their inhibitory control by raphe magnus stimulation. *Brain Res.,* 176: 355–364.

Rivot, J.P., Calvino, B. and Besson, J.M. (1987) Is there a serotonergic tonic descending inhibition on the responses of dorsal horn convergent neurons to C-fibre inputs. *Brain Res.,* 403: 142–146.

Ross, C.A., Ruggiero, D.A., Joh, T.H., Park, D.H. and Reis, D.J. (1984) Rostral ventrolateral medulla: selective projections to the thoracic autonomic cell column from the region containing C1 adrenaline neurons. *J. Comp. Neurol.,* 228: 168–185.

Ruda, M.A. and Gobel, S. (1980) Ultrastructural characterization of axonal endings in the substantia gelatinosa which take up ^{3}H-serotonin. *Brain Res.,* 184: 57–84.

Sagen, J. and Proudfit, H.K. (1984) Effects of intrathecally administered noradrenergic antagonists on nociception in the rat. *Brain Res.,* 310: 295–301.

Sherrington, C.S. (1906) *The Integrative Action of the Nervous System,* Constable and Co. Ltd., London.

Sinclair, J.G., Fox, R.E., Mokha, S.S. and Iggo, A. (1980) The effect of naloxone on the inhibition of nociceptor driven neurones in the cat spinal cord. *Quart. J. Exp. Physiol.,* 65: 181–188.

Soja, P.J. and Sinclair, J.G. (1980) Evidence against a serotonin involvement in the tonic descending inhibition of nociceptor-driven neurons in the cat spinal cord. *Brain Res.,* 199: 225–230.

Soja, P.J. and Sinclair, J.G. (1983a) Tonic descending influences on cat spinal cord dorsal horn neurons. *Somatosens. Res.,* 1: 83–93.

Soja, P. and Sinclair, J.G. (1983b) Evidence that noradrenaline reduces tonic descending inhibition of cat spinal cord nociceptor-driven neurones. *Pain,* 15: 71–81.

Torebjörk, E. (1985) Nociceptor activation and pain. *Phil. Trans. Roy. Soc. Lond. B,* 308: 227–231.

Vidal, C. and Jacob, J. (1980) The effect of medial hypothalamus lesions on pain control. *Brain Res.,* 199: 89–100.

Vierck, C.J. Jr., Hamilton, D.M. and Thornby, J.I. (1971) Pain reactivity of monkeys after lesions to the dorsal and lateral columns of the spinal cord. *Exp. Brain Res.,* 13: 140–158.

Wall, P.D. (1967) The laminar organization of dorsal horn neurones and effects of descending impulses. *J. Physiol.,* 188: 403–423.

Willis, W.D., Haber, L.H. and Martin, R.F. (1977) Inhibition of spinothalamic tract cells and interneurones by brain stem stimulation in the monkey. *J. Neurophysiol.,* 40: 968–981.

Wolstencroft, J.H. and West, D.C. (1982) Functional characteristics of raphe spinal and other projections from nucleus raphe magnus. In B. Sjölund and A. Björklund (Eds.), *Brain Stem Control of Spinal Mechanisms,* Elsevier Biomedical Press, Amsterdam, pp. 359–380.

Woolf, C.J., Mitchell, D. and Barrett, G.D. (1980) Antinociceptive effect of peripheral segmental electrical stimulation in the rat. *Pain,* 8: 237–252.

Yaksh, T.L., Jessell, T.M., Gamse, R., Mudge, A.W. and Leeman, S.F. (1980) Intrathecal morphine inhibits substance P release from mammalian spinal cord in vivo. *Nature,* 286: 155–156.

Yezierski, R.P., Wilcox, R.K. and Willis, W.D. (1982) The effects of serotonin antagonists on the inhibition of primate spinothalamic tract cells produced by stimulation in nucleus raphe magnus or periaqueductal gray. *J. Pharmacol. Exp. Ther.,* 220: 266–277.

Zhu, C.E., Saudri, C. and Akert, K. (1981) Morphological identification of axo-axonic and dendro-dendritic synapses in the rat substantia gelatinosa. *Brain Res.,* 230: 25–40.

H.L. Fields and J.-M. Besson (Eds.)
Progress in Brain Research, Vol. 77
© 1988 Elsevier Science Publishers B.V. (Biomedical Division)

CHAPTER 12

Discussion of the paper by A.W. Duggan and C.R. Morton, entitled 'Tonic descending inhibition and spinal nociceptive transmission'

J.G. Collins

Department of Anesthesiology, Yale University School of Medicine, New Haven, CT 06510, USA

Dr. Duggan presents a timely interpretation of a way in which we may view tonic descending inhibition as being more global than just a pain suppressing mechanism. We are not being told that the systems are not involved in pain modulation, but rather that diminished pain perception may be only one aspect of the effect of tonic descending inhibitory systems acting at a given point in time.

As part of his presentation, Dr. Duggan raised the following question concerning tonic inhibition in awake animals, a question that warrants further discussion. Is tonic descending inhibition, the existence of which has been suggested by a large number of studies in acute preparations (e.g. Brown, 1971; Handwerker et al., 1975; Wall, 1967), an entity that exists in conscious animals, or is it just an artifact of the experimental preparation?

It is clear from studies conducted in awake animals that there are mechanisms in the conscious animal that are capable of profoundly influencing the response properties of neurons in either the spinal or medullary dorsal horn. Descending inhibition is not an artifact of acute preparations, it does exist in conscious animals. We must consider however, if this descending modulation is tonically active at all times. To do that, we should remember that the nature of the preparation itself, especially in the conscious animal where the behavioral state

of the animal can alter very quickly, will determine the relative level of modulation present at any point in time.

In an acute preparation, with the exception of slowly changing levels of anesthesia, most parameters that would be likely to alter descending modulatory systems are fairly constant or at least under some degree of experimenter control. As such, a relatively steady-state level may be achieved, and many of the response properties of neurons to peripheral stimulation are maintained constant over long periods of time. In acute preparations receptive field size and sensivity, stimulus-response functions and other measures of the organism's response to a stimulus appear to be very constant in the absence of some intentional perturbation of the system by the experimenter. This is not the case for similar studies conducted in awake animals. One of the most obvious differences between the acute preparation and neurophysiologic studies in conscious animals is the greater variability of response profiles of an individual neuron to a series of stimuli in the awake animal. This variability is due in part, or so we assume, to changes in the tone of descending influences.

The literature contains several examples of the moment-to-moment variability in modulation of dorsal horn neuronal activity in conscious animals (e.g. Duncan et al., 1987; Hayes et al., 1981; Sorkin, 1983). To me, the most striking example of this varying tone was contained in a 1981 publication by Hayes, Dubner and Hoffman (Hayes et al., 1981). By altering behavioral paradigms they were able to significantly influence activity of medullary dorsal horn neurons in the awake monkey. They reported, among other findings, one medullary dorsal horn neuron that responded to noxious stimulation on either side of the face but with a selectivity that was dependent upon the behavioral significance of the stimulus. Presentation of a 49°C stimulus to one side of the face raised neuronal activity above the baseline only if the stimulus was relevant to the behavioral paradigm being employed at the time. Experiments of this type clearly demonstrate the existence of systems that are capable of modulating dorsal horn neuronal activity in conscious animals.

Experiments like the one described above tell us that behavioral paradigms may influence the modulation of dorsal horn neurons, but we also need to know to what degree this modulation is tonically active in the absence of behavioral training that emphasizes detection of noxious stimuli. Work in our laboratory has begun to provide evidence of tonic inhibition of noxiously evoked activity in some spinal dorsal horn neurons in conscious, behaviorally naive cats. The i.v. administration of pentobarbital (Collins and Ren, 1987) or methysergide (unpublished observations) unmasks the response of some spinal dorsal horn neurons to noxious mechanical or thermal stimuli. This unmasking is evident because prior to drug administration, although the animals reflexly withdraw from the noxious stimulus, the neurons are not activated to a level above that produced by non-noxious stimulation. After drug administration, however, cells that are unmasked demonstrate a significant increase in their response to the noxious stimulation. The change is such that the classification of the neuron is altered. Prior to drug administration, the lack of response to noxious stimulation causes the cells to be classified as low threshold neurons. Following drug administra-

tion, their response profile is better described as that of a wide dynamic range (WDR) neuron. We interpret these findings to mean that tonic inhibition exists in the conscious animal. Prior to drug administration that inhibition limits the response of some neurons to noxious stimulation. It is likely that serotonin is involved in the tonic modulation since the non-specific 5HT antagonist, methysergide, appears to release it. The pentobarbital action is likely to be due to an inhibition of descending inhibitory systems.

We have also observed that methysergide seems to alter some response properties that are evoked by non-noxious stimuli. Thus, the tonic inhibition seen in our preparation seems to have a more global influence than just the modulation of noxiously evoked activity.

It is clear that tonic inhibitory systems do influence dorsal horn neurons in awake animals. It is not yet possible, however, to accurately define, at any point in time, which component of a system may be active, or more importantly, what effect the tonic activity is likely to have upon the response properties of an individual, or a population of neurons, under study.

Although for the sake of this discussion the desired effect of descending modulatory systems that alter pain sensation is to inhibit the transmission of information about pain, we must not fall into the trap of assuming that all descending systems are inhibitory. As demonstrated in this volume (see Chapter 17 by Fields, Barbaro and Heinricher), as well as elsewhere, the inhibition of pain may result from both excitatory and inhibitory activity within the nervous system. We must also remember that the suppression of nociceptor transmission is not dependent solely upon descending systems. Although emphasis at this meeting has been placed upon descending systems arising in the brain stem we must not forget potential actions in the periphery, at supraspinal sites outside of the brain stem or at intrinsic loci within the cord.

The waxing and waning of modulatory influences on dorsal horn neurons points out two crucial aspects of neuronal responsivity that must be kept in mind as we continue to attempt to understand how modulatory systems are likely to control nociceptive transmission. First, we need to realize that in any preparation, the presence or absence of a particular response to a noxious stimulus does not define all possible response profiles of that neuron. Rather, it simply tells us that under those specific conditions, this is the way that the neuron is going to respond to the stimulus. We must always keep in mind that, for at least some neurons in the dorsal horn, there appears to be a continuum of responses and that at any particular point in time, only one segment of that continuum will be evident. Thus, our attempts to classify neurons as low threshold, high threshold and wide dynamic range (convergent, multi-receptive, etc.), although certainly helpful in allowing us to conceptualize how information is transmitted, must be recognized as a construct of a particular set of circumstances from which the neuron is being recorded, rather than a true representation of the total responsivity of the neuron.

The second, and perhaps more important, implication of this waxing and waning is the realization that the state of the animal is capable of increasing a neuron's (and therefore neuronal populations') response to noxious stimulation. It is possible that the presence of an injury enhances the ability of the nervous system to signal the presence of subsequent tissue-damaging stimulation. If previous tissue damage is capable of causing such changes, then we need to recognize the fact that our attempts to understand the neurophysiology of chronic pain may be influenced by our expectation of certain response profiles that have been seen in acute preparations – response profiles that may not accurately reflect the neurophysiologic responses to similar stimuli in a chronic pain state. We must be aware of the potential for moment-to-moment changes in the response profiles of individual neurons and must develop humane means of studying the impact of such changes on sensory processing in awake animals.

References

Brown, A.G. (1971) Effects of descending impulses on transmission through the spinocervical tract. *J. Physiol. (Lond.)*, 219: 103–125.

Collins, J.G. and Ren, K. (1987) WDR response profiles of spinal dorsal horn neurons may be unmasked by bariturate anesthesia. *Pain*, 28: 369–378.

Duncan, G.H., Bushnell, M.C., Bates, R. and Dubner, R. (1987) Task-related responses of monkey medullary dorsal horn neurons. *J. Neurophysiol.*, 57: 289–310.

Handwerker, H.O., Iggo, A. and Zimmerman, M. (1975) Segmental and supraspinal actions on dorsal horn neurons responding to noxious and non-noxious skin stimuli. *Pain*, 1: 147–165.

Hayes, R.L., Dubner, R. and Hoffman, D.S. (1981) Neuronal activity in medullary dorsal horn of awake monkeys trained in a thermal discrimination task. II. Behavioral modulation of responses to thermal and mechanical stimuli. *J. Neurophysiol.*, 46: 428–443.

Sorkin, L.S. (1983) Spinal cord unit activity in the awake cat. *Doctoral Dissertation*, University of Michigan.

Wall, P.D. (1967) The laminar organization of dorsal horn and effects of descending impulses. *J. Physiol. (Lond.)*, 188: 403–423.

H.L. Fields and J.-M. Besson (Eds.)
Progress in Brain Research, Vol. 77
© 1988 Elsevier Science Publishers B.V. (Biomedical Division)

CHAPTER 13

The effect of behavioral state on the sensory processing of nociceptive and non-nociceptive information

Ronald Dubner

Neurobiology and Anesthesiology Branch, National Institute of Dental Research, National Institutes of Health, Bethesda, MD 20892, USA

Introduction

We are continuously bombarded with sensory stimuli in our environment, yet only a fraction of these signals reach our awareness. We attend to sensory cues that are behaviorally significant and ignore most others. For example, we are rarely conscious of stimuli produced by the contact of different textured clothing on our skin. Eye movements made to fixate on a new stimulus in our visual space result in a wave of visual signals that are ignored. In manipulating an unfamiliar object, we attend to only a fraction of the tactile input activating our peripheral mechanoreceptors. Our ability to focus on significant stimuli in our environment is commonly referred to as selective attention and represents one form of behavioral modulation of what we perceive in our environment. Behavioral modulation reveals that sensation is an active process. What we perceive depends on the behavioral context in which a sensory signal is received.

The neural mechanisms responsible for our ability to extract useful information from the environment are largely unknown. As an animal participates in goal-directed behavior, it searches its environment for relevant stimuli. These stimuli trigger pre-planned sensory and motor responses. Such mechanisms permit a relevant stimulus to guide behavior depending upon the expectations or 'set' of the animal. The concept of set is useful in describing behavior produced by significant stimuli. Woodworth (1958) defined set as a state of readiness to receive a stimulus that had not yet arrived, or a state of readiness to make a movement. This definition involves preparation to receive the particular stimulus, preparation to execute a particular movement, and preparation to execute the movement upon reception of the stimulus. In other words, both sensory and motor preparation are components of neural processing associated with behaviorally relevant sensory cues. Hebb (1959) provided some of the early formulations of the role of behavioral state in neural transmission. He proposed that significant sensory events result in associations of sensory neurons with one another and with particular motor-related assemblies of neurons. His ideas led to a model in which a particular sensory event could lead to different sensory processing and motor responses depending on behavioral state. How are sensory and motor neural pathways 'primed' to respond differentially depending upon behavioral context? What are the neural mechanisms that account for the recognition of behaviorally relevant signals? These are the questions to be addressed in this paper.

Modulation of movement-induced sensory stimulation

A relatively simple example of the effect of behavior on sensory responses is the modulation

214

following jaw or limb movement. These simple motor behaviors activate sensory receptors, and an animal must distinguish between sensory input from the environment and that produced by the motor act itself. Sensory signals produced by motor behavior can be modified in the central nervous system. Fig. 1 is an example of such an effect in the rostral part of the trigeminal brainstem sensory nucleus of the rabbit (Olsson et al., 1986). The neuron illustrated responded to low-threshold mechanical stimulation on the whisker pad and exhibited spontaneous activity of 15 – 20 impulses per s. This neuron was silenced during mastication

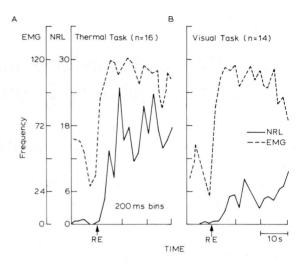

Fig. 2. Peristimulus histograms comparing responses to mechanical stimuli of a WDR neuron while the monkey performed the thermal task (A) or the visual task (B). Movement of the probe on the face during reception of the water reward produced increases in neuronal activity. The ordinate plots the neuronal responses (NRL) as well as the EMG activity recorded from the lip musculature averaged for the same trials. Arrow indicates the delivery of the water reward at the end of the trial. Note the larger neuronal discharge during the thermal task than during the visual task, whereas the lip movements are equivalent. (From Hayes et al., 1981.)

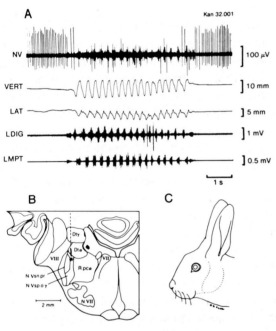

Fig. 1. (A) Record showing the cessation of spontaneous firing of a trigeminal neuron during mastication. The upper record shows the neuronal discharge followed in sequence by records of vertical movements of the mandibular symphysis (VERT), lateral movements of the mandibular symphysis (LAT), left digastris EMG (LDIG) and left medial pterygoid EMG (LMPT). (B) Drawing of a coronal section of the brain stem showing the position (∗) where the neuron was recorded in the trigeminal subnucleus oralis. Dt, Dieter's nucleus, subdivisions alpha and gamma; VII, facial nerve; VIII, vestibular nerve; R. pcα, nucleus reticularis parvocellularis, pars alpha; N.Vsn.pr, principal trigeminal nucleus; N.Vsp.oγ, trigeminal nucleus oralis, pars gamma. (C). Receptive field of the neuron on the vibrissae pad. (From Olsson et al., 1986.)

produced by insertion of a rubber tube in the rabbit's mouth. Spontaneous firing began again at the end of the chewing movements. The neuronal modulation in this example may be due to activity in other afferents with resultant afferent inhibition, or it may have originated from the central pattern generator responsible for the repetitive masticatory movements.

Another example of modulation of sensory responses associated with movement is shown in Fig. 2. In this example, a monkey performed a complex reaction time task and lip movements during reception of a liquid reward activated a wide-dynamic-range neuron in the medullary dorsal horn (Hayes et al., 1981). The lip movements apparently activated low-threshold mechanoreceptive afferents providing input to the neuron. The activity of the neuron was reduced in a visual task as compared to a task in which thermal stimuli were applied to the face. The electromyographic (EMG) activity was the same in both tasks, indicating that sensory afferents were activated similarly by the lip movements. This modulation likely is related to the greater relevance of facial mechanical input in the thermal task, since proper thermode contact on the face was critical for its execution. This type of modulation most likely is related to central nervous system (CNS) mechanisms since the afferent input produced by the movement appeared to be the same in both tasks. The origin of such central modulation is unknown.

A similar type of modulation can be found in the superficial gray and optic layers of the monkey superior colliculus (Richmond and Wurtz, 1980). In this region, cells respond to a moving stimulus when the eye is stationary, but not when the monkey makes a saccadic eye movement across the same, but stationary, stimulus. These cells show a suppression of activity following the onset of saccadic eye movements, and the suppression persists in total darkness. Furthermore, the suppression persists when peripheral feedback from the orbit or from head movements is blocked, suggesting that the modulation is of CNS origin and probably involves input from the oculomotor system.

Similar observations have been made in other sensory systems and in other animal invertebrate and vertebrate species (Richmond and Wurtz, 1980; Bell, 1984; Gellman et al., 1985). Thus, such a non-specific suppression or modulation of sensory input produced as a consequence of an animal's own movement is a common feature of sensory modulation in many species and sensory systems, and is likely an evolutionary important one.

Modulation of behaviorally-significant environmental stimuli

Numerous studies in monkeys have correlated behavior with neuronal activity in what is commonly referred to as a delayed-response task (Evarts et al., 1984). The animal is given an instructional sensory cue indicating which response must be executed when a second, trigger stimulus

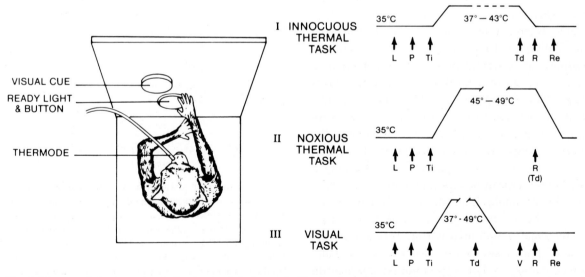

Fig. 3. Diagram of the thermal and visual tasks. L indicates the illumination of the panel button signaling that the monkey could initiate a trial; P represents the monkey pressing the panel button; R represents the monkey releasing the button. Ti and Td show, respectively, the increase and decrease to baseline (35°C) of the thermode temperature. The ranges of temperatures in each task are shown. V indicates the onset of the visual cue in the visual task. The monkey received a reward for correct detection of Td in the innocuous thermal task and V in the visual task. No reward was received in the noxious thermal task but release of the button immediately terminated the noxious temperature. (From Duncan et al., 1987.)

is presented. Fig. 3 is a diagram of a typical delayed response task. A light appears on a panel button indicating that the monkey can initiate a trial. The monkey presses the panel button and at the same time a temperature increase occurs beneath a contact probe located above the monkey's lip. This temperature change is an instructional stimulus indicating to the monkey that the trigger stimulus will be a second temperature change occurring some random time after pressing the panel button. The trigger stimulus then occurs, in this case a temperature decrease, and the monkey executes the appropriate motor behavior, release of the button, followed by reinforcement delivery. Three patterns of neuronal modulation have been observed in neurons while monkeys perform such a task (Evarts et al., 1984; Duncan et al., 1987). First, there may be phasic modulations associated with the presentation of the instructional cues (light onset or temperature increase). Second, there may be changes in activity while the animal awaits the trigger stimulus and prepares to execute the appropriate motor behavior. Third, there may be phasic modulation associated with the trigger stimulus and the motor response.

Studies have shown that one type of behavioral modulation in delayed-response tasks occurs in response to instructional stimuli presented in a neuron's receptive field (Wurtz et al., 1980; Hayes et al., 1981; Bushnell et al., 1984). The 'receptive field' of such a neuron is defined as that receptive zone in which an adequate stimulus activates the neuron, irrespective of the behavioral state, i.e., waking, sleeping, anesthetized, or performing a task. In this type of behavioral modulation, the instructional stimulus is an adequate stimulus for activating the neuron. However, as described later, instructional stimuli need not always be adequate stimuli. Fig. 4 shows the responses of a wide-dynamic-range (WDR) trigeminothalamic neuron in the medullary dorsal horn that responded to graded increases in noxious heat stimuli between 43°C and 49°C (Bushnell et al., 1984). In the behavioral task, this temperature increase was an instructional stimulus that indicated whether the

trigger stimulus (a temperature decrease) would or would not occur. The monkey was required to discriminate the intensity of the instructional stimulus in order to determine whether the trigger stimulus would occur. The peristimulus histogram in Fig. 4 shows the response of the neuron to a 49°C temperature presented during the thermal

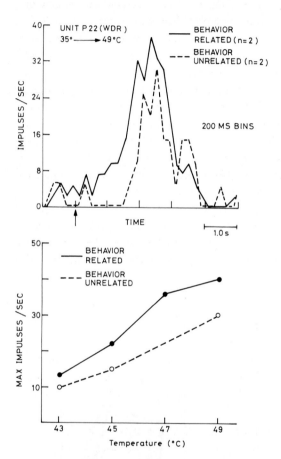

Fig. 4. Responses of a wide-dynamic-range (WDR) thalamic projection neuron to thermal stimuli presented during the thermal task (behavior related) and presented during the intertrial interval (behavior unrelated). The top portion is a perihistogram of the response to 49°C stimuli. The arrow indicates stimulus onset. The bottom graph shows stimulus-response functions in the two behavioral conditions for suprathreshold stimuli. Each point represents one to five trials. The ordinate indicates the peak discharge rate. These differences were not statistically significant ($p < 0.08$), but when the same cell was tested comparing thermal and visual trials, differences were significant ($p < 0.03$). (From Bushnell et al., 1984.)

task and presented unexpectedly between trials. When the monkey was using the stimulus as a discriminative cue during the task, the neuronal response magnitude was greater and the neuronal response latency was shorter than when the stimulus was presented between trials and unrelated to the monkey's behavior. The lower portion of Fig. 4 shows that the response of the neuron was enhanced for all suprathreshold thermal stimuli when the monkey was using the stimulus for discriminative information.

Such a difference in thermal responsivity in and out of a task could be related to differences in arousal, attention, or motivation. In order to control for general arousal and motivational effects, Bushnell et al. (1984) compared neuronal responses to thermal stimuli presented in the thermal task with those responses to behaviorally irrelevant thermal stimuli presented during a similar visual task. In the visual task, there was usually no change in temperature when the monkey pressed the panel button. The absence of a temperature change indicated to the monkey that the trigger stimulus would be the onset of a light on the response panel (Fig. 3). Blocks of visual trials were presented together, and on some of these trials a thermal stimulus occurred while the monkey awaited the visual trigger stimulus. The monkeys appeared to ignore the thermal stimulus, and executed the same latency motor response on visual trials with and without irrelevant thermal stimuli. Fig. 5 shows the stimulus-response functions of a WDR thalamic projection neuron to behaviorally relevant temperatures presented during the thermal task and to behaviorally irrelevant temperatures presented during the visual task. The neuronal response magnitude was enhanced in the thermal task relative to the visual task in two ways: the thermal threshold was lower in the the thermal task (43°C) than in the visual task (45°C), and at every temperature above threshold, the response magnitude was greater in the thermal task than in the visual task.

These data suggest that the enhancement of activity in response to stimuli in the neuron's receptive field is related to differences in the monkey's

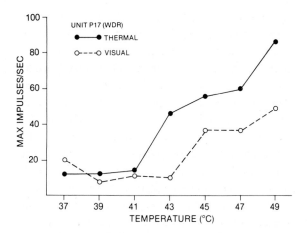

Fig. 5. Stimulus-response functions for a WDR thalamic projection neuron during the thermal and visual tasks. Each point represents two to seven trials. Higher response rates occurred in the thermal task than in the visual task for every temperature above threshold ($p < 0.01$). Response rates were the same below threshold. The data were obtained within a 2–3 h period. (From Bushnell et al., 1984.)

selective attention to the relevant thermal stimuli. General arousal probably contributed little since the two tasks were similar in difficulty, ruling out different states of arousal. Differences in motivational significance of the thermal stimulus in the two tasks also is unlikely because for temperatures above 43°C, the thermal stimuli were not directly associated with liquid reward in either task. Furthermore, it is unlikely that the monkey attended to the thermal stimuli equally in both tasks. The monkey was required to attend to the temperature in the thermal task in order to perform correctly, but was required to ignore it in the visual task. Thus, differences in the level of attention probably are responsible for the modulation of responses to instructional thermal stimuli presented in the receptive fields of medullary dorsal horn neurons.

Since medullary dorsal horn neurons project to the thalamus, it is reasonable to suggest that the perceived intensity of noxious thermal stimuli may be affected by changes in the animal's attentional state. Bushnell et al. (1984) performed experiments that suggest this is the case. Human subjects and monkeys were trained to detect a noxious thermal stimulus when their attention was directed to that stimulus by an instructional signal. These trials were compared to trials in which no attention-directing instructional signal was provided. Both the monkeys and the humans responded more accurately and faster to the noxious thermal stimulus in the signaled as opposed to the unsignaled condition. These findings support the conclusion that selective attentional mechanisms can alter the perceived intensity of environmental stimuli, presumably via the enhancement of neuronal responses of stimulus-intensity encoding neurons.

The enhancement of responses to behaviorally relevant stimuli presented in the receptive field of neurons also has been reported at several levels of the visual (Wurtz et al., 1980) and auditory (Ryan and Miller, 1977) systems. In the visual system, three types of enhancement have been demonstrated (Wurtz et al., 1980). Neurons in the striate cortex exhibit enhanced responsiveness that is independent of the location of the stimulus (inside or outside the receptive field of the neuron), and unrelated to the initiation and guidance of specific eye movements. This first type of enhancement, likely, is related to general arousal and alerting functions that influence the processing of all types of stimuli equally. In the superior colliculus, a second type of enhancement occurs when the monkey uses the visual stimulus as a target for a saccade. When the monkey fixates its attention at a central point of light and a spot is flashed in the neuron's receptive field, some neurons in the deeper layers of the superior colliculus exhibit a weak response. In this task, the fixation point is an instructional stimulus that informs the monkey to continue to fixate until the point dims (the trigger stimulus). The spot in the neuron's receptive field is an irrelevant visual stimulus, similar to the thermal stimuli in the visual task described above in the studies of enhancement in the medullary dorsal horn (Hayes et al., 1981; Bushnell et al., 1984). However, when the spot of light in the cell's receptive field is the target for a saccade, there is an enhancement of the response preceding the saccade. In this situation, the spot in the neuron's receptive field is an instructional stimulus informing the monkey to sac-

cade to this new spot and fixate until it dims. The spot in the receptive field of the neuron is now a relevant stimulus. It results in an enhanced response similar to that produced by thermal stimuli in the thermal task described above. This enhanced response is spatially selective, since it does not occur when a spot of light outside the cell's receptive field is the target for the saccade. The response is dependent on the stimulus occurring in the neuron's receptive field, again similar to the studies in the medullary dorsal horn. However, this enhanced response is not present when the monkey attends to the spot in the receptive field, but does not make an eye movement to it. Thus, this second type of enhancement cannot be dissociated from the motor response and, likely, is related to the initiation and execution of specific eye movements and is not involved in visual attention.

In the visual system, the third type of enhancement is found in the pulvinar and the posterior parietal cortex (Wurtz et al., 1980; Petersen et al., 1987) and likely is involved in mechanisms underlying attention. The enhancement in the pulvinar is spatially selective, and can be dissociated from any motor response the monkey makes toward the stimulus. There is enhancement when the monkey makes a saccade towards, or merely attends to, the light in the neuron's receptive field. This enhancement is absent when the monkey attends to a light outside of the visual receptive field of the neuron. Thus, the enhancement in the pulvinar is akin to that found in the medullary dorsal horn (Hayes et al., 1981; Bushnell et al., 1984). It is in response to an instructional stimulus only in the neuron's receptive field and it is dissociable from the motor behavior leading to reinforcement.

Behavioral context can also result in the suppression of irrelevant environmental stimuli that are present in the receptive field of a neuron (Dubner et al., 1980). Fig. 6 illustrates the suppression of activity of a medullary dorsal horn neuron whose receptive field was located under the thermal probe providing signals in the thermal task (Fig. 3). This neuron exhibited maintained discharge to the

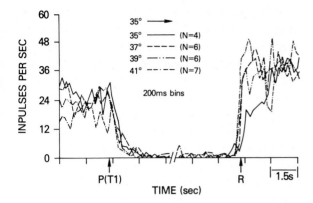

Fig. 6. Suppression of activity of a low-threshold mechano-receptive neuron in the medullary dorsal horn while the monkey waited for the trigger stimulus. The histograms are plotted relative to press of the panel button [P(T1)] on the left and release (R) on the right. N refers to the number of trials averaged in each pair of histograms. (From Dubner et al., 1980.)

placement of the contact probe and presumably received input from slowly adapting, low-threshold mechanoreceptive afferents innervating the face. The maintained activity was totally suppressed soon after the monkey initiated the trial and pressed the panel button. Activity returned to previous levels following panel button release, the motor behavior leading to successful execution of the task. The suppression of activity was unrelated to the thermal stimulus accompanying panel button press, since it occurred in the absence of any thermal stimulation. Suppression was absent outside of the behavioral task. These findings suggest that selective attention to appropriate sensory cues can influence the responsivity of neurons to irrelevant as well as relevant stimuli.

The encoding of behavioral set

Behavioral modulation of neuronal activity, as mentioned above, can be associated with instructional stimuli, sensory and motor preparation for trigger stimuli, and the execution of the motor behavior following the trigger stimulus. Changes in neuronal discharge can occur to stimuli that pro-

duce no response of the neuron outside of the behavioral task. For example, in the thermal and visual tasks shown in Fig. 3, the illumination of the panel button is an instructional cue that is clearly not an adequate stimulus for activating medullary dorsal horn neurons under other circumstances. However, in the behavioral task, some neurons exhibit responses to such instructional stimuli. These responses appear to encode behavioral set rather than any features of the stimulus. They represent a state of readiness or preparation associated with the occurrence of behaviorally significant stimuli. Dubner et al. (1981) have referred to such neuronal activity as task-related responses in the medullary

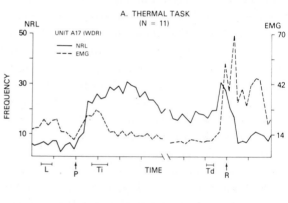

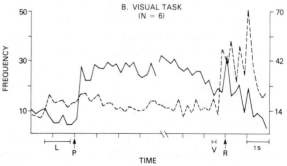

Fig. 7. Peristimulus histograms of the response of a WDR thalamic projection neuron (solid line) and of the EMG activity (broken line) recorded from the lip musculature during the thermal (A) and visual (B) tasks. All temperatures were below threshold for activation of the neuron. The histograms are averaged around button press (P) and button release (R). Brackets under the abscissa mark the time period of the button illumination to start the trial (L), the temperature increase (Ti), the temperature decrease (Td) and the visual stimulus (V). (From Bushnell et al., 1984.)

dorsal horn. Approximately 45 to 65% of the medullary dorsal horn neurons studied, exhibited task-related responses (Dubner et al., 1981; Duncan et al., 1987).

Fig. 7 is an example of task-related responses of a WDR thalamic projection neuron in the monkey medullary dorsal horn during the performance of the thermal and visual tasks (Bushnell et al., 1984). The cell did not exhibit graded responses to innocuous or noxious thermal stimuli. However, when the monkey pressed the panel button following its illumination, there was an increase in neuronal discharge in the thermal task (Fig. 7, A) that persisted while the monkey awaited the trigger stimulus. The trigger stimulus, in this instance a decrease in temperature, produced a phasic neuronal discharge that returned to pretrial levels following execution of the motor response, the release of the button. Similar tonic and phasic responses occurred in the visual task (Fig. 7, B). These responses were independent of the magnitude of the temperature changes occurring during the trials. In other experiments, the phasic response following the trigger stimulus has been dissociated from lip and arm movements, providing evidence that these responses are related to sensory preparation rather than the initiation and execution of specific movements (Dubner et al., 1981). Fig. 7 also shows that there was little relationship between lip EMG activity and neuronal discharge frequency. Therefore, it is unlikely that this task-related activity was an artifact caused by mechanical stimulation of the face.

The presence of task-related responses in both the visual and thermal tasks indicates that they are independent of stimulus modality. They also are independent of specific stimulus features (Dubner et al., 1981). Inhibitory responses are also common in the thermal and visual tasks (Duncan et al., 1987). Inhibitory task-related responses were associated with instructional stimuli, preparation for trigger stimuli, and the execution of motor behavior following the trigger stimulus. Most commonly, they occurred in conjunction with a contiguous excitatory task-related response.

There have been numerous investigations in monkey cerebral cortex of neuronal activity associated with instructional stimuli in which the monkey awaits a trigger sensory cue before executing an appropriate motor response. These responses only occur during the tasks and are related to behavioral set. Such activity is usually interpreted according to the presumed functional attributes of the given cortical area. Thus, the activity is thought to be associated with short-term memory in the inferotemporal cortex (Fuster and Jervey, 1982), visual fixation in the posterior parietal cortex (Mountcastle et al., 1975), and sensorimotor association in the auditory cortex (Vaadia et al., 1982). In these areas, as in the medullary dorsal horn, the activity is linked to sensory readiness or preparation. In the premotor (Weinrich and Wise, 1982), supplementary motor (Tanji et al., 1980) and precentral motor (Tanji and Evarts, 1976) cortex, the activity has been linked to motor preparation. Fig. 8 illustrates the responses of a neuron in the premotor cortex that exhibited sustained activity following an instructional stimulus indicating where the next target key was located. The monkey, after a signaled delay period, was required to depress the new target key. Note the increase in activity while the monkey waited for the trigger stimulus to move to the new target.

It would appear that neuronal activity related to behaviorally relevant information plays a variety of roles, depending on where it occurs in the brain. Relevant information related to the animal's environment is disseminated to numerous parts of the nervous system involved in the animal's ongoing guided behavior. The studies in the medullary dorsal horn (Dubner et al., 1981; Bushnell et al., 1984; Duncan et al., 1987) are the first demonstrations of task-related activity in a non-cortical receiving area involved in the extraction of stimulus feature information. Such findings suggest that neuronal activity related to sensory mechanisms needs to be examined along a behavioral dimension as well as a stimulus-feature extraction dimension.

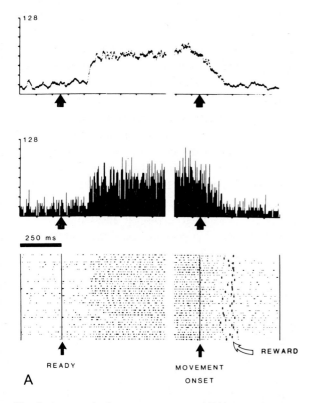

Fig. 8. A neuron in the premotor cortex exhibiting sustained activity while the monkey waited for the trigger stimulus following the occurrence of an instructional stimulus which tells the monkey that the next movement would be to the left-most target. The histograms and dot rasters are synchronized around the occurrence of the instructional or ready cue on the left, and the onset of the movement on the right. Note the similarity of this sustained activity to that found in the thermal and visual tasks shown in Fig. 7. (From Weinrich and Wise, 1982.)

Neuronal pathways mediating behavioral set

Delayed response tasks involve sequential sensory and motor responding that is subject to temporal analysis by the nervous system. These tasks probably activate specific descending control systems that are capable of modulating or gating aggregates of neurons so that the time of occurrence of a sensory event determines its source and significance to the animal. In the medullary dorsal horn, such modulation likely has its origin from multiple sites in the cerebral cortex and medial

brain stem nuclei. Electrical stimulation of the postcentral gyri in monkey preferentially inhibits activity of dorsal horn thalamic projection neurons, whereas stimulation of motor cortex results in excitation (Coulter et al., 1976; Yezierski et al., 1983). Cortical stimulation of postcentral cortex in cat inhibits the evoked responses of low-threshold neurons more effectively than those of nociceptive neurons in the medullary dorsal horn (Sessle et al., 1981). Although such modulation probably involves mainly polysynaptic pathways relaying through medial reticular nuclei (Dubner et al., 1981), direct corticotrigeminal and corticospinal pathways to the dorsal horn exist.

There are multiple descending pathways originating in the midbrain, pons and medulla that have direct and indirect effects on the response of spinal and medullary dorsal horn neurons (Basbaum and Fields, 1978; Willis, 1982). Although these effects are often related only to analgesia, it is likely that they play a role in more fundamental processing of sensory information. The recent studies of 'on' and 'off' cells in the raphe magnus and surrounding nuclei in the brain stem (H. Fields, in this volume) suggest that these neurons may be involved in sensory and motor preparation leading to activation of the tail-flick response following heat stimulation.

The chemical mediators participating in these pathways are of great interest. The ability to modulate responses in the medullary dorsal horn probably involves the multiplicity of chemical mediators located at that site. Opioid peptides such as enkephalin and dynorphin are contained in dorsal horn local circuit neurons and projection neurons and their effects are mimicked by exogenous opiate compounds. Morphine, when microinjected into the monkey medullary dorsal horn, reduces the perceived intensity of noxious heat stimuli (Oliveras et al., 1986). Morphine acts directly on the nociceptive neurons that encode stimulus intensity information and exhibit behavioral enhancement and task-related responses. The effect is likely on all components of the response at this early level of sensory processing. Oliveras et al. (1986) showed that the effect on the perceived intensity of the stimulus was independent of any general attentional, motivational or motoric effects of the drug. In the thalamic pulvinar nucleus, the microinjection of GABA agonists leads to slower reaction times associated with a slowing of the shift of attention to visual stimuli (Petersen et al., 1987). In contrast, bicuculline, a GABA antagonist, produces a small decrease in reaction times in the same attentional task when microinjected into the same sites. GABA is found in local circuit neurons in the pulvinar and has an inhibitory effect on sensory transmission. Ascending norepinephrine pathways originating from the locus coeruleus, have been shown to amplify novel and behaviorally relevant signals in the cerebral cortex (Foote et al., 1983). The multitargeted effects of descending monoaminergic pathways, originating in the pons and medulla, suggest that they may provide a global enhancement or suppression of activity associated with behavioral tasks, in which sensory and motor preparation are critical to correct performance.

Summary

From this brief review, it can be seen that behavioral modulation of sensory responsiveness is prevalent in different sensory and motor systems and at different levels of the nervous system. It occurs in response to self-generated stimuli, environmental stimuli in the receptive field of sensory neurons, and following sensory events that provide instructional information in a task or are trigger stimuli leading to goal-directed behavior. In all cases, this neural modulation is essential for the extraction of relevant sensory cues from the surrounding environment. Iterative behavioral tasks such as those described above probably activate specific descending control systems that modulate neuronal activity so that the time of occurrence of a sensory event determines its source and significance to the animal. In the medullary dorsal horn, such modulation likely has its origin from multiple sites in the cerebral cortex and medial brain stem nuclei.

The chemical mediators participating in these pathways are of great interest. There is evidence that all three major classes of chemical mediators, amino acids, monoamines and peptides, participate in the modulation of sensory information association with behavior. Opiates modify the perceived intensity of noxious stimuli in the dorsal horn, GABA alters attentional mechanisms in the thalamic pulvinar nucleus, and monoamines amplify novel and behaviorally significant stimuli in the cerebral cortex. Future studies are needed to determine the role of different descending control pathways and their chemical messengers in an animal's ability to prepare for significant sensory events in its environment.

References

Basbaum, A.I. and Fields, H.L. (1978) Endogenous pain control mechanisms: review and hypothesis. *Ann. Neurol.*, 4: 451–462.

Bell, C.C. (1984) Effects of motor commands on sensory inflow, with examples from electric fish. In L. Bolis, R.D. Keynes and S.H.P. Maddrell (Eds.), *Comparative Physiology of Sensory Systems*, Cambridge University Press, Cambridge, pp. 637–646.

Bushnell, M.C., Duncan, G.H., Dubner, R. and He, L.F. (1984) Activity of trigeminothalamic neurons in medullary dorsal horn of awake monkeys trained in a thermal discrimination task. *J. Neurophysiol.*, 52: 170–187.

Coulter, J.D., Foreman, R.D., Beall, J.E. and Willis, W.D. (1976) Cerebral cortical modulation of primate spinothalamic neurons. In J.J. Bonica and D. Albe-Fessard (Eds.), *Advances in Pain Research and Therapy, Vol. 1*, Raven Press, New York, pp. 271–277.

Dubner, R., Hayes, R.L. and Hoffman, D.S. (1980) Neural and behavioral correlates of pain in the trigeminal system. In J.J. Bonica (Ed.), *Pain, Association for Research in Nervous and Mental Disease, Vol. 58*, Raven Press, New York, pp. 63–72.

Dubner, R., Hoffman, D.S. and Hayes, R.L. (1981) Neuronal activity in medullary dorsal horn of awake monkeys trained in a thermal discrimination task. III. Task-related responses and their functional role. *J. Neurophysiol.*, 46: 444–464.

Duncan, G.H., Bushnell, M.C., Bates, R. and Dubner, R. (1987) Task-related responses of monkey medullary dorsal horn neurons. *J. Neurophysiol.*, 57: 289–310.

Evarts, E.V., Shinoda, Y. and Wise, S.P. (1984) *Neurophysiological Approaches to Higher Brain Functions*, Wiley, New York, 198 pp.

Foote, S.L., Bloom, F.E. and Aston-Jones, G. (1983) The

nucleus locus coeruleus: new evidence of anatomical and physiological specificity. *Physiol. Rev.,* 63: 844 – 914.

Fuster, J.M. and Jervey, J.P. (1982) Neuronal firing in the inferotemporal cortex of the monkey in a visual memory task. *J. Neurosci.,* 2: 361 – 375.

Gellman, R., Gibson, A.R. and Houk, J.C. (1985) Inferior olivary neurons in the awake cat: detection of contact and passive body displacement. *J. Neurophysiol.,* 54: 40 – 60.

Hayes, R.L., Dubner, R., Hoffman, D.S. (1981) Neuronal activity in medullary dorsal horn of awake monkeys trained in a thermal discrimination task. II. Behavioral modulation of responses to thermal and mechanical stimuli. *J. Neurophysiol.,* 46: 428 – 443.

Hebb, D.O. (1959) A neuropsychological theory. In S. Koch (Ed.), *Psychology: A Study of Science, Vol. 1, Sensory, Perceptual and Physiological Formulations,* McGraw-Hill, New York, pp. 622 – 643.

Mountcastle, V.B., Lynch, J.C., Georgopoulos, A., Sakata, H. and Acuna, C. (1975) Posterior parietal cortex of the monkey: command functions for operations within extrapersonal space. *J. Neurophysiol.,* 38: 871 – 908.

Oliveras, J.-L., Maixner, W., Dubner, R., Bushnell, M.C., Kenshalo, Jr., D.R., Duncan, G.H., Thomas, D.A. and Bates, R. (1986) The medullary dorsal horn: a target for the expression of opiate effects on the perceived intensity of noxious heat. *J. Neurosci.,* 6: 3086 – 3093.

Olsson, K.A., Sasamoto, K. and Lund, J.P. (1986) Modulation of transmission in rostral sensory nuclei during chewing. *J. Neurophysiol.,* 55: 56 – 75.

Petersen, S.E., Robinson, D.L. and Morris, J.D. (1987) Contributions of the pulvinar to visual spatial attention. *Neuropsychologia,* 25: 97 – 105.

Richmond, B.J. and Wurtz, R.H. (1980) Vision during saccadic eye movements. II. A corollary discharge to monkey superior colliculus. *J. Neurophysiol.,* 43: 1156 – 1167.

Ryan, A. and Miller, J. (1977) Effects of behavioral performance on single unit firing patterns in inferior colliculus of the rhesus monkey. *J. Neurophysiol.,* 40: 943 – 956.

Sessle, B.J., Hu, J.W., Dubner, R. and Lucier, G.E. (1981) Functional properties of neurons in cat trigeminal subnucleus caudalis (medullary dorsal horn). II. Modulation of responses to noxious and nonnoxious stimuli by periaqueductal gray, nucleus raphe magnus, cerebral cortex, and afferent influences, and effect of naloxone. *J. Neurophysiol.,* 45: 193 – 207.

Vaadia, E., Gottlieb, Y. and Abeles, M. (1982) Single-unit activity related to sensorimotor association in auditory cortex of a monkey. *J. Neurophysiol.,* 48: 1201 – 1213.

Weinrich, M. and Wise, S.P. (1982) The pre-motor cortex of the monkey. *J. Neurosci.,* 2: 1329 – 1345.

Willis, W.D. (1982) Control of nociceptive transmission in the spinal cord. In D. Ottoson (Ed.), *Progress in Sensory Physiology,* Springer-Verlag, Heidelberg, pp. 1 – 159.

Woodworth, R.S. (1958) *Dynamics of Behavior,* Holt, Rinehart and Winston, New York.

Wurtz, R.H., Goldberg, M.E. and Robinson, D.L. (1980) Behavioral modulation of visual responses in the monkey: stimulus selection for attention and movement. In J. Sprague and A.N. Epstein (Eds.), *Progress in Psychobiology and Physiological Psychology, Vol. 9,* Academic Press, New York, pp. 43 – 83.

Yezierski, R.P., Gerhart, K.D., Schrock, B.J. and Willis, W.D. (1983) A further examination of effects of cortical stimulation on primate spinothalamic tract cells. *J. Neurophysiol.,* 49: 424 – 441.

H.L. Fields and J.-M. Besson (Eds.)
Progress in Brain Research, Vol. 77
© 1988 Elsevier Science Publishers B.V. (Biomedical Division)

CHAPTER 14

Discussion: Descending modulation in the trigeminal system

B.J. Sessle

Faculty of Dentistry, University of Toronto, Toronto, Ontario, M5G 1G6, Canada

In view of the insights and comprehensive review provided by Dr. Willis of spinal nociceptive control, I will emphasize descending modulation in the trigeminal (V) brain stem complex. The raphe magnus (NRM), periaqueductal gray (PAG) and adjacent reticular formation have also been the focus of the limited amount of study of descending modulatory influences on V-nociceptive transmission (for review, see Dubner et al., 1978; Basbaum, 1985; Sessle, 1987). Stimulation of PAG or NRM can suppress the digastric jaw-opening reflex (JOR) in the awake, decerebrate or anaesthetized animal, and also reduce nociceptive behavioural responses to noxious facial or tooth pulp stimuli. A major factor in these suppressive effects is the demonstrated inhibitory influence exerted by PAG and NRM on the tooth pulp, cutaneous, visceral or muscle afferent-evoked responses in nociceptive V brain stem neurons, since many of these neurons serve as reflex interneurons or as projection neurons to higher levels of the brain. These effects may also be partly related to the changes demonstrated by Dubner and his colleagues in the nociceptive response properties of brain stem neurons in V subnucleus caudalis that can be induced by different behavioural contingencies which an awake animal may be carrying out, and so may contribute to the well-recognized effects that motivation, anxiety, attention, distraction, etc. may have on pain.

Postsynaptic inhibition, which appears to be involved in raphe-induced suppression of spinal nociceptive neurons, may underlie some of the suppressive effects, since PAG or NRM stimulation blocks antidromic invasion and glutamate-evoked activity of V neurons. Because primary afferent depolarization (PAD) is thought to underlie presynaptic inhibition, presynaptic regulatory mechanisms may also be involved: PAG or NRM stimulation induces PAD in the brain stem terminals of tooth pulp and facial primary afferents. Dr. Willis cited a study reporting that NRM produces a decreased excitability of C fibre afferents, although it inhibits nociceptive afferent input to spinal dorsal horn neurons. Our studies, however, have noted a correlation between the effects of NRM stimulation on V primary afferent input and V brain stem neuronal activity, since NRM induces inhibition of the brain stem neurons and a correlated PAD in the brain stem endings of nociceptive (and non-nociceptive) facial afferents.

Peptides, noradrenaline, and 5HT-containing terminals, possibly originating from the raphe and other brain stem loci, have been described within the V complex, especially subnucleus caudalis, and have been implicated in these descending influences. Nonetheless, it should be noted that some of these effects appear to involve the neural circuitry which is intrinsic to the V complex and which may involve local interneurons containing these substances and other neurochemicals such as GABA. These same local or segmental circuits and neurochemicals might also be brought into operation by other descending influences, as well as by sensory inputs that can induce analgesia.

It should also be emphasized that, as in the spinal somatosensory system, the effects of PAG or NRM stimulation are not limited to V nociceptive transmission; indeed, other functions (e.g. motor control, autonomic regulation, sleep) can also be modulated. In the V system, stimulation of PAG or NRM profoundly suppresses JOR responses evoked by low-threshold afferent inputs, inhibits the majority of low-threshold mechanosensitive (LTM) neurons throughout the V brain stem complex that are excited by nonnoxious orofacial stimuli, and produces PAD of non-nociceptive V afferents. Our studies have also shown that PAG and NRM influence both threshold and suprathreshold responses of the neuronal responses, which contrasts with some of the work cited by Dr. Willis on changes in threshold and gain in the spinal system. We have also documented that NRM-induced inhibition of V neurons may be associated with a reduction in mechanoreceptive field size, an effect not apparently investigated in the spinal system.

In keeping with the concept raised by Dr. Willis that there are multiple descending influences modulating nociceptive transmission, it has been shown that JOR and V brain stem neuronal responses to both noxious and non-noxious orofacial stimuli can also be suppressed by stimulation of the somatosensory cerebral cortex; cortical stimulation also induces PAD in the brain stem endings of V primary afferents. Stimulation of a number of reticular formation sites in the brain stem can also suppress the JOR and both nociceptive and non-nociceptive V brain stem neurons, and produces PAD of the brain stem endings of V afferents. Other effective sites include locus coeruleus, cerebellum, orbital cortex, and a number of thalamic areas; we have also recently found that the anterior pretectal nucleus exerts an inhibitory influence on the JOR and V brain stem neurons. A particular challenge, facing both the V and the spinal neuroscientist, is to delineate the functional circumstance(s) in which each of these multiple descending influences operates.

References

Basbaum, A.I. (1985) Functional analysis of the cytochemistry of the spinal dorsal horn. *Adv. Pain Res. Ther.,* 9: 149 – 175.

Dubner, R., Sessle, B.J. and Storey, A.T. (1978) *The Neural Basis of Oral and Facial Function,* Plenum Press, NY.

Sessle, B.J. (1987) The neurobiology of facial and dental pain: present knowledge, future directions. *J. Dent. Res.,* 66: 962 – 981.

H.L. Fields and J.-M. Besson (Eds.)
Progress in Brain Research, Vol. 77
© 1988 Elsevier Science Publishers B.V. (Biomedical Division)

CHAPTER 15

Discussion of the paper by Ronald Dubner: The effect of behavioral state on the sensory processing of nociceptive and non-nociceptive information

Kenneth L. Casey

University of Michigan Medical Center, Neurology Service, Veterans Administration Medical Center, Ann Arbor, MI 48105, USA

Dr. Dubner has outlined several ways in which behavior modifies sensory processing in the somatosensory system. Movements generate peripheral inputs that guide ongoing behavior. Activation of voluntary movement mechanisms in the central nervous system may modulate central sensory transmission. Motivationally significant environmental stimuli selectively modify sensory processing in several sensory systems. Finally, some neurons that respond to sensory stimuli appear to encode behavioral state. Dr. Dubner showed examples of these effects from the work of others and from the excellent work generated in his laboratory at the National Institutes of Health in Bethesda. The work from that laboratory sets very high standards for the conduct of behavioral neurophysiological experiments, especially in the primate.

The work of Dubner's group clearly shows the nature and degree of modulation of excitability of medullary dorsal horn cells and emphasizes the observation that wide dynamic range or multireceptive neurons appear to encode stimulus intensity within the noxious range; nociceptive-specific cells appear to have some other role. This work also shows the marked alteration in the activity of some of these dorsal horn cells related specifically to the behavioral task required of the animal.

Behavioral neurophysiology is a demanding field of neuroscience. However, it provides essential information about the functioning of the normal brain at levels ranging from the multicellular to the molecular; it is the only way we will really be able to address the issue of the functional significance of neuronal activity. At this conference, for example, Bill Willis showed how a motor neuron recorded from an anesthetized animal could easily be mistaken for a nociceptive-specific sensory cell. Certainly, there is much information yet to be obtained from experiments in anesthetized preparations, and the massive amount of data being generated in the field of chemohodology will ultimately add to our understanding of how various neural systems function. However, the speculations generated by such information must ultimately be put to the test in the context of behavioral neurophysiology.

Dr. Dubner's presentation touched upon some general problems in behavioral neurophysiology. One of these is the role of learning in determining the properties of neurons. Highly trained animals have highly trained neurons, and the physiological properties they manifest will almost certainly depend on the behavioral context in which they are studied. This issue will deserve more serious consideration as the field grows and the results of different studies are compared. For example, in our studies of untrained squirrel monkeys, Dr. Thomas

Morrow and I find that approximately 50% of the cells in the ventrobasal thalamus show excitability changes related to behavioral state, but the remaining cells appear to show very stable responses, even when drugs are used to modify profoundly the animal's responsiveness. This raises the related question of the neurophysiological basis for neuronal mutability or immutability in sensory systems.

We need to think carefully about the need to develop a new nomenclature to describe some of the complex properties of these cells. We can no longer refer to neural activity as simply sensory or motor, but our thinking seems too often guided by terms derived from reflexive behavioral paradigms. As Lewis Carroll reminded us, names are important. In the case of neuroscience, the name may strongly imply an understanding of a mechanism or of a role in behavior. Descriptors of neuronal properties will have to rely upon an unambiguous identification of behavioral state, and take into account the possibility that the degree and the type of modulation may vary with behavioral state and with the site of recording.

The future seems very exciting because we are entering into an era in which the results of behavioral neurophysiological experiments might be related rather directly to clinical neurology. The new neuroimaging techniques such as computerized tomography, magnetic resonance imagery, and positron emission tomography, provide us with the opportunity to identify focal structural and even metabolic changes in the central nervous system, and to relate these changes to alterations in sensory, motor, or higher integrative functions. Undoubtedly, the imaging techniques will improve in both spatial and temporal resolution so that more sophisticated questions can be asked and answered. Equally critical will be the continued development of standardized and quantitative examination techniques that will reveal the behavioral alterations associated with focal lesions. During these evolutionary developments, there should be a strong facilitatory interaction between behavioral neurophysiological experiments in animals and clinical neurological observation.

Reference

Carroll, L. (1946) *Through the Looking Glass and What Alice Found There.* Random House, New York.

H.L. Fields and J.-M. Besson (Eds.)
Progress in Brain Research, Vol. 77
© 1988 Elsevier Science Publishers B.V. (Biomedical Division)

CHAPTER 16

Effects of morphine given in the brain stem on the activity of dorsal horn nociceptive neurons

G.F. Gebhart and S.L. Jones

Department of Pharmacology, College of Medicine, University of Iowa, Iowa City, IA 52242, USA

Introduction

It is generally held that morphine activates descending systems of inhibition, contributing significantly to the analgesia produced. Whether given intracerebroventricularly or intracerebrally, morphine inhibits responses to nociceptive stimuli, including nociceptive withdrawal reflexes organized segmentally (e.g., the hindlimb withdrawal and tail flick reflexes), consistent with activation by morphine of a descending system(s) of inhibition. For example, it is well documented that microinjection of morphine into the midbrain periaqueductal gray (PAG) or medullary nucleus raphe magnus (NRM), two sites in the brain stem considered important to endogenous systems of pain control, inhibits responses in analgesiometric tests organized either spinally or supraspinally (see Gebhart, 1982, and Yaksh and Rudy, 1978, for reviews). In addition, bulbospinal monoaminergic systems are activated by morphine microinjected into either the PAG or NRM and antinociceptive effects of morphine, whether given systemically or intracerebrally, are attenuated by lesions in the medulla or spinal cord and by receptor antagonists administered into the intrathecal space. These and other data are briefly reviewed below and would seem to establish clearly that a significant part of the analgesia/antinociception produced by morphine and other opioids arises by activation of centrifugal modulatory systems.

Activation of descending systems

The microinjection of morphine into the PAG was first reported by Yaksh and Tyce (1979) to evoke the release of serotonin from the spinal cord in the rat. Similarly, the microinjection of morphine into the NRM increases the synthesis of serotonin in the spinal cord (Sukuki and Taguchi, 1986; Vasko et al., 1984). Focal electrical stimulation in the PAG or NRM likewise releases serotonin at the level of the spinal cord (Hammond and Yaksh, 1985; Sorkin et al., 1987). Since the serotonergic innervation of the spinal cord arises from the caudal medullary raphe group, including the NRM, these neurochemical data demonstrate an activation by morphine (or stimulation) of bulbospinal serotonergic neurons presumably involved in the modulation of spinal nociceptive processing. Complementary electrophysiologic studies have demonstrated that the microinjection of morphine into the PAG activates neurons in the NRM (Behbehani and Pomeroy, 1978; Fields and Anderson, 1978), specifically those neurons hypothesized to mediate descending inhibition of spinal nociceptive transmission (Cheng et al., 1986). In support, the microinjection of the excitatory amino acid glutamate into the PAG has also been shown to activate neurons in the NRM (Behbehani and Fields, 1979). In analgesiometric tests, it has been widely documented that morphine or glutamate, when microinjected into the PAG or NRM, reliably produce an antinociception (e.g., Aimone and Gebhart, 1986; Behbehani and Fields, 1979; Jensen and Yaksh, 1984, 1986a). Finally, the intrathecal administration of pharmacologic antagonists of serotonin and/or adrenergic receptors in the lumbar spinal cord significantly attenuates the antinociceptive effects of morphine in the tail flick test when morphine is administered into the PAG (Camarata and Yaksh, 1985; Jensen and Yaksh, 1986b; Yaksh, 1979) or NRM (Jensen and Yaksh, 1986b).

That morphine activates descending systems of inhibition when microinjected into the brain stem is also supported by studies examining the effects of stimulation or glutamate microinjected into the same sites. Stimulation-produced descending inhibition of the nociceptive tail flick reflex from the PAG or NRM is attenuated by methysergide and yohimbine, serotonin and α_2-adrenergic receptor antagonists, respectively (e.g., Aimone et al., 1987; Barbaro et al., 1985). Similarly, glutamate-produced descending inhibition from the PAG and NRM has been reported to be mediated by the same spinal receptors (Jensen and Yaksh, 1984; Satoh et al., 1983). Thus, converging evidence from a large body of literature, recently reviewed by Besson and Chaouch (1987), provides strong support for the activation by morphine of centrifugal inhibitory systems from the brain stem. That the descending inhibitory effects of morphine, focal electrical stimulation and glutamate are mediated by the same spinal receptors is telling since glutamate and stimulation undeniably *activate* neurons when applied in the PAG or NRM.

While it may be questioned whether an effect by morphine (or stimulation or glutamate) on a segmentally-organized withdrawal reflex represents antinociception, electrophysiologic investigations of spinal nociceptive transmission provide complementary support. The centrifugal modulation of dorsal horn neuronal responses to nociceptive stimuli by focal electrical stimulation in the PAG or NRM is well documented (see Gebhart, 1986, for a review). Similarly, activation of neurons in the PAG or NRM by glutamate also significantly at-

tenuates spinal nociceptive transmission (Jones and Gebhart, 1987; Ness and Gebhart, 1987). While analgesiometric tests employing reflex or escape measures leave uncertain the extent to which the antinociceptive manipulation influences a sensory and/or motor component of the response, electrophysiologic studies clearly establish that such manipulations engage descending systems that inhibit sensory transmission. Thus, activation of neurons in the PAG or NRM by electrical stimulation or microinjection of glutamate provides strong support for inhibition of spinal nociceptive transmission by engaging descending systems of inhibition. These same medullary and midbrain sites from which centrifugal modulatory influences are activated by electrical or chemical stimulation have also been demonstrated to be activated by morphine, although the data from such experiments are not wholly consistent. These data are reviewed below and are summarized in Table I.

Morphine effects on spinal nociceptive transmission

Bennett and Mayer (1979) first reported that morphine (4 – 16 μg) or etorphine (0.25 – 0.5 μg) microinjected into the midbrain of rats significantly attenuated responses of lumbar spinal neurons to nociceptive stimuli. The responses of a population of class 2 spinal neurons ('wide dynamic range' type), recorded in rats in which the antinociceptive efficacy of the opioids had been previously documented, were shown to be attenuated at times following drug microinjection consistent with the time of peak effect of the drugs in the antinociceptive test (tail flick test). Control experiments established that the inhibitory effects produced by morphine did not arise from diffusion of drug to a spinal site of action nor were the effects of morphine non-specific since naloxone was shown to antagonize them. While Bennett and Mayer (1979) reported that morphine or etorphine markedly inhibited (i.e., >25%) 27 of 42 spinal units studied and had no effect on eight others, the responses of four units were facilitated by morphine. Interestingly, they report that two of these four units were recorded in rats which had previously exhibited hyperreactivity following the microinjection of morphine into the midbrain. Ryall and co-workers (Clark and Ryall, 1983; Clark et al., 1983) also observed inhibitory effects of morphine and etorphine on lumbar spinal neurons when microinjected into the midbrain or medulla of the cat. However, they report that relatively large doses of morphine were required (mean 93 μg) and produced only modest inhibition

TABLE I

Effects of morphine administered intracerebrally on spinal unit responses to nociceptive stimuli

Site[a]	Species/Anesthetic[b]	Dose (μg)	Stimulus[c]	n[d]	Inhibited[d]	Facilitated[d]	No effect[d]	References
PAG/DR	Rat – Pb, α-chl	4 – 16	Heat	20	11 (> 20%)	4 (26 – 116%)	5	Bennett and Mayer, 1979
NRM	Rat – Hal/N$_2$O	5	Elec-A	14			14	LeBars et al., 1980a
			Elec-C	14		6	8	
PAG	Cat – Pb	28 – 171	Heat	11	7 (21%)		4	Clark et al., 1983
VMM		28 – 285	Heat	30	22 (52%)		8	
PAG	Rat – Hal/N$_2$O	5	Elec-C	33	4	11	18	Dickenson and LeBars, 1983
		20	Elec-C	18		5	13	
PAG	Cat – Pb/N$_2$O	10 – 20	Heat	18	14 (57%)		4	Gebhart et al., 1984
LRF		10 – 20	Heat	5			5	
NRM	Cat – Pb/N$_2$O	10 – 20	Heat	8	8 (75%)			Du et al., 1984
			Elec-A	8	8 (26%)			
			Elec-C	8	8 (44%)			
ICV	Cat – Hal, α-chl	10^{-5} M	Heat	2			2	Sinclair, 1986
		10^{-4} M	Heat	2			2	
		10^{-3} M	Heat	6		6		
NRM	Rat – Hal	5	Heat	27	4	18	5	Llewelyn et al., 1986
PAG/DR	Rat – Hal/N$_2$O	5	Elec-C	39	7 (50%)	20 (50%)	12	Dickenson and LeBars, 1987
PAG	Rat – Pb	10 – 20	Heat	12	8 (36%)		4	Jones and Gebhart, 1988
NRM		10 – 20	Heat	11	8 (40%)		3	

[a] Site of microinjection: DR, dorsal raphe nucleus; ICV, intracerebroventricular; LRF, lateral (midbrain) reticular formation; NRM, nucleus raphe magnus; PAG, periaqueductal gray; VMM, ventromedial medulla.
[b] Anesthetics: α-chl, α-chloralose; Hal, halothane; N$_2$O, nitrous oxide; Pb, pentobarbital.
[c] Nociceptive stimuli: Heat, usually radiant, 45 – 53°C, or transcutaneous electrical (Elec) nerve stimulation at intensities supramaximal for activation of A or A and C fibers.
[d] n, number of spinal units studied and number in which responses to the nociceptive stimulus were inhibited, facilitated or unaffected following administration of morphine. Numbers in parenthesis represent reported or estimated magnitude by which responses were changed.

(mean 21%) of spinal unit responses to noxious heat (Clark et al., 1983). In the same report, greater doses of morphine microinjected into the NRM or adjacent medullary reticular formation (121 μg and 137 μg mean doses, respectively) produced significantly greater inhibition (mean 47% and 57%, respectively). Still greater doses of morphine (mean 1015 μg), injected into the NRM of four cats in which the spinal cord was transected, were required to inhibit (mean 28%) spinal unit responses to noxious heat. Based on the magnitude of effects produced, doses of morphine required, volumes of microinjection (0.5 – 5.0 μl), calculations of drug concentration and distance of diffusion, and recording preparation (i.e. spinalized versus intact), they conclude that the descending inhibition produced by morphine microinjected into the brain stem is due in part to a local (brain stem) effect at lesser doses, but due to general systemic effects at greater doses.

Lesser doses of morphine (mean 15.5 μg) microinjected into the PAG of the cat have, however, been reported to produce potent descending inhibitory effects on responses of 14 of 18 class 2 lumbar spinal neurons to noxious heating of the skin (to 43% of control; i.e. 57% inhibition) (Gebhart et al., 1984). Contrary to the report of Clark et al. (1983), no evidence was found in this study for a systemic effect of morphine following its intracerebral administration. Systemic (intravenous) doses of 100 μg of morphine, 5 – 10 times greater than given into the PAG, failed to affect spinal unit responses to heat; a greater 1 mg/kg dose of morphine, however, did attenuate unit responses to about 50% of control. The effects of morphine also were demonstrated to be specific. Naloxone reversed the effects of morphine, but was most efficacious in doing so when microinjected into the same site as morphine, suggesting that morphine's activation of descending inhibition was receptor-mediated at the locus of microinjection in the PAG. It is noteworthy in this report that the microinjection of morphine into nine sites greater than 2.0 mm lateral to the midline and extending into the lateral mesencephalic

reticular formation, was without effect on unit responses thus supporting the selectivity of the PAG as one locus of morphine's action (see Yaksh and Rudy, 1978). When microinjected into the NRM of the cat, similar doses of morphine (10 – 20 μg) have been reported to attenuate responses of spinal neurons evoked by afferent A and C fiber electrical stimulation (74% and 56% of control, respectively) as well as responses evoked by noxious heating of the skin (38% of control) (Du et al., 1984). In this report, morphine's effects were also demonstrated to be antagonized by naloxone, and not to be reproduced by systemic administration of a 100-μg dose of morphine.

In a recent study in the rat, we examined the effects of morphine microinjected into the PAG or NRM on responses of lumbar spinal units to noxious heat, comparing effects with glutamate microinjected into the same sites (Jones and Gebhart, 1987). The experiments were performed in adult, male Sprague-Dawley rats anesthetized with pentobarbital and paralyzed with pancuronium bromide. The effects of morphine (10 – 20 μg in 0.5 μl) or glutamate (50 nmol in 0.5 μl) microinjected into the PAG or NRM were studied on the responses of class 2 lumbar dorsal horn neurons to noxious radiant heating (50°C) of the plantar surface of the hindfoot. Heat stimuli were feedback-controlled by a thermocouple placed in the center of the field of heat stimulation and presented at 3-min intervals. This paradigm results in stable unit responses to heating (see Jones and Gebhart, 1986, and Fig. 2 below) as defined by requiring that consecutive responses to heat fall within 10% of the mean (i.e., the number of unit discharges was required to be within 10% of the unit's response to heating 3 min prior to and 3 min following the heat stimulus).

Morphine was microinjected into 15 sites in the midbrain, 12 of which were in the PAG, and 11 sites in and adjacent to the NRM. Histologically reconstructed sites of microinjection of morphine and glutamate are summarized in Fig. 1. Unit responses to heating of the skin were generally inhibited by morphine microinjected into the PAG. Results representative of the effects of morphine, glutamate and focal electrical stimulation given at the same sites in the PAG are illustrated in Fig. 2. In this experiment, the effects of electrical and chemical stimulation at three sites in the PAG, separated dorsoventrally 0.5 mm and labeled a, b and c in panel (B), were examined on responses of the same dorsal horn unit to noxious heating of the foot (note that time is continuous in the three panels in (A)). While electrical stimulation was efficacious at site a, glutamate was not; the effects of morphine were not tested at this site. In this example, and in these experiments, glutamate was always microinjected first, followed by morphine. It was not 'required', however, that glutamate be effective before morphine was tested; it *was* necessary for focal electrical stimulation to be effective before glutamate and morphine were microinjected. At sites b and c, glutamate and morphine both significantly attenuated spinal unit responses to heat. Note that the efficacy of stimulation at site b was not affected by the microinjection of glutamate, indicating that the site of microinjection was not damaged. The inhibitory effect of glutamate was typically shortlived (see also Jones and Gebhart, 1986; Ness and Gebhart, 1987), while the onset and effect of morphine was gradual, peaking at 15 – 18 min after its microinjection. Morphine inhibited unit responses to

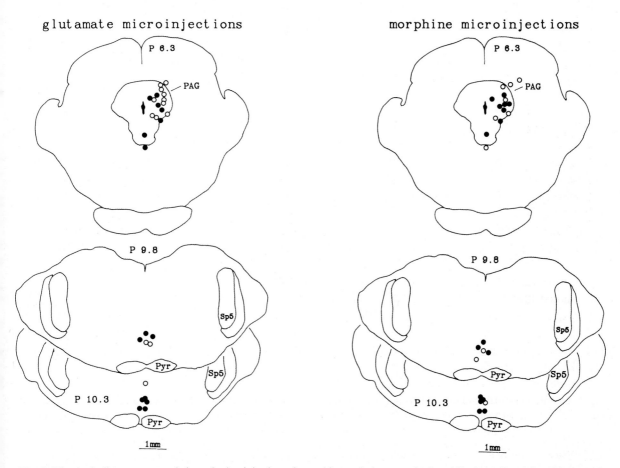

Fig. 1. Histologically reconstructed sites of microinjection of morphine and glutamate in the midbrain and medulla. Filled circles represent sites of microinjection where unit responses to heat were attenuated; unfilled circles represent sites where drug microinjections had no effect.

73.5% and 72.7% of control at sites b and c, respectively. Morphine's inhibitory effects here and in other experiments (see below) were shown to be reversed by naloxone. A final comment about this example and the use of controlled radiant heat as a nociceptive stimulus bears emphasizing. Note the stability of the unit's response over time (mean, 1226 ± 65 sd impulses in 20 s, $n = 21$) to heat (50°C) applied at 3 min intervals. Peristimulus time histograms, corresponding to ef-

fects at site b in panel (A), are illustrated in panel (C).

At eight of 12 sites in the PAG, morphine attenuated unit responses to a mean 64.3 ± 7.6% of control (i.e., 36% inhibition) at a mean time to maximum effect of 11.9 ± 3.4 min. Morphine had no effect at three sites in the PAG and reduced unit responses to heat to 91% of control at one site, an effect not considered significant. The time course of effect is consistent with literature reports on

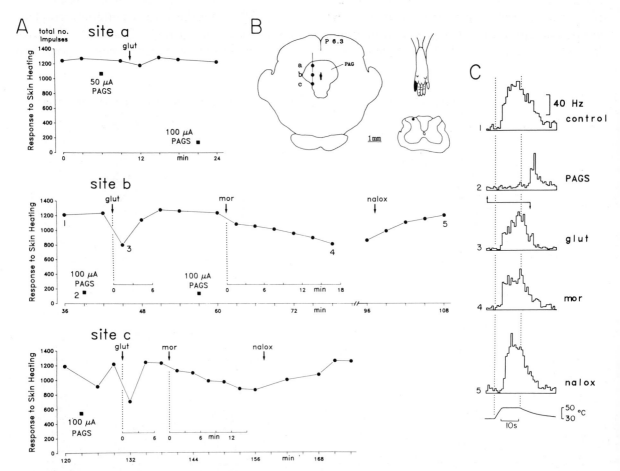

Fig. 2. Example of the effects of stimulation, glutamate (50 nmol in 0.5 μl) and morphine (20 μg in 0.5 μl) given in the periaqueductal gray (PAG) on a dorsal horn unit's response to 50°C heating of the skin. (A) The unit's response to heat is represented on the ordinate as the total number of impulses (in 20 s) against time (min) on the abcissa; time is continuous in the three panels. Morphine (mor), glutamate (glut) and naloxone (nalox; 2 μg in 0.5 μl) were given in the same sites as stimulation in the PAG (PAGS, ■; intensity given). (B) Sites of PAGS and drug microinjections (a – c correspond to the panels in (A)), recording site and peripheral receptive field. (C) Peristimulus time histograms (1 s bin width) of the same unit's responses to heating of the skin during stimulation (PAGS; period of stimulation is indicated) and following microinjection of glutamate, morphine and naloxone into the PAGS at site b; a control histogram is illustrated topmost and the period of heating below. Numbers correspond to numbers in (A), site b.

times to antinociceptive effects following microinjection of morphine into the PAG (e.g., see Jensen and Yaksh, 1986a). Morphine was without effect on unit responses to heat when microinjected into four sites in the PAG or three sites adjacent to, but outside of the PAG (Fig. 1). There was no apparent difference in the magnitude of inhibition produced by microinjection of 10 µg versus 20 µg

of morphine ($n = 6$ for each dose; mean 29% versus 38% inhibition, respectively), and data reported above (and below) have been pooled for the two doses tested. This is perhaps not surprising, given the size of the sample and the distribution of sites of microinjection; the site of microinjection of morphine within the PAG (dorsal versus ventral) apparently was not a determining factor with

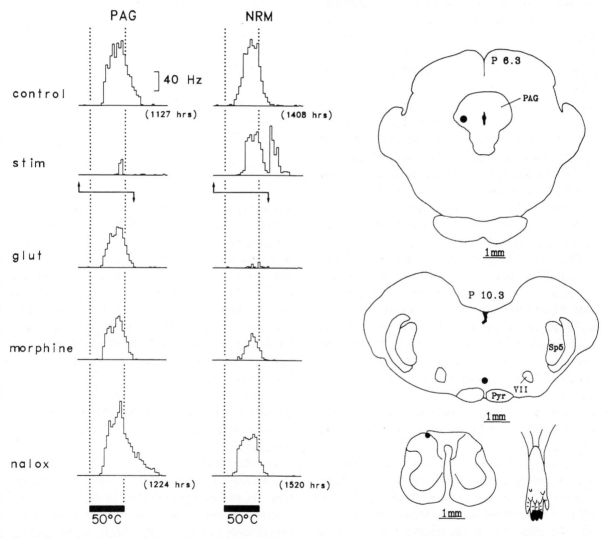

Fig. 3. Examples of effects of stimulation and drugs microinjected into the periaqueductal gray (PAG) and nucleus raphe magnus (NRM) on a unit's responses to 50°C heating of the skin. Data are portrayed as peristimulus time histograms (1 s bin width) for the same unit's responses to heat during stimulation (stim, 75 µA; period of stimulation is indicated) and following administration of glutamate (glut, 50 nmol), morphine (20 µg) and naloxone (nalox, 1 mg/kg i.v.); control histograms are illustrated topmost in each column. The time course of the experiment (parentheses) and the period of heating (15 s) are indicated. Sites of stimulation and recording and the receptive field are illustrated to the right.

regard to morphine's inhibitory effects on unit responses to heat.

In the NRM, morphine inhibited unit responses to heating of the skin to 59.8 ± 5.9% of control (i.e., 40% inhibition) when microinjected into 8/11 sites; morphine did not affect unit responses when microinjected into two sites in the NRM, and insignificantly attenuated responses to 92% of control at one site. An example of the inhibitory effect of morphine when microinjected into the NRM is illustrated in Fig. 3. In this experiment, the effects of stimulation, glutamate and morphine given in the PAG preceded an examination of their effects on the same spinal unit when given in the NRM. The unit's response to heating of the skin was attenuated to 52% of control at 15 min and 27% of control at 12 min following the microinjection of morphine into the PAG and NRM, respectively. The average time to morphine's maximum effect after microinjection into the NRM was 14.7 ± 2.4 min, which was not different from the time to maximum effect when morphine was microinjected into the PAG.

Thus, morphine microinjected into the midbrain or medulla produced only inhibitory or no effects on spinal unit responses to heating of the hindfoot. Morphine microinjected into three sites in the midbrain outside of the PAG was without effect as were vehicle microinjections into the brain stem (see also Gebhart et al., 1984). Naloxone, given systemically in five experiments (1 mg/kg i.v.) and into the PAG in four experiments (2 μg in 0.5 μl) at the same site as morphine had been microinjected, antagonized the effects of morphine in all cases but one.

Glutamate (50 nmol in 0.5 μl) was microinjected into 13 and eight of the same sites in the midbrain and NRM, respectively, as morphine (Fig. 1). The effects of morphine and glutamate microinjected into the same sites in the midbrain and medulla were highly complementary and are summarized in Table II. In five sites in the PAG, both morphine and glutamate attenuated unit responses to heating of the skin, and in six sites in the midbrain (four in the PAG) neither morphine nor glutamate pro-

TABLE II

Effects of morphine and glutamate microinjected into the same sites in the brain stem on unit responses to heating of the skin

		n	Effect of morphine	
			inhibition	none
Midbrain	*Effect of glutamate*	13		
	inhibition		5	0
	none		2	6
Medulla	inhibition	8	5	1
	none		1	1

duced any effect. In the remaining two sites in the midbrain, morphine attenuated unit responses while glutamate did not. When both glutamate and morphine were microinjected into the NRM, inhibition of unit responses was produced from five of eight sites by both morphine and glutamate. In one site, neither drug influenced unit responses to heat and in the remaining sites of microinjection, glutamate produced an inhibitory effect while morphine did not in one site and glutamate had no effect while morphine produced an inhibition in the other. Thus, the effects of glutamate and morphine when microinjected into the midbrain or medulla were the same in 11/13 and 6/8 cases, respectively.

To address the question of the possibility that the effects of morphine arose due to diffusion from the site of microinjection to the systemic circulation, morphine was given intravenously in ten experiments. In two experiments where the intravenous dose of morphine was 100 μg (5 – 10 times that microinjected intracerebrally), morphine failed to influence unit responses to heating of the skin. However, greater doses of morphine given intravenously (3 mg/kg) produced significant inhibition of unit responses in all experiments (to 53% of control). See Fig. 4 for examples. These results further support the hypothesis that morphine acts supraspinally to modulate spinal nociceptive transmission by activating (a) descending inhibitory system(s). Morphine's effects were shown: (1) not to arise due to redistribution from the site of microinjection, (2) to occur at a time consistent with antinociception produced when microinjected into the midbrain or medulla, (3) to be antagonized by naloxone, and (4) to be duplicated by glutamate microinjected into the same sites.

Thus, notwithstanding the relatively few numbers of studies reported, it would appear that morphine, like electrical stimulation or glutamate, engages descending systems of inhibition by local actions in the PAG and NRM. There is, however, surprising disagreement on this point. LeBars and co-workers have reported that morphine (5 μg) microinjected into the PAG (Dickenson and LeBars, 1983, 1987) or NRM (LeBars et al., 1980a) of the rat *facilitates* spinal unit responses to transcutaneous (percutaneous?) electrical stimulation supramaximal for activation of C fibers, thus *decreasing* descending inhibition. Also in the rat,

Llewelyn et al. (1986) reported that morphine (5 μg) microinjected into the NRM increased the responses of 67% of 27 spinal neurons to noxious heating of the foot. In the cat, Sinclair (1986) reported that perfusion between the third ventricle and cisterna magna with morphine in a concentration of 10^{-3}, but not in concentrations of 10^{-4} or 10^{-5}, increased responses of spinal neurons to noxious radiant heat applied in the receptive field. The emphasis here on facilitation of responses by morphine obscures the fact that in many studies where morphine facilitated spinal unit responses, a significant proportion of the neuronal sample was unaffected by morphine (e.g., 57% in LeBars et al., 1980a; 55% in Dickenson and LeBars, 1983; and 31% in Dickenson and LeBars, 1987). Regardless, the failure of morphine to inhibit spinal unit responses in these studies, in addition to the facilitatory effects reported, also argues against the hypothesis that morphine activates a descending system(s) of inhibition. These reports are supported by others, employing different approaches, which also conclude that morphine, while possessing powerful inhibitory effects on nociceptive transmission at the level of the spinal cord, does not produce its inhibitory effects by activation of

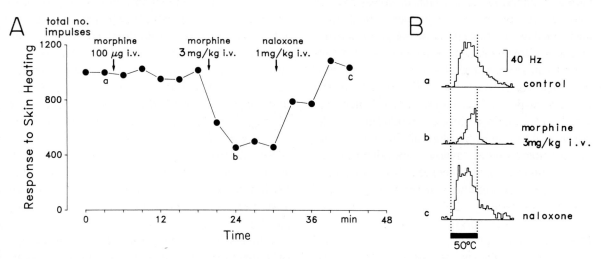

Fig. 4. Example of the effects of morphine administered intravenously on a unit's responses to 50°C heating of the skin. (A) The unit's response to heat is represented on the ordinate as the total number of impulses (in 20 s) against time (min) on the abcissa. Times of administration of morphine and naloxone are indicated. (B) Peristimulus time histograms (1 s bin width) correspond to data in (A). The period of heating (15 s) is indicated.

a descending system of inhibition (e.g., Duggan et al., 1980; Jurna and Grossman, 1976; LeBars et al., 1980b). Thus, although a potent analgetic at both spinal and supraspinal sites in man, whether morphine's analgetic efficacy arises from activation of descending systems of nociceptive control is a topic of controversy.

In the aggregate, the pharmacological, behavioral and neurochemical data cited here and reviewed elsewhere (Besson and Chaouch, 1987) are consistent in support of the hypothesis that morphine activates descending systems of inhibition. The electrophysiological data reviewed here, to the contrary, are markedly divergent on this point. About half of the studies conclude that morphine does not engage a system(s) of descending inhibition since morphine facilitates spinal unit responses, or produces no effect, following its administration intracerebrally or intracerebroventricularly. Naloxone reversibility of morphine's facilitatory effect was not established in many of these studies, and the work can be criticized on these grounds. However, that doses in the antinociceptive range consistently facilitated spinal nociceptive transmission cannot be simply dismissed as non-specific. There is not a readily apparent explanation for the lack of consistency of findings. As Besson and Chaouch (1987) comment, differences in preparations (e.g., anesthetic) or species are inadequate explanations. Both inhibitory and facilitatory effects of morphine have been reported in both cats and rats, and in the presence of the same anesthetics. How, then, can the electrophysiologic data be reconciled with the larger body of pharmacological, behavioral and neurochemical data? Below, consideration of dose, temporal relation between dose and effect, and nociceptive stimulus will serve to provide a basis for discussion.

Dose

A wide range of concentrations of morphine, usually contained in 0.5 μl, has been tested for antinociceptive effects when microinjected intracerebrally (see Yaksh and Rudy, 1978, for review). The 'standard' antinociceptive dose of morphine is 5 μg. In unanesthetized rats, an antinociception is reliably produced by this dose when microinjected into the PAG or NRM (e.g., see Jensen and Yaksh, 1986a). In rats lightly anesthetized with a barbiturate, however, the potency of morphine has been demonstrated to be reduced (Ossipov and Gebhart, 1984; Aimone and Gebhart, 1986). The efficacy of morphine is apparently unaffected by anesthetics since the antinociceptive effect of morphine is dose-dependent when microinjected into the PAG or NRM, whether in unanesthetized rats or rats lightly anesthetized with pentobarbital (Ossipov and Gebhart, 1984; Aimone and Gebhart, 1986). Since barbiturates enhance the physiological effects of GABA, it should not be surprising that barbiturate anesthesia reduces the potency of morphine, particularly in light of data by Moreau and Fields (1986) which suggest that opioids produce their antinociceptive effects in part by inhibiting GABAergic inhibitory interneurons in the midbrain PAG. Thus, an argument that doses of morphine (10 – 20 μg) were excessive in those studies where morphine attenuated spinal unit responses (Du et al., 1984; Gebhart et al., 1984; Jones and Gebhart, 1987), compared to doses of 5 μg in other studies where morphine's effect was none or facilitatory (Dickenson and LeBars, 1987; LeBars et al., 1980a; Llewelyn et al., 1986), cannot account for the different effects reported. Both LeBars et al. (1980a) and Bennett and Mayer (1979) established the antinociceptive efficacy of morphine microinjected into the PAG and NRM, respectively, in doses up to 16 μg, before electrophysiologic studies in the same rats; Bennett and Mayer (1979) reported that facilitatory effects of morphine were associated with behavioral hyperreactivity in two of four cases.

Conversely, the facilitatory effect of morphine on spinal unit responses may arise, due to an insufficient dose. While there is no direct evidence in any of the studies reviewed that this may be so, lesser or greater doses of morphine have not been widely tested in those studies finding facilitation of spinal unit responses by morphine. A *decrease* in descending inhibition could conceivably arise from somewhat selective inhibition of excitatory interneurons in the PAG by low doses of morphine, resulting, for example, in a local inhibition and consequent facilitation of spinal nociceptive transmission by decreasing 'tone' in a descending inhibitory system(s). Greater doses of morphine are also locally inhibitory, but, as suggested by Moreau and Fields (1986), disinhibit *inhibitory* interneurons (as well as excitatory interneurons), resulting in a net excitation of neurons at the locus of microinjection and consequent increase in descending modulatory influences.

Time to effect

When microinjected in 'active' sites in the PAG or NRM, the standard 5 µg dose of morphine produces antinociceptive effects which are maximal by 10 – 20 min (e.g., see Jensen and Yaksh, 1986a). In those studies where time to inhibitory effect of morphine on unit responses has been reported, the time has been consistent with what one would expect based on results from analgesiometric tests (e.g., mean 12 and 15 min, respectively, following microinjection of morphine into the PAG or NRM, Jones and Gebhart, 1987; see also Bennett and Mayer, 1979; Du et al., 1984; Gebhart et al., 1984). Similarly, the time to effect of facilitation of unit responses by morphine is generally consistent with morphine-produced antinociception. For example, LeBars et al. (1980a) reported that the responses of six of 14 spinal units which were facilitated following the microinjection of morphine into the NRM, exhibited a 'striking parallelism between time course curves' (of antinociception and facilitation). The time to peak effect of morphine (facilitation) was 60 min in a more recent report from the same investigators (Dickenson and LeBars, 1987), although an effect was apparent at 10 min following the microinjection of morphine into the PAG. Interestingly, the time to peak effect of *inhibition* of unit responses

by morphine in this study occurred earlier (30 min).

Thus, there are no notable discrepancies apparent in the literature which suggests that the inhibitory or facilitatory effects of morphine on unit responses, when microinjected into either the PAG or NRM, occurs in a temporal relation inconsistent with the antinociception produced by morphine when given in the same sites.

Nociceptive stimulus

With one exception (Llewelyn et al., 1986), studies reporting facilitation of responses by morphine microinjected into the brain stem have employed transcutaneous electrical nerve stimulation (Dickenson and LeBars, 1983, 1987; LeBars et al., 1980a). Studies reporting inhibition of unit responses by morphine, on the other hand, have employed noxious radiant heat. Thus, while considerations of dose and time to effect appear not to help reconcile the differences reported, we believe that the nature of the nociceptive stimulus employed and, moreover, the manner in which it is employed, may be critical to the effects described following the intracerebral microinjection of morphine.

Noxious radiant heat is a natural stimulus which produces reliable responses throughout the course of an experiment (e.g., see Fig. 2, and Jones and Gebhart, 1986). When applied appropriately (e.g., 3-min intervals), sensitization or desensitization of the peripheral receptive field does not occur. Electrical nerve stimulation, on the other hand, does not reproduce a natural stimulus; it is synchronous in nature and instantaneous in onset. In the study of Du et al. (1984), where the microinjection of morphine into the NRM was shown to reduce unit responses to electrical stimulation of the isolated tibial nerve, a standard conditioning-test paradigm was employed rather than repetitive transcutaneous electrical stimulation. In other studies, transcutaneous electrical stimulation, at intensities 2 – 8 times threshold for activation of C fibers, delivered at a frequency of 0.6 Hz, 50 – 150 times every 5–10 min, was employed. The authors acknowledge that 'wind up' results from repetitive stimulation, and thus the effects of morphine, are assessed from peristimulus histograms generated from unit responses accumulated after the initial period of wind up (e.g., after 20 stimuli). In addition, unit responses to repetitive transcutaneous electrical stimulation do not appear to exhibit the same stability as do spinal unit responses to heat. For example, examination of published figures shows variability of responses estimated as great as 20–40% in the 'control' periods immediately preceding administration of morphine (e.g., see Dickenson and LeBars, 1987, Figs. 2 and 3). Finally, electrical stimulation is not selective, bypassing peripheral receptor sensitivities and stimulus transduction, and activating simultaneously all fiber types. Transcutaneous electrical stimulation is likely even less selective inasmuch as afferents contained in several nerves, including afferents from muscles and joints, may be affected to an unknown extent. It has also been noted that some dorsal horn neurons, responsive to natural cutaneous stimuli, were unresponsive to intense electrical stimulation of dorsal roots (Light et al., 1979). The extent to which different populations of spinal units might have contributed to the results of studies reviewed, cannot be determined.

Since radiant heat, by comparison, is a very selective stimulus, the nature of the nociceptive stimulus employed in the studies reviewed is an important consideration relative to the results reported. The mode of application of these two stimuli also clearly differs between those supporting inhibitory as opposed to no or facilitatory effects of morphine. As indicated above, transcutaneous electrical stimulation is repetitive; between 50–150 pulses are given at 0.6 Hz. Radiant heat is applied at much greater, fixed intervals, and produces stable responses to heat over the course of an experiment. Thus, among the factors of dose, time to effect and nociceptive stimulus, the prominent feature of the studies reviewed which distinguishes one group of results from another is the nociceptive stimulus – its nature, its selectivity, and inter- and intra-animal reproducibility, particularly with respect to the stability of unit responses.

Conclusion

As a focus for discussion, we propose that additional, indirect effects of the nociceptive stimulus, contribute to the results reported. For example, repetitive, high-intensity transcutaneous electrical stimulation likely affects both blood pressure and heart rate. It has been well documented that activation of afferent fibers in the vagus nerve is capable of modulating spinal nociceptive reflexes and spinal nociceptive transmission (see Randich and Maixner, 1984, for review and Ren et al., 1988, for a parametric study). The inhibitory effects of vagal afferent stimulation are believed to be due to activation of C fibers in the vagus nerve. Subthreshold vagal afferent stimulation, however, *facilitates* the nociceptive tail flick reflex (Ren et al., 1988) and also the responses of some thoracic (Thies and Foreman, 1981) and lumbar (Ren and Gebhart, unpublished) spinal units. The effects of transcutaneous electrical stimulation on blood pressure and heart rate are not reported in any studies reviewed here. It is conceivable that transcutaneous electrical stimulation indirectly activates lower threshold cardiopulmonary afferents, or a component of the baroreceptor reflex arc, even if changes in blood pressure or heart rate are not great in magnitude and contribute to facilitation of spinal unit responses to activation of C fibers in the hindlimb by transcutaneous electrical stimulation.

Alternatively, high intensity, repetitive transcutaneous electrical stimulation may directly or indirectly influence sympathetic afferents. The simultaneous activation, either directly or indirectly, of sympathetic, and/or parasympathetic (i.e., visceral), and possibly deep (e.g., joint and muscle) afferents, in addition to cutaneous afferents, can lead to modification of spinal unit responses at the segmental level or by descending influences after a rostral, supraspinal loop. For example, Foreman et al. (1987) report differential modulation of thoracic (inhibited) and lumbar (excited) spinothalamic tract neurons during stimulation of cardiopulmonary sympathetic afferents. They suggest that such inhibition may function to increase the contrast between cells that are excited and those not excited by nociceptive input. Indeed, a similar principle underlies the proposed mechanism(s) of diffuse noxious inhibitory controls (e.g., see LeBars et al., 1983).

In addition, it is also possible that the administration of opioids intracerebrally may be additive to indirect effects of transcutaneous electrical stimulation mediated by changes in heart rate or blood pressure. For example, opioids seem to facilitate the baroreceptor reflex by enhancing synaptic transmission in the brain stem (e.g., nucleus tractus solitarius, Laubie et al., 1977; see also Arndt, 1987, and Szilagyi, 1987). Opioid effects in this regard are notably biphasic and related to dose: excitation is associated with low doses, along with tachycardia and hypertension, while inhibition is associated with high doses, along with bradycardia and hypertension (see Arndt, 1978).

Such speculation is, of course, experimentally testable. First, it would seem appropriate to examine the effects of morphine microinjected into the PAG or NRM on the same spinal units' responses to heat and repetitive transcutaneous electrical stimulation. One could also ask what effect morphine has on unit responses to heat or transcutaneous electrical stimulation in sinoaortic deafferented or vagotomized preparations. The primary objective of such experiments would be to address whether it is the nociceptive stimulus that leads to the present controversy in the literature with respect to the effect of morphine given in the brain stem on spinal nociceptive neurons.

In summary, only speculation can be offered as to why divergent effects on spinal nociceptive neurons by morphine given in the brain stem characterize electrophysiologic studies (reviewed here), but not neurochemical, behavioral or pharmacological studies. The nociceptive stimuli employed are distinctly different in many respects,

and generally correlate with results obtained: transcutaneous electrical nerve stimulation with facilitatory or no effect of morphine, and radiant heat with inhibitory effects of morphine. We speculate that the nociceptive stimulus indirectly and/or directly, for example, by an effect on heart rate and/or blood pressure, may alter centrifugal modulatory systems by affecting the interface in the brain stem of cardiovascular and pain regulatory systems and their interactions, an interaction not presently well understood. The net result, whether effected by direct or indirect influences of repetitive, high intensity transcutaneous electrical nerve stimulation, may not differ from what has been proposed with respect to contrast and extraction of signal from noise (e.g., see LeBars et al., 1983), but interpretation of experimental results suggesting a decrease, rather than an increase, of descending inhibition by morphine, may require reevaluation.

Acknowledgements

The excellent secretarial assistance of Teresa Fulton and graphics assistance of Michael Burcham are gratefully acknowledged. Special thanks are extended to Alan Randich for thoughtful and provocative discussions on cardiopulmonary-nociceptive interactions.

The author's data reported here was supported by USPHS awards DA 02879 and NS 19912.

References

Aimone, L.D. and Gebhart, G.F. (1986) Stimulation-produced spinal inhibition from the midbrain in the rat is mediated by an excitatory amino acid neurotransmitter in the medial medulla. *J. Neurosci.,* 6: 1803–1813.

Aimone, L.D., Jones, S.L. and Gebhart, G.F. (1987) Stimulation-produced descending inhibition from the periaqueductal gray and nucleus raphe magnus in the rat: mediation by spinal monoamines but not opioids. *Pain,* 31: 123–136.

Arndt, J.O. (1987) Opiate receptors in the CNS and their possible role in cardiovascular control. In J.P. Buckley and C.M. Ferrario (Eds.), *Brain Peptides and Catecholamines in Cardiovascular Regulation,* Raven Press, New York, pp. 137–151.

242

Barbaro, N.M., Hammond, D.L. and Fields, H.L. (1985) Effects of intrathecally administered methysergide and yohimbine on microstimulation-produced antinociception in the rat. *Brain Res.,* 343: 223 – 229.

Behbehani, M.M. and Fields, H.L. (1979) Evidence that an excitatory connection between periaqueductal gray and the nucleus raphe magnus mediates stimulation-produced analgesia. *Brain Res.,* 170: 85 – 93.

Behbehani, M.M. and Pomeroy, S.L. (1978) Effects of morphine injected in periaqueductal gray on the activity of single units in nucleus raphe magnus of the rat. *Brain Res.,* 149: 266 – 269.

Bennett, G.J. and Mayer, D.J. (1979) Inhibition of spinal cord interneurons by narcotic microinjection and focal electrical stimulation in the periaqueductal gray matter. *Brain Res.,* 172: 243 – 257.

Besson, J.M. and Chaouch, A. (1987) Peripheral and spinal mechanisms of nociception. *Physiol. Rev.,* 67: 67 – 186.

Camarata, P.J. and Yaksh, T.L. (1985) Characterization of the spinal adrenergic receptors mediating the spinal effects produced by the microinjection of morphine into the PAG. *Brain Res.,* 336: 133 – 142.

Cheng, Z-F, Fields, H.L. and Heinricher, M.M. (1986) Morphine microinjected into the periaqueductal gray has differential effects on three classes of medullary neurons. *Brain Res.,* 375: 57 – 65.

Clark, S.L. and Ryall, R.W. (1983) The antinociceptive action of etorphine in the dorsal horn is due to a direct spinal action and not to activation of descending inhibition. *Br. J. Pharmacol.,* 78: 307 – 319.

Clark, S.L., Edeson, R.O. and Ryall, R.W. (1983) The relative significance of spinal and supraspinal actions in the antinociceptive effect of morphine in the dorsal horn: an evaluation of the microinjection technique. *Br. J. Pharmacol.,* 79: 807 – 818.

Dickenson, A.H. and LeBars, D. (1983) Morphine microinjections in periaqueductal gray matter of the rat: Effects on dorsal horn neuronal responses to C-fibre activity and diffuse noxious inhibitory controls. *Life Sci.,* 33: 549 – 552.

Dickenson, A.H. and LeBars, D. (1987) Supraspinal morphine and descending inhibition acting on the dorsal horn of the rat. *J. Physiol. (Lond.),* 384: 81 – 107.

Du, H.J., Kitahata, L.M., Thalhammer, J.G. and Zimmermann, M. (1984) Inhibition of nociceptive neuronal responses in the cat's spinal dorsal horn by electrical stimulation and morphine microinjection in nucleus raphe magnus. *Pain,* 19: 249 – 257.

Duggan, A.W., Griersmith, B.T. and North, R.A. (1980) Morphine and supraspinal inhibition of spinal neurons. Evidence that morphine decreases tonic descending inhibition in the anesthetized cat. *Br. J. Pharmacol.,* 69: 461 – 466.

Fields, H.L. and Anderson, S.D. (1978) Evidence that raphe-spinal neurons mediate opiate and midbrain stimulation-produced analgesia. *Pain,,* 5: 333 – 349.

Foreman, R.D., Hobbs, S.F., Oh, U.T. and Chandler, M.J. (1987) Differential modulation of thoracic and lumbar spinothalamic tract cell activation during stimulation of cardiopulmonary sympathetic afferent fibers in the primate. A new concept for visceral pain? *Pain,* Suppl., 4: S23.

Gebhart, G.F. (1982) Opiate and opioid effects on brainstem neurons: Relevance to nociception and antinociceptive mechanisms. *Pain,* 2: 93 – 140.

Gebhart, G.F. (1986) Modulatory effects of descending systems on spinal dorsal horn neurons. In T.L. Yaksh (Ed.), *Spinal Afferent Processing,* Plenum Press, New York, pp. 391 – 416.

Gebhart, G.F., Sandkühler, J., Thalhammer, J.G. and Zimmermann, M. (1984) Stimulation and morphine in the PAG: inhibition in the spinal cord of nociceptive information by electrical stimulation and morphine microinjection at identical sites in the midbrain of the cat. *J. Neurophysiol.,* 51: 75 – 89.

Hammond, D.L. and Yaksh, T.L. (1985) Efflux of 5-hydroxytryptamine and noradrenaline into spinal cord superfusates during stimulation of the rat medulla. *J. Physiol. (Lond.),* 359: 151 – 162.

Jensen, T.S. and Yaksh, T.L. (1984) Spinal monoamine and opioid systems partially mediate the analgesia produced by glutamate at brainstem sites. *Brain Res.,* 321: 287 – 298.

Jensen, T.S. and Yaksh, T.L. (1986a) I. Comparison of antinociceptive action of morphine in the periaqueductal gray, medial and perimedial medulla in rat. *Brain Res.,* 363: 99 – 113.

Jensen, T.S. and Yaksh, T.L. (1986b) II. Examination of spinal monamine receptors through which brainstem opiate-sensitive systems act in the rat. *Brain Res.,* 363: 114 – 127.

Jones, S.L. and Gebhart, G.F. (1986) Quantitative characterization of ceruleospinal inhibition of nociceptive transmission in the rat. *J. Neurophysiol.,* 56: 1397 – 1410.

Jones, S.L. and Gebhart, G.F. (1987) Chemical vs. electrical inhibition of dorsal horn neurons from the brainstem in the rat. *Soc. Neurosci. Abs.,* 13: 300.

Jurna, I. and Grossmann, W. (1976) The effect of morphine on the activity evoked in ventrolateral tract axions of the cat spinal cord. *Expt. Brain Res.,* 24: 473 – 484.

Laubie, M., Schmitt, H. and Drouillat, M. (1977) Central sites and mechanisms of the hypotensive and bradycardic effects of the narcotic analgesic agent, fentanyl. *Naun.-Schmiedeb. Arch. Pharmacol.,* 296: 255 – 261.

LeBars, D., Dickenson, A.H. and Besson, J.M. (1980a) Microinjection of morphine within nucleus raphe magnus and dorsal horn neurone activities related to nociception in the rat. *Brain Res.,* 189: 467 – 481.

LeBars, D., Guilbaud, G., Chitour, D. and Besson, J.M. (1980b) Does system morphine increase descending inhibitory controls of dorsal horn neurones involved in nociception? *Brain Res.,* 202: 223 – 228.

LeBars, D., Dickenson, A.H. and Besson, J.M. (1983) Opiate

analgesia and descending control systems. In J.J. Bonica, U. Lindblom and A. Iggo (Eds.), *Advances in Pain Research and Therapy, Vol. 5,* Raven Press, New York, pp. 341 – 372.

Light, A.R., Trevino, D.L. and Perl, E.R. (1979) Morphological features of functionally defined neurons in the marginal zone and substantia gelatinosa of the spinal dorsal horn. *J. Comp. Neurol.,* 186: 151 – 172.

Llewelyn, M.B., Azami, J. and Roberts, M.H.T. (1986) Brainstem mechanisms of antinociception: Effects of electrical stimulation and injection of morphine into the nucleus raphe magnus. *Neuropharmacology,* 25: 727 – 735.

Moreau, J.L. and Fields, H.L. (1986) Evidence for GABA involvement in midbrain control of medulla neurons that modulate nociceptive transmission. *Brain Res.,* 397: 37 – 46.

Ness, T.J. and Gebhart, G.F. (1987) Quantitative comparison of inhibition of visceral and cutaneous spinal nociceptive transmission from the midbrain and medulla in the rat. *J. Neurophysiol.,* 58: 850 – 865.

Ossipov, M.H. and Gebhart, G.F. (1984) Light pentobarbital anesthesia diminishes the antinociceptive potency of morphine administered intracranially but not intrathecally in the rat. *Eur. J. Pharmacol.,* 97: 137 – 140.

Randich, A. and Maixner, W. (1984) Interactions between cardiovascular and pain regulatory systems. *Neurosci. Biol. Behav. Rev.,* 8: 343 – 367.

Ren, K., Randich, A. and Gebhart, G.F. (1988) Vagal afferent modulation of a nociceptive reflex in rats: involvement of spinal opioid and monoamine receptors. *Brain Res.,* 446: 285 – 294.

Satoh, M., Oku, R. and Akaike, A. (1983) Analgesia induced by microinjection of L-glutamate into the rostral ventral medial bulbar nuclei of the rat and its inhibition by intrathecal α-adrenergic blocking agents. *Brain Res.,* 261: 361 – 364.

Sinclair, J.G. (1986) The failure of morphine to attenuate spinal cord nociceptive transmission through supraspinal actions in the cat. *Gen. Pharmacol.,* 17: 351 – 354.

Sorkin, L.S., Hughes, M.G., Willis, W.D. and McAdoo, D.J. (1987) Midbrain stimulation induced serotonin (5-HT) release in discrete regions of primate spinal cord recovered with dialysis. *Pain,* Suppl., 4: S29.

Sukuki, Y. and Taguchi, K. (1986) In vitro voltammetric studies of the effect of morphine on the serotonergic system in the cat spinal cord. *Brain Res.,* 398: 413 – 418.

Szilagyi, J. (1987) Opiates and hypertension. In J.P. Buckley and C.M. Ferrario (Eds.), *Brain Peptides and Catecholamines in Cardiovascular Regulation,* Raven Press, New York, pp. 191 – 199.

Thies, R. and Foreman, R.D. (1981) Descending inhibition of spinal neurons in the cardiopulmonary region by electrical stimulation of vagal afferent nerves. *Brain Res.,* 207: 178 – 183.

Vasko, M.R., Pang, I.H. and Vogt, M. (1984) Involvement of 5-hydroxytryptamine-containing neurons in antinociception produced by injection of morphine into nucleus raphe magnus or onto spinal cord. *Brain Res.,* 306: 341 – 348.

Yaksh, T.L. (1979) Direct evidence that spinal serotonin and noradrenaline terminals mediate the spinal antinociceptive effects of morphine in the PAG. *Brain Res.,* 160: 180 – 185.

Yaksh, T.L. and Rudy, T.A. (1978) Narcotic analgesics: CNS site and mechanisms of action as revealed by intracerebral injection techniques. *Pain,* 4: 299 – 359.

Yaksh, T.L. and Tyce, G.M. (1979) Microinjection of morphine into the PAG evokes the release of serotonin from spinal cord. *Brain Res.,* 171: 176 – 181.

H.L. Fields and J.-M. Besson (Eds.)
Progress in Brain Research, Vol. 77
© 1988 Elsevier Science Publishers B.V. (Biomedical Division)

CHAPTER 17

Brain stem neuronal circuitry underlying the antinociceptive action of opiates

H.L. Fields, N.M. Barbaro and M.M. Heinricher

Departments of Neurology, Neurosurgery and Physiology, University of California San Francisco, San Francisco, CA 94143, USA

Introduction

Opiates are the most potent and reliable analgesic agents presently available. They are of great clinical value because their action on pain is relatively selective: consciousness, motor function, and sensory function other than pain are spared at the usual analgesic doses. Over the past two decades our understanding of opiate analgesia has progressed remarkably (Fields, 1985). It is now clear that opiates produce analgesia by an action at highly selective receptors located at specific anatomical sites within the central nervous system. This chapter will review evidence relating to the contribution of particular classes of brain stem neurons to opiate analgesia.

As discussed at length elsewhere in this volume, the midbrain periaqueductal gray (PAG) and the rostral ventromedial medulla (RVM, which includes the nucleus raphe magnus and the laterally adjacent reticular formation) are brain stem components of a network which controls nociceptive transmission at the level of the spinal cord. This network was proposed to underlie the antinociceptive actions of opiates, and this idea was strongly supported by the observation that direct application of minute quantities of opiates in the PAG and in the RVM produces analgesia. However, the reports by Yaksh and his colleagues (1981) that opiates can act directly at the spinal level to block nociceptive transmission raised the possibility that

systemically administered opiates produce analgesia by an action at the spinal level. If this were the case, a supraspinal action might not be necessary.

Although subsequent work has amply confirmed that a direct spinal action of opiates contributes to antinociception, the weight of evidence supports a crucial role for the PAG and RVM. First, opiates injected at the brain stem elicit analgesia at doses that are orders of magnitude lower than those required to elicit an equianalgesic effect by systemic administration (Yaksh, 1979). Second, cutting the spinal dorsolateral funiculus, which contains descending projections from the RVM, reduces the effectiveness of a given dose of systemically administered morphine (Barton et al., 1980). Finally, injection of the opiate antagonist naloxone into the RVM reverses the analgesic effect of systemically administered opiates (Dickenson et al., 1979; Azami et al., 1982). A major step toward understanding the relative brain stem and spinal contributions to opiate analgesia was the finding that concurrent injections of morphine at spinal and supraspinal sites result in a multiplicative interaction, i.e., a much lower total dose is required than if a single large injection were made at either site (Yeung and Rudy, 1980). Thus, it is reasonable to conclude that the RVM and PAG normally contribute to the analgesic effect of systemically administered opiates.

How do opiates act at these sites to produce

analgesia? This question might be easiest to answer at the RVM, because a significant number of RVM neurons project directly to those laminae of the dorsal horn that contain nociceptive transmission neurons. Opiates could act in the RVM to modify nociceptive transmission at the spinal cord by *activating* RVM output neurons that inhibit nociceptive transmission or by *inhibiting* RVM neurons that facilitate nociceptive processing.

The observations that antinociception is produced by electrical stimulation (Fields and Basbaum, 1978; Basbaum and Fields, 1984) and by microinjection of glutamate (Satoh et al., 1983; Jensen and Yaksh, 1984) in RVM, both of which are thought to have purely excitatory effects, indicated that one opiate action relevant to analgesia is activation of RVM output neurons that inhibit nociceptive transmission. In fact, in early work, RVM neurons, including some shown to project to the spinal cord, were predominantly excited by opiates given systemically or microinjected into the PAG (Fields and Anderson, 1978). Furthermore, Satoh et al. (1979) reported that microiontophoretic application of opiates produced excitation of most RVM neurons.

Despite these encouraging findings, problems began to emerge. Although the excitatory effect observed in these studies was reversed by naloxone in some cases, there were many exceptions. Furthermore, most investigators found that a significant percentage of RVM cells were either inhibited or unaffected by opiates (Anderson et al., 1977; Deakin et al., 1977, Behbehani and Pomeroy, 1978; Fields and Anderson, 1978; Toda, 1982; see Gebhart, 1982, and Duggan and North, 1984 for reviews). A significant difficulty arising from the early studies was that there seemed to be no way to predict whether a given RVM cell would be excited by morphine. A different conceptual framework for understanding the physiological properties of RVM neurons was clearly needed.

Classification of brain stem nociceptive modulating neurons

Investigators studying the properties of RVM neurons initially approached them as if they were sensory relay neurons. Using adequate stimuli, receptive fields were found to be large, often (though not invariably) covering the whole body surface and, in the rat and cat, usually requiring stimuli of noxious intensity for activation. In addition to RVM cells with excitatory receptive fields, many RVM cells were inhibited by noxious stimuli over a wide area of the body surface (Fields and Anderson, 1978; Guilbaud et al., 1980; Eisenhart et al., 1983; Auerbach et al., 1985). The lack of spatial boundaries for a 'receptive field' raises an important conceptual issue, because the cell's discharge may be more closely related to a general behavioral function such as escape or arousal than to the signalling of specific sensory information. Because of this, an approach to the study of RVM neurons which recognizes their proposed modulatory role is required. With this in mind, we correlated activity in RVM cells with both a reproducible noxious stimulus (controlled heat to the tail) and with the behavioral response to that stimulus (Fig. 1) (Fields et al., 1983a). The tail flick response (TF) evoked by noxious heat has several advantages as a model for studying nocifensive behavior and opiate function. It is a simple, all-or-none response, its latency can be accurately timed, and its blockade by an opiate is a good predictor of that drug's clinical analgesic potency (D'Amour and Smith, 1941; Grumbach and Chernov, 1965).

A further advantage is that the TF occurs and can be blocked by opiates in rats maintained under light barbiturate anesthesia; thus, acute neurophysiological studies are feasible. In our experiments, rats are maintained in a lightly anesthetized state by a continuous infusion of methohexital, a short-acting barbiturate. The infusion rate is adjusted so that the TF response can be obtained with a stable latency and so that the animal shows no signs of discomfort, such as spontaneous movement, vocalization, or excessive or prolonged withdrawal responses following noxious pinch to the limbs.

A feedback-controlled projector lamp focused on the blackened ventral surface of the tail is used to elicit the TF (Fig. 1). A thermistor probe placed

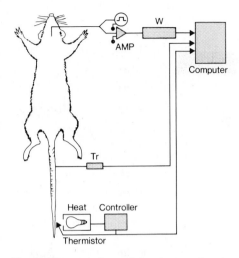

Fig. 1. Diagram of experimental set-up for simultaneous recording of tail flick, tail temperature and unit activity. A metal
microelectrode is stereotactically placed in the appropriate
region. If electrical stimulation blocks the tail flick using currents of 10 μA or less, the electrode is switched to the recording
mode (connection to amplifier (AMP) and window
discriminator (W)). Unit data are stored on computer along
with the tail temperature (measured using a thermistor) and the
time of occurrence of the tail flick (measured by the force
transducer (Tr)).

in contact with the tail provides the feedback signal
for control of the heat stimulus, and a mechano-
electric transducer attached to the tail allows
precise timing of the TF latency. Tail temperature
is maintained at 35°C between TF trials, and the
heat stimulus consists of a temperature ramp with
a 1.8°/s rate of rise. The heat is turned off auto-
matically as soon as the TF occurs, or, in the
absence of a TF, after 10 s have elapsed. In this
preparation, the TF usually occurs when the tail
temperature is between 43 and 45°C, at a latency
of 4 to 5 s.

A gold- and platinum-plated stainless-steel microelectrode is placed stereotactically, and advanced
toward the RVM until a site is located at which the
TF can be inhibited (10 s cut-off) with a current of
no more than 10 μA (400 μs cathodal pulses, 50 Hz
continuous trains applied beginning 3 s prior to the
heat stimulus). At this point, the electrode is connected to an amplifier, and the search for units
with TF-related changes in activity is begun. Cell

activity, tail temperature and TF latency are collected concurrently, and the activity of a given cell
is analyzed with respect to both tail temperature
and the time of occurrence of the TF.

Two classes of neurons with TF-related changes
in activity can be identified in RVM using this approach. 'Off-cells' show an abrupt pause, and 'on-
cells' a sudden acceleration just prior to the TF
(Fig. 2). Cells of a third class, 'neutral cells', show
no discernible change in activity at the time of the
TF (Fields et al., 1983a).

Off-cells

In the lightly anesthetized rat, the off-cell usually
shows a periodic pattern of spontaneous activity.
The active phases range in duration from a few
seconds to several minutes, and alternate with
similar periods of silence. Off-cell activity is usually inhibited by noxious stimuli anywhere on the
body surface.

When the activity of the off-cell is correlated
with a behavioral response such as the TF, there is
a much closer temporal correlation of the off-cell
pause with the time of occurrence of the TF than
with the heat stimulus that induces it (Fig. 2, A).
This casts further doubt on the notion that the
discharge of the off-cell represents a sensory signal
in the traditional sense.

The off-cell as the RVM inhibitory output neuron

The firing properties of the off-cell implicate it
as the RVM inhibitory output cell. Thus, while firing, an inhibitory output cell would be expected to
suppress the activity of a population of spinal
neurons that underlie the TF reflex, and a pause in
the firing of the inhibitory neuron would be required to permit the TF to occur in response to
noxious heat. The off-cell fits this description in
that it shows an abrupt cessation of firing *before*
the occurrence of the reflex. Presumably, electrical
stimulation and glutamate microinjection would
block the TF by causing the off-cell to fire continuously. It is relevant to this idea that if noxious
heat is maintained, the latency to flick following

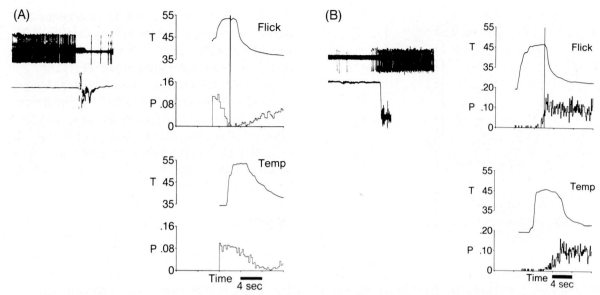

Fig. 2. Characterization of on- and off-cells. (A) Typical off-cell. Left: single oscilloscope sweep showing discharge of the off-cell on the upper trace and the tail flick on the lower trace. The pause in off-cell firing clearly precedes first detectable movement. The duration of the full oscilloscope sweep is 10 s. Right: data averaged from multiple trials ($n = 8$). Upper plot, the data averaged with respect to time of the occurrence of the tail flick (the vertical line in mid-trace). Temperature is shown above (T) and the probability of spike occurrence is plotted below (P). Lower plot, the same unit data are displayed with respect to the time of occurrence of the heat stimulus. The fall-off in unit firing is much more abrupt when the data are aligned with respect to the tail flick than when the temperature stimulus is used as the reference time. (B) Typical on-cell. Upper left shows the sharp increase in unit firing at time of occurrence of the tail flick. All scales are the same as in (A). The impression obtained from examination of single-trace data is confirmed by averaging multiple trials which shows, similar to the off-cell shown in (A), that the abrupt increase in on-cell activity is correlated more closely with the time of occurrence of the tail flick than with the temperature stimulus.

cessation of electrical stimulation in RVM is similar to its usual latency from the beginning of the off-cell pause (approximately 350 ms).

Our observations that a significant number of off-cells project to the spinal cord (Vanegas et al., 1984b) and that they are excited by electrical stimulation of the PAG (Vanegas et al., 1984a), provide crucial support for the hypothesis that off-cells are RVM inhibitory output neurons. The most convincing evidence for this is that off-cells are the only class of RVM neuron that is excited by analgesic doses of morphine given systemically or microinjected into the PAG (Fields et al., 1983b; Barbaro et al., 1986; Cheng et al., 1986). Morphine has the same effect on all off-cells that we have studied: a shift from periodic to continuous firing (i.e. an increase in average discharge frequency) and a block of the TF-related pause (Figs. 3, 4). The increase in off-cell discharge precedes

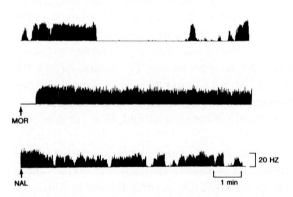

Fig. 3. Off-cells fire continuously following administration of morphine. Ratemeter record shows spontaneous activity of an off-cell before (top trace) and after microinjection of morphine into the PAG (5.0 µg morphine sulfate in 0.3 µl). Periodic cycling is lost, but returns following administration of naloxone (0.25 mg/kg, i.v.). Times of administration are shown for morphine (MOR) and naloxone (NAL).

the increase in TF latency produced by morphine. Thus, the off-cell fills the requirement for an output cell that is activated by opiates and inhibits nociceptive transmission at the spinal level.

In addition to satisfying the circuit logic de-manded by the electrical stimulation and glutamate microinjection results, the description of the off-cell and the demonstration that off-cells are uni-formly activated by morphine also provided an im-mediate resolution of the problem of the unpre-

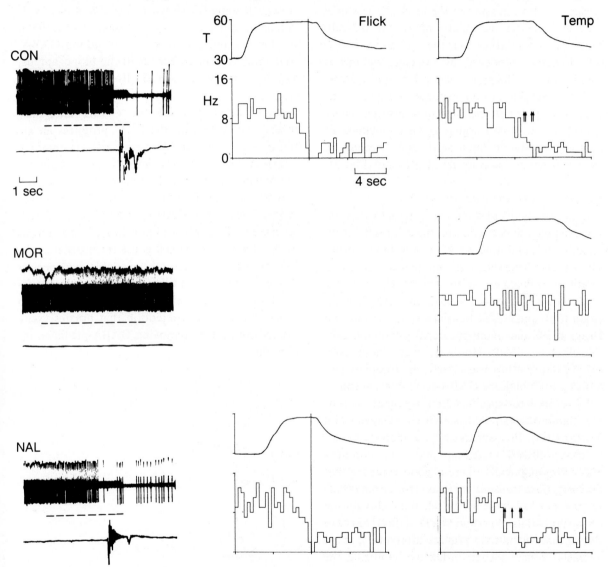

Fig. 4. Effect of morphine on TF-related activity of an off-cell.

CON (Left) Single oscilloscope sweep showing control response of an off-cell (upper trace) with typical pause preceding the TF; lower trace is tail position, heat was applied during period indicated by dashed line, sweep length is 10 s. (Middle) Averaged response of same cell over five TF trials. Cell activity is aligned with occurrence of the TF (vertical line). (Right) Same data aligned according to tail temperature. Arrows indicate occurrence of TF on individual trials.

MOR (Left) Cell firing continues without pause following morphine administration (5 mg/kg, i.v.). (Right) Averaged response during five tail heat trials shows that application of heat to the tail no longer elicits a decrease in cell activity.

NAL (Left) Return of typical off-cell pause after systemic administration of naloxone (1 mg/kg, i.v.). (Middle) Averaged response of the cell over five TF trials. (Right) Same data aligned according to tail temperature.

dictability of opiate effects on putative pain inhibitory neurons, since off-cells are the only RVM neurons excited by morphine.

The mechanism of the effect of systemic opiates is somewhat uncertain because opiates can block nociceptive transmission at the level of the spinal cord and nociceptive inputs inhibit the off-cell. Thus, one could argue that the excitation of off-cell discharge produced by systemic opiates is simply due to blocking nociceptive input. However, the fact that morphine microinjected into the PAG also excites off-cells and prevents their pause (Cheng et al., 1986) argues against blockade of nociceptive afferent input as the sole mechanism by which opiates activate RVM off-cells (Fig. 3).

How do opiates activate off-cells?

In theory there are several ways to activate CNS neurons: by a direct action on the cell itself, or indirectly, by inhibiting an inhibitory interneuron. There is very little evidence that opiates exert direct receptor-mediated excitatory actions. Opiates have been shown to produce a naloxone-reversible excitation of spinal cord Renshaw cells (Davies and Dray, 1978) and of hippocampal pyramidal cells (Nicoll et al., 1980). However, in the latter case, the excitatory effect was clearly due to opiates inhibiting an inhibitory GABA-ergic interneuron.

Direct receptor-specific inhibitory opiate actions are ubiquitous and well-established (Duggan and North, 1984). Post-synaptically, μ agonists hyperpolarize cells by increasing potassium conductance. Presynaptically, there is good evidence that opiates reduce transmitter release from primary afferents, possibly by reducing calcium influx during action potentials. Werz and MacDonald (1983) have shown that, in cultured primary afferents, μ and δ agonists reduce calcium influx by stabilizing the membrane potential through an increase in potassium conductance. $\varkappa$ agonists seem to have a direct blocking action on a voltage-dependent calcium channel (MacDonald and Werz, 1986).

Because of the lack of convincing evidence for a direct excitatory opiate effect on neurons, and the fact that the best-studied example of an excitatory

effect of opiates on CNS neurons was due to disinhibition, we have begun to explore the hypothesis that the opiate-induced excitation of the RVM off-cell is also due to disinhibition (Fig. 5). Because the inhibitory neurotransmitter GABA is present in some RVM neurons (Belin et al., 1983; Mugnaini and Oertel, 1985; Nagai et al., 1985), and because opiates are known to inhibit GABA-ergic inhibitory interneurons in the hippocampus, we chose to focus specifically on the role of GABA.

Direct application of the GABA antagonist bicuculline (BIC) into the RVM produces an antinociceptive action (Drower and Hammond, 1985). At the single unit level, we have obtained preliminary data showing that off-cells are consistently and profoundly inhibited by iontophoretic application of GABA, and that this effect is reversed by BIC. Most importantly, iontophoresis of BIC blocks the off-cell pause (Heinricher et al., 1987b). Thus, all presently available evidence indicates that there is a significant GABA-ergic contribution to the off-cell pause. These data are also consistent with the contention that opiates excite off-cells in part by removing GABA-mediated inhibition.

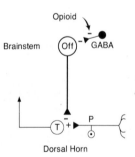

Fig. 5. Diagram of proposed model for the role of the RVM inhibitory output neuron (off-cell) in opiate analgesia. According to this model, the off-cell projects to the spinal cord dorsal horn where it depresses transmission from the primary afferent (P) to the nociceptive transmission cell (C). At the brain stem level, off-cell activation depends on opioid inhibition of a GABA-ergic inhibitory interneuron, thus indirectly increasing off-cell discharge and inhibiting dorsal horn nociceptive transmission.

The on-cell: evidence for brain stem facilitation of nociceptive transmission

On-cells are defined by the acceleration of their firing that precedes the TF. As with the off-cell pause, the on-cell acceleration has a better temporal correlation with the flick than with the antecedent thermal stimulus (Fig. 2, B). Under light barbiturate anesthesia, and in the absence of somatic stimuli or pharmacological manipulation, on-cells show periodic alternation between brisk activity and silence. Noxious stimuli usually do not elicit a further increase in on-cell discharge during active periods, so that excitatory responses are most clearly observed during silent periods (Barbaro et al., 1986). During these silent periods on-cells can be excited by noxious stimuli virtually anywhere on the body surface.

What is the role of the on-cell in the nociceptive modulating function of the RVM? In early studies, electrical stimulation in the RVM was shown to produce inhibition of dorsal horn nociceptive transmission as well as suppression of nocifensive reflexes (Mayer and Price, 1976; Basbaum and Fields, 1984). Because of this, the RVM has usually been considered to exert a purely inhibitory effect on nociceptive transmission. However, if one accepts this view, the firing pattern of the on-cell is paradoxical. The fact that its discharge rate accelerates just prior to the occurrence of the TF is inconsistent with the on-cell having an inhibitory action on nociceptive transmission. If the on-cell were inhibitory, such an increase in activity would block the TF. If anything, its firing pattern suggests that the on-cell has a facilitating effect on nociception. The idea that the RVM may contain neural elements that facilitate nociceptive transmission, is supported by the recent intracellular studies of dorsal horn neurons by Light and his colleagues (1986) who demonstrated that, although electrical stimulation of RVM has a purely inhibitory effect on nociceptive-specific cells, it has a mixed excitatory-inhibitory effect on multireceptive dorsal horn cells.

Noradrenergic actions on the on-cell

Is there any evidence, other than the TF-related increase in firing rate, to support the idea that the on-cell facilitates nociceptive transmission? Some progress has recently been made on this issue using pharmacologic methods. Because there is a significant noradrenergic projection to RVM, Hammond et al. (1980) reasoned that direct application of adrenergic antagonists in RVM should have an effect on nociceptive transmission. They showed that microinjection of the alpha-adrenergic antagonist phentolamine produced an increase in TF latency. In subsequent work, Sagen and Proudfit (1985) demonstrated that microinjection of an α_2 receptor agonist resulted in an increase in TF latency (hypoalgesia), whereas an α_1 receptor agonist had the opposite effect (hyperalgesia).

In order to understand how these behavioral effects come about, we applied norepinephrine (NE) and the selective α_2 agonist clonidine to identified RVM neurons using microiontophoretic techniques (Heinricher et al., 1987c). Norepinephrine consistently and selectively excited on-cells, an effect attenuated by iontophoresis of the α_1 antagonist, prazosin. Clonidine selectively inhibited on-cells, an effect blocked by the α_2 antagonist yohimbine. Neither norepinephrine nor clonidine had any effects on off-cells. Although iontophoretic application is not strictly comparable to microinjection of behaviorally significant doses of the same drugs, the results are consistent with the idea that on-cells facilitate nociceptive transmission. An action at the α_1 receptor is associated with hyperalgesia and with on-cell excitation. Conversely, an action at the α_2 receptor is associated with hypoalgesia and with suppression of on-cell activity.

Morphine actions on the on-cell

Another pharmacological line of evidence supporting a facilitating role for the on-cell derives from the effects of morphine. When morphine is given systemically or microinjected into the PAG, the on-cell becomes completely silent, and no longer shows any active periods (Fig. 6). The on-cell acceleration that precedes the TF is also reduced and then blocked as the TF latency increases (Fig. 7) (Barbaro et al., 1986; Cheng et al., 1986). These results are consistent with a facilitatory influence of the on-cell on the TF.

If on-cells do facilitate nociception, one could argue that morphine blockade of the TF is due to both acceleration of the inhibitory off-cell and to suppression of the facilitatory on-cell. However, because the TF persists in spinalized rats, removal of RVM on-cell facilitation would not be sufficient to explain morphine's inhibition of the reflex.

When morphine-induced analgesia is acutely reversed by naloxone in lightly anesthetized rats, the TF latency falls below baseline levels, i.e. there is hyperalgesia. This shortening of TF latency is accompanied by off-cell silence and very high discharge rates in the on-cell. The fact that TF latency falls below its baseline level during a period of very high on-cell discharge provides further support for the hypothesis that the on-cell facilitates nociceptive transmission (Bederson et al., 1987).

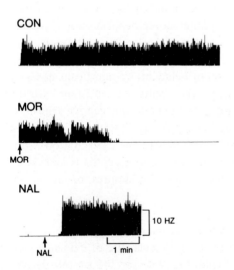

Fig. 6. Morphine inhibition of RVM on-cell. Ratemeter record shows spontaneous activity of an on-cell before and after microinjection of morphine into the PAG (5.0 μg morphine sulfate in 0.3 μl). There is a gradual cessation of activity. The spontaneous activity returns following naloxone administration (0.25 mg/kg, i.v.).

The likelihood of bidirectional control by two populations of RVM neurons demands a careful assessment of studies which investigate the effect of RVM manipulations (e.g. electrical stimulation, lesion, or drug injection) on dorsal horn function. This issue is also discussed by Gebhart in this volume. For example, when the RVM is stimulated electrically or by glutamate, both on- and off-cells should be excited, yet the inhibitory effects predominate. Although it may simply be that the inhibitory effect of the off-cell is more powerful than the putative facilitatory effect of the on-cell, this observation casts some doubt on a direct facilitatory influence of RVM neurons on nociceptive transmission. Thus, it could be that on-cells have nothing to do with nociceptive control, although the correlation of their discharge with a nocifensive reflex makes this unlikely. Another possibility is that on-cells function primarily as intrinsic interneurons that inhibit off-cells (thus indirectly facilitating nociceptive transmission, vide infra). In fact, if there are interneurons in RVM that inhibit off-cells, they would be expected to display the firing pattern of on-cells. However, although some on-cells may be inhibitory interneurons, a significant number of on-cells has been shown to project to the spinal cord (Vanegas et al., 1984b), and thus the possibility that they contribute directly to nociceptive control at the level of the spinal cord must be given serious consideration.

In summary, the weight of evidence supports the concept that RVM neurons exert bidirectional control over nociceptive transmission at the spinal level (Fig. 8). Off-cells inhibit and on-cells facilitate nociceptive transmission. Morphine's analgesic effect derives in part from activation of off-cells, and there is some evidence that this excitation is produced indirectly, by inhibition of GABA-containing inhibitory neurons. It is also likely that suppression of on-cell activity makes some contribution to opiate analgesia.

Functional relationships between on- and off-cells, and implications for the intrinsic circuitry of RVM

We would like to consider the question of whether

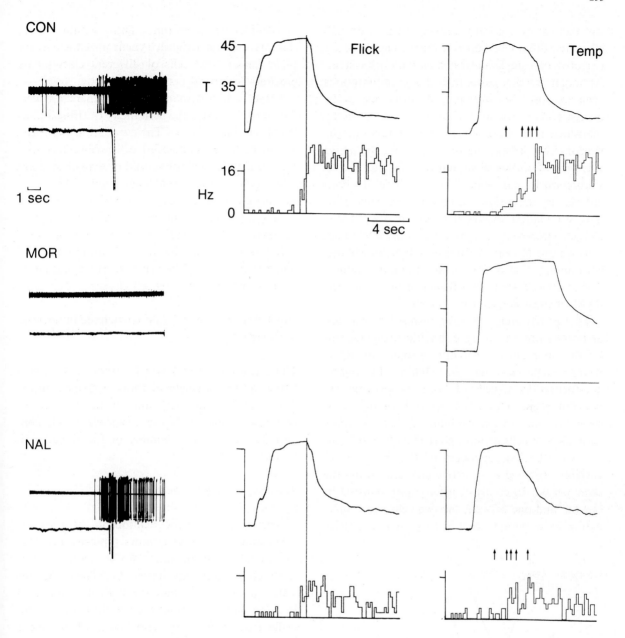

Fig. 7. Effect of morphine on TF-related activity of an on-cell.

CON (Left) Single oscilloscope sweep showing control response of an on-cell with typical burst beginning just prior to the TF; lower trace is tail position, heat onset was at beginning of trace, sweep length is 10 s. (Middle) Averaged response of same cell over five TF trials. Cell activity is aligned with occurrence of the TF (vertical line). (Right) Same data aligned according to tail temperature. Arrows indicate occurrence of TF on individual trials.

MOR (Left) Both the TF response and TF-related burst of the on-cell are completely suppressed following administration of morphine (1.25 mg/kg, i.v.). (Right) Averaged response during five tail heat trials shows that application of heat of the tail no longer elicits an increase in cell activity.

NAL (Left) Return of typical on-cell response after administration of naloxone (1 mg/kg, i.v.). (Middle) Averaged response of the cell over five TF trials. (Right) Same data aligned according to tail temperature.

the facilitating (on-cell) and inhibiting (off-cell) elements within RVM operate independently or are two arms of a single integrated modulatory system. Although we recognize that it is presumptuous even to pose this question, it turns out to be heuristic. For example, if off-cell activation by morphine is a consequence of disinhibition, the neurons that inhibit the off-cell should be active when the off-cell is silent and have activity that is suppressed by morphine. The on-cell fulfills both criteria. By definition, all on-cells fire when noxious stimulation evokes a pause in off-cell discharge. Moreover, on-cells are the only RVM neurons whose activity is suppressed by morphine. This implies that if there is an inhibitory connection to off-cells that arises from neurons within the RVM, it must derive from on-cells.

To further study the relationship between on- and off-cell firing, we have simultaneously recorded the spontaneous activity of pairs of RVM neurons (Barbaro et al., 1985). In lightly anesthetized rats, cells of both classes alternate between silent and active periods lasting from several seconds to a few minutes. When recording from pairs of cells within a given class (two on-cells or two off-cells), members of the pair are invariably observed to be active or silent during the same period. In contrast, when a pair consists of one on- and one off-cell, the two cells show alternating active periods, that is, they are never active

or silent at the same time. Thus, within a given class, all cells have tightly synchronized active and silent phases, and cells of different classes have precisely reciprocal periods of activity.

These results demonstrate that there are very tight correlations in the periodicity of firing among RVM on- and off-cells. The correlation is positive within a cell class and negative between cell classes. The positive correlations could be explained if like cells receive a common afferent input. They could also arise from excitatory connections among cells of a given class. Similarly, negative correlations between on- and off-cell active periods could derive from extrinsic inputs, or from inhibition of cells of one class by the other, or from mutual inhibition between the two cell classes.

Other brainstem nuclei that participate in nociceptive control

The major input to RVM is from the ventrolateral PAG and the adjacent midbrain reticular formation, including nucleus cuneiformis. In fact the two brain stem areas are reciprocally interconnected, and display a number of functional similarities.

The PAG to RVM connection

In early studies of the relationship between the PAG and RVM, investigators typically recorded extracellularly from single RVM neurons while stimulating electrically in the PAG. The RVM cells were characterized mainly by their anatomical location and by whether they could be antidromically activated from the spinal cord. These studies demonstrated that the predominant effect of electrical stimulation of the PAG is excitation of RVM cells. No differences were observed between raphespinal neurons and those raphe magnus neurons which could not be antidromically activated from the spinal cord (Fields and Anderson, 1978). Recent studies, using intracellular recording and single pulse stimulation of the PAG, are consistent with a predominantly excitatory effect upon RVM

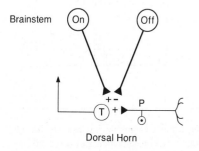

Fig. 8. Diagram of bi-directional control of nociceptive transmission. Both the on-cell and the off-cell contribute to nociceptive modulation at the level of the dorsal horn. The off-cell has a suppressive effect, while the on-cell facilitates transmission from the primary afferent (P) to the nociceptive transmission cell (T).

neurons (Mason et al., 1986). Glutamate microinjection into PAG also excites RVM neurons, implicating cells, as opposed to fibers of passage (Behbehani and Fields, 1979).

We re-investigated the issue of PAG control of RVM neurons using the methods of RVM cell recording and identification described above (Vanegas et al., 1984a). In these experiments, continuous trains of square wave pulses (50 Hz, 400 μs) were delivered to PAG. Stimulation intensity was increased in a stepwise fashion. We observed that such stimulation produces powerful, continuous driving of both on- and off-cells. The threshold for excitation of RVM cells by continuous electrical stimulation of PAG was indistinguishable from that for inhibiting the TF reflex. This finding directly supports the hypothesis that the antinociceptive effect of electrical stimulation in the PAG is mediated, at least in part, by activation of RVM neurons.

Microinjection of morphine and GABA antagonists in the PAG

Morphine microinjected into the PAG in doses sufficient to block the TF (5 – 10 μg in 0.3 μl over 60 – 90 s), has a consistent and differential effect on the activity of the two classes of TF-related neurons in RVM: off-cells become continuously active and on-cells become silent. These effects are indistinguishable from those of systemically administered morphine. Furthermore, the changes in cell activity precede the increase in TF latency (Cheng et al., 1986).

Like morphine microinjection, direct application of GABA antagonists in the PAG activates RVM off-cells, inhibits on-cells, and blocks the TF. Thus, opiates may exert their effect in the PAG by inhibiting cells which release GABA. This suggestion is supported by the observation that microinjection of the GABA agonist muscimol into the PAG can reverse the TF blockade produced by injection of morphine at the same site (Moreau and Fields, 1986).

Thus, the RVM and PAG region are reciprocally

interconnected, and the two regions display significant functional similarities. Electrical stimulation and morphine microinjection in either region results in antinociception, and we have recently identified both on- and off-cells in the PAG and adjacent reticular formation (Heinricher et al. 1987a; Haws et al., 1987). It would be important to determine whether PAG on- and off-cells respond to opiates as do on- and off-cells in RVM, and whether the on- and off-cells in the midbrain project to on- and off-cells in the RVM, and vice-versa. At present, the known similarities between the two regions, and the observations that direct application of morphine and GABA antagonists in the PAG consistently and differentially affect the activity of RVM on- and off-cells while producing TF inhibition, make it reasonable to consider that the populations of on- and off-cells in the midbrain and RVM constitute a functional entity, with the RVM serving as the output to the spinal cord.

Conclusions

Thus, the presently available evidence indicates that on- and off-cells in RVM are involved in the antinociceptive action of opiates. Off-cells, the putative RVM inhibitory output neurons, are uniformly excited by administration of morphine. The activity of on-cells is consistently suppressed by morphine, and it is difficult to explain the role of this cell class except in terms of a facilitatory influence. Correlative evidence indicates that increases in on-cell activity are associated with enhanced nociceptive responsiveness, whereas decreases are associated with depressed nociceptive responsiveness.

On-cells could facilitate nociceptive transmission indirectly, by inhibiting off-cells. There is some evidence that this is the case. Opiate-induced excitation of off-cells may derive from inhibition of a GABA-containing interneuron. Since any inhibitory connection to off-cells from within the RVM probably derives from on-cells, at least some of the proposed GABA-containing interneurons in RVM should be on-cells. If so, iontophoretically applied opiates should inhibit at least a subpopulation of on-cells. It is, however, unlikely that the role of the on-cell is restricted to that of an inhibitory interneuron, because a significant number of on-cells project to the spinal cord, an observation consistent with a direct influence at spinal levels.

Thus, the weight of evidence indicates that off-cells exert an inhibitory influence and on-cells exert both a direct and indirect facilitatory influence on dorsal horn nociceptive transmission. If so, opiates could inhibit dorsal horn nociceptive transmission in two complementary ways: by releasing the off-cell from inhibition and by suppressing the facilitatory influence of the on-cell.

Acknowledgements

Research support from N.I.D.A. (DA 01949), N.I.N.C.D.S. (NS 21445, NS 07265) and the National Headache Foundation. Technical support — Pat Littlefield; editorial assistance — Susan Elliott, Wendy Ng. Helpful comments — Christine Haws and Peggy Mason.

References

Anderson, S.D., Basbaum, A.I. and Fields, H.L. (1977) Response of medullary raphe neurons to peripheral stimulation and to systemic opiates. *Brain Res.,* 123: 363 – 368.

Auerbach, S., Fornal, C. and Jacobs, B.L. (1985) Response of serotonin-containing neurons in nucleus raphe magnus to morphine, noxious stimuli, and periaqueductal gray stimulation in freely moving cats. *Exp. Neurol.,* 88: 609 – 628.

Azami, J., Llewelyn, M.B. and Roberts, M.H.T. (1982) The contribution of nucleus reticularis paragigantocellularis and nucleus raphe magnus to the analgesia produced by systematically administered morphine, investigated with the microinjection technique. *Pain,* 12: 229 – 246.

Barbaro, N.M., Fields, H.L. and Heinricher, M.M. (1985) Reciprocal activity in on- and off-cells in the rostral ventromedial medulla of the rat. *Soc. Neurosci. Abstr.,* 11: 1180.

Barbaro, N.M., Heinricher, M.M. and Fields, H.L. (1986) Putative pain modulating neurons in the rostral ventral medulla: reflex related activity predicts effects of morphine. *Brain Res.,* 366: 203 – 210.

Barton, C., Basbaum, A.I. and Fields, H.L. (1980) Dissociation of supraspinal and spinal actions of morphine: a quantitative evaluation. *Brain Res.,* 188: 487 – 498.

Basbaum, A.I. and Fields, H.L. (1984) Endogenous pain control systems: brainstem spinal pathways and endorphin circuitry. *Annu. Rev. Neurosci.,* 7: 309 – 338.

Bederson, J.B., Fields, H.L. and Barbaro, N.M. (1987) Naloxone-precipitated hyperalgesia following single morphine dose is correlated with increased on-cell activity in rostroventral medulla. *Pain,* Suppl. 4, S113.

Behbehani, M.M. and Fields, H.L. (1979) Evidence that an excitatory connection between the periaqueductal gray and nucleus raphe magnus mediates stimulation produced analgesia. *Brain Res.,* 170: 85 – 93.

Behbehani, M.M. and Pomeroy, S.L. (1978) Effect of morphine injected in periaqueductal gray on the activity of single units in nucleus raphe magnus of the rat. *Brain Res.,* 149: 266 – 269.

Belin, M.F., Nanopoulos, D., Didier, M., Aguera, M., Steinbusch, H., Verhofstad, A., Maitre, M. and Pujol, J.F. (1983) Immunohistochemical evidence for the presence of γ-aminobutyric acid and serotonin in one nerve cell. A study of the raphe nuclei of the rat using antibodies to glutamate decarboxylase and serotonin. *Brain Res.,* 275: 329 – 339.

Cheng, Z.F., Fields, H.L. and Heinricher, M.M. (1986) Morphine microinjected into the periaqueductal gray has differential effects on 3 classes of medullary neurons. *Brain Res.,* 375: 57 – 65.

D'Amour, F.E. and Smith, D.L. (1941) A method for determining loss of pain sensation. *J. Pharmacol. Exp. Ther.,* 72: 74 – 79.

Davies, J. and Dray, A. (1978) Pharmacological and electrophysiological studies of morphine and enkephalin on rat supraspinal neurones and cat spinal neurones. *Br. J. Pharmacol.,* 63: 87 – 96.

Deakin, J.F.W., Dickenson, A.H. and Dostrovsky, J.O. (1977) Morphine effects on rat raphe magnus neurones. *J. Physiol.,* 267: 43 – 44P.

Dickenson, A.H., Oliveras, J.-L. and Besson, J.-M. (1979) Role of the nucleus raphe magnus in opiate analgesia as studied by the microinjection technique in the rat. *Brain Res.,* 170: 95 – 111.

Drower, E. and Hammond, D. (1985) Effects on nociceptive threshold of THIP and bicuculline microinjected in the nucleus raphe magnus. *Soc. Neurosci. Abstr.,* 11: 1179.

Duggan, A.W. and North, R.A. (1984) Electrophysiology of opioids. *Pharmacol. Rev.,* 35: 219 – 281.

Eisenhart, S.F., Morrow, T.J. and Casey, K.L. (1983) Sensory and motor properties of bulboreticular and raphe neurons in awake and anesthetized cats. In J.J. Bonica et al. (Eds.), *Advances in Pain Research and Therapy, Vol. 5,* Raven Press, New York, pp. 161 – 168.

Fields, H.L. (1985) Neural mechanisms of opiate analgesia. In H.L. Fields et al. (Eds.), *Advances in Pain Research and Therapy, Vol. 9,* Raven Press, New York, pp. 479 – 486.

Fields, H.L. and Anderson, S.D. (1978) Evidence that raphe-spinal neurons mediate opiate and midbrain stimulation-produced analgesias. *Pain,* 5: 333 – 349.

Fields, H.L. and Basbaum, A.I. (1978) Brainstem control of spinal pain-transmission neurons. *Annu. Rev. Physiol.,* 40: 217 – 248.

Fields, H.L., Bry, J., Hentall, I. and Zorman, G. (1983a) The activity of neurons in the rostral medulla of the rat during withdrawal from noxious heat. *J. Neurosci.,* 3: 2545 – 2552.

Fields, H.L., Vanegas, H., Hentall, I. and Zorman, G. (1983b) Evidence that disinhibition of brain stem neurones contributes to morphine analgesia. *Nature,* 306: 684 – 686.

Grumbach, L. and Chernov, H.I. (1965) The analgesic effect of opiate-opiate antagonist combinations in the rat. *J. Pharmacol. Exp. Ther.,* 149: 385 – 396.

Gebhart, G.F. (1982) Opiate and opioid peptide effects on brain stem neurons: relevance to nociception and antinociceptive mechanisms. *Pain,* 12: 93 – 140.

Guilbaud, G., Peschanski, M. and Binder, D. (1980) Responses of neurons of the nucleus raphe magnus to noxious stimuli. *Neurosci. Lett.,* 17: 149 – 154.

Hammond, D.L., Levy, R.A. and Proudfit, H.K. (1980) Hypoalgesia following microinjection of noradrenergic antagonists in the nucleus raphe magnus. *Pain,* 9: 85 – 101.

Haws, C.M., Williamson, A.M. and Fields, H.L. (1987) Putative pain-modulating neurons in the mesencephalic and pontine reticular formation. *Pain,* Suppl. 4, S29.

Heinricher, M.M., Cheng, Z.F. and Fields, H.L. (1987a) Evidence for two classes of nociceptive modulating neurons in the periaqueductal gray. *J. Neurosci.,* 7: 271 – 278.

Heinricher, M.M., Haws, C.M. and Fields, H.L. (1987b) Iontophoresis of the GABA antagonist bicuculline blocks off-cell pause: evidence for GABA-mediated control of putative pain modulating neurons in the rostral ventromedial medulla. *Soc. Neurosci. Abstr.,* 13.

Heinricher, M.M., Haws, C.M. and Fields, H.L. (1987c) Opposing actions of norepinephrine and clonidine on single pain-modulating neurons in rostral ventromedial medulla. *Pain,* Suppl. 4: S28.

Jensen, T.S. and Yaksh, T.L. (1984) Spinal monoamine and opiate systems partly mediate the antinociceptive effects produced by glutamate at brainstem sites. *Brain Res.,* 321: 287 – 297.

Light, A.R., Casale, E.J. and Menetrey, D.M. (1986) The effects of focal stimulation in nucleus raphe magnus and periaqueductal gray on intracellularly recorded neurons in spinal laminae I and II. *J. Neurophysiol.,* 56: 555 – 571.

MacDonald, R.L. and Werz, M.A. (1986) Dynorphin A decreases voltage-dependent calcium conductance of mouse dorsal root ganglion neurones. *J. Physiol.,* 377: 237 – 249.

Mason, P., Strassman, A. and Maciewicz, R. (1986) Intracellular responses of raphe magnus neurons during the jaw-opening reflex evoked by tooth pulp stimulation. *Brain Res.,* 379: 232 – 241.

Mayer, D.J. and Price, D.D. (1976) Central nervous system mechanisms of analgesia. *Pain,* 2: 379 – 404.

Moreau, J.L. and Fields, H.L. (1986) Evidence for GABA involvement in midbrain control of medullary neurons that modulate nociceptive transmission. *Brain Res.,* 397: 37 – 46.

Mugnaini, E. and Oertel, W. (1985) An atlas of the distribution of GABA-ergic neurons and terminals in the rat CNS as revealed by GAD immunohistochemistry. In A. Björklund and T. Hökfelt (Eds.), *Handbook of Chemical Neuroanatomy, Vol. 4, Part 1,* Elsevier, Amsterdam, pp. 436 – 608.

Nicoll, R.A., Alger, B.E. and Jahr, C.E. (1980) Enkephalin blocks inhibitory pathways in the vertebrate CNS. *Nature,* 287: 22 – 25.

Nagai, T., Maeda, T., Imai, H., McGeer, P. and McGeer, E. (1985) Distribution of GABA-T-intensive neurons in the rat hindbrain. *J. Comp. Neurol.,* 231: 260 – 269.

Sagen, J. and Proudfit, H.K. (1985) Evidence for pain modulation by pre- and postsynaptic noradrenergic receptors in the medulla oblongata. *Brain Res.,* 331: 285 – 293.

Satoh, M., Akaike, A. and Takagi, H. (1979) Excitation by morphine and enkephalin of single neurons of nucleus reticularis paragigantocellularis in the rat: a probable mechanism of analgesic action of opioids. *Brain Res.,* 169: 406 – 410.

Satoh, M., Oku, R. and Akaike, A. (1983) Analgesia produced by microinjection of L-glutamate into the rostral ventromedial bulbar nuclei of the rat and its inhibition by intrathecal alpha-adrenergic blocking agents. *Brain Res.,* 261: 361 – 364.

Toda, K. (1982) Responses of raphe magnus neurons to systemic morphine in rats. *Brain Res. Bull.,* 8: 101 – 103.

Vanegas, H., Barbaro, N.M. and Fields, H.L. (1984a) Midbrain stimulation inhibits tail-flick only at currents sufficient to excite rostral medullary neurons. *Brain Res.,* 321: 127 – 133.

Vanegas, H., Barbaro, N.M. and Fields, H.L. (1984b) Tail-flick related activity in medullospinal neurons. *Brain Res.,* 321: 135 – 141.

Werz, M.A. and MacDonald, R.L. (1983) Opioid peptides selective for mu- and delta-opiate receptors reduce calcium-dependent action potential duration by increasing potassium conductance. *Neurosci. Lett.,* 42: 173 – 178.

Yaksh, T.L. (1979) Central nervous system sites mediating opiate analgesia. *Adv. Pain Res. Ther.,* 3: 411 – 426.

Yaksh, T.L. (1981) Spinal opiate analgesia: characteristics and principles of action. *Pain,* 11: 293 – 346.

Yeung, J.C. and Rudy, R.A. (1980) Multiplicative interaction between narcotic agonisms expressed at spinal and supraspinal sites of antinociceptive action as revealed by concurrent injections of morphine. *J. Pharmacol. Exp. Ther.,* 215: 633 – 642.

H.L. Fields and J.-M. Besson (Eds.)
Progress in Brain Research, Vol. 77
© 1988 Elsevier Science Publishers B.V. (Biomedical Division)

CHAPTER 18

Some views on the influence of morphine on brain stem pain modulating neurons and descending controls acting on the spinal cord

Anthony Dickenson

Department of Pharmacology, University College London, London, UK

Introduction

It is clear that morphine can markedly alter the activity of brain stem neurons implicated in the modulation of pain both in terms of the sensory and motor components of nociception. However, it is equally clear that there is, at present, little overall consensus as to the direction of effect of morphine on descending controls (see Gebhart, this volume) emanating from these neurons. I wish here to propose some possible resolutions of these differences of opinion, concentrating on the descending controls emanating from the nucleus raphe magnus (NRM) and adjacent zones.

Serotonin and brain stem neurons

A first possibility for disparate findings is that 5HT systems may differ from non-5HT processes in terms of location, adequate stimuli for activation and final effects on the spinal cord. Many studies, over the years, have been based on counts of 5HT-containing cells in the NRM, and estimates range from early studies indicating only 15% (Wiklund et al., 1980) to a recent study where about 75% NRM-spinal cells were judged to be serotoninergic (Bowker, this volume). In a study in normal and 5HT-depleted rats we gauged that about 60% of neurons were unresponsive to pe-

ripheral noxious stimuli in the depleted animals compared to only 10% in normal animals (Dickenson and Goldsmith, 1986). Furthermore, 75% of neurons tested with metergoline, a 5HT antagonist, had their responses attenuated. In both conditions, cells responding to the peripheral stimuli with either increased or decreased activity were presumed to be serotoninergic.

The coexistence of 5HT with substance P, thyrotropin-releasing hormone (TRH) and enkephalins in descending fibres means that interpretation of the final effect of activation or inhibition of these systems is not easy (Basbaum, Ruda, Bowker, 1988, this volume). If the pharmacology of peripheral peptide neurons relates to the CNS, then prolonged stimulation of these systems containing 5HT and a peptide may lead to a depletion of the peptide before the monoamine (Lundberg and Hökfelt, 1983). Thus, acute and more prolonged pain may have different effects on co-transmission in these descending controls.

Effects of morphine

In nearly all studies on the effects of morphine applied systemically on either the resting activity or noxious evoked activity of NRM cells, dual effects, namely inhibition or facilitation have been seen. Fields et al. (this volume) have demonstrated that cells switched off by noxious stimuli (off-cells) are facilitated whilst on-cells are inhibited by systemic and periaqueductal gray (PAG) morphine.

Indirect studies, but based on the solid partial involvement of 5HT in diffuse noxious inhibitory controls (DNIC) (Le Bars et al., 1982), would indicate that low doses of systemic morphine, with no spinal actions decrease these 5HT descending inhibitions (Le Bars et al., 1981), which would be compatible with the on-cell population. PAG microinjection of morphine produces similar effects when sites include nucleus raphe dorsalis and further emphasises the brain stem site of action (Dickenson and Le Bars, 1987). Other indirect studies have found either decreased or unaltered descending tonic inhibition after morphine (Duggan et al., 1979; Sinclair, 1984). However, other studies have found the opposite, so that PAG morphine and NRM morphine seem to enhance descending inhibitions (Gebhart, this volume).

Neurochemical studies have addressed this problem by gauging the effect of morphine on spinal 5HT levels. However, again the problem of the logical impasse of morphine studied in the absence of pain turns up, and in a recent study, where noxious stimuli have been used, morphine reduces the increased 5HT levels induced by a noxious stimulus, whilst also slightly increasing the resting levels of 5HT (Weil-Fugazza et al., 1984). The former finding is clearly of much greater relevance to the physiological role of these systems in nociception, and indicates that tonic and evoked descending inhibitions may be differentially altered by opiates.

In all these studies with morphine, with the exception of microinjection studies, a potential problem in interpretation resides in the site of action of morphine. Given that the 5HT descending controls can be triggered by a noxious input, if morphine has a direct spinal inhibitory action then the descending control will be reduced at its source. This has been shown for DNIC following intrathecal morphine (Le Bars et al., 1986), and must be borne in mind in studies using systemic opiates.

Are there dual effects in the spinal cord?

If the effects of morphine on descending controls are to increase them in some studies yet to decrease them in others, if both directions of effect have functional relevance, and if both the on-cells and the off-cells participate in modulation of nociceptive processes, then effects at the spinal level in opposing directions should be observed. Although there are reports of increases in activity of some neurons following morphine and decreased responses in other cells (Woolf and Fitzgerald, 1981), these effects are seen with spinal application of opiates (Dickenson and Sullivan, 1986), and so are unlikely to involve only brain stem mechanisms.

However, with regard to the on- and off-cells, activation of DNIC markedly simultaneously inhibits both the activity of dorsal horn convergent neurons (Le Bars et al., 1979) and also the nociceptive flexion reflex produced by C fibre and natural noxious stimulation (Schouenborg and Dickenson, 1985). At the same time, without any increase in activity of other dorsal horn cells, a novel released C fibre reflex is observed. We have proposed that the inhibition of the convergent neurons reduces the flexion reflex but also causes a disinhibition of a nociceptive specific neuron-driven reflex which disappears again when DNIC have worn off (Schouenborg and Dickenson, 1985).

Another possibility could be that different components of descending projections activate different subclasses of the 5HT receptor and, interestingly, the $5HT_{1A}$ type in the rat has been reported to predominate in the dorsal horn whereas the $5HT_{1B}$ type is located in ventral zones (Pazos and Palacios, 1985). Confirmation of the role of the $5HT_1$ types in modulation of nociception has come from behavioural studies following intrathecal application (Schmauss et al., 1983; Zemlan et al., 1983). In human spinal cord, high levels of $5HT_1$ receptors are found dorsally and $5HT_2$ types are densely packed in ventral zones (Pazos et al., 1987a,b).

Finally, it should also be considered that both PAG morphine and electrical stimulation can give rise to mixed effects whereby analgesia, aversive reactions, escape and hyperalgesia can be elicited from different sites (Jacquet and Lajtha, 1974; Yaksh, 1987). Some of the discrepancies in the various studies may result from different sites of opiate microinjection sites, so influencing different zones of the PAG mediating quite different effects (see Dickenson and Le Bars, 1987).

A concensus

The basic premise behind DNIC and opiates is that the activation of descending inhibitory controls in the dorsolateral funiculus (DLF) is required for elaboration of a pain signal by dorsal horn convergent cells, since DNIC will produce a means of distinguishing noxious from innocuous messages (Le Bars et al., 1986; Le Bars, this volume). Low doses of systemic morphine (without any spinal action), PAG microinjections and i.c.v. morphine reduce DNIC, with the latter also being observed in man. A projection of the on-cells to the dorsal horn would be compatible with this, since these on-cells are inhibited by morphine, so the opiate would decrease descending inhibitions. Thus, both the on-cells and DNIC have been proposed to facilitate nociception and both processes are reduced by morphine.

If $5HT_1$ and $5HT_2$ receptors have a differential localization in dorsal and ventral horns, as would seem to be the case, then use of various agonists and antagonists should allow $5HT_1$- and $5HT_2$-mediated effects to be differentiated (Roberts, this volume). This, and other attempts to dissect out the complex anatomy, pharmacology and physiology of the descending controls and opiate influences thereon, would seem useful objectives for future experiments on these systems.

Acknowledgements

The author's work is supported by the Medical Research Council and the Wellcome Trust.

References

Dickenson, A.H. and Goldsmith, G. (1986) Evidence for a role of 5-hydroxytryptamine in the responses of rat raphe neurones to peripheral noxious stimuli. *Neuropharmacology,* 25: 863 – 868.

Dickenson, A.H. and Le Bars, D. (1987) Supraspinal morphine and descending inhibitions acting on the dorsal horn of the rat. *J. Physiol.,* 384: 81 – 107.

Dickenson, A.H. and Sullivan, A.F. (1986) Electrophysiological studies on the effects of intrathecal morphine on nociceptive neurones in the rat dorsal horn. *Pain,* 24: 211 – 222.

Duggan, A.W., Griersmith, B.T. and North, R.A. (1980) Morphine and supraspinal inhibitions of spinal neurones: evidence that morphine decreases tonic descending inhibition in the anaesthetized cat. *Br. J. Pharmacol.,* 69: 461 – 466.

Jacquet, Y.F. and Lajtha, A. (1974) Paradoxical effects following morphine microinjection in the periaqueductal grey matter in the rat. *Science,* 185: 1055 – 1057.

Le Bars, D., Chitour, D., Kraus, E., Clot, A.M., Dickenson, A.H. and Besson, J.M. (1981) The effects of systemic morphine upon diffuse noxious inhibitory controls (DNIC) in the rat: evidence for lighting of certain descending inhibitory controls of dorsal horn convergent neurones. *Brain Res.,* 215: 257 – 274.

Le Bars, D., Dickenson, A.H. and Besson, J.M. (1982) The triggering of bulbo-spinal serotonergic inhibitory controls by noxious peripheral inputs. In B. Sjölund and A. Björklund (Eds.), *Brain Stem Control of Spinal Mechanisms.* Elsevier Biomedical Press, Amsterdam, pp. 381 – 410.

Lundberg, J.M. and Hökfelt, T. (1983) Coexistence of peptides and classical transmitters. *Trends Neurol. Sci.,* 6: 325 – 333.

Pazos, A. and Palacios, J.M. (1985) Quantitative autoradiographic mapping of serotonin receptors in the rat brain. I. Serotonin-I receptors. *Brain Res.,* 346: 205 – 230.

Pazos, A., Probst, A. and Palacios, J.M. (1987) Serotonin receptors in the human brain. III. Autoradiographic mapping of serotonin-1 receptors. *Neuroscience,* 21: 97 – 122.

Pazos, A., Probst, A. and Palacios, J.M. (1987) Serotonin receptors in the human brain. IV. Autoradiographic mapping of serotonin-2 receptors. *Neuroscience,* 21: 123 – 139.

Schmauss, C., Hammond, D.L., Ochi, J.W. and Yaksh, T.L. (1983) Pharmacological antagonism of the antinociceptive effects of serotonin in the rat spinal cord. *Eur. J. Pharmacol.,* 90: 349 – 357.

Schouenborg, J. and Dickenson, A. (1985) The effects of a distant noxious stimulation on A and C fibre evoked flexion reflexes and neuronal activity on the dorsal horn of the rat. *Brain Res.,* 328: 23 – 32.

Sinclair, J.G. (1984) Evidence against a supraspinal-mediated spinal action of morphine in cats. *Pain,* Suppl. 2: 330.

Villaneuva, L. and Le Bars, D. (1986) Indirect effects of intrathecal morphine upon diffuse noxious inhibitory controls (DNIC) in the rat. *Pain,* 26: 233 – 244.

Wiklund, L., Leger, L. and Persson, M. (1980) Monoamine cell distribution in the cat brain stem. A fluorescence histochemical study with quantification of indolaminergic and locus coereleus cell groups. *J. Comp. Neurol.,* 203: 613 – 647.

Woolf, C.J. and Fitzgerald, M. (1981) Lamina specific alteration of C fibre evoked activity by morphine in the dorsal horn of the rat spinal cord. *Neurosci. Lett.,* 25: 37 – 41.

Zemlan, F.P., Kow, L-M, and Pfaff, D.W. (1983) Spinal serotonin (5HT) receptor subtypes and nociception. *J. Pharmacol. Exp. Ther.,* 226: 477 – 485.

H.L. Fields and J.-M. Besson (Eds.)
Progress in Brain Research, Vol. 77
© 1988 Elsevier Science Publishers B.V. (Biomedical Division)

CHAPTER 19

Endogenous opioid peptides in the descending control of nociceptive responses of spinal dorsal horn neurons

Albert Herz and Mark J. Millan

Department of Neuropharmacology, Max-Planck-Institut für Psychiatrie, D-8033 Planegg-Martinsried, FRG

Introduction

The identification of opioid receptors and detection of endogenous ligands of these receptors opened a new era of pain research. The differentiation of several types of opiate receptors and the characterization of a series of opioid peptides illustrates the striking complexity of opioid systems. The implications of this multiplicity for neurobiology in general and for pain control in particular are presently not fully understood. It is the purpose of the present article to analyse the significance of these opioid systems for the descending control of nociceptive responses of spinal dorsal horn neurons.

Multiple opioid peptide families

On the basis of their derivation from three distinct precursor molecules (corresponding to three different genes) three families of endogenous opioid peptides may be distinguished (Fig. 1) (Höllt, 1983; Millan, 1987).

Pro-opiomelanocortin (POMC): precursor for β-lipotropin, β-endorphin (β-EP), adrenocorticotropin (ACTH) and α-melanocyte-stimulating hormone (α-MSH). (The latter two peptides are not opioids.) β-EP bears a met-enkephalin (ME) sequence at its N-terminus: however, physiologically ME is not derived from POMC.

Whether smaller fragments of β-EP such as α- or γ-endorphin are cleaved in vivo in the CNS is not established.

Pro-enkephalin A (PEA): PEA yields four MEs, one leu-enkephalin (LE), one heptapeptide (ME-Arg^6-Phe^7) and one octapeptide (ME-Arg^6-Gly^7-Phe^8). Larger peptides bearing these ME sequences at their N-termini may also be generated; these include peptides E and F (Fig. 1).

Pro-enkephalin B (PEB) or pro-dynorphin: source of three opioids bearing LE at their N-termini: dynorphin (DYN), dynorphin B and α-neo-endorphin. Smaller or larger fragments of these peptides are also formed and stored.

This multiplicity of opioid peptides (see Fig. 1) may appear bewilderingly complex. Nevertheless, it is sufficient to concentrate on β-EP, ME and DYN, since these can be considered as representatives of the three opioid peptide families and the majority of work on pain has been undertaken with these peptides.

Organization of multiple opioid peptide networks

In the brain, β-EP synthesizing nerve cells are (with the exception of a minor cell group in the nucleus tractus solitarius) confined to the arcuate region of the hypothalamus; they project from there to many brain regions, including those implicated in nociceptive processes such as the peri-

264

aqueductal grey (PAG) and adjacent regions and the thalamus (Watson et al., 1984). No somata containing β-EP are detectable in the mature spinal cord, wherein authentic β-EP has not unequivocally been shown to exist. In contrast, ME-containing somata and fibre networks are widely distributed in brain and spinal cord; of particular relevance in the present context is the presence of ME in, for example, the amygdala, thalamus, dorsal raphe, PAG and the nucleus raphe magnus. DYN also is widely distributed and is found for example in the PAG, the limbic system and the thalamus. Thus, although there are differences in the precise distribution of the various opioid peptides, each of these characteristic peptides is represented in regions involved in pain control.

Pre–Pro–Opiomelanocortin (265 residues)

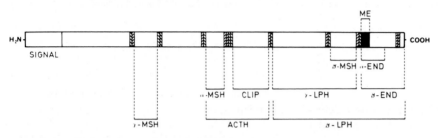

Pre–Pro–Enkephalin A (263 residues)

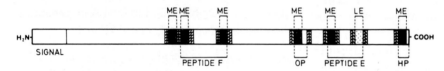

Pre–Pro–Enkephalin B = Pre–Pro–Dynorphin (256 residues)

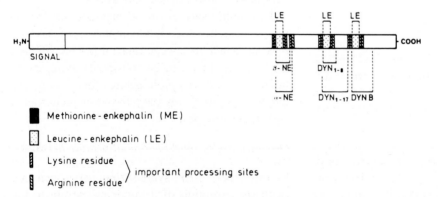

Methionine-enkephalin (ME)

Leucine-enkephalin (LE)

Lysine residue
Arginine residue } important processing sites

Fig. 1. Simplified schematic representation of the structures of bovine pre-pro-opiomelanocortin, bovine pre-pro-enkephalin A and ovine pre-pro-enkephalin B = pre-pro-dynorphin. These are the three precursors from which all as yet known endogenous opioid peptides are derived. Most met-enkephalin and leu-enkephalin sequences are flanked by the basic amino acids, lysine and arginine, major processing sites for trypsin-like enzymes. Abbreviations as follows: ACTH, adrenocorticotropin; CLIP, corticotropin-like intermediate lobe peptide; DYN, dynorphin; END, endorphin; HP, heptapeptide: LPH, lipotropin; MSH, melanocyte-stimulating hormone; NE, neo-endorphin; OP, octapeptide.

Multiple opioid receptors

In the course of the last decade an abundance of evidence for the existence of multiple classes of opioid receptors has accumulated (Zukin and Zukin, 1984; Herz, 1983). The concept of a multiplicity of opioid receptors originally emerged from studies of synthetic opiates in the chronic spinal dog; the differential pharmacological spectra of activity and their inability to substitute for each other in the suppression of abstinence symptoms following discontinuation of long-term treatment, favoured such a multiplicity. The prototype ligands for the thereby specified μ, $\varkappa$ and σ receptors were, respectively, morphine, ketocyclazocine and N-allylnormetazocine (Martin et al., 1976). Subsequently, a receptor with high affinity for the enkephalins and termed δ receptor was identified in the mouse vas deferens. Furthermore, on the basis of the high potency of β-EP in the rat vas deferens, the existence of ϵ receptors has been postulated (Schulz et al., 1981). Extensive studies on the pharmacological properties of various natural and synthetic opioid ligands in vivo, radioligand studies of the binding of these to nervous tissue together with analyses of cross-tolerance between receptor classes in vitro and in vivo, has resulted in the general acceptance of the existence of μ, δ and $\varkappa$ receptors (Magnan et al., 1982; Paterson et al., 1984; Höllt, 1986). The more recently proposed ϵ receptor still requires more comprehensive characterization, while the σ receptor seems not to be an opioid receptor in the strict sense as binding to it is not reversible by naloxone (Zukin and Zukin, 1984).

Both radioligand binding and autoradiographic studies employing highly selective ligands for the various receptor types, together with functional studies, have suggested the presence of μ, δ and $\varkappa$ receptors in the CNS. These mapping studies yielded the picture of a differential distribution of particular types in mammals including humans (Pfeiffer et al., 1982; Tempel and Zukin, 1987). μ Sites are predominant, for example, in patches of the striatum, laminae III and IV of the cortex,

habenula, thalamus and PAG. Particularly high amounts of $\varkappa$ receptors are occurring in the hypothalamus, PAG and claustrum. In comparison to μ and $\varkappa$ receptors, there is a relative paucity of δ receptors in most brain areas, including the PAG. Both μ and δ receptors are present in high concentrations in the superficial layers of the spinal cord dorsal horn.

Clearly, there are significant differences between the opioid receptor types as regards their distribution in structures of significance in the modulation of nociception. There are only low levels of each type in, for example, the nucleus raphe magnus and gigantocellularis pars α of the medulla, areas assumed to be important links in descending brain stem control. However, it must be stressed, that a low level of receptor density does not necessarily indicate a lack of functional significance. A few strategically located receptors may be sufficient to exert a decisive action.

Correspondence between multiple opioid ligands and multiple receptor types

The correspondence between the multiplicity of opioid ligands and opioid receptors is not clear (Höllt, 1986). Thus, DYN (and peptides of equivalent size deriving from PEB) exhibit a pronounced preference for the $\varkappa$ receptor as evaluated by the use of in vitro tissue preparations, binding experiments and cross-tolerance studies. That DYN represents an endogenous ligand for $\varkappa$ receptor is, thus, very probable (Chavkin et al., 1982; Wüster et al., 1981; Schulz et al., 1981a). β-EP, in contrast, shows a weak affinity for $\varkappa$ receptors but binds well not only to ϵ but also to μ and δ receptor types (Magnan et al., 1982). Opioid peptides deriving from PEA display a complicated pattern of preferences; the long-chain products of this precursor exhibit preference for the μ and for the $\varkappa$ receptor, while the processing products with short chain lengths, in particular the enkephalins, exhibit preference for the δ receptor (Höllt, 1986). This might indicate that the enkephalins are physiological ligands of the δ receptors. In the case of the μ receptor this is an open question although long-chain PEA peptides may be considered. There are other aspects which render the question of the physiological ligands of the various receptor types a very difficult one (see Millan, 1986).

Multiple opioid systems and the modulation of nociception at the cerebral level

It is well established that periventricular brain stem areas are important sites for the antinociceptive effects of opioids. Microinjection of low doses of morphine into the PAG or into the isolated mesencephalic aqueduct induces a strong antinociception (Tsou and Jang, 1964; Herz et al., 1970; Teschemacher et al., 1973; Pert and Yaksh, 1974). As spinally mediated nociceptive reflexes are inhibited after the cerebral application of morphine, it is clear that descending opioidergic control is activated from these sites. The raphe system may represent one link in these (apparently multiple) descending pathways (Basbaum and Fields, 1984; Gebhart, 1982).

In view of the identification of multiple endogenous opioid systems the question arises as to the particular roles of the various endogenous ligands and receptors in this descending brain stem control of nociception.

Effects comparable to those obtained by intracerebral injection of morphine are obtained by i.c.v. application of β-EP (Tseng et al., 1976). In more recent experiments a series of opioid peptides deriving from the three opioid peptide precursors were injected i.c.v. in mice (Höllt et al., 1982); besides β-EP, the long-chain peptides derived from PEA also caused a strong inhibition of the tail flick reflex while peptides deriving from PEB, the dynorphins, were relatively ineffective, indicating that μ receptor ligands (possibly also ϵ receptor ligands), but not $\varkappa$ receptor ligands are able to activate descending inhibition. This latter assumption is supported by the finding that spinalization in rats largely reduces the antinociceptive effect of morphine, but not that of the ligand ethylketacyclazocine (EKC) which acts at $\varkappa$ receptors (Wood et al., 1981).

Stimulation-produced antinociception (SPA) — mediation by an opioidergic mechanism

Electrical brain stem stimulation in rats induces antinociception by activating descending inhibitory mechanisms (Liebeskind et al., 1973; see Oliveras, this volume). Depending on the particular experimental conditions, e.g. site of stimulation, opioidergic mechanisms may have a large contribution to this effect (Akil et al., 1976; Lewis and Gebhart, 1977; Cannon et al., 1982; Gebhart et al., 1984). In the experiments in freely moving rats described here, the electrodes were located in the ventral PAG and around the dorsal raphe. The stimulation resulted in a pronounced antinociception against noxious heat and noxious

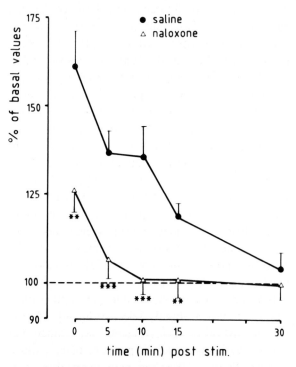

Fig. 2. The opioid antagonist, naloxone, attenuates the antinociception evoked by stimulation of the PAG in freely-moving rats. Stimulation by bipolar, stereotaxically-implanted stainless-steel electrodes in the ventral PAG in the region of the dorsal raphe; 350 μAmp, constant current. Tail flick test, naloxone 2 mg/kg (s.c.). The asterisks in this and the following Figs. refer to the level of significance in the Student's two-tailed t test: * < 0.05, ** < 0.01, *** < 0.001.

pressure. This effect could be powerfully attenuated by pre-treatment with 2 mg/kg naloxone. This indicates that SPA is at least partially mediated by opioids. Naloxone, however, did not affect basal nociceptive thresholds. PAG stimulation also induced some locomotor effects such as ipsilateral rotation; these effects were not antagonized by naloxone. Further, the hyperthermia seen with stimulation was resistant to naloxone. These data show that naloxone selectively antagonizes the antinociceptive effect of electrical stimulation and may not be regarded as a simple stress phenomenon (Millan et al., 1985).

Role of β-endorphin in stimulation-produced antinociception

The slow return of the nociceptive threshold to baseline within 30 min after cessation of the current, together with the naloxone sensitivity of the antinociception, indicates that electrical stimulation releases an opioid. Further experiments were performed to evaluate whether β-EP may be a candidate. Several aspects point to such a possibility: β-EP neurons originating from the arcuate nucleus of the hypothalamus (Finley et al., 1981) provide a heavy innervation of the PAG area; there are some (controversial) indications that β-EP is released into the CSF upon brain stimulation (Akil et al., 1978; Hosobuchi et al., 1979; Fessler et al., 1984; Dionne et al., 1984); finally β-EP injected into the PAG induces strong antinociception (Jacquet, 1978).

Several approaches were used to address the question of a role of β-EP in SPA. Bilateral radiofrequency destruction of the arcuate nucleus from which the β-EP-containing fibres originate, led to a dramatic depletion of levels of β-EP throughout the brain, but did not change plasma levels. These rats revealed a marked reduction in the magnitude of SPA, comparable to the effect of naloxone in intact rats. The other ('unspecific') effects of stimulation (rotation, hyperthermia) were unchanged (Millan et al., 1986).

In further experiments, the effect of acute

stimulation of the PAG upon discrete pools of β-EP (in addition to other opioid peptides) in the PAG and other regions of the brain and spinal cord, the pituitary and the systemic circulation was investigated. SPA was associated with a significant fall in the levels of β-EP in the PAG while the levels of other opioid peptides therein, dynorphin, met-enkephalin, and leu-enkephalin were not significantly affected. Further, the influence on β-EP was restricted to the PAG. There was no difference between control and stimulated rats in other regions of the brain, the pituitary or the

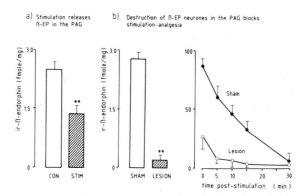

Fig. 3. β-Endorphin mediates stimulation-produced analgesia from the periaqueductal grey. Radiofrequency destruction of the hypothalamic arcuate nucleus depletes β-EP in the brain (e.g. septum) but not in the circulation (plasma) and attenuates SPA from the PAG. S = sham; L = lesion. For further details see Fig. 1. (From Millan et al., 1986.)

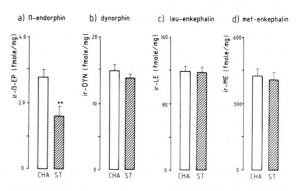

Fig. 4. Stimulation of the PAG selectively depletes levels of ir-β-EP therein. CHA refers to rats placed in the chamber and which are not stimulated, and ST to stimulated rats.

plasma (Millan et al., 1987a). Although it is difficult to definitively interpret the significance of changes in tissue levels of a peptide, the depletion seen immediately after stimulation may reasonably be attributed to the activation of terminals of β-EP neurons in the PAG and the release of β-EP therein. In summary, these data suggest that electrical stimulation of the PAG activates β-EP neurons and that the increase in nociceptive threshold is a direct (or indirect) consequence of this activation.

Which receptor(s) mediate(s) stimulation-produced antinociception?

As mentioned earlier, there are indications for a particular type of receptor for β-EP in the rat vas deferens (ϵ receptors) (Schulz et al., 1981). Concerning the central nervous system, the data for its occurrence are ambiguous (Goodman et al., 1983; Houghton et al., 1984). β-EP possesses a high affinity for μ receptors and also displays a considerable affinity for δ receptors while its affinity for $\varkappa$ receptors is weak (Magnan et al., 1982). Thus, the opioid receptor type involved in β-EP-mediated SPA is an open question – although there is evidence that supraspinal μ opioid receptors play a decisive role in antinociceptive processes at the level of the brain (see Millan, 1986). Thus, a systematic effort was undertaken to elucidate their significance in SPA.

Previous studies indicated that even very low doses of naloxone may attenuate the SPA elicited from the PAG (Cannon et al., 1982). This is of importance in as much as the affinity of naloxone for μ receptors is at least 10-fold higher than its affinity for δ and $\varkappa$ receptors. In recent studies, employing functional and autoradiographic approaches, we have demonstrated that it is possible to selectively block μ receptors by infusion of rats with a low dose of naloxone (0.5 mg $\cdot$ kg^{-1} $\cdot$ h^{-1}) via subcutaneously implanted osmotic minipumps. In the presence of the pumps – which remain in place for a week – the antinociceptive action of the selective μ agonist, morphine, is completely

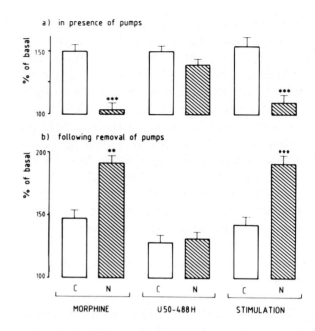

Fig. 5. Infusion of naloxone via minipumps (0.5 mg $\cdot$ kg^{-1} $\cdot$ h^{-1}, 7 days) blocks SPA from the PAG and antinociception evoked by morphine, but not U50,488H. After removing the pumps, SPA and morphine (but not U50,488H) antinociception is potentiated.

eliminated, whereas that of a selective $\varkappa$ agonist, U50,488H, is not modified (Millan et al., 1987b). Following removal of the pumps, the antinociceptive action of morphine is potentiated, whereas that of U50,488H remains unchanged. This facilitation reflects the up-regulation of μ receptors (Tempel et al., 1985). Evidently, this procedure allows for the selective blockade and up-regulation of μ receptors. Rats receiving this low dose of naloxone via minipumps revealed a pronounced reduction in SPA. In analogy, the antinociceptive effect of morphine, but not that of U50,488H, was abolished. Following removal of the pumps, SPA was enhanced, as was the antinociceptive effect of morphine, but not that of U50,488H. Thus, these data provide strong evidence for a mediation of the SPA evoked from the PAG by μ receptors (Millan et al., 1987b).

Tolerance phenomena in stimulation-produced antinociception

A characteristic property of μ agonists, such as morphine, is that, upon repeated administration, tolerance develops to its specific (antinociceptive) actions. One may therefore predict that tolerance to SPA would develop upon repetitive PAG stimulation. In fact, previous authors have found that repetitive stimulation is accompanied by a progressive decline in its antinociceptive efficacy (Mayer and Hayes, 1975; Mayer and Murgin, 1976; Lewis and Gebhart, 1977b). Tolerance in a pharmacological sense, however, is a strictly defined phenomenon; it implies that the dose response curve should be shifted to the right and that the effect should be reinstated upon increasing the dose (current). Fig. 6 shows that this is the case, and that the reinstatement of SPA by higher currents can be blocked by naloxone (Millan et al., 1987c). Thus, essential criteria for the development of tolerance in the strict sense are fulfilled, and conditioning phenomena or tissue damage were shown not to be the cause of the decreasing effects upon repeated stimulation. Also an exhaustion of transmitter seems improbable, since levels of β-EP (and other opioids) are unchanged in the PAG of

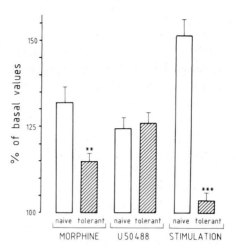

Fig. 7. Rats rendered tolerant to SPA are cross-tolerant to morphine, but not to U50,488H.

chronically stimulated rats and it is reasonable to suggest that this reflects a tolerance at the level of the μ receptor.

Consistent with this supposition and offering further support for the hypothesis of the mediation of SPA by μ receptors are data obtained in experiments in which the rats were stimulated repeatedly, twice daily for 7 days; tolerance had developed at that time and stimulation no longer elicited antinociception. In a subsequent session it became obvious that there was an attenuation of the action of the μ agonist, morphine, but not that of the $\varkappa$ agonist U50,488H. This evidence of a cross-tolerance between SPA- and morphine-antinociception provides further evidence for the involvement of μ receptors in the generation of SPA. This cross-tolerance between SPA- and morphine-antinociception appears to be bilateral, since SPA was found to be reduced in rats rendered tolerant to morphine (Millan et al., 1987c).

Stress-induced antinociception and acupuncture

Acute foot-shock stress and acupuncture are other pain models in which opioidergic brain mechanisms seem to be involved; in addition, there are indications that these procedures also activate

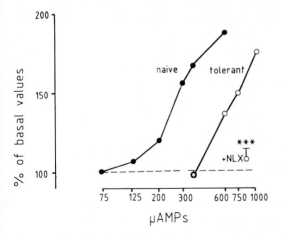

Fig. 6. In rats subjected to recurrent stimulation of the PAG, the current intensity-antinociception curve is shifted to the right; the reinstatement of SPA can be blocked by naloxone (NLX).

cerebral β-EP. Rats, in which by lesioning of the hypothalamic arcuate nucleus β-EP neurons were destroyed, displayed no pronounced, permanent alterations in basal nociceptive threshold (tail flick) but showed an attenuation of the antinociception elicited by acute stress (Millan et al., 1981). Further, microinjections of antibodies against β-EP into the PAG attenuated the antinociception elicited by electroacupuncture in the absence of an action upon basal nociceptive thresholds (Xie et al., 1983). These data suggest that cerebral β-EP plays no major role in the determination of basal nociceptive thresholds but that it participates in the antinociception (in each case, at least partially, naloxone-sensitive) evoked by stress and electroacupuncture. In the case of stress, such data are reinforced by studies indicating a mobilization of central (including PAG) pools of β-EP in response to it (Millan et al., 1981). Techniques such as hypophysectomy (or selective ablation of individual pituitary lobes), adrenalectomy and pharmacological modulation of circulating corticosteroid levels have been attempted for an evaluation of the functional roles of hypophyseal pools of β-EP. In general, such approaches have not convincingly indicated any role of hypophyseal β-EP released into the systemic circulation in the control of nociception. Thus, it is cerebral rather than hypophyseal β-EP which is critical (see Millan, 1986).

Role of δ and $\varkappa$ opioid receptors

As regards δ receptors, though in mice they do seem of importance, for pain modulation at the cerebral level, the problem is still not finally resolved in rats (Galligan et al., 1984; Hynes and Frederickson, 1982; Schulz et al., 1981). Certain data do point to a role at the cerebral level in inducing antinociception, but there are also contradictory data. One special problem here is the limited selectivity of the ligands used, DPDPE and DPLPE: the only selective δ receptor ligands known, have very weak antinociceptive effects upon administration into the brain. Their potency is far less than would be expected from studies on NG108-15 cells or peripheral tissue preparations. It has even been argued that a residual μ activity could account for their antinociceptive effects. Nevertheless, the work of Jensen and Yaksh (1986) suggests that there exist structures in which δ but not μ preferential ligands are active. This supports a role of cerebral δ receptors, but final conclusive evidence is still lacking as regards rats.

The problem of a cerebrally mediated antinociceptive effect of $\varkappa$ opioid receptor ligands was already addressed above when discussing the experiments of Wood (1981) which indicate the lack of an effect of EKC at the cerebral level. Relatively few novel data are available as concerns cerebral antinociceptive actions mediated by $\varkappa$ receptors. Indeed, there is still a need to perform careful experiments with highly selective $\varkappa$ agonists, e.g. U50,488H, against various types of noxious stimuli. One potential problem in establishing an antinociceptive action of $\varkappa$ receptors may be the intensity of noxious stimulus used. It has recently been observed that $\varkappa$ agonists act powerfully against low-intensity but not high-intensity thermal stimuli (Headley et al., 1984; Millan, unpublished). Moreover, as yet no microinjection studies have been reported in which $\varkappa$ agonists have been applied directly into brain regions involved in antinociceptive processes. In recent work, we and others (Hill, unpublished) have reexamined the issue of cerebral $\varkappa$ receptor mediated antinociception and indicated that there may indeed be a component of $\varkappa$ analgesia exerted supraspinally which is probably expressed via descending mechanisms. However, possibly due to its aversive actions (Mucha and Herz, 1985), $\varkappa$ agonists do *not* affect nociceptive measures (such as vocalization) in which there is a strong affective component.

Finally, in considering the roles of opioid systems at the cerebral level, one should be aware that they may not necessarily be expressed independently of those of their spinal counterparts. It is possible that certain networks may be 'in series': i.e. an opioidergic link at the segmental level may mediate the antinociceptive action of an opioid at the suprasegmental level. This possibility has been raised by Tseng et al. (1985) regarding the antinociceptive action of β-EP in the brain: it has been speculated that this is effected via a met-enkephalin neuron in the cord. In this respect, a distinction was drawn to the prototypic μ agonist, morphine. One implication would be that β-EP does not act at μ receptors, an argument supported by the ability of β-EP$_{1-27}$ to block β-EP but not morphine antinociception. These data pointing to a particular (ϵ) receptor for β-EP are of interest. However, the data are not conclusive and pertain to *exo*genously applied β-EP. As discussed, above there is evidence that *endo*genous β-EP may exert antinociceptive effects via μ receptors.

Conclusion

It is apparent that opioid systems play an important role in the engagement of centrifugal networks that inhibit the flow of nociceptive information to the brain. A major problem is to establish the identity, location and mechanisms of action of the opioid peptides and the opioid receptor types involved. In this respect, one should be aware that these are independent, though interrelated questions, owing to our current limited knowledge of the correspondence between the multiplicity of opioid peptides on the one hand and receptor types on the other. The future resolution of such problems should contribute to the development of opioid-based strategies of pain relief specifically targeted on the systems which play a decisive role in the physiological activation of descending inhibition.

Acknowledgement

This work was supported by Deutsche Forschungs-gemeinschaft, Bonn.

References

Akil, H., Mayer, D.J. and Liebeskind, J.C. (1976) Antagonism of stimulation-produced analgesia by naloxone, a narcotic antagonist. *Science*, 191: 961 – 962.

Akil, H., Richardson, D.E., Barchas, J.D. and Li, C.H. (1978) Appearance of β-endorphin-like immunoreactivity in human ventricular fluid upon analgesic electrical stimulation. *Proc. Natl. Acad. Sci. (Wash.)*, 75: 5170 – 5172.

Basbaum, A.I. and Fields, H.L. (1984) Endogenous pain control systems: brainstem spinal pathways and endorphin circuitry. *Annu. Rev. Neurosci.*, 7: 309 – 338.

Cannon, J.T., Prieto, G.J., Lee, A. and Liebeskind, J.C. (1982) Evidence for opioid and non-opioid forms of stimulation-produced analgesia in the rat. *Brain Res.*, 243: 315 – 321.

Chavkin, C., James, I.F. and Goldstein, A. (1982) Dynorphin is a selective endogenous ligand of the $\varkappa$-opiate receptor. *Science*, 215: 413 – 415.

Dionne, R.A., Mueller, G.P., Young, R.F., Greenberg, R.P., Hargreaves, R.M., Gracely, R. and Dubner, R. (1984) Contrast medium causes the apparent increase in β-endorphin levels in human cerebrospinal fluid following brain stimulation. *Pain*, 20: 313 – 321.

Fessler, R.G., Brown, F.D., Rachlin, J.R. and Mullan, S. (1984) Levels of β-endorphin in cerebrospinal fluid after electrical brain stimulation: artifact of contrast infusion? *Science*, 224: 1017 – 1019.

Finley, C.C.W., Lindström, P. and Petrucz, P. (1984) Immunocytochemical localization of β-endorphin containing neurones in the rat brain. *Neuroendocrinology*, 32: 28 – 42.

Galligan, J.L., Mosberg, H.I., Hurst, R., Hruby, V.I. and Burks, T.F. (1984) Cerebral delta opioid receptors mediate analgesia but not intestinal motility effects of intracerebroventricularly administered opioids. *J. Pharmacol. Exp. Ther.*, 229: 641 – 648.

Gebhart, G.F. (1982) Opiate and opioid peptide effects on brain stem neurones: relevance to nociception and antinociceptive mechanisms. *Pain*, 12: 93 – 140.

Gebhart, G.F., Sandkühler, J., Thalhammer, J.C. and Zimmermann, M. (1984) Inhibition in spinal cord of nociceptive information by electrical stimulation and morphine microinjection at identical sites in the midbrain of the rat. *J. Neurophysiol.*, 51: 75 – 89.

Goodman, R.R., Houghten, R.A. and Pasternak, G.W. (1983) Autoradiography of [^{3}H]β-endorphin binding in brain. *Brain Res.*, 288: 334 – 337.

Headley, P.M., Parsons, C.G. and West, D.C. (1984) Comparison of μ-, $\varkappa$- and σ-preferring agonists for effects on spinal nociceptive and other responses in rat. *Neuropeptides*, 5: 249 – 252.

Herz, A. (1983) Multiple opiate receptors and their functional significance. *J. Neural Transmis.*, Suppl. 18: 227 – 233.

Herz, A., Albus, K., Metys, J., Schubert, P. and Teschemacher Hj. (1970) On the central sites for the antinociceptive action of morphine and fentanyl. *Neuropharmacology*, 9: 539 – 551.

Herz, A., Millan, M.J. and Shippenberg (1987) Cerebral opioid systems in pain modulation and motivational processes. *NIDA Research Monography*, in press.

Höllt, V. (1983) Opioid peptide processing and receptor selectivity (1986) *Annu. Rev. Pharmacol. Toxicol.,* 26: 59 – 77.

Höllt, V., Tulunay, F.C., Woo, S.K., Loh, H.H. and Herz, A. (1982) Opioid peptides derived from pro-enkephalin A but not from pro-enkephalin B are substantial analgesics after administration into brain of mice. *Eur. J. Pharmacol.,* 85: 355 – 356.

Höllt, V., Sanchez-Blazquez, P. and Garzón, J. (1985) Multiple opioid ligands and receptors in the control of nociception. *Phil. Trans. R. Soc. London, B,* 308: 299 – 310.

Hosobuchi, Y., Rossier, J., Bloom, F.E. and Guillemin, R. (1979) Stimulation of human periaqueductal grey for pain-relief increases immunoreactive β-endorphin in ventricular fluid. *Science,* 203: 279 – 281.

Houghton, R.A., Johnson, N. and Pasternak, G.W. (1984) [^{3}H]-β-endorphin binding in rat brain. *J. Neurosci.,* 4: 2460 – 2465.

Hynes, M.D. and Frederickson, C.A. (1982) Cross-tolerance studies distinguish morphine- and metkophamid-induced analgesia. *Life Sci.,* 31: 1201 – 1204.

Jacquet, Y. (1978) Opiate effects after adrenocorticotropin or β-endorphin injection in the periaqueductal gray matter of rats. *Science,* 201: 1032 – 1034.

Jensen, T.S. and Yaksh, T.L. (1986) Comparison of the antinociceptive action of μ and δ opioid receptor ligands in the periaqueductal grey matter, medial and paramedial ventral medulla in the rat studied by the microinjection technique. *Brain Res.,* 372: 301 – 312.

Lewis, V.A. and Gebhart, G.F. (1977a) Evaluation of the periaqueductal cerebral grey (PAG) as a morphine-specific locus of actions and examination of morphine-induced and stimulation-produced analgesia at coincident PAG loci. *Brain Res.,* 124: 283 – 303.

Lewis, V.A. and Gebhart, G.F. (1977b) Morphine-induced and stimulation-produced analgesia at coincident periaqueductal central grey loci: evaluation of analgesic congruence, tolerance and cross-tolerance. *Exp. Neurol.,* 57: 934 – 955.

Liebeskind, J.C., Guilbaud, G., Besson, J.M. and Oliveras, J.L. (1973) Analgesia from electrical stimulation of the periaqueductal grey matter in the cat: behavioural observations and inhibitory effects on spinal and interneurones. *Brain Res.,* 50: 441 – 446.

Magnan, J., Paterson, S.J., Tavani, A. and Kosterlitz, M.W. (1982) The binding spectrum of narcotic analgesic drugs with different agonist and antagonist properties. *Naunyn-Schmiedeb. Arch. Pharmacol.,* 319: 197 – 205.

Martin, W.R., Eades, C.G., Thompson, J.A., Huppler, R.E. and Gilbert, P.E. (1976) The effects of morphine- and nalorphine-like drugs in the non-dependent and morphine-dependent chronic spinal dog. *J. Pharmacol. Exp. Ther.,* 198: 66 – 82.

Mayer, D.J. and Hayes, R.L. (1975) Stimulation-produced analgesia: development of tolerance and cross-tolerance to morphine. *Science,* 188: 941 – 943.

Mayer, D. and Murgin, R. (1976) Stimulation-produced analgesia (SPA) and morphine analgesia (MA): cross-tolerance from application at the same brain site. *Fed. Proc.,* 35: 385.

Millan, M.H., Millan, M.J. and Herz, A. (1985) Midbrain stimulation induced antinociception in the rat: characterization of the role of β-endorphin. In Fields et al. (Eds.), *Advances in Pain Research and Therapy, Vol. 9,* Raven Press, New York, pp. 483 – 498.

Millan, M.H., Millan, M.J. and Herz, A. (1986) Depletion of central β-endorphin blocks midbrain stimulation produced analgesia in the rat. *Neuroscience,* 18: 641 – 649.

Millan, M.J. (1986) Multiple opioid systems and pain. *Pain,* 27: 303 – 347.

Millan, M.J., Przewłocki, R., Jerlicz, M.H., Gramsch, C., Höllt, V. and Herz, A. (1981) Stress-induced release of brain and pituitary β-endorphin: major role of endorphins in generation of hyperthermia not analgesia. *Brain Res.,* 208: 325 – 328.

Millan, M.J., Członkowski, A., Millan, M.H. and Herz, A. (1987a) Activation of periaqueductal grey pools of β-endorphin by analgetic electrical stimulation in freely-moving rats. *Brain Res.,* 407: 199 – 203.

Millan, M.J., Członkowski, A. and Herz, A. (1987b) Evidence that μ-opioid receptors mediate midbrain stimulation produced analgesia in the rat. *Neuroscience,* 22: 885 – 896.

Millan, M.J., Członkowski, A. and Herz, A. (1987c) An analysis of the 'tolerance' which develops to analgetic electrical stimulation of the midbrain periaqueductal grey in freely-moving rat. *Brain Res.,* 435: 97 – 111.

Mucha, R. and Herz, A. (1985) Motivational properties of kappa and mu opioid receptor agonists studied with place and taste preference conditioning. *Psychopharmacology,* 86: 274.

Paterson, S.J., Robson, L.E. and Kosterlitz, H.W. (1984) Opioid receptors. In S. Udenfriend and J. Meierhofer (Eds.), *The Peptides, Vol. 6,* Academic Press, New York, pp. 147 – 189.

Pert, A. and Yaksh, T. (1974) Sites of morphine-induced analgesia in the primate brain: relation to pain pathways. *Brain Res.,* 80: 135 – 140.

Pfeiffer, A., Pasi, A., Mehraein, P. and Herz, A. (1982) Opiate receptor binding sites in human brain. *Brain Res.,* 248: 87 – 96.

Schulz, R., Wüster, M. and Herz, A. (1981a) Pharmacological characterization of the ε-opiate receptor. *J. Pharmacol. Exp. Ther.,* 216: 604 – 616.

Schulz, R., Wüster, M. and Herz, A. (1981b) Differentiation of opiate receptors in the brain by the selective development of tolerance. *Pharmacol. Biochem. Behav.,* 14: 75 – 79.

Tempel, A., Gardner, E.L. and Zukin, R.S. (1985) Neurochemical and functional correlates of naltrexone-induced opiate receptor up-regulation. *J. Pharmacol. Exp. Ther.,* 232: 439 – 444.

Tempel, A. and Zukin, R.S. (1987) Neuroanatomical patterns of μ, δ, and κ opioid receptors of rat brain as determined by quantitative in vitro autoradiography. *Proc. Natl. Acad. Sci. USA,* 84: 4308 – 4312.

Teschemacher, Hj., Schubert, P. and Herz, A. (1973) Autoradiographic studies concerning the supraspinal sites of the antinociceptive action of morphine when inhibiting the hind leg reflexor reflex in rabbits. *Neuropharmacology,* 12: 123 – 131.

Tseng, L.-F., Loh, H.H. and Li, C.H. (1976) β-Endorphin: cross-tolerance to and cross-physical dependence of morphine. *Proc. Natl. Acad. Sci. USA,* 73: 4187 – 4189.

Tseng, L.-F., Higgins, M.J., Hong, J.-S., Hudson, P.M. and Fujimoto, J.M. (1985) Release of immunoreactive metenkephalin from the spinal cord by intraventricular β-endorphin but not morphine in anesthetized rats. *Brain Res.,* 343: 60 – 69.

Tsou, K. and Jang, C.S. (1964) Studies on the sites of analgetic action of morphine by intracerebral micro-injection. *Sci. Sinica,* 8: 1099 – 1109.

Watson, S.J., Akil, H., Khachaturian, H., Young, E. and Lewis, M.E. (1984) Opioid systems: anatomy, physiological and clinical prespectives. In J. Hughes, H.O.J. Collier, M.J. Rance and M.B. Tyers (Eds.), *Opioids: Past, Present and Future,* Taylor and Francis, London, pp. 145 – 178.

Wood, P.L., Rackham, A. and Richard, J. (1981) Spinal analgesia: comparison of the mu agonist morphine and the kappa agonist ethylketacyclazocine. *Life Sci.,* 28: 2119 – 2225.

Wüster, M., Rubini, P. and Schulz, R. (1981) The preference of putative proenkephalins for different types of opiate receptors. *Life Sci.* 29: 1219 – 1227.

Xie, G.X., Han, J.S. and Höllt, V. (1983) Electroacupuncture analgesia blocked by microinjection of anti-beta-endorphin antiserum into periaqueductal grey of the rabbit. *Int. J. Neurosci.,* 18: 287 – 292.

Zukin, R.S. and Zukin, S.R. (1984) The case of multiple opiate receptors. *Trends Neurosci.,* 7: 160 – 162.

H.L. Fields and J.-M. Besson (Eds.)
Progress in Brain Research, Vol. 77
© 1988 Elsevier Science Publishers B.V. (Biomedical Division)

CHAPTER 20

Electrophysiological evidence for the activation of descending inhibitory controls by nociceptive afferent pathways

Daniel Le Bars and Luis Villanueva

Unité de Recherches de Neurophysiologie Pharmacologique de l'INSERM (U. 161), 75014 Paris, France

Introduction

During the last decade, our knowledge of processes involved in the transmission and integration of nociceptive signals within the central nervous system has made great strides forward. Most studies in this field have been devoted to the elucidation of the mechanisms by which spinal and trigeminal nociceptive neurons are activated and modulated; indeed, it is a current concept today that, as early as this level, powerful controls are able to modify nociceptive information, more particularly through mechanisms involving segmental and propriospinal circuits and others which originate from supraspinal levels. Owing to their remarkable efficacy, the latter have been the subject of numerous studies which are reviewed in the present volume. Most of these studies have been carried out by investigating the effects of central electrical stimulation; these have testified without doubt to the existence of descending inhibitory pathways capable of modulating the spinal processing of nociceptive information but have not allowed any conclusions to be reached as to the physiological meaning of these controls and especially to the circumstances under which they would be activated physiologically. In fact, the manner in which such systems are triggered during stimulation-produced analgesia almost certainly constitutes an artificial situation in which parts of a more complex circuit are by-passed.

Some authors have maintained that these systems are part of an 'intrinsic analgesic system', the final function of which would seem to be to produce analgesia (Liebeskind et al., 1976; Mayer and Price, 1976; Fields and Basbaum, 1978; Mayer, 1979). The existence of anatomical links between ascending pain pathways and bulbo-spinal inhibitory pathways has been emphasized; such a configuration, which allows the possibility of these being a complex regulatory mechanism, has been interpreted as a simple negative feed-back loop by which nociceptive messages may attenuate themselves (Basbaum and Fields, 1978, 1980; Fields and Basbaum, 1978, 1984).

In the rat, a painful focus does actually trigger widespread inhibitory phenomena acting upon some neurons of the dorsal horn, namely the convergent neurons (Le Bars et al., 1979a,b); these phenomena have been termed 'diffuse noxious inhibitory controls' (DNIC). However, as will be seen, such controls cannot be explained by the triggering of negative feed-back loops since heterotopic nociceptive stimuli are effective. Incidently, it should also be noted that electrophysiological studies in the monkey and the cat have also suggested the existence of spino-bulbo-spinal positive feed-back loops (Giesler et al., 1981a; Cervero and Wolstencroft, 1984).

DNIC affect the whole population of convergent

276

neurons whether recorded in the superficial or deeper layers within the dorsal horn in various segments of the spinal cord (Le Bars et al., 1979a; Calvino et al., 1984) or in trigeminal nucleus caudalis (Dickenson et al., 1980a). By contrast, DNIC do not affect the other neuronal types that are found within the dorsal horn or nucleus caudalis, i.e. noxious-specific, non-noxious specific, cold responsive and proprioceptive neurons (Le Bars et al., 1979b; Dickenson et al., 1980a).

The main feature of DNIC is that they can be triggered from any part of the body, distant from the excitatory receptive field of the neuron under study (heterotopic stimulation) provided that this conditioning stimulus is clearly noxious. Indeed, DNIC can be triggered by any heterotopic nocicep-

tive stimulus whatever its type − mechanical, thermal, chemical or electrical − whereas non-noxious stimuli are completely ineffective. For strong stimuli, the inhibitory effects are powerful and following by long-lasting post stimulation effects which can last for several minutes.

One striking feature of DNIC is their capacity to affect the activity of convergent neurons whether evoked from the periphery by noxious or non-noxious, natural or electrical stimuli or directly by the microelectrophoretic application of excitatory amino acids (Villanueva et al., 1984a,1984b). Examples are given of recordings from convergent neurons with activities evoked by noxious radiant heat (Fig. 1) or moderate pinch (Fig. 2) applied to the receptive field. Transcutaneous electrical stimuli applied to the receptive field of convergent

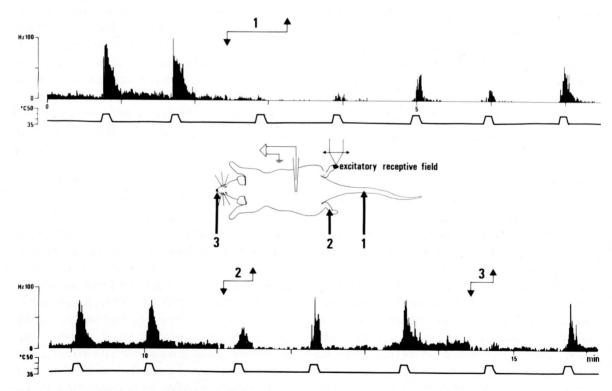

Fig. 1. Effects of noxious pinches applied to various parts of the body (1, 2, 3) on the activity of a lumbar dorsal horn convergent neuron evoked by noxious radiant heat applied on its peripheral excitatory receptive field (temperatures indicated below the histograms), in the intact anaesthetized rat (continuous record). Note that both the evoked responses and the spontaneous activity of the neuron were subject to the inhibitory effects and that post-effects occurred when the conditioning stimulus was applied for a long period (upper histogram). (From Le Bars et al., 1981d.)

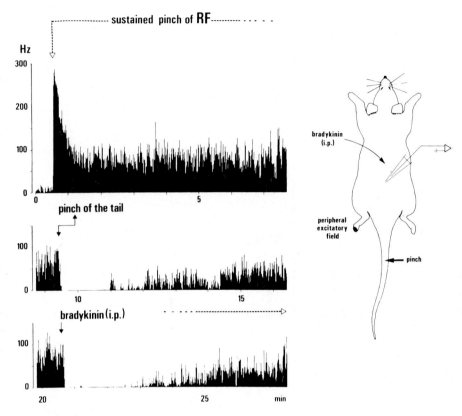

Fig. 2. Inhibitory effects induced by two heterotopic noxious stimuli in the intact anaesthetized rat (continuous record). The application of sustained pinch (open arrowhead, broken line) to the peripheral excitatory field of the convergent neuron resulted in a phasic response followed by a tonic discharge (upper histogram). A pinch applied to the tail (middle histogram) or an intraperitoneal injection of bradykinin (8 μg in 1 ml saline, lower trace) both resulted in a blockade of firing. Note the long-lasting post-effects (full recovery in about 5 min). (From Le Bars et al., 1986.)

neurons produce an activation of large (Aα) and fine (C) fibres and in systematic studies of DNIC, supra-threshold currents have been employed because these evoke a reproducible 'C-fibre response' from convergent neurons. All noxious conditioning stimuli tested have induced marked inhibition of such responses. Fig. 3 summarizes these findings using a single modality of conditioning stimulation, namely, pinch of the hindpaw. This Fig. is based on four experiments in which four convergent cells were recorded in four different loci: nucleus caudalis ipsilateral and contralateral to the site of pinch application, the lumbar cord contralateral to the site of pinch application and the sacral spinal cord. Note how the con-

ditioning stimuli blocked the evoked response irrespective of the recording site. That DNIC influences the transmission of information from convergent neurons to the brain has been verified in the rat by demonstrating that DNIC affect identified spino-thalamic and trigemino-thalamic convergent neurons (Dickenson and Le Bars, 1983b). No obvious difference in the characteristics of DNIC was seen between projecting and non-projecting convergent neurons.

The studies cited so far illustrated the profound inhibition of convergent neurons produced by noxious stimuli of diverse areas of the body. Although these observations did not seem to have been reported previously, there were hints in the

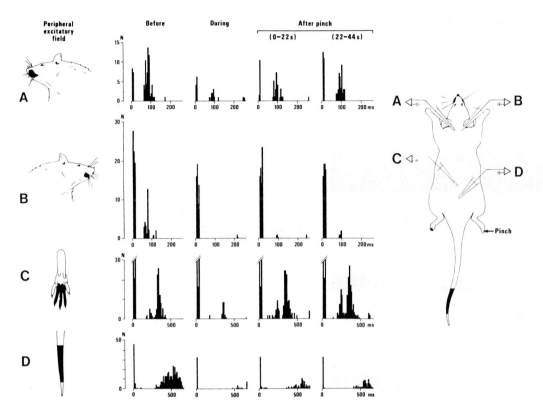

Fig. 3. Examples of inhibitory effects induced by pinches applied to the right hindpaw on the responses of four convergent neurons (A, B, C, D) to suprathreshold transcutaneous electrical stimulation of their excitatory fields (depicted on the left). Poststimulus histograms (PSH; 15 trials; bin width 2 ms for neurons A and B and 5 ms for neurons C and D) built just before (left PSH), during (middle PSH), and after (two right PSHs) the application of a strong pinch to the right hindpaw. Each neuron responded with a short-latency A-fibre response (truncated for neuron C) followed by a long-latency C-fibre response. Note that this latter response disappeared almost completely during the application of the pinch; because of the supramaximal nature of the electrical shocks, A responses were affected to a lesser extent. (From Le Bars et al., 1986.)

literature of electrophysiological findings that may well have been related. For example, stimulation of the infraorbital nerve can inhibit some mechanical responses of spinothalamic neurons in the cat (Mc Creary and Bloedel, 1976). Recently the existence of DNIC has been demonstrated in the cat (Morton et al., 1987).

'Diffuse noxious inhibitory controls' cannot be demonstrated in anaesthetized or decerebrate animals in which the spinal cord has been sectioned (Le Bars et al., 1979b; Cadden et al., 1983; Morton et al., 1987). The mechanisms underlying DNIC are therefore not confined to the spinal cord and thus supraspinal structures must be implicated in

the circuits. In this respect, it is important to note that such a system differs from segmental inhibitory systems, since segmental inhibitory receptive fields are found in both intact and spinal animals. Furthermore, this latter type of inhibition can be triggered by the activation of low threshold afferents. DNIC are also different from propriospinal inhibitory processes triggered by noxious inputs (Gerhart et al., 1981; Fitzgerald, 1982; Cadden et al., 1983).

In the present review we will successively present evidence for the specific triggering of DNIC by nociceptive events and for the involvement of bulbo-spinal inhibitory controls in such processes.

In a third section we will put forward hypotheses regarding the functional significance of the DNIC circuitry.

I. Specific triggering of 'diffuse noxious inhibitory controls' (DNIC) by nociceptive events

(1) Encoding of nociceptive stimuli by DNIC

A clear correlation between the intensity of a noxious stimulus and the resultant strength of DNIC would seem to be an important piece of evidence

for the possibility of a coding of nociceptive information by inhibitory phenomena such as DNIC (see Section III, 1). For simplicity and technical ease, we have considered the effect of various temperatures applied to the tail on the responses of lumbar and trigeminal convergent neurons activated by transcutaneous electrical stimulation of their hindpaw and facial receptive fields (Le Bars et al., 1981a; Villanueva and Le Bars, 1985). These studies are summarized in Fig. 4. It should be noted that the threshold for producing DNIC is between 40 and 44°C, and above this temperature

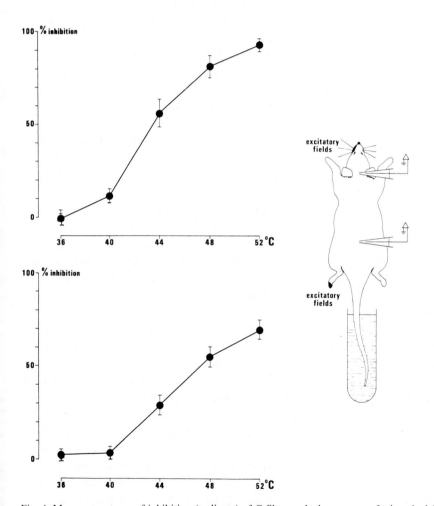

Fig. 4. Mean percentages of inhibition (ordinate) of C fibre evoked responses of trigeminal (upper curve) and lumbar (lower curve) convergent neurons induced by the immersion of the tail in water baths at various temperatures (abscissa). Note that no significant effects were observed when 36°C or 40°C was applied to the tail but that there was a highly significant correlation between noxious temperatures (44 – 52°C) and the degree of inhibition. (From Le Bars et al., 1986.)

(in the range 44 – 52°C), a highly significant correlation exists between the conditioning temperature and the degree of inhibition. In addition, analogous results have been obtained when identical thermal stimuli have been tested against activities evoked by microelectrophoresis of an excitatory amino acid (Villanueva and Le Bars, 1985).

These data reinforce the hypothesis that DNIC are triggered specifically by the activation of peripheral nociceptors whose signals are carried by Aδ and C fibres. C-polymodal nociceptors have been described in the cat, rat, monkey, rabbit and man (see Refs. in Villanueva and Le Bars, 1985). They constitute a large proportion of the total population of C fibre afferents in these species and it is important to note that, to date, all C fibres recorded in man have shown the characteristics of polymodal nociceptors (Van Hees and Gybels, 1981; Torebjörk et al., 1984). In addition, a population of Aδ-polymodal nociceptors responding to thermal stimuli exists and these have electrophysiological characteristics essentially similar to those of C-polymodal nociceptors; they have been described in monkey and man (see Refs. in Villanueva and Le Bars, 1985). Both types of polymodal nociceptors increase their discharge when the temperatures applied to their receptive fields increase, especially in the 45 – 51°C range. According to Lamotte and Campbell (1978), their mean threshold for activation is 43.6°C.

In man, the pain threshold induced by thermal stimulation is achieved when the skin temperature reaches 45°C (Hardy et al., 1951). In addition, a linear dolorimetric scale is only apparent in the 44 – 50°C range (Adair et al., 1968; Lamotte and Campbell, 1978). Furthermore, Gybels et al. (1979) have demonstrated a good correlation between the activity of polymodal nociceptors triggered by thermal stimulation and the subject's assessment of the resultant sensation on a dolorimetric scale. Finally, Dubner and Beitel (1976) have reported an analogous correlation between such activity and escape behaviour in the monkey.

Taken together, these data illustrate the close parallels between the strength of DNIC, pain sensations in man and the firing of polymodal nociceptors recorded in man and animals; this strongly suggests that DNIC are specifically triggered by the activation of nociceptors.

(2) Activation of Aδ and C fibres triggers DNIC

We investigated the mechanisms underlying the inhibition triggered by heterotopic percutaneous electrical stimulation and by so doing clarified some points regarding the peripheral part of the loop which subserves DNIC (Bouhassira et al., 1987).

For this purpose, we took advantage of the facts that trigeminal and spinal dorsal horn neurons respond with relatively steady discharges to the electrophoretic application of excitatory amino acids and that DNIC act on convergent neurons by a final post-synaptic inhibitory mechanism involving hyperpolarisation of the neuronal membrane (see Section II, 3). During recordings of trigeminal convergent neurons directly excited by the electrophoretic application of DL-homocysteate (DLH), the percutaneous electrical application of single square-wave stimuli (10 mA; 2 ms) to the tail always induced a biphasic depression of such activity. Both the early and late components of this inhibition occurred at shorter latencies when the base rather than the tip of the tail was stimulated (Fig. 5). Since the two stimulation sites were 100 mm apart, it was possible to use these differences in latencies from the two sites to estimate the conduction velocities of the peripheral fibres which were triggering the inhibitions. For the onset of the earlier and later components of the inhibition, the mean differences between the latencies from the two sites of stimulation were 13.6 and 147.7 ms respectively, corresponding to peripheral conduction velocities of 7.3 and 0.68 m/s, respectively. According to Gasser and Erlanger (1927) and Burgess and Perl (1973), these values correspond to peripheral conduction velocities in the Aδ and C fibre ranges, respectively.

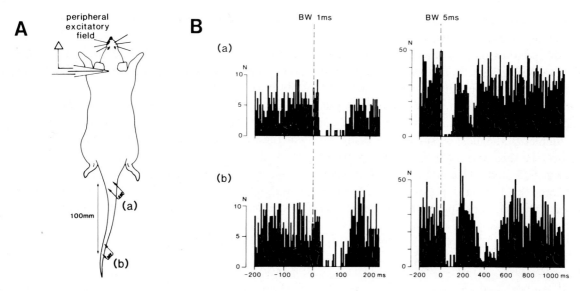

Fig. 5. (A) Schematic representation of the experimental design. Neurons with receptive fields located ipsilaterally on the muzzle were recorded in trigeminal nucleus caudalis. The continuous electrophoretic application of an excitatory amino acid, DL-homocysteic acid (DLH), induced a steady discharge from the neuron under study. The repetitive application of single percutaneous electrical stimuli of adequate intensities to the base (a) or the tip (b) of the tail induced biphasic depressions of activity which exclusively affected convergent neurons. (B) Individual example of the biphasic inhibitory processes triggered by repetitive single percutaneous electrical stimuli (10 mA; 0.66 Hz; 2 ms duration; 200 ms delay) applied to the base (a) or the tip (b) of the tail, on the discharge of a trigeminal convergent neuron evoked by the continuous electrophoretic application of DLH (17 nA). Post-stimulus histograms (bin width 1 ms, left; 5 ms, right) were built from 100 trials. The earlier component is detailed in the left part of the Fig. while the whole biphasic inhibition is shown on the right. Note that both components appeared earlier when the base (a) rather than the tip (b) of the tail was stimulated. (From Bouhassira et al., 1987.)

Although peripheral unmyelinated and thin myelinated fibres can respond to stimuli below the pain threshold, the relationship between the activation of such fibres and nociceptive reactions or pain is a classical one (see Refs. in Bouhassira et al., 1987).

(3) The threshold for triggering DNIC is lowered in an animal model of chronic pain

The studies cited so far involved the use of acute stimuli and it seemed essential to also investigate the way in which DNIC act in situations more relevant to clinical pain. Rats rendered arthritic by intradermal injection of Freund's adjuvant into the tail (Pearson and Wood, 1959) are considered to be a model of chronic pain relevant to human rheumatoid arthritis (Pircio et al., 1975; De Castro Costa et al., 1981; Colpaert et al., 1982). We chose to record dorsal horn neurons between the 3rd and the 4th week following the adjuvant inoculation since in a recent study (Calvino et al., 1987a), we found that such a period is critical in the disease both in terms of clinical observations, including radiological analyses, and behavioural data, including pain-related tests.

As facial areas are not affected by arthritis, we recorded from trigeminal nucleus caudalis neurons in order to investigate the effects of heterotopically applied stimuli of various intensities on the responses of convergent neurons whose receptive fields were not in regions affected by the disease (Calvino et al., 1987c). All convergent neurons were inhibited by heterotopic stimuli whether noxious (52°C, pinch) or non-noxious (light and mild pressure) applied to inflamed areas. While the inhibition triggered by noxious stimuli was similar to that observed in healthy rats, the inhibition triggered by non-noxious mechanical stimuli had never previously been found when such stimuli were applied heterotopically in healthy animals. Moreover, the strength of these inhibitions was related to the inflammatory state of the part of the body stimulated, the most sensitive areas being the hindpaws; in this case light and mild pressure resulted in 60% and 100% inhibitions, respectively, followed by long-lasting post-effects (several minutes). The relationship between conditioning

strength and degree of inhibition was clear; such a correlation is reminiscent of one of the main characteristics of DNIC, although a shift towards the range of non-noxious mechanical stimuli was observed in arthritic rats.

The increase in peripheral sensitivity induced by arthritis could account for such an augmentation of the heterotopic inhibitory phenomena. Peripheral changes induced by arthritis have been described: joint capsule receptors, which have non-myelinated or poorly myelinated axons, have lower thresholds to mechanical stimulation (Guilbaud et

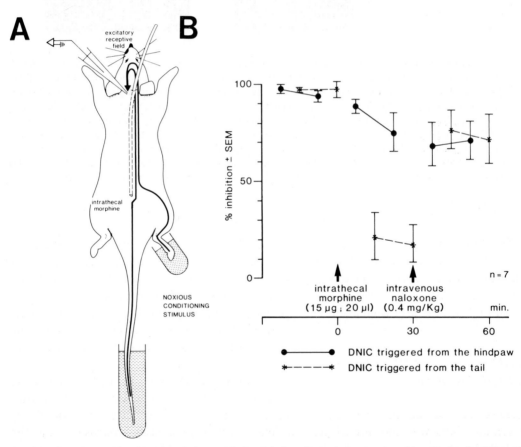

Fig. 6. (A) Schematic representation of the experimental design. Convergent neurons with receptive fields located ipsilaterally on the muzzle were recorded in the left trigeminal nucleus caudalis. Their C-fibre evoked responses were conditioned by immersion of the hind paw or tail in a 52°C waterbath. During the surgical preparation, a nylon catheter connected to a Hamilton microlitre syringe containing morphine sulphate solution was placed in the subarachnoid space so that its tip reached the sacrococcygeal level. (B) Mean results. These are expressed in terms of the percentage inhibition of C-fibre responses induced by noxious thermal conditioning (*n*, number of cells). Note the differential effect of intrathecal morphine, and that the lifting of the inhibition triggered from the tail was reversed by systemic naloxone. (From Villanueva and Le Bars, 1986.)

al., 1985) and some dorsal horn neurons exhibit exaggerated responses to light mechanical stimulation (Menétrey and Besson, 1982; Calvino et al., 1987b).

Light and mild pressure are non-noxious but probably painful stimuli in arthritic rats as shown in behavioural experiments: the threshold for struggle or vocalization triggered by calibrated pressure applied to one of the inflamed hindpaws – the Randall-Selitto test (1957) – is strongly depressed (50%) during the 3 – 4 weeks post inoculation (Kayser and Guilbaud, 1981; Calvino and Le Bars, 1986; Calvino et al., 1987a), a finding which clearly demonstrates hyperalgesia during this period.

(4) Blockade of DNIC by intrathecal morphine

If DNIC are specifically triggered by noxious peripheral inputs, then specific pharmacological manipulations of the spinal processing of nociceptive information would also be expected to influence these controls by interfering with the early stages of the looped pathway which subserves them. We aimed to test this hypothesis by making use of the well-known anti-nociceptive action of morphine at the spinal level (Yaksh, 1981).

We, therefore, chose an experimental procedure (Fig. 6, A) in which the effects of DNIC triggered by noxious thermal stimulation of caudal regions of the body, were monitored at the trigeminal level (Villanueva and Le Bars, 1986). In such a preparation, spinal blockade of nociceptive transmission by intrathecal morphine would be expected to result in a concomitant blockade of the effects of DNIC on the remote, i.e., trigeminal, neuronal population. This was actually the case since intrathecal morphine (15 μg; 20 μl), administered over the coccygeal segments, strongly reduced the effects of DNIC at the trigeminal level when these controls were triggered by noxious thermal stimulation of the tail, without significantly affecting analogous inhibitions triggered from the hindpaw; importantly, this reduction was reversed by naloxone (Fig. 6, B). Thus, intrathecal morphine

induced a segmental depression of nociceptive signals strong enough to prevent the spinal initiation of DNIC.

Knowing that intrathecal morphine specifically blocks pain, leaving other somaesthetic sensations intact, and that morphine depresses the neuronal responses in the dorsal horn to noxious but not to innocuous stimuli, this finding further emphasises the close relationship between DNIC and nociception.

(5) The ascending signals triggering DNIC are confined to the ventrolateral quadrants

We have already mentioned that DNIC acting on convergent lumbar neurons are abolished by a total section of the (cervical) spinal cord. It appears, therefore, that the involvement of a supraspinal loop is an essential characteristic in the triggering of DNIC. To determine the anatomical profile of the ascending limb of the loop subserving DNIC, we made use of the fact that DNIC act on nucleus caudalis convergent neurons. By triggering DNIC from a posterior part of the body, we were able to undertake the study of a model in which the circuitry of the involved loop is successively organized in long ascending (Fig. 7, left: A) and short descending (Fig. 7, left: B) pathways (Villanueva et al., 1986a). In such a situation, a blockade of DNIC by subtotal spinal section would have to be due to the impairment of nociceptive transmission in ascending spinal pathways rather than of transmission in descending pathways to the trigeminal system. The use of a thermal nociceptive conditioning stimulus applied to either the left or right hindpaw allowed us to compare the strength of DNIC before and following: (1) lumbar commissurotomy (Fig. 7, a); (2) restricted lesions of the cervical spinal cord corresponding to various sensory ascending pathways; (3) unilateral and bilateral sections of the ventrolateral quadrant at the cervical level (Fig. 7, b) and 4) thalamic lesions (Fig. 7, c).

To ascertain the possible crossed nature of the pathways responsible for the heterotopic processes, the effects of lumbar commissurotomy were investigated. As shown in Fig. 7(a), the inhibitory processes, whether triggered from the left or right hindpaw, were strongly depressed in all the experiments. However, this depression was not complete, suggesting that both crossed and uncrossed components play a role.

Lesioning dorsal, dorsolateral, and ventromedial parts of the cervical cord was found not to affect inhibitory processes triggered from either hindpaw. It appeared therefore that several sensory pathways for which roles in nociception have been suggested could not have been involved, namely: the postsynaptic fibres of the dorsal col-

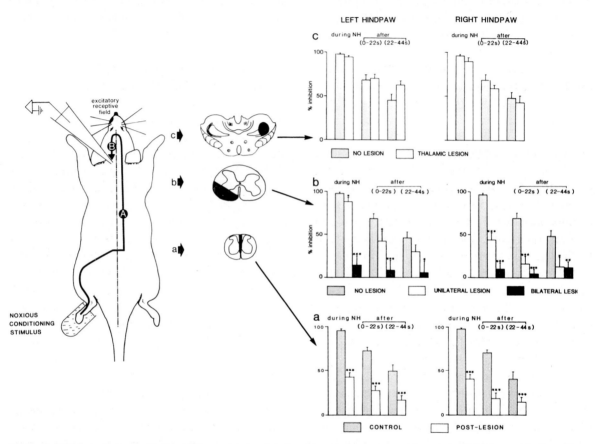

Fig. 7. (Left) Schematic representation of the experimental design. Convergent neurons with receptive fields located ipsilaterally on the muzzle were recorded in the left trigeminal nucleus caudalis. C-fibre responses were conditioned by immersion of either hindpaw in a 52°C water bath. With this experimental arrangement the supraspinal loop sustaining DNIC comprised a long ascending (A) and a short descending (B) pathway. The effects of three types of CNS lesions were studied: (a) lumbar commissurotomy, (b) cervical sections, and (c) destruction of the right ventrobasal thalamic complex. (Right) Summary of results. Histograms represent the percentage inhibitions observed during ('during NH') and within the 44 s after ('after 0 – 22 s', 'after 22 – 44 s') the immersion of the left (left histograms) or the right (right histograms) hindpaws. Controls are shown as hatched columns. (a) Lumbar commissurotomy. Note the symmetrical nature of the reductions of the inhibitions triggered from either hindpaw, which were induced by the commissurotomy (open columns). (b) Ventrolateral lesions. Inhibitions observed in rats with unilateral (open columns) or bilateral lesions (dark columns) are compared with those observed in untransected animals. Note that (1) in unilateral lesions, inhibitory processes triggered from the right hindpaw were strongly reduced, with the poststimulus effects disappearing almost completely; inhibitory processes triggered from the left hindpaw were slightly decreased and (2) in bilateral lesions, the inhibitions, whether triggered from the left or the right handpaw, disappeared almost completely. (c) Lesion of the right ventrobasal thalamic complex. Note that the inhibitions could be triggered equally from either hindpaw (open columns); they did not differ significantly from those observed in control situations in intact rats. (From Villanueva et al., 1986a.)

umns (Uddenberg, 1968; Angaut-Petit, 1975a, 1975b; Giesler et al., 1984; Giesler and Cliffer, 1985), the spinocervical tract which travels through the dorsolateral funiculus (Morin, 1955; Lundberg and Oscarsson, 1961; Craig and Tapper, 1978; Giesler et al., 1979), part of the spinothalamic tract, i.e. those fibres projecting to the medial and intralaminar thalamus and travelling through the ventromedial funiculus (Giesler et al., 1979).

On the other hand, our results did underline an essential role for the ventrolateral quadrant in the triggering of DNIC, since it was this single region that remained undamaged when the overlap of the lesions that did not attenuate DNIC was considered. Conversely, all lesions that reduced DNIC triggered from the hindpaw included the ventrolateral region of the opposite side or at least the lateral part of that region.

Furthermore, unilateral lesions of the left ventrolateral quadrant resulted in a strong reduction of inhibitory processes triggered from the right hindpaw, whereas inhibition triggered from the left hindpaw was slightly, albeit significantly, decreased (Fig. 7, b, open columns). Bilateral lesions of the ventrolateral quadrant resulted in a complete disappearance of inhibition, whether triggered from the right or left hindpaw (Fig. 7, b, black columns). Thus, the lateral spinothalamic tract (Mehler et al., 1960; Kerr, 1975; Boivie, 1979; Giesler et al., 1979, 1981b) and the part of the spinoreticular system which travels within the ventrolateral quadrant (Mehler et al., 1960; Mehler, 1969; Zemlan et al., 1978) could have been involved.

The mainly crossed nature of the ascending pathways subserving DNIC could suggest the participation of spinothalamic neurons in these processes. It has been shown, in the rat, that ascending projections reaching the lateral thalamus are completely crossed (Peschanski et al., 1983), and the axons of spinothalamic neurons are classically described as crossing the midline at the level of the segment containing the cell body (Foerster and Gagel, 1931; Willis et al., 1979). All these considerations prompted us to undertake the last series

of experiments in which the neurons of the right lateral thalamus were destroyed by prior microinjection of kainic acid. The results were unambiguous: DNIC were triggered equally well from either hindpaw after large lesions involving the right ventrobasal thalamic complex (Fig. 7, c). These experiments eliminate a possible lateral thalamic link in the loop subserving DNIC.

The remaining candidate for a role in triggering DNIC was the spinoreticular tract, since it has been clearly established that its axons are located in the ventrolateral region of the spinal cord (Mehler et al., 1960; Mehler, 1969; Kerr, 1975). Interestingly, in the rat, these pathways have been shown to comprise a crossed and an uncrossed component (Mehler et al., 1960; Mehler, 1969; Zemlan et al., 1978).

II. The triggering of bulbo-spinal inhibitory controls by noxious peripheral inputs

(1) Involvement of a serotonergic link in the loop subserving DNIC

Due to the ascending/descending nature of the inhibitory loop activated by peripheral nociceptors, one can speculate that DNIC involve brain stem structures such as the nucleus raphe magnus (NRM), electrical stimulation of which inhibits the activities of convergent neurons (see Oliveras, Willis in this volume). Considering that the NRM is rich in serotonin-containing cell bodies, and since serotonin (5HT) plays a major role in descending control systems (see Basbaum, Bowker, Willis in this volume), the effect of various manipulations of serotonergic systems on DNIC were studied. These included the depletion of 5HT by *p*-chlorophenylalanine (pCPA), blockade of 5HT receptors and administration of the precursor of 5HT, 5-hydroxytryptophan (5-HTP).

Pretreatment with pCPA (300 mg/kg, i.p., 3 days) strongly reduced DNIC (Dickenson et al., 1981); the post-effects were also reduced in terms of magnitude and duration. Although our pretreatment procedure induced a total 5HT depletion at the spinal level, the blockade of DNIC was not complete. This observation suggests that additional non-serotonergic mechanisms are involved in DNIC. In fact, in pCPA-pretreated rats, the effects of noxious peripheral conditioning stimulation exhibited a great variability, ranging from the absence of any inhibition to some strong inhibitory effects equivalent to those observed in normal animals.

This is in keeping with a study devoted to the effects of electrical stimulation of the NRM, where such a variability was found in pCPA-pretreated rats (Rivot et al., 1980). We therefore undertook a comparison of the effects of peripheral and central conditioning stimuli on the same convergent neurons in pCPA pretreated rats (Le Bars et al., 1982): a good correlation was found between the degree of inhibition induced by a calibrated noxious pinch applied to the tail and by the electrical stimulation of NRM. The parallels between both types of inhibition were further emphasized by the fact that excitatory effects, both during and immediately following the conditioning noxious stimuli and following NRM stimulation, were observed in pCPA pretreated rats.

The results presented above needed further confirmation since the effect of pCPA is not totally restricted to 5HT depletion. We therefore utilized complementary pharmacological tools, i.e. 5HT receptor blockers (cinanserin and metergoline) and a precursor of 5HT synthesis. Both systemic cinanserin and metergoline strongly reduced DNIC, whereas 5HTP increased these inhibitory effects (Chitour et al., 1982).

Although the most likely site of action for the effects we have reported with systematically administered drugs is on serotonergic bulbo-spinal descending inhibitory pathways, we cannot rule out the possibility that the effects reported above may have involved serotonergic systems other than the bulbo-spinal pathways.

The idea of descending serotonergic pathways being activated by noxious stimuli is supported by biochemical evidence. Bilateral high intensity − but not low intensity − stimulation of the sciatic nerve induces a release of 5HT in superfusates from the spinal cord of the cat; thoracic cord cold block prevented this effect (Tyce and Yaksh, 1981). Since a rise in 5HT release was also observed following stimulation of the infraorbital branch of the trigeminal nerve, there may be a diffuse release of the monoamine within the cord no matter what part of the body is stimulated. Interestingly, 5HT release could be induced by electrical stimulation of the dorsolateral funiculus (DLF) (Tyce and Yaksh, 1981), the NRM or the nucleus reticularis paragigantocellularis (Rivot et al., 1982; Hammond et al., 1985; Pilowsky et al., 1986). In addition, the prolonged application of intense nociceptive electrical stimuli to the tail of anaesthetized rats induced a rise in 5HT synthesis in the dorsal part of the cord; by contrast the prolonged application of innocuous electrical stimuli to the tail was not followed by any detectable change in 5HT synthesis (Weil-Fugazza et al., 1984). Interestingly, electrical stimulation of the NRM also produced an increased synthesis of 5HT within the cord (Bourgoin et al., 1980).

(2) Involvement of an opioidergic link in the loop subserving DNIC

The parallels between NRM- and DNIC-mediated inhibition are further emphasized by the fact that both are decreased to a comparable extent by the opiate antagonist naloxone, at least in the rat and when experiments are performed under identical conditions. Indeed, comparison of the results related to DNIC in the rat (Le Bars et al., 1981c) with those of Rivot et al. (1979) in the same species, shows that the antagonistic effect of systemic naloxone was of the same order of magnitude for NRM- and DNIC-mediated inhibition. Naloxone could antagonize DNIC at supraspinal and/or spinal sites, strongly suggesting the participation of endogenous opioids.

A possible participation of spinal opioids in DNIC is supported by our biochemical data showing that a noxious mechanical stimulus does not alter the release of metenkephalin-like material (MELM) from neuronal segments related to the stimulated area of the body, but does increase its release from other segments (Le Bars et al., 1987a). Interestingly, in an additional study we demonstrated that this heterosegmental release of MELM is sustained by activity in descending pathways travelling in the DLF (Le Bars et al., 1987b). This probably implies that the release of MELM is sustained by a supraspinal loop since a large number of studies have implicated the DLF as the descending part of an inhibitory system originating from the brain stem (see Willis in this volume, and Section II, 5).

(3) Hyperpolarization of convergent neurons by DNIC

DNIC is equally effective against all responses of convergent neurons evoked from the periphery (for instance whether produced by A or C fiber stimulation). These properties of DNIC suggest a postsynaptic inhibitory influence.

As an alternative to recording intracellularly from dorsal horn neurons, we used the microelectrophoretic application of glutamate ions (see Puil, 1981) to excite identified neurons and then investigated the effects of noxious conditioning stimuli applied to various parts of the body (Villanueva et al., 1984a, 1984b; Villanueva and Le Bars, 1985). DNIC very markedly reduced the excitation produced by glutamate in all the covergent neurons whether recorded in the spinal dorsal horn or in trigeminal nucleus caudalis. In contrast, no effects of the conditioning stimuli were obtained for the glutamate-evoked activity of other types of neurons.

It seems likely that the neuronal processes responsible for the effects observed on convergent neurons involve postsynaptic inhibitory mechanisms (Curtis et al., 1959; see Besson et al., 1974; Belcher et al., 1978; Jordan et al., 1978), but in order to obtain further support for such a proposition, we tested the effect of noxious conditioning stimuli during periods of excessive depolarization (Curtis et al., 1960): the fact that heterotopic noxious stimuli were able to restore extracellularly recorded spike discharges, most probably reflecting a repolarization of the neuronal membrane, strongly suggests that inhibitory postsynaptic potentials were being triggered by such stimuli.

Here again, the parallel between DNIC- and NRM-mediated inhibitions has to be emphasized, since inhibitory post-synaptic potentials evoked by stimulation of this nucleus have been recorded in convergent neurons at the origin of the spinothalamic tract in the monkey (Giesler et al., 1981c; see also Belcher et al., 1978). However, we cannot exclude the participation of other complementary mechanisms in DNIC, since signs of presynaptic inhibition mechanisms have been reported after NRM stimulation (see Willis, this volume).

(4) Involvement of nucleus raphe magnus (NRM) in the loop subserving DNIC

Since there are striking similarities between the inhibition produced by DNIC and those elicited by stimulation of the NRM, we have directly investigated the involvement of NRM in DNIC by comparing the inhibitory effects of DNIC on trigeminal nucleus caudalis and dorsal horn convergent neurons before and after electrolytic lesions of the NRM (Dickenson et al., 1980b). In most neurons recorded in a group of rats in which the cumulative lesions destroyed areas of the brain stem including the NRM, the ventral part of nucleus reticularis paragigantocellularis (NRPG) and the midline reticular formation immediately dorsal to the NRM, a strong reduction of DNIC was apparent, both immediately after the lesion and also in later tests. Due to the difficulty in confining lesions to the NRM, we cannot rule out a participation of the medial part of the NRPG in some of the effects. However, this medial area and the region of the NRPG overlying the pyramidal tract also contain serotonergic cell bodies, and these areas together with NRM coincide with the original nucleus B3 of Dahlström and Fuxe (1965),

288

in their first description of serotonergic cell areas (see Bowker, this volume).

(5) The descending signals triggering DNIC are confined to the dorso-lateral funiculus.

To analyze the anatomical profile of the descending tracts of the loop subserving DNIC, inhibitions were triggered from a rostral part of the body and recordings were made from lumbar dorsal horn convergent neurons (Villanueva et al., 1986b). In this situation the circuitry of the loop is organized in short ascending (Fig. 8, a: A) and long descending (Fig. 8, a: B) pathways. In such a situation, a blockade of DNIC by a subtotal spinal section would have to be due to the impairment of transmission in the descending part of the loop. A thermal nociceptive conditioning stimulus (52°C)

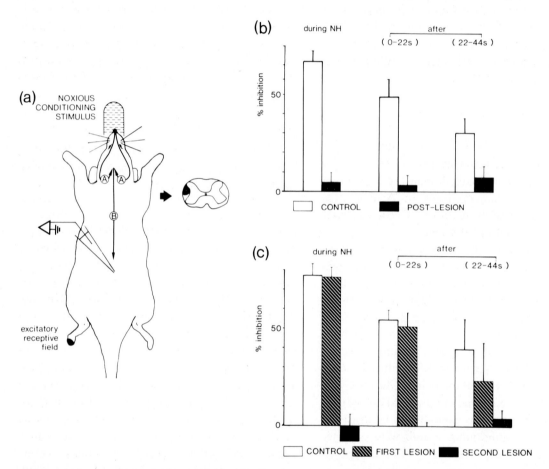

Fig. 8. (a) Schematic representations of the experimental design. Convergent neurons with receptive fields located on the extremity of the ipsilateral hindpaw were recorded in the dorsal horn of the lumbar spinal cord. C-fibre responses were conditioned by immersion of the muzzle in a 52°C waterbath. With this experimental arrangement, the loop sustaining DNIC comprised a short ascending (A) and a long descending (B) pathway. Effects of restricted cervical lesions involving the dorsolateral funiculus were studied. (b) Summary of experiments involving a single ipsilateral dorsolateral funiculus (DLF) lesion. Histograms represent the percentage inhibition observed during ('during NH') and within the 44 s following ('after 0 – 22 s'; 'after 22 – 44 s') the immersion of the muzzle in a 52°C waterbath. Note that the inhibitory processes (open columns) disappeared after the DLF lesions (black columns). (c) Summary of the experiments involving two consecutive dorsolateral funiculus lesions. Note that inhibitory processes were not essentially different before (open columns) and after (hatched columns) the contralateral DLF lesions. In contrast, after ipsilateral DLF lesions (black columns) the inhibitory processes were abolished. (From Villanueva et al., 1986b.)

applied to the muzzle allowed us to compare the strength of DNIC before and after DLF lesions of the cervical spinal cord. Such an experimental design was chosen to answer the question of whether the DLF ipsilateral and/or contralateral to the recording site carries signals responsible for DNIC.

As shown in Fig. 8(b), a lesion including the DLF ipsilateral to the neurons under study, completely abolished the inhibitory processes triggered from the muzzle. To further ascertain the principal, if not exclusive, participation of the ipsilateral DLF in the descending projections responsible for DNIC, the effects of a lesion of the contralateral DLF were investigated. Neither the inhibitory processes nor the unconditioned C fibre responses were altered by this procedure; again, a second lesion including the ipsilateral DLF induced a blockade of DNIC (Fig. 8, c).

One can therefore conclude that the descending projections involved in the triggering of DNIC are mainly, if not entirely, confined to the DLF ipsilateral to the neuron under study.

This is consistent with a role for 5HT containing axons in DNIC. In fact, Skagerberg and Björklund (1985) showed that most of the 5HT axons originating from the brain stem descend ipsilaterally in the DLF, whereas the descending, non-5HT projections are bilateral.

III. Functional significance

The fact that a noxious stimulus activates certain brain stem structures which in turn leads to hyperpolarization of spinal and trigeminal convergent neurons but only when the stimulus is such as to be perceived as noxious by the experimenter, suggests that DNIC could play a role in nociception. What then could be the mechanism(s) by which DNIC could code nociceptive information (see Section I, 1)? In other words, how can descending inhibitory controls, the functional role of which would intuitively seem to be their involvement in analgesic phenomena, play a role in nociception?

(1) DNIC and the processing of nociceptive information

This proposition, which at first might seem illogical, becomes realistic when one considers a paradoxical property of convergent neurons, i.e. the ease with which convergent neurons can be activated by innocuous stimuli (Le Bars and Chitour, 1983). Since such stimuli are a common and frequent occurrence in everyday life, one can confidently predict that the total population of spinal and trigeminal convergent neurons will be active to a marked degree as a result of activity in cutaneous mechanoreceptors. This activity can be considered as a 'somaesthetic background activity' from within which the higher centres must attempt to recognize a significant nociceptive message.

'Diffuse noxious inhibitory controls' may provide a means by which an unequivocal nociceptive signal can be recognized from the non-specific somaesthetic activity arising from convergent neurons (Le Bars et al., 1979b, 1983, 1986). As detailed earlier, DNIC inhibit all activities of these convergent cells, notably in this context, the spontaneous and innocuous activities. If one accepts the existence of a relatively high order of background somesthetic activity in the absence of a noxious stimulus (Fig. 9, A), the experimental situations can be interpreted in the following way: as an intense noxious stimulus is applied to an area of the body, the convergent and nociceptive-specific neurons in the corresponding segmental zone will be activated (Fig. 9, B) and then give rise to excitatory signals transmitted to higher centres (Fig. 9, C). This signal will then, in turn, induce DNIC (Fig. 9, D), which will inhibit those convergent spinal and trigeminal neurons not directly influenced by the initial stimulus (Fig. 9, E). By these means, a high level of contrast will be attained between the activities of the excited segmental neurons and the depressed activity of the other convergent cells.

The facts which remain unknown are the mechanisms for recognition and eventually for processing of this signal at higher centres. We have proposed that the brain is able to recognize this contrast signal and that DNIC can consequently be interpreted as a filter, allowing the extraction of a nociceptive message from the overall activity of convergent neurons. If the brain is able to recognize such a contrasted picture as a signal of pain, then DNIC could be interpreted not only as a filter that allows the extraction of a meaningful nociceptive message from the nonspecific activities of convergent neurons but also, and perhaps more importantly, as an additional amplifier favouring the basic gain system and, therefore, the 'alarm' function of nociceptive messages.

It is obviously extremely difficult to directly verify this model of pain transmission. One can, however, derive certain theoretical implications of the model that can then be tested experimentally. The following sections consider first clinical and behavioural and then pharmacological evidence for this proposition.

(2) DNIC and the phenomenon of counterirritation

We have already stressed the effects of DNIC on all activities of convergent neurons including those produced by noxious stimuli: quite simply, when two noxious stimuli are applied to two distant areas of the body, the pool of neurons activated by the weaker stimulus is inhibited. If, as seems likely, these convergent neurons are involved in the transmission of a nociceptive signal towards supraspinal structures, the result of the simultaneous applica-

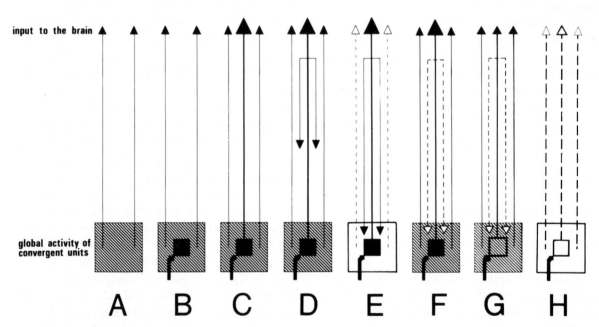

Fig. 9. Hypothetical interpretation of the global activity of convergent neurons involved in nociception at spinal and trigeminal levels. Taken as a whole, this activity would be of a reasonably high order in freely moving animals because of the properties of convergent neurons, sending a basic somaesthetic activity toward the brain (A). A noxious stimulus activates both noxious-only and convergent neurons (B), which send an excitatory input to the brain (C). These inputs trigger the DNIC system (D), with a consequent reduction of the activity of the remaining nonsegmental convergent units not directly affected by the initial stimulus; hence, a contrast signal is set up (E). Morphine whether administered systemically in low doses, intracerebrally or intracerebroventricularly, blocks DNIC and restores the background activity (F). Morphine whether administered systemically in high doses or intrathecally, blocks the spinal transmission of nociceptive information, further reducing the contrast (G). Electrical stimulation of brain sites inhibits the entire population of neurons, resulting in powerful analgesia (H).

tion of two noxious stimuli will, in terms of pain sensation, depend on a balance between the activities of the two pools of active neurons, the net result being an attenuation of the pain produced by the weaker stimulus.

This prediction of our model has its roots in historical observations and can be expressed as 'one pain can mask another'. A good number of practices in popular medicine are founded on this principle (counterirritation), which most probably dates from ancient times (see Le Bars et al., 1984). More recently, these traditional practices have been reintroduced under the term 'hyperstimulation analgesia', to cover certain therapeutic methods (Melzack, 1984). It is also of great interest to note the parallels between the phenomenon of counterirritation and the hypoalgesic effects obtained using both traditional forms of acupuncture and contemporary electroacupuncture (see Refs. in Han and Terenius, 1982; Le Bars et al., 1984; Melzack, 1984). The conclusions reached by Mann (1974) and Andersson et al. (1977) on the basis of a large number of clinical observations were that acupunctural stimuli must be painful or even only just tolerable by the subject to be effective. Furthermore, it has been reported that organic pain is accompanied by an elevation of the threshold for experimental pain applied elsewhere on the body (Hazouri and Mueller, 1950; Merskey and Evans, 1975; Lipman et al., 1987).

These clinical observations are corroborated by studies in animals. In the rat, for example, it has been shown that various nociceptive stimuli produce a reduction in the responses of the animals to noxious stimuli applied to other areas of the body (see Le Bars et al., 1984; Calvino and Le Bars, 1986). Similarly, in the cat, electrical stimulation of tooth pulp produces a considerable increase in the threshold for escape behaviour induced by electrical stimulation of the paws (Anderson et al., 1976).

The last but not least observation (see Section I, 2) lies in the importance of Aδ fibre activation in the production of analgesia or antinociceptive effects by somatic electrical stimulation which has been suggested by several authors (e.g. Woolf et al., 1980; Kawakita and Funakoshi, 1982; Chung et al., 1984; Lee et al., 1985; Sjölund, 1985).

We believe that DNIC could be one of the neuronal substrates for these hypoalgesic effects (Le Bars et al., 1979b, 1984; Calvino et al., 1984). This proposition is borne out not only by the preceding analysis but also by the fact that, in man, the pain-relieving effects of heterotopic nociceptive stimuli are extremely well correlated with a concomitant depression of a spinal nociceptive reflex (Willer et al., 1984, 1987). In an electrophysiological and psychophysiological study of these phenomena in man, the sural nerve was stimulated, and the variations in the resulting pain sensation and nociceptive reflex (flexion reflex RIII), produced by various noxious conditioning stimuli applied elsewhere on the body were studied. It was found, for example, that the thresholds for sensation and the reflex were highly significantly increased in a correlated fashion by hot water ($\geqslant 45°C$) applied to the hand contralateral to the foot in which the sural nerve was being stimulated. Interestingly, such inhibitory effects were not observed on the RIII reflex recorded in patients suffering from a total cervical spinal cord section of traumatic origin (Roby-Brami et al., 1987). These data suggest that the modulation of pain by heterotopic nociceptive stimuli is sustained by supraspinal structures and can be explained, at least in part, by a depression in the transmission of nociceptive signals at the spinal level. Related results have been obtained in the rat, where concurrent with the depression by tail or nose pinch of convergent neuronal activity produced by C-fibre-strength stimulation of the sural nerve, flexion reflex activity was similarly reduced by the conditioning stimulus (Schouenborg and Dickenson, 1985).

It is apparent, then, that as two noxious stimuli are applied to distinct areas of the body, a competitive effect is induced, with the stronger stimulus able to limit the perceptual and motor responses induced by the second stimulus.

(3) DNIC and morphine analgesia

We have explained the reasons for believing that DNIC may be involved in the coding of nociceptive information. On the basis of the hypothesis that certain neural events leading to recognition of a painful sensation could be induced by a gradient of activity between a pool of activated neurons and the relative silence of the rest of the population of cells, one could envisage that any enhancement of this contrast would result in hyperalgesia, whereas

interfering with the contrast would lead to hypoalgesia or even analgesia if the contrast were abolished. A direct consequence of this model is that pharmacological manipulations of this gradient of activity should lead to corresponding changes in pain sensations. These manipulations could equally involve the active pool and/or the concomitantly inhibited pool of neurons. Thus, a depression of the signals emanating from the activated cells could lead to hypoalgesia, and a facilitation could correspondingly result in hyperalgesia; an increase in the 'background somaesthetic activity' (by a reduction in DNIC) could produce hypoalgesia (see below), and a decrease in this activity (by a facilitation of DNIC)

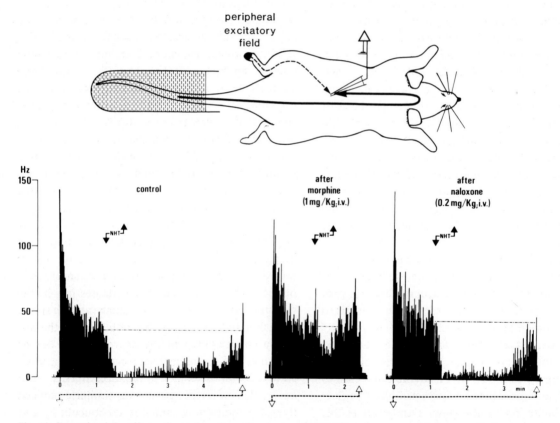

Fig. 10. Example of the effects of morphine (1 mg/kg, i.v.) on DNIC. The neuron responded to sustained pressure (open arrows) applied on its receptive field located on the ipsilateral hindpaw extremity with a steady discharge which followed a short adapting period. The dashed lines indicate the firing level of this unit in the absence of conditioning stimuli. Note, in the control sequence, the pronounced inhibitory effects followed by long-lasting post-effects induced by the immersion of the tail in water at 52°C for 30 s (filled arrow; NHT). The DNIC-mediated inhibitions were profoundly lifted by morphine, these effects being reversed by naloxone. (From Le Bars et al., 1981b.)

could result in hyperalgesia (see Section I, 3).

We have reported (Le Bars et al., 1981b) that DNIC are highly sensitive to the administration of low doses of morphine (0.1 – 1 mg/kg, i.v.). An example is provided in Fig. 10. This effect is dose-dependent, stereospecific and naloxone-reversible. These results show that descending inhibitory controls from the brain stem are reduced by morphine, at least when these controls are activated by a nociceptive peripheral stimulus. Supplementary biochemical evidence matches this interpretation of these electrophysiological studies: the increase in the synthesis of serotonin in the dorsal horn produced by a nociceptive stimulus is very significantly reduced by morphine (1 mg/kg, i.v.), an effect which is naloxone-reversible (Weil-Fugazza et al., 1984). The conclusion then is that a nociceptive stimulus activates bulbospinal serotoninergic controls and that morphine blocks this effect. Finally, psychophysical experiments in man and behavioural experiments in the rat have also shown that morphine decreases inhibitory controls elicited by noxious stimuli (Wolff et al., 1940; Kraus and Le Bars, 1986).

We have also studied the effects of morphine microinjected (5 μg, 0.2 μl) into the PAG. Injection sites in the medioventral PAG including the dorsal raphe nucleus significantly blocked DNIC (but see Gebhart, this volume). The time course of this effect was identical to that seen in behavioural studies involving monitoring the effect of microinjection of morphine on the vocalization test (Dickenson and Le Bars, 1983a, 1987). Furthermore, we have observed that morphine injected into the third ventricle also blocks DNIC in a dose-related (range 0.6 – 2.5 μg) and naloxone-reversible fashion (Bouhassira et al., 1986, 1988).

It is worth referring to some results obtained when recording from neurons in the lower medulla (see Fields, this volume). It was emphasized that the inhibition induced by noxious heating of the tail in some cells (called 'off-cells') was blocked by morphine (5 mg/kg, i.v.) and it was suggested that such a disinhibition of off-cells is a primary process contributing to opiate inhibition of nocicep-

tor-induced reflexes (Fields et al., 1983). However, the excitation induced by noxious heating of the tail in another group of cells (called 'on-cells') was blocked by a lower dose (1.25 – 2.5 mg/kg, i.v.) of systemic morphine (Barbaro et al., 1986). All these effects of systemic morphine were mimicked by microinjections of morphine (5 μg) into the ventral PAG (Cheng et al., 1986). Although there is evidence that these on-cells are facilitatory, it is possible that they are inhibitory. Thus, while the off-cell result could provide an argument for the hypothesis that morphine increases descending inhibitory controls, the on-cell findings could provide a key neuronal link for the inhibition of DNIC by low systemic doses of morphine.

Overall then, the studies discussed here are difficult to interpret in terms of the existing hypothesis for morphine analgesia (see Fields, Gebhart and Jones, in this volume). By contrast they are perfectly compatible with the model we have proposed where the contrast effect between the two pools of neurons is at the origin of processes underlying pain (Fig. 9, E).

Low doses of morphine reduce the contrast by restoring the background noise (Fig. 9, F), and this is likely to be a supraspinal action since intracerebral or ICV morphine also act in this fashion. Then, as doses are increased, an additional mechanism is brought into play, the reduction in contrast by the direct spinal action of the opiate (Fig. 9, G).

It should be noted that our interpretation does not preclude the fact that analgesia can be obtained by electrical stimulation of supraspinal sites (see Barbaro, Hosobuchi, Meyerson, Oliveras et al., Willis in this volume), since in this case all the neurons will be inhibited, thus completely abolishing the contrast and resulting in a powerful analgesia (Fig. 9, H). What our interpretation does question however, is the idea that these systems constitute an intrinsic analgesic system. Although the effects produced by electrical stimulation of these structures can reveal a potential function of these systems, it does not necessarily imply a physiological mechanism, since electrical stimulation ignores the natural conditions under which these systems are activated which our results would suggest as being in the processes giving rise to pain. In our hypothesis, it is not contradictory, only superficially paradoxical, that electrical stimulation of a structure artificially gives rise to an analgesia, whereas in reality this area is functionally involved in nociception.

In any case, our view is in accord with clinical and behavioural studies of the characteristics of morphine analgesia. In man, morphine is analgesic at low doses (0.15 mg/kg) similar to those that lift DNIC (ED_{50} about 0.6 mg/kg) and almost identical to the doses that block the inhibitory postaffects (ED_{50} 0.13 mg/kg). It is interesting to note that these low doses are without effect on the behavioural tests in animals in which threshold measurements are made using acute cutaneous nociceptive stimuli, but they are clearly effective against nociceptive reactions induced by prolonged stimuli from deep structures such as experimental arthritis (Pircio et al., 1975; Kayser and Guilbaud, 1983) or intraperitoneal injections of algogenic agents (Niemegeers et al., 1975). Additionally, the direct spinal action of morphine, far from counteracting the supraspinal action, tends to amplify it for two major reasons. It is generally agreed that morphine acts on the noxious-related activities of convergent cells without altering their responses to innocuous stimuli (Le Bars et al., 1987c). This property would not have functional significance if the convergent neurons were able to discriminate the two types of information. In contrast, this observation is particularly significant in the light of our hypothesis, as the spinal action will not hinder or counteract the supraspinal effect of morphine in restoring the 'background' somaesthetic activity' from the sensory milieu. Furthermore, it is clear that the direct depression of activity in the spinal cord by morphine will lead to a reduced activation of the loop subserving DNIC, and so result in a recovery of the level of somaesthetic activity. Our results, showing that intrathecal morphine is able to block DNIC (see Section I, 4), provide evidence to support this premise.

Effects such as this will facilitate the supraspinal effect of lifting DNIC and signify that the spinal and supraspinal actions will not be simply additive but synergistic. Consistent with this hypothesis, behavioural studies (Yeung and Rudy, 1980) have clearly demonstrated that the analgesia produced by intracerebroventricular administration of morphine is potentiated by intrathecal injection of morphine.

(4) Concluding remarks

The results reported above indicate that the three routes of administration of morphine which are used for alleviating pain in man − systemic, intrathecal, ICV − can be correlated with a reduction of DNIC. It is hard to believe that such an action could have no functional meaning.

However, it could be rather disconcerting that two opposite manipulations, the activation of DNIC by counterirritation procedures and its blocking by morphine, lead in therapeutic terms to the same end point, i.e. hypoalgesia. We feel, however, that this seeming anomaly reflects the complexity of the spinal systems and provides an insight into the likely role of the convergent neurons in the encoding of nociceptive and non-nociceptive sensory information. In this context, it appears to us that the existence within a neuronal population, of gradients of activity, the existence of which cannot be doubted when a painful focus occurs, at least for convergent cells in the rat, should be taken into consideration in pharmacological and biochemical studies concerning nociceptive transmission towards higher centres.

In any case, the future trends of our research undoubtedly lie in determining the supraspinal circuitry which subserves DNIC.

Acknowledgements

This work was supported by l'Institut National de la Santé et de la Recherche Médicale (INSERM) and la Direction des Recherches et Etudes Techniques (DRET).

The authors are very grateful to Drs. Besson, Bouhassira, Cadden, Calvino, Chaouch, Chitour, Dickenson, Kraus, Peschanski and Rivot, for their contribution to some aspects of this work, to Dr. Cadden for advice in the preparation of the manuscript, to Mrs. M. Cayla and M. Hoch for the dactylography, to E. Dehausse for the drawings and H. de Pommery for the photography.

References

Adair, E.E., Stevens, J.C. and Marks, L.E. (1968) Thermally induced pain: the dol scale and the psychological power law. *Am. J. Psychol.,* 81: 147 – 164.

Anderson, K.V., Pearl, G.S. and Honeycutt, C. (1976) Behavioural evidence showing the predominance of diffuse pain stimuli over discrete stimuli in influencing pain perception. *J. Neurosci. Res.,* 2: 283 – 289.

Andersson, S.A., Holmgren, E. and Roos, A. (1977) Analgesic effects of peripheral conditioning stimulation - II. Importance of certain stimulation parameters. Acupunct. *Electro-Ther. Res. Int. J.,* 2: 237 – 246.

Angaut-Petit, D. (1975a) The dorsal column system. I. Existence of long ascending post-synaptic fibres of the cat's fasciculus gracilis. *Exp. Brain Res.,* 22: 457 – 470.

Angaut-Petit, D. (1975b) The dorsal column system. II. Functional properties and bulbar relay of the post-synaptic fibres of the cat's fasciculus gracilis. *Exp. Brain Res.,* 22: 471 – 493.

Barbaro, N.H., Heinricher, M.M. and Fields, H.L. (1986) Putative pain modulating neurons in the rostral ventral medulla: reflex-related activity predicts effects of morphine. *Brain Res.* 366: 203 – 210.

Basbaum, A.I. and Fields, H.L. (1978) Endogenous pain control mechanisms: review and hypothesis. *Ann. Neurol.,* 4: 451 – 462.

Basbaum, A.I. and Fields, H.L. (1980) Pain control: a new role for the medullary reticular formation. In J.A. Hobson and M.A.B. Brazier (Eds.), *The Reticular Formation Revisited,* Raven Press, New York, pp. 329 – 348.

Belcher, G., Ryall, R.W. and Schaffner, R. (1978) The differential effects of 5-hydroxytryptamine, noradrenaline and raphe stimulation on nociceptive and non nociceptive dorsal horn interneurons in the cat. *Brain Res.,* 151: 307 – 321.

Besson, J.M., Catchlove, R.F.H., Feltz, P. and Le Bars, D. (1974) Further evidence for post-synaptic inhibitions on lamina V dorsal horn interneurons. *Brain Res.,* 66: 531 – 536.

Boivie, J. (1979) An anatomical reinvestigation of the termination of the spinothalamic tract in the monkey. *J. Comp. Neurol.,* 186: 343 – 370.

Bouhassira, D., Villanueva, L. and Le Bars, D. (1986) Effects of intraventricular (i.c.v.) morphine upon Diffuse Noxious Inhibitory Controls (DNIC) in the rat. *Neurosci. Lett.,* Suppl. 26: S140.

Bouhassira, D., Le Bars, D. and Villanueva, L. (1988) Heterotopic activation of Aδ and C fibres triggers inhibition of trigeminal and spinal convergent neurones in the rat. *J. Physiol. (Lond.),* 389: 301 – 317.

Bouhassira, D., Villanueva, L. and Le Bars, D. (1987b) Intracerebroventricular morphine restores the basic somesthetic activity of dorsal horn convergent neurones in the rat. *Eur. J. Pharmacol.,* in prress.

Bourgoin, S., Oliveras, J.L., Bruxelle, J., Hamon, M. and Besson, J.M. (1980) Electrical stimulation of the nucleus raphe magnus in the rat: effects on 5-HT metabolism in the spinal cord. *Brain Res.,* 194: 377 – 389.

Burgess, P.R. and Perl, E.R. (1973) Cutaneous mechanoreceptors and nociceptors. In A. Iggo (Ed.), *Handbook of Sensory Physiology,* Springer, Berlin, pp. 29 – 78.

Cadden, S.W., Villanueva, L., Chitour, D. and Le Bars, D. (1983) Depression of activities of dorsal horn convergent neurones by propriospinal mechanisms triggered by noxious inputs; comparison with Diffuse Noxious Inhibitory Controls (DNIC). *Brain Res.,* 275: 1 – 11.

Calvino, B. and Le Bars, D. (1986) The response to visceroperitoneal nociceptive stimuli is reduced in experimental arthritic rat. *Brain Res.,* 370: 191 – 195.

Calvino, B., Villanueva, L. and Le Bars, D. (1984) The heterotopic effects of visceral pain: behavioural and electrophysiological approaches in the rat. *Pain,* 20: 261 – 271.

Calvino, B., Crepon-Bernard, M.O. and Le Bars, D. (1987a) Parallel clinical and behavioural studies of adjuvant-induced arthritis in the rat: possible relationship with 'chronic pain'. *Behav. Brain Res.,* 24: 11 – 29.

Calvino, B., Villanueva, L. and Le Bars, D. (1987b) Dorsal horn (convergent) neurons in the intact anaesthetized arthritic rat. I. Segmental excitatory influences. *Pain,* 28: 81 – 98.

Calvino, B., Villanueva, L. and Le Bars, D. (1987c) Dorsal horn (convergent) neurons in the intact anaesthetized arthritic rat. II. Heterotopic inhibitory influences. *Pain,* 31: 359 – 379.

Cervero, F. and Wolstencroft, J.H (1984) A positive feedback loop between spinal cord nociceptive pathways and antinociceptive areas of the cat's brainstem. *Pain,* 20: 125 – 138.

Cheng, Z.F., Fields, H.L. and Heinricher, M.M. (1986) Morphine microinjected into the periaqueductal gray has differential effects on 3 classes of medullary neurons. *Brain Res.,* 375: 57 – 65.

Chitour, D., Dickenson, A.H. and Le Bars, D. (1982) Pharmacological evidence for the involvement of serotonergic mechanisms in Diffuse Noxious Inhibitory Controls (DNIC). *Brain Res.,* 236: 329 – 337.

Chung, J.M., Lee, K.H., Hori, Y., Endo, K. and Willis, W.D. (1984) Factors influencing peripheral nerve stimulation produced inhibition of primate spinothalamic tract cells. *Pain,* 19: 277 – 293.

Colpaert, F.C., Meert, T.H., De Witte, P.H. and Schmitt, P. (1982) Further evidence validating adjuvant arthritis as an experimental model of chronic pain in the rat. *Life Sci.,* 31: 67 – 75.

Craig, A.D. Jr. and Tapper, D.N. (1978) Lateral cervical nucleus in the cat: functional organization and characteristics. *J. Neurophysiol.,* 41: 1511 – 1534.

Curtis, D.R., Phillis, J.W. and Watkins, J.C. (1959) Chemical excitation of spinal neurons. *Nature (Lond.),* 183: 611 – 612.

Curtis, D.R., Phillis, J.W. and Watkins, J.C. (1960) The chemical excitation of spinal neurones by certain acidic amino-acids. *J. Physiol. (Lond.),* 150: 656 – 682.

Dahlström, A. and Fuxe, K. (1965) Evidence for the existence of monoamine neuron in the central nervous system. II. Experimentally induced changes in the intraneuronal amine levels of bulbospinal neuron system. *Acta Physiol. Scand.,* 64, Suppl. 247: 1 – 36.

De Castro Costa, M., De Sutter, P., Gybels, J. and Van Hees, J. (1981) Adjuvant induced arthritis in rats; a possible model of chronic pain. *Pain,* 10: 173 – 186.

Dickenson, A.H. and Le Bars, D. (1983a) Morphine microinjections into periaqueductal grey matter of the rat: effects on dorsal horn neuronal responses to C-fibre activity and diffuse Noxious Inhibitory Controls. *Life Sci.,* 33S1: 549 – 554.

Dickenson, A.H. and Le Bars, D. (1983b) Diffuse Noxious Inhibitory Controls (DNIC) involve trigeminothalamic and spinothalamic neurons in the rat. *Exp. Brain Res.,* 49: 174 – 180.

Dickenson, A.H. and Le Bars, D. (1987) Supraspinal morphine and descending inhibitions acting on the dorsal horn of the rat. *J. Physiol. (Lond.),* 384: 81 – 107.

Dickenson, A.H., Le Bars, D. and Besson, J.M. (1980a) Diffuse Noxious Inhibitory Controls (DNIC). Effects on trigeminal nucleus caudalis neurons in the rat. *Brain Res.,* 200: 293 – 305.

Dickenson, A.H., Le Bars, D. and Besson, J.M. (1980b) An involvement of nucleus raphe magnus in diffuse noxious inhibitory controls (DNIC) in the rat. *Neurosci. Lett.,* Suppl. 5: S375.

Dickenson, A.H., Rivot, J.P., Chaouch, A., Besson, J.M. and Le Bars, D. (1981) Diffuse Noxious Inhibitory Controls (DNIC) in the rat with or without pCPA pretreatment. *Brain Res.,* 216: 313 – 321.

Dubner, R. and Beitel, E. (1976) Peripheral neural correlates of escape behavior in rhesus monkey to noxious heat applied to the face. In: J.J. Bonica and D. Albe-Fessard (Eds.), *Advances in Pain Research and Therapy, Vol. 1,* Raven Press, New York, pp. 155 – 160.

Fields, H.L. and Basbaum, A.I. (1978) Brain stem control of spinal pain transmission neurons. *Annu. Rev. Physiol.,* 40: 193 – 221.

Fields, H.L. and Basbaum, A.I. (1984) Endogenous pain control mechanisms. In P.D. Wall and R. Melzack (Eds.), *Textbook of Pain,* Churchill Livingstone, Edinburgh, pp. 142 – 152.

Fields, H.L., Vanegas, H., Hentall, I.D. and Zorman, G. (1983) Evidence that disinhibition of brain stem neurones contributes to morphine analgesia. *Nature,* 306: 684 – 686.

Fitzgerald, M. (1982) The contralateral input to the dorsal horn of the spinal cord in the decerebrate spinal rat. *Brain Res.,* 236: 275 – 287.

Foerster, O. and Gagel, O. (1931) Die Vorderseitenstrangdurchschneidung beim Menschen. Eine Klinisch-pathophysiologische-anatomische Studie. *Z. Ges. Neurol. Psychiat.,* 138: 1 – 92.

Gasser, H.S. and Erlanger, J. (1927) The role played by the sizes of the constituent fibers of a nerve trunk in determining the form of its action potential wave. *Am. J. Physiol.,* 80: 522 – 547.

Gerhart, K.D., Yezierski, R.P., Giesler, G.J. Jr. and Willis, W.D. (1981) Inhibitory receptive fields of primate spinothalamic tract cells. *J. Neurophysiol.,* 46: 1309 – 1325.

Giesler, G.J. Jr. and Cliffer, K.D. (1985) Post-synaptic dorsal column pathway of the rat. II. Evidence against an important role in nociception. *Brain Res.,* 326: 347 – 356.

Giesler, G.J. Jr., Menetrey, D. and Basbaum, A.I. (1979) Differential origins of spinothalamic tract projections to medial and lateral thalamus in the rat. *J. Comp. Neurol.,* 184: 107 – 126.

Giesler, G.J. Jr., Yezierski, R.P., Gerhart, K.D. and Willis, W.D. (1981a) Spinothalamic tract neurons that project to medial and/or lateral thalamic nuclei: evidence for a physiologically novel population of spinal cord neurons. *J. Neurophysiol.,* 46: 1285 – 1308.

Giesler, G.J. Jr., Spiel, H.R. and Willis, W.D. (1981b) Organization of spinothalamic tract axons within the rat spinal cord. *J. Comp. Neurol.,* 195: 243 – 252.

Giesler, G.J. Jr., Gerhart, K.D., Yezierski, R.P., Wilcox, T.K. and Willis, W.D. (1981c) Postsynaptic inhibition of primate spinothalamic neurons by stimulation in nucleus raphe magnus. *Brain Res.,* 204: 184 – 188.

Giesler, G.J. Jr., Nahin, R.L. and Madsen, A. (1984) Postsynaptic dorsal column pathway of the rat. I. Anatomical studies. *J. Neurophysiol.,* 51: 260 – 275.

Guilbaud, G., Iggo, A. and Tegner, R. (1985) Sensory receptors in ankle joint capsules of normal and arthritic rats. *Exp. Brain Res.,* 58: 29 – 40.

Gybels, J., Handwerker, H.O. and Van Hees, J. (1979) Comparison between the discharges of human nociceptive nerve fibres and the subject's rating of his sensation. *J. Physiol., (Lond.),* 292: 193 – 206.

Hammond, D.L., Tyce, G.M. and Yaksh, T.L. (1985) Efflux of 5-hydroxytryptamine and noradrenaline into spinal cord superfusates during stimulation of the rat medulla. *J. Physiol. (Lond.),* 359: 151 – 162.

Han, J.S. and Terenius, L. (1982) Neurochemical basis of

acupuncture analgesia. Annu. Rev. Pharmacol. Toxicol., 22: 193 – 220.

Hardy, J.D., Goodell, H. and Wolff, H.G. (1951) The influence of skin temperature upon the pain threshold as evoked by thermal radiation. Science, 114: 149 – 150.

Hazouri, L.A. and Mueller, A.D. (1950) Pain threshold studies on paraplegic patients. Arch. Neurol. Psychiat., 64: 607 – 613.

Jordan, L.M., Kenshalo, D.R., Martin, R.F., Haber, L.H. and Willis, W.D. (1978) Depression of primate spinothalamic tract neurons by iontophoretic application of 5-hydroxytryptamine. Pain, 5: 135 – 142.

Kawakita, K. and Funakoshi, M. (1982) Suppression of the jaw-opening reflex by conditioning A-delta fiber stimulation and electroacupuncture in the rat. Exp. Neurol., 78: 461 – 465.

Kayser, V. and Guilbaud, G. (1981) Dose-dependent analgesic and hyperalgesic effects of systemic naloxone in arthritic rats. Brain Res., 226: 344 – 348.

Kayser, V. and Guilbaud, G. (1983) The analgesic effects of morphine, but not those of the enkephalinase inhibitor Thiorphan, are enhanced in arthritic rats. Brain Res., 267: 131 – 138.

Kerr, F.W.L. (1975) The ventral spinothalamic tract and other ascending systems of the ventral funiculus of the spinal cord. J. Comp. Neurol., 159: 335 – 356.

Kraus, E. and Le Bars, D. (1986) Morphine antagonizes inhibitory controls of nociceptive reactions, triggered by visceral pain in the rat. Brain Res., 379: 151 – 156.

Lamotte, R.H. and Campbell, J.N. (1978) Comparison of responses of warm and nociceptive C fiber afferent in monkey with human judgements of thermal pain. J. Neurophysiol., 41: 509 – 528.

Le Bars, D. and Chitour, D. (1983) Do convergent neurones in the spinal cord discriminate nociceptive from non-nociceptive information? Pain, 17: 1 – 19.

Le Bars, D., Dickenson, A.H. and Besson, J.M. (1979a) Diffuse Noxious Inhibitory Controls (DNIC). 1. Effects on dorsal horn convergent neurons in the rat. Pain, 6: 283 – 304.

Le Bars, D., Dickenson, A.H. and Besson, J.M. (1979b) Diffuse Noxious Inhibitory Controls (DNIC). II. Lack of effect on non convergent neurons, supraspinal involvement and theoretical implications. Pain, 6: 305 – 327.

Le Bars, D., Chitour, D. and Clot, A.M. (1981a) The encoding of thermal stimuli by Diffuse Noxious Inhibitory Controls (DNIC). Brain Res., 230: 394 – 399.

Le Bars, D., Chitour, D., Kraus, E., Clot, A.M., Dickenson, A.H. and Besson, J.M. (1981b) The effect of systemic morphine upon Diffuse Noxious Inhibitory Controls (DNIC) in the rat: evidence for a lifting of certain descending inhibitory controls of dorsal horn convergent neurons. Brain Res., 215: 257 – 274.

Le Bars, D., Chitour, D., Kraus, E., Dickenson, A.H. and Besson, J.M. (1981c) Effect of naloxone upon Diffuse Noxious Inhibitory Controls (DNIC) in the rat. Brain Res., 204: 387 – 402.

Le Bars, D., Dickenson, A.H., Rivot, J.P., Chitour, D., Chaouch, A., Kraus, E. and Besson, J.M. (1981d) Les systèmes sérotonergiques bulbo-spinaux jouent-ils un rôle dans la détection des messages nociceptifs? J. Physiol. (Paris), 77: 463 – 471.

Le Bars, D., Dickenson, A.H. and Besson, J.M. (1982) The triggering of bulbo-spinal serotonergic inhibitory controls by noxious peripheral inputs. In B. Sjölund and A. Björklund (Eds.), Brain Stem Control of Spinal Mechanisms, Fernström Foundation, Series 1, Elsevier, Amsterdam, pp. 381 – 340.

Le Bars, D., Dickenson, A.H. and Besson, J.M. (1983) Opiate analgesia and descending control systems. In J.J. Bonica, U. Lindblom and A. Iggo (Eds.), Advances in Pain Research and Therapy, Vol. 5, Raven Press, New York, pp. 341 – 372.

Le Bars, D., Calvino, B., Villanueva, L. and Cadden, S. (1984) Physiological approaches to counter-irritation phenomena. In M.D. Tricklebank and G. Curzon (Eds.), Stress-induced Analgesia, John Wiley, Chichester, pp. 67 – 101.

Le Bars, D., Dickenson, A., Besson, J.M. and Villanueva, L. (1986) Aspects of sensory processing through convergent neurons. In T.L. Yaksh (Ed.), Spinal Afferent Processing, Plenum Publishing Corporation, New York, pp. 467 – 504.

Le Bars, D., Bourgoin, S., Clot, A.M., Hamon, M. and Cesselin, F. (1987a) Noxious mechanical stimuli increase the release of Met-enkephalin-like material heterosegmentally in the rat spinal cord. Brain Res., 402: 188 – 192.

Le Bars, D., Bourgoin, S., Villanueva, L., Clot, A.M., Hamon, M. and Cesselin, F. (1987b) Involvement of the dorsolateral funiculi in the spinal release of Met-enkephalin-like material triggered by heterosegmental noxious mechanical stimuli. Brain Res., 412: 190 – 195.

Le Bars, D., Dickenson, A.H., Villanueva, L. and Bouhassira, D. (1987c) Electrophysiological studies on the mechanism of action of opiates. In P. Scherpereel, J. Meynadier and S. Blond (Eds.), The Pain Clinic, II, VNU Science Press, Utrecht, pp. 35 – 67.

Lee, H.K., Chung, J.M. and Willis, W.D. (1985) Inhibition of primate spinothalamic tract cells by TENS. J. Neurosurg., 2: 276 – 287.

Liebeskind, J.C., Giesler, G.J. Jr. and Urca, G. (1976) Evidence pertaining to an endogenous mechanism of pain inhibition in the central nervous system. In I. Zotterman (Ed.), Sensory Functions of the Skin in Primates, Pergamon Press, Oxford, pp. 561 – 573.

Lipman, J.J., Blumenkopf, B. and Parris, W.C.V. (1987) Chronic pain assessment using heat beam dolorimetry. Pain, 30: 59 – 67.

Lundberg, A. and Oscarsson, O. (1961) Three ascending spinal pathways in the dorsal part of the lateral funiculus. Acta Physiol. Scand. 51: 1 – 16.

Mc Creery, D. and Bloedel, J.R. (1976) Effect of trigeminal

298

stimulation on the excitability of cat spinothalamic neurons. *Brain Res.,* 117: 136–140.

Mann, F. (1974) Acupuncture analgesia, report of 100 experiments. *Br. J. Anaesth.,* 46: 361–364.

Mayer, D.J. (1979) Endogenous analgesia systems: neural and behavioral mechanisms. In J.J. Bonica, J.C. Liebeskind and D. Albe-Fessard (Eds.), *Advances in Pain Research and Therapy, Vol. 3,* Raven Press, New York, pp. 385–410.

Mayer, D.J. and Price, D.D. (1976) Central nervous system mechanisms of analgesia. *Pain,* 2: 379–404.

Mehler, W.R. (1969) Some neurological species differences – a posteriori. *Ann. NY Acad. Sci.,* 167: 424–468.

Mehler, W.R., Feferman, M.E. and Nauta, W.J.H. (1960) Ascending axon degeneration following anterolateral cordotomy: an experimental study in monkey. *Brain,* 83: 718–750.

Melzack, R. (1984) Acupuncture and related forms of folk medicine. In P.D. Wall and R. Melzack (Eds.), *Textbook of Pain,* Churchill Livingstone, Edinburgh, pp. 691–700.

Menétrey, D. and Besson, J.M. (1982) Electrophysiological characteristics of dorsal horn cells in rats with cutaneous inflammation resulting from chronic arthritis. *Pain,* 13: 343–364.

Merskey, H. and Evans, P.R. (1975) Variations in pain complaint threshold in psychiatric and neurological patients with pain. *Pain,* 1: 73–79.

Morin, F. (1955) A new spinal pathway for cutaneous impulses. *Am. J. Physiol.,* 183: 245–252.

Morton, C.R., Maisch, B. and Zimmerman, M.(1987) Diffuse noxious inhibitory controls of lumbar spinal neurons involve a supraspinal loop in the cat. *Brain Res.,* 410: 347–352.

Niemegeers, C.J.E., Van Bruggen, J.A.A. and Janssen, P.A.J. (1975) Suprofen, a potent antagonist of acetic-induced writhing in rat. *Arzneim. Forsch.,* 25: 1505–1509.

Pearson, C.M. and Wood, F.D. (1959) Studies of polyarthritis and other lesions induced in rats by injection of mycobacterial adjuvant. I. General clinical and pathological characteristics and some modifying factors. *Arthr. Rheum.,* 2: 440–459.

Peschanski, M., Guilbaud, G., Lam Lee, C. and Mantyh, P.W. (1983) Involvement of the rat ventrobasal thalamic complex in the sensory-discriminative aspects of pain: electrophysiological and anatomical data. In G. Macchi, A. Rustioni and R. Spreafico (Eds.), *Somatosensory Integration in the Thalamus,* Elsevier, Amsterdam, pp. 147–163.

Pilowsky, P.M., Kapour, V., Minson, J.B., West, M.J. and Chalmers, J.P. (1986) Spinal cord serotonin release and raised blood pressure after brainstem kainic acid injection. *Brain Res.,* 366: 354–357.

Pircio, A., Fedele, C.T. and Bierwagen, M.E. (1975) A new method for the evaluation of analgesic activity using adjuvant induced arthritis in the rat. *Eur. J. Pharmacol.,* 31: 207–215.

Puil, E. (1981) S-glutamate: its interactions with spinal

neurons. *Brain Res. Rev.* 3: 229–322.

Randall, L.O. and Selitto, J.J. (1957) A method for measurement of analgesic activity on inflamed tissue. *Arch. Int. Pharmacodyn.,* 151: 409–419.

Rivot, J.P., Chaouch, A. and Besson, J.M. (1979) The influence of naloxone on the C-fiber response of dorsal horn neurons and their inhibitory control by raphe magnus stimulation. *Brain Res.,* 176: 355–364.

Rivot, J.P., Chaouch, A. and Besson, J.M. (1980) Nucleus raphé magnus modulation of response of rat dorsal horn neurons to unmyelinated fiber inputs: partial involvement of serotonergic pathways. *J. Neurophysiol.,* 44: 1039–1057.

Rivot, J.P., Chiang, C.Y. and Besson, J.M. (1982) Increase in serotonin metabolism within the dorsal horn of the spinal cord during nucleus raphé magnus stimulation, as revealed by in vivo electrochemical detection. *Brain Res.,* 238: 117–126.

Roby-Brami, A., Bussel, B., Willer, J.C. and Le Bars, D. (1987) An electrophysiological investigation into the pain-relieving effects of heterotopic nociceptive stimuli: possible involvement of a supraspinal loop. *Brain,* 110: 69–80.

Schouenborg, J. and Dickenson, A. (1985) The effects of a distant noxious stimulation on A and C fibre evoked flexion reflexes and neuronal activity in dorsal horn of the rat. *Brain Res.,* 328: 23–32.

Sjölund, B.H. (1985) Peripheral nerve suppression of C-fiber-evoked flexion reflex in rats. I. parameters of continuous stimulation. *J. Neurosurg.,* 63: 612–616.

Skagerberg, G. and Björklund, A. (1985) Topographic principles in the spinal projections of serotonergic and non-serotonergic brainstem neurons in the rat. *Neuroscience,* 15: 445–480.

Torebjörk, H.E., Lamotte, R.H. and Robinson, C. (1984) Peripheral neural correlates of magnitude of cutaneous pain and hyperalgesia: simultaneous recordings in humans of sensory judgements of pain and evoked responses in nociceptors with C-fibers. *J. Neurophysiol.,* 51: 325–329.

Tyce, G.M. and Yaksh, T.L. (1981) Monoamine release from cat spinal cord by somatic stimuli: an intrinsic modulatory system. *J. Physiol. (Lond.),* 314: 513–529.

Uddenberg, N. (1968) Functional organization of long, second-order afferents in the dorsal funiculus. *Exp. Brain Res.,* 4: 377–382.

Van Hees, J. and Gybels, J. (1981) C-nociceptor activity in human nerve during painful and non painful skin stimulation. *J. Neurol. Psychiat.,* 44: 600–607.

Villanueva, L. and Le Bars, D. (1985) The encoding of thermal stimuli applied to the tail of the rat by lowering the excitability of trigeminal convergent neurones. *Brain Res.,* 330: 245–251.

Villanueva, L. and Le Bars, D. (1986) Indirect effects of intrathecal morphine upon Diffuse Noxious Inhibitory Controls (DNIC) in the rat. *Pain,* 26: 233–243.

Villanueva, L., Cadden, S.W. and Le Bars, D. (1984a)

Evidence that Diffuse Noxious Inhibitory Controls (DNIC) are mediated by a final post-synaptic inhibitory mechanism. *Brain Res.,* 298: 67 – 74.

Villanueva, L., Cadden, S.W. and Le Bars, D. (1984b) Diffuse Noxious Inhibitory Controls (DNIC): evidence for post-synaptic inhibition of trigeminal nucleus caudalis convergent neurons. *Brain Res.,* 321: 165 – 168.

Villanueva, L., Peschanski, M., Calvino, B. and Le Bars, D. (1986a) Ascending pathways in the spinal cord involved in triggering of Diffuse Noxious Inhibitory Controls (DNIC) in the rat. *J. Neurophysiol.,* 55: 34 – 55.

Villanueva, L., Chitour, D. and Le Bars, D. (1986b) Involvement of the dorsolateral funiculus in the descending spinal projections responsible for Diffuse Noxious Inhibitory Controls in the rat. *J. Neurophysiol.,* 56: 1185 – 1195.

Weil-Fugazza, J., Godefroy, F. and Le Bars, D. (1984) Increase in 5-HT synthesis in the dorsal part of the spinal cord, induced by a nociceptive stimulus: blockade by morphine. *Brain Res.,* 297: 247 – 264.

Willer, J.C., Roby, A. and Le Bars, D. (1984) Psychophysical and electrophysiological approaches to the pain relieving effect of heterotopic nociceptive stimuli. *Brain,* 107: 1095 – 1112.

Willer, J.C., Barranquero, A., Kahn, M.F. and Salliere, D. (1987) Pain in sciatica depresses lower limb cutaneous reflexes to sural nerve stimulation. *J. Neurol. Neurosurg. Psychiat.,* 50: 1 – 5.

Willis, W.D., Kenshalo, D.R. Jr. and Leonard, R.B. (1979) The cells of origin of the primate spinothalamic tract. *J. Comp. Neurol.,* 188: 543 – 574.

Wolff, H.G., Hardy, J.D. and Goodell, H. (1940) Studies on pain. Measurement of the effect of morphine, codeine and other opiates on the pain threshold, and an analysis of their relation to the pain experience. *J. Clin. Invest.,* 19: 659 – 680.

Woolf, C.J., Mitchell, D. and Barrett, G.D. (1980) Antinociceptive effect of peripheral segmental electrical stimulation in the rat. *Pain,* 8: 237 – 252.

Yaksh, T.L. (1981) Spinal opiate analgesia: characteristics and principles of action. *Pain,* 11: 293 – 346.

Yeung, J.C. and Rudy, T.A. (1980) Multiplicative interaction between narcotic agonisms expressed at spinal and supraspinal sites of antinociceptive action as revealed by concurrent intrathecal and intracerebroventricular injections of morphine. *J. Pharmacol. Exp. Ther.,* 215: 633 – 642.

Zemlan, F.P., Leonard, C.M., Kuw, L.M. and Pfaff, D.W. (1978) Ascending tracts of the lateral columns of the rat spinal cord: a study using the silver impregnation and horseradish peroxidase techniques. *Exp. Neurol.,* 62: 298 – 334.

H.L. Fields and J.-M. Besson (Eds.)
Progress in Brain Research, Vol. 77
© 1988 Elsevier Science Publishers B.V. (Biomedical Division)

301

Paradoxical effects of low doses of naloxone in experimental models of inflammatory pain

V. Kayser, J.-M. Besson and G. Guilbaud

Unité de Recherches de Neurophysiologie Pharmacologique, INSERM, U. 161, 75014 Paris, France

Introduction

The major problem related to the functional significance of the endogenous opioid systems is to understand how they are triggered. Many questions remain to be answered, including their possible tonic activity.

In order to establish a possible involvement of these systems in the modulation of pain, numerous studies have been based upon the effects of the opiate receptor antagonist naloxone on various behavioural tests in animals or pain perception in humans. Contradictory results have been reported, some authors finding the expected hyperalgesic effects (Lasagna, 1965; Jacob et al., 1974; Frederickson et al., 1976; Pomeranz and Chiu, 1976; Berntson and Walker, 1977; Grevert and Goldstein, 1977; Kokka and Fairhurst, 1977; Walker et al., 1977; Amir and Amit, 1978; Grevert et al., 1978; Jacob and Ramabadran, 1978; Levine et al., 1978; Carmody et al., 1979; Dehen et al., 1979; Levine et al., 1979; Ramabadran and Jacob, 1979; Coderre and Rollman, 1983; Gracely et al., 1983; Costentin et al., 1986; Ueda et al., 1986), others claiming a lack of effect (Evans et al., 1974; Tulunay et al., 1975; Elliot et al., 1976; El Sobky et al., 1976; Goldstein et al., 1976; Pert and Walter, 1976; Yaksh et al., 1976, Berntson and Walker, 1977; Dykstra and Mc Millan, 1977; Grevert and Goldstein, 1977, 1978; Amir and Amit, 1978; North, 1978; Kaplan and Glick, 1979;

Lindblom and Tegner, 1979; Rosenfeld and Rice, 1979; Satoh et al., 1979; Millan et al., 1987) or, more rarely, a hypoalgesic effect (Lasagna, 1965; Sewell and Spencer, 1976; Buchsbaum et al., 1977; Chesher and Chan, 1977; Pinski et al., 1978; Ferreira and Nakamura, 1979; Levine et al., 1979; Woolf, 1980; Dickenson et al., 1981; Rios and Jacob, 1983; Levine and Gordon, 1986; Ueda et al., 1986). It was suggested that the controversy may be partly due to a disregard of individual variations in pain responsiveness either in man (Buchsbaum et al., 1977; Dehen et al., 1979; Levine et al., 1979) or in animals (Satoh et al., 1979). However, such a discrepancy has also been reported in various electrophysiological investigations, including studies with spinalized animals (see Refs. in Duggan and North, 1984; Besson and Chaouch, 1987).

The aim of the present study was to evaluate the effects of naloxone in an experimental model of chronic inflammatory pain in rats rendered polyarthritic by the injection of Freund's adjuvant into the tail (Pearson et al., 1961; Gouret et al., 1976). Interestingly, in these animals, which experience a diffuse, persistent inflammatory state, there are changes in endogenous opioid peptides: their levels are increased in the central nervous system, mainly in the spinal cord (Cesselin et al., 1980; Faccini et al., 1984; Przewlocki et al., 1985; Höllt et al., 1987), while their release into the CSF is apparently diminished (Cesselin et al., 1984). In addition, in these animals, the antinociceptive effects of morphine are more pronounced than in normal rats (Pircio et al., 1975; Colpaert, 1979; Kayser and Guilbaud, 1983).

Further, we examined the effects of naloxone in another model of inflammation induced by the intraplantar injection of carrageenin (Winter et al., 1962; Vinegar et al., 1969; Di Rosa et al., 1971; Roch-Arveiller et al., 1977). By contrast to arthritic animals, this model exhibits a localized and acute inflammatory process with a brief time course which can be followed over a few hours.

As a nociceptive test, we used the measure of the vocalization threshold to paw pressure. This test, commonly used to evaluate the activity of anti-inflammatory and antinociceptive drugs, appeared particularly well suited to assess drug effects in arthritic and carrageenin-injected rats, which exhibit an hyperalgesic inflammation.

Some of this data have previously been published (Kayser and Guilbaud, 1981, 1987a; Kayser et al., 1986a).

Methods

Experiments were performed in male Sprague-Dawley arthritic rats and normal rats, all 9 – 10 weeks old, weighing respectively 200 – 225 g and 250 – 290 g, obtained from Charles River, France.

The rats were allowed to habituate to the colony room for at least 7 days before the experiments.

Arthritic rats were used 21 days after the induction of arthritis by inoculation at the breeding center (Charles River, France) of Freund's adjuvant at the base of the tail. At this time, the arthritic lesions and the concomitant humoral changes are at a stable maximum (Gouret et al., 1976; Calvino et al., 1987). In addition, as previously described (Kayser and Guilbaud, 1981), the rats exhibited a clear decrease in vocalization threshold to paw pressure in comparison with normal rats. Since these conditions induce a certain amount of suffering, the guidelines proposed by the Committee for Research and Ethical Issues of the IASP (1980) have been followed. In particular,

the experiment duration was as short as possible and the number of rats used was kept to a minimum. In addition to the general housing conditions used for the normal rats (animal room at a constant temperature of 22°C with a 12-h alternating light-dark cycle), particular dispositions were kept. The rats were housed 4 – 5 to a large cage, the floor of which was covered with sawdust; this arrangement minimised the possibility of painful interactions between rats placed in closed contact. The food was directly available on the sawdust in the cages to minimise the need for the animals to make potentially painful movements to obtain food that they could receive ad libitum. Indeed, although the arthritic animals were less active than normal rats, they ate and drank unaided.

The vocalization threshold to paw pressure was measured using the Basile analgesimeter (Apelex). Increasing pressure was applied to the hindpaw, until an audible squeak was elicited. Prior to the test phase, rats had no experience with the testing apparatus.

For each rat, preliminary threshold determinations spaced by at least 5 min were carried out, until two consecutive tests with thresholds varying by not more than 10% were obtained (the mean of these served as baseline), then naloxone or morphine was injected intravenously into the tail. Nociceptive pressure thresholds were then determined every 5 or 10 min after the drug injection for a period of at least 30 min. Results are expressed as a percentage of the control (mean of the two control values measured before the acute injection). Statistical analyses were carried out with the Student's t test. When p values were greater than 0.05, differences were not considered to be significant.

Arthritic animals

The effects of an acute injection of naloxone (1 to 3000 μg/kg) administered intravenously into the tail were determined in arthritic animals. The effects of the same doses of naloxone were also determined in normal rats.

Control arthritic and normal rats received an acute injection either of saline or Fixanal (a buffer solution with a pH = 6 equivalent to that of the naloxone solution).

The effects of the same doses of naloxone were also examined in arthritic animals rendered tolerant with repeated large or low doses of subcutaneous (s.c.) morphine. In the first case, treatment consisted of administering increasing doses in a sustained release preparation according to the technique of Collier et al. (1972) with minor modifications. A single dose of morphine was administered every day for 4 days (40 mg/kg on day 1, 80 mg/kg on day 2, 120 mg/kg on day 3 and 160 mg/kg on day 4). It has previously been shown that this morphine pretreatment renders arthritic rats tolerant to morphine (the mean peak value of the antinociceptive effect of 1 mg/kg i.v. morphine decreased by about 60% in these morphine pretreated animals; Kayser and Guilbaud, 1985). Control arthritic rats were injected with the vehicle only, for 4 consecutive days.

In the second case, arthritic animals were pretreated with morphine 3 000 μg/kg s.c. It has been shown that this dose induces antinociceptive effects roughly similar to those observed with 1 mg/kg i.v. morphine, and is sufficient to induce tolerance, when injected twice daily over 4 days in arthritic rats (mean peak value of the analgesic effect of 1 mg/kg i.v. morphine decreased by 54% in these pretreated animals as extensively described by Kayser et al., 1986b). Control arthritic animals were injected twice daily for 4 days with saline. The repeated large or low doses of morphine used did not affect weight development or initial nociceptive thresholds (Kayser and Guilbaud, 1985, 1986b).

The effects of naloxone were determined on day 5, 24 h after the last s.c. morphine or saline injection. The higher doses of naloxone induced some signs of withdrawal such as diarrhoea in morphine-pretreated rats.

Since low doses of naloxone (as detailed further) induce paradoxical antinociceptive effects which peak at 3 μg/kg i.v. in naive arthritic rats, further experiments were devoted to the following questions: (a) is chronic pretreatment with low doses of naloxone able to reduce the paradoxical antinociceptive effect of this drug? (b) what is the antinociceptive effect of morphine in these naloxone-pretreated rats?

In these two experimental series, rats were pretreated with 9 μg/kg naloxone s.c. twice daily during 4 days. This 9 μg/kg dose of naloxone s.c. was chosen since it induces an antinociceptive effect roughly equivalent to that obtained in these rats with 3 μg/kg i.v. Control arthritic animals were pretreated with Fixanal (a buffer solution with a pH = 6 equivalent to that of naloxone solution).

The effects of naloxone (3 μg/kg i.v.) or morphine (1 mg/kg i.v.) were evaluated in these animals on day 5, 24 h after the last chronic naloxone or Fixanal injection.

Carrageenin-injected animals

For each rat, preliminary threshold determinations were performed as described above in the methods, then λ-carrageenin (Satia Laboratory, Paris) (0.2 ml of 1% solution) or saline was injected subcutaneously in the right plantar area of the hindpaw. Vocalization thresholds were then determined 1, 4 or 24 h after injection of carrageenin. Thereafter, naloxone or saline in the same volume was administered i.v. and thresholds for vocalization were measured every 5 min for at least 30 min. Thresholds were expressed as a percentage of pre-naloxone control values.

Taking into account the results obtained in arthritic rats, only one dose of naloxone (3 μg/kg i.v.) was tested in these carrageenin-injected rats.

Results

For the whole experimental series, these various doses of naloxone did not induce significant modifications of the vocalization threshold in normal naive rats (Fig. 1, E and F).

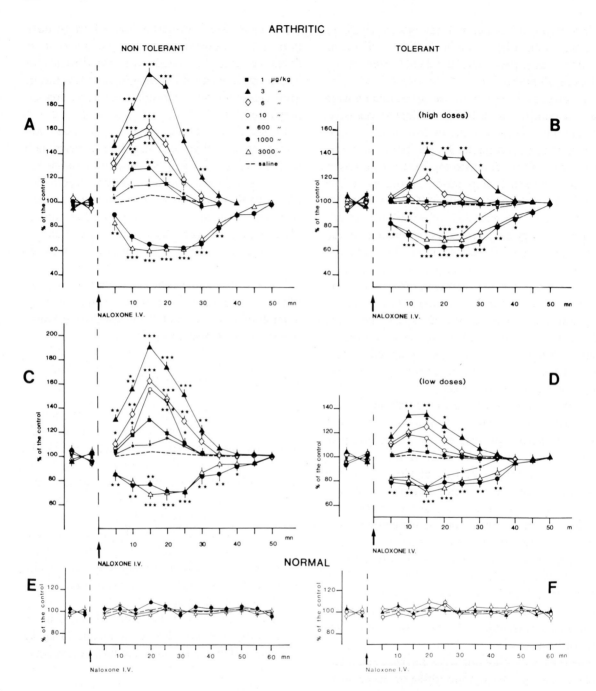

Fig. 1. Mean curves of naloxone effects upon the threshold for vocalization ($\pm$ SEM) expressed as percentages of the control in tolerant and non-tolerant arthritic rats and in normal rats. The arthritic rats were rendered tolerant with repeated administration of high doses (B) or low (D) doses of morphine. Non-tolerant arthritic rats were pretreated with vehicle (A) or saline (C) ($n = 9$ in each group of rats). The mean curves obtained with Fixanal (pH equivalent to that of the naloxone solution), not illustrated in the Fig., were similar to those of saline. * $p < 0.05$; ** $p < 0.01$; *** $p < 0.001$; Student's t test.

Arthritic rats

Effects of naloxone

The effects of naloxone were determined in various successive experimental series using a large range of doses (1, 3, 6, 10, 600, 1 000 and 3 000 μg/kg i.v.) (Fig. 1).

A bi-directional effect of naloxone was clearly observed in naive rats. Hyperalgesia was observed for high doses (1 000 and 3 000 μg/kg i.v.). For both doses, the vocalization threshold to paw pressure was decreased by about 30% at the moment of maximum effect (Fig. 1, A and C). Such a decrease coexisted with behavioural manifestations, the rats being more reactive to the manipulations, and vocalizing loudly in response to touch.

By contrast, lower doses of naloxone produced a paradoxical antinociceptive effect. Already significant at 600 μg/kg i.v., this antinociceptive effect progressively increased as the naloxone dose was decreased. It peaked at 3 μg/kg i.v. For this latter dose, the antinociceptive effect was potent, with an increased threshold of about 90%. This was comparable to the antinociceptive effect induced by morphine 1 mg/kg i.v. in arthritic rats. As is shown in the two large series of experiments we have performed (Fig. 1, A and C), the effects are reproducible when considering the dose-response relationship and the time-course of the effect. For example, for the two series at the 3 μg/kg dose of naloxone, the maximum increases in threshold were of 107.1 ± 5.8% and 90.5 ± 4.3%, respectively ($n = 9$ in each group).

Effects of naloxone in morphine-tolerant rats

In the rats rendered tolerant to morphine's antinociceptive effects with repeated administration of high (Fig. 1, B) or low (Fig. 1, D) doses of morphine, the paradoxical antinociceptive effects of naloxone (1, 3, 6, 10 μg/kg i.v.) were significantly reduced in a dose-dependent manner. The linear regression from 10 to 3 μg/kg i.v. after pretreatment with low doses of morphine was $r = 0.97$, $n = 27$, $p < 0.001$. For example, in the two series, the paradoxical antinociceptive effects of naloxone

with the dose of 3 μg/kg i.v. were decreased by 33% and 29%, respectively (Fig. 1, B and D).

In contrast, the hyperalgesic effect induced by higher doses of naloxone (1 000 and 3 000 μg/kg i.v.) remained unmodified by morphine pretreatment in comparison with saline-pretreated rats. This was observed whether the rats were rendered tolerant using high or low doses of morphine (Fig. 1, B and D).

Effects of naloxone in 'naloxone-tolerant' rats

In rats pretreated with naloxone (9 μg/kg s.c.) twice daily for 4 days, the paradoxical antinociceptive effect of naloxone (3 μg/kg i.v.) was almost abolished. The increase in vocalization threshold dropped from 88% in control animals to 16% of the control value in naloxone-pretreated rats (Fig. 2). Moreover, a detailed analysis of the time-course of the effects of this dose of naloxone revealed that the initial increase in vocalization threshold was followed by a significant decrease in the vocalization threshold to paw pressure. Interestingly, the doses of 10 and 600 μg/kg i.v.

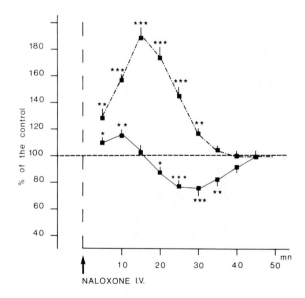

Fig. 2. Mean curves of the effects of naloxone (2 μg/kg i.v.) in arthritic rats pretreated twice daily for 4 days either with naloxone 9 μg/kg s.c. (continuous lines) or Fixanal (discontinuous lines) administered in same volume ($n = 9$ in each dose). * $p < 0.05$; ** $p < 0.01$; *** $p < 0.001$; Student's t test.

naloxone, which induced an increase in threshold in naive arthritic rats, elicited a significant decrease in threshold in naloxone-pretreated rats (Kayser and Guilbaud, 1987a).

Effects of morphine in 'naloxone-tolerant' rats

In these experimental conditions, the classical potent antinociceptive effects of morphine (100 to 1 000 μg/kg i.v.) were significantly and dose-dependently decreased (Fig. 3). With 1 mg/kg of morphine, the mean elevation in threshold dropped from 104% in the naive to 44% in the naloxone-pretreated rats. The linear regression from 100, 300, 500 and 1 000 μg/kg i.v. morphine was $r = 0.94$, $n = 36$, $p < 0.001$.

Since the paradoxical antinociceptive effects of naloxone were not observed in normal rats, they appear to be related to the fact that the arthritic animals are in a state of persistent inflammation. This led us to determine if such a modification could also be exhibited in another model of inflammatory pain, the carrageenin-induced rat paw oedema.

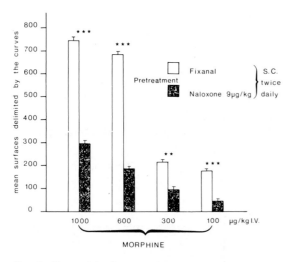

Fig. 3. Comparison between the mean surfaces (± SEM) calculated for four doses of morphine in Fixanal- and naloxone-pretreated arthritic rats. Each mean surface was calculated from the individual curves obtained for each group of rats (n = 9 in naloxone-pretreated and n = 6 in Fixanal-pretreated rats). ** $p < 0.01$; *** $p < 0.001$ Student's t test.

Carrageenin-injected rats

As previously described (Kayser and Guilbaud, 1987b), the plantar injection of carrageenin induces a decrease in pain threshold to paw pressure which can be followed for several hours, until 24 h for some rats. All rats tested 1 and 4 h after injection of carrageenin exhibited a significant decrease in vocalization threshold to paw pressure, by comparison with the pre-carrageenin control values. By contrast, for some rats (13/34 rats) tested 24 h after injection of carrageenin, the vocalization threshold was not significantly decreased.

In a first part of the study, only rats with a significant decrease of the vocalization threshold compared to the pre-carrageenin control values were considered. In these rats, the mean decreases in vocalization threshold to paw pressure were 24 ± 1.5% (n = 10), 34 ± 3.6% (n = 10) and 30 ± 2.9% (n = 21), respectively, for the rats tested 1 h, 4 h and 24 h after injection of carrageenin (Fig. 4, B).

In the group of rats tested 1 h after injection of carrageenin, naloxone (3 μg/kg i.v.) induced a slight and transient antinociceptive effect (the mean peak value expressed as percentage of pre-naloxone control was 121.6 ± 1.9%, n = 10; Fig. 4, A). This paradoxical antinociceptive effect of naloxone increased progressively over the following 4 and 24 h (the mean peak values of the antinociceptive effects of naloxone were 139.6 ± 6.3%, n = 10 and 151.4 ± 5.5%; n = 34, respectively, for rats tested 4 h and 24 h after injection of carrageenin; Fig. 4, A). When the mean surfaces were calculated from the individual curves of naloxone's effects obtained for each group of rats (Fig. 4, B), it appears that the paradoxical antinociceptive effect of naloxone was about two times greater in rats tested 24 h than in those tested 4 h after injection of carrageenin. This suggests that the antinociceptive effect of naloxone was related to the duration of carrageenin-induced hyperalgesia.

In a second part of the study, the effects of naloxone were also tested in rats which did not ex-

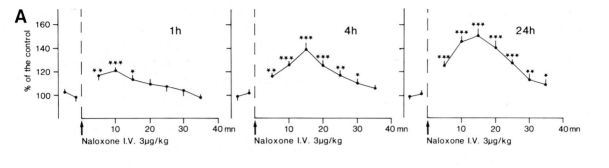

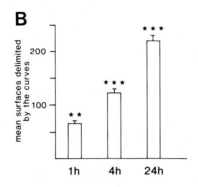

Fig. 4. Effects of naloxone in carrageenin-injected rats. (A) Mean curves of the effects of naloxone (3 µg/kg i.v.) in rats tested 1 h ($n = 10$), 4 h ($n = 10$) and 24 h ($n = 21$) after injection of carrageenin. All rats selected exhibited a significant decrease in vocalization threshold to paw pressure by comparison with pre-carrageenin control values. $* p < 0.05$; $** p < 0.01$; $*** p < 0.001$; Student's t test. (B) Mean surfaces ($\pm$ SEM) calculated from the individual curves obtained for each group of rats for naloxone 3 µg/kg i.v. $** p < 0.01$; $*** p < 0.01$; Student's t test.

hibit a significant decrease in vocalization threshold to paw pressure 24 h after injection of carrageenin. Comparing the effects of naloxone in these rats and those obtained in hyperalgesic rats, it appears that the antinociceptive effect of naloxone was clearly related to the vocalization threshold determined before the injection of naloxone (Fig. 5).

Conclusion – discussion

From various experiments performed in experimentally induced arthritic animals since 1981 (Kayser and Guilbaud, 1981, 1987a; Kayser et al., 1986b), it is clear that naloxone at extremely low doses can have a paradoxical antinociceptive effect, while high doses induce the expected

hyperalgesia. An analogous biphasic effect of naloxone has been reported in animals in certain experimental conditions after its intrathecal injection (Woolf, 1980; Dickenson et al., 1981) and interestingly also in clinical postoperative pain in humans (Lasagna, 1965; Levine et al., 1979).

These results suggest the existence of two different systems which might underly the two opposite effects of naloxone in this model of inflammatory pain. The experiments using morphine-tolerant arthritic rats tend to support such an hypothesis. Indeed, whatever the dose used to render rats tolerant to morphine, the paradoxical antinociceptive effects induced by low doses of naloxone are significantly attenuated in these animals. By contrast, the hyperalgesia induced by higher doses of naloxone persists. Another argu-

308

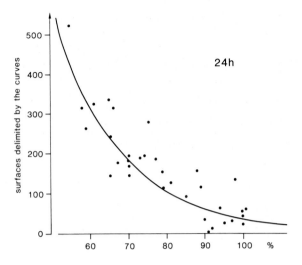

Fig. 5. Relation between the antinociceptive effect of naloxone (surfaces delimited by the curves) and the vocalization threshold to paw pressure (expressed as percentage of pre-carrageenin control values) in rats tested 24 h after injection of carrageenin. Each point represents an individual animal. $r = 0.77$; $\alpha < 0.01$; $n = 34$.

ment is that in naloxone-pretreated rats, the paradoxical antinociceptive effect of 3 μg/kg i.v. naloxone almost disappeared, while other doses (10 and 600 μg/kg i.v.), which were antinociceptive in naive arthritic rats became hyperalgesic in the naloxone-pretreated rats (Kayser and Guilbaud, 1987a).

This complex reactivity of endogenous opioid systems seems to be related to the disease since in preliminary experiments performed 8 weeks after the induction of arthritis, both the antinociceptive and hyperalgesic effects of naloxone were not observed. Interestingly, at this time of the disease, the threshold for struggle (Calvino et al., 1987) and the threshold for vocalization (personal observation), which were maximally decreased between 3 and 5 weeks, were close to those observed in normal rats.

We were also able to demonstrate the paradoxical antinociceptive effects of naloxone using another model of inflammatory pain, carrageenin-induced rat paw oedema (see also Rios and Jacob, 1983). This model allows us to determine the onset

and the development of naloxone's paradoxical effect which seems related to the degree and the duration of carrageenin-induced hyperalgesia. However, the antinociceptive effect observed in such a model is much less than that induced by the same dose of naloxone in rats which have arthritis for 3 weeks. It is important to emphasize that the increase in pain threshold obtained in arthritic rats with 3 μg/kg i.v. naloxone is comparable to that induced by 1 mg/kg i.v. morphine, the antinociceptive effect of which has been shown to be enhanced in these arthritic rats (Pircio et al., 1975; Colpaert, 1979; Kayser and Guilbaud, 1983).

As to the mechanism(s) involved in the paradoxical antinociceptive effect of low doses of naloxone, we suggest the possibility of an interaction with putative presynaptic opiate receptors which could be specially sensitive to this drug in arthritic rats. The existence of such a receptor has been hypothesized in different studies (Kosterlitz and Hughes, 1975; Goldstein and Cox, 1977; Hagan and Hughes, 1984) and has been demonstrated for other neuromediators (Langer, 1981; Starke, 1981; Arrang et al.,1983). According to such an hypothesis, low doses of naloxone would increase the spontaneous release of endogenous opioids modulated by these receptors and thus generate an antinociceptive effect. One could speculate that in morphine-tolerant arthritic rats, these receptors would already be occupied, and thus extremely low doses of naloxone would be ineffective. By contrast, the hyperalgesic effect induced by high doses of naloxone remained unmodified in morphine-pretreated arthritic rats. This persistence, while the antinociceptive effect of low doses declined, emphasizes the involvement of opiate receptors different in their sensitivity and/or in their functions in the opposite effects of naloxone. In this respect, in both morphine-pretreated and naloxone-pretreated arthritic rats, certain doses of naloxone which induced antinociceptive effects in naive animals became hyperalgesic.

These observations emphasize the complexity of endogenous opioid systems. They might explain the controversial reports in the literature concerning its use as an antagonist of endogenous opioids. Indeed, our study demonstrates that the effects of naloxone seem to be dependent on the experimental conditions and doses used. This could be the source of contradictory results in acute experiments which are invasive and prolonged.

Summary

Rats rendered polyarthritic by the injection of Freund's adjuvant at the base of the tail were used as a model of chronic inflammatory pain. In these animals which are particularly sensitive to morphine, the opiate antagonist naloxone induced a bidirectional dose-dependent effect as gauged by the vocalization threshold to paw pressure. Paradoxical antinociceptive effect occurred with low doses $(3-10 \ \mu g/kg$ i.v.), hyperalgesia with high doses $(1-3$ mg/kg i.v.). The paradoxical antinociceptive effect almost disappeared in morphine-tolerant arthritic rats, while the hyperalgesic effect was not affected. In addition, cross-tolerance between low antinociceptive doses of naloxone and low doses of morphine could be demonstrated in these arthritic animals.

In a further study, rats injected with carrageenin were used as a model of acute inflammatory pain. In these hyperalgesic animals, the effects of low doses of naloxone were tested at different times following injection of carrageenin in the plantar hindpaw. A paradoxical antinociceptive effect of naloxone could also be observed. It appeared clearly 4 h after the injection of carrageenin and was more potent 24 h after. In addition, this further study provided evidence that the antinociceptive effect of naloxone was related to the degree and the duration of hyperalgesia.

The complexity of this effect underlines the difficulties in understanding the activity of endogenous opioid systems and our results could explain the various discrepancies reported in the literature with naloxone.

Acknowledgements

The authors wish to thank Dr. A. H. Dickenson, Mrs. M. Gautron and Mr. E. Dehausse for technical assistance.

References

Amir, S. and Amit, Z. (1978) Endogenous opioid ligands may mediate stress-induced changes in the affective properties of pain-related behavior in rats. *Life Sci.,* 23: 1143–1152.

Arrang, J.M., Garbarg, M. and Schwartz, J.C. (1983) Autoinhibition of brain histamine release mediated by a novel class (H3) of histamine receptors. *Nature (Lond.),* 302: 832–837.

Berntson, C.G. and Walker, J.M. (1977) Effect of opiate receptor blockade on pain sensitivity in the rat. *Brain Res. Bull.,* 2: 157–159.

Besson, J.M. and Chaouch, A. (1987) Peripheral and spinal mechanisms of nociception. *Physiol. Rev.,* 67: 67–186.

Buchsbaum, M.S., Davis, G.C. and Bunney, W.E. (1977) Naloxone alters pain perception and somatosensory evoked potentials in normal subjects. *Nature,* 270: 620–622.

Calvino, B., Crepon-Bernard, M.O. and Le Bars, D. (1987) Parallel clinical and behavioural studies of adjuvant-induced arthritis in the rat: possible relationship with 'chronic pain'. *Behav. Brain Res.,* 24: 11–29.

Carmody, J.J., Caroll, P.R. and Morgans, D. (1979) Naloxone increases pain perception in rats and mice. *Life Sci.,* 24: 1149–1152.

Cesselin, F., Montastruc, J.L., Gros, C., Bourgoin, S. and Hamon, M. (1980) Met-enkephalin levels and opiate receptors in the spinal cord of chronic suffering rats. *Brain Res.,* 191: 289–293.

Cesselin, F., Bourgoin, S., Artaud, F., Gozlan, H., Le Bars, D., Clot, A.M., Besson, J.M. and Hamon, M. (1984) The release of met-enkephalin-like material at the spinal level, in vivo and in vitro studies. In J.M. Besson and Y. Lazorthes (Eds.), *Spinal Opioids and the Relief of Pain,* INSERM, Paris, pp. 241–263.

Chesher, G.B. and Chan, B. (1977) Footshock induced analgesia in mice: its reversal by naloxone and cross tolerance with morphine. *Life Sci.,* 21: 1569–1574.

Coderre, T.J. and Rollman, G.B. (1983) Naloxone hyperalgesia and stress-induced analgesia in rats. *Life Sci.,* 32: 2139–2146.

Collier, H.O.J., Francis, D.L. and Schneider, C. (1972) Modifications of morphine withdrawal by drugs interacting

310

with humoral mechanisms: some contradictions and their interpretation. *Nature (Lond.),* 237: 220–223.

Colpaert, F.C. (1979) Can chronic pain be suppressed despite purported tolerance to narcotic analgesia. *Life Sci.,* 24: 1201–1210.

Costentin, J., Vlaiculescu, A., Chaillet, P., Ben Natan, L., Aveaux, D. and Schwartz, J.C. (1986) Dissociated effects of inhibitors of enkephalin-metabolising peptidases or naloxone on various nociceptive responses. *Eur. J. Pharmacol.,* 123: 37–44.

Dehen, H., Willer, J.C. and Cambier, J. (1979) Congenital indifference to pain and endogenous morphine-like system. In J.J. Bonica et al. (Eds.), *Advances in Pain Research and Therapy, Vol. 3,* Raven Press, New York, pp. 553–557.

Dickenson, A.H., Le Bars, D. and Besson, J.M. (1981) Endogenous opiates and nociception: a possible functional role in both pain inhibition and detection as revealed by intrathecal naloxone. *Neurosci. Lett.,* 24: 161–164.

Di Rosa, M. Giroud, J.P. and Willoughby, D.A. (1971) Studies of the mediators of the acute inflammatory response induced in rats in different sites by carrageenin and turpentine. *J. Pathol.,* 104: 15–29.

Duggan, A.W. and North, R.A. (1983) Electrophysiology of opioids. *Pharmacol. Rev.,* 35: 219–281.

Dykstra, L.A. and Mc Millan, D.E. (1977) Electric shock titration: effects of morphine, methadone, pentazocine, nalorphine, naloxone, diazepam and amphetamine. *J. Pharmacol. Exp. Ther.,* 202: 660–669.

Elliott, H.W., Spiehler, V. and Navarro, G. (1976) Effect of naloxone on anti-nociceptive activity of phenoxybenzamine. *Life Sci.,* 19: 1637–1644.

El-Sobky, A., Dostrovsky, J.O. and Wall, P.D. (1976) Lack of effect of naloxone on pain perception in humans. *Nature (Lond.),* 263: 783–784.

Evans, J.M., Hogg, M.I.J., Lunn, J.N. and Rosen, M. (1974) A comparative study of the narcotic antagonist activity of naloxone and levallorphan. *Anesthesia,* 29: 721–727.

Faccini, E., Uzumaki, H., Govoni, S., Missale, C., Spano, P.F., Covelli, V. and Trabucchi, M. (1984) Afferent fibers mediate the increase of met-enkephalin elicited in rat spinal cord by localized pain. *Pain,* 18: 25–31.

Ferreira, S. H. and Nakamura, M. (1979) Prostaglandin hyperalgesia: the peripheral analgesic activity of morphine, enkephalins and opioid antagonists. *Prostaglandins,* 18: 191–200.

Fredrickson, R.C.A., Nickander, R., Smithwick, E.L., Schumann, R. and Norris, F.H. (1976) Pharmacological activity of met-enkephalin and analogs in vitro and in vivo. Depression of single neuronal activity in specific brain regions. In H.W. Kosterlitz (Ed.), *Opiates and Endogenous Opiate Peptides.* Elsevier/North-Holland, Amsterdam, pp. 239–246.

Goldstein, A. and Cox, B.M. (1977) Opioid peptides (endorphins) in pituitary and brain. *Psychoneuroendocrinology,* 2: 11–16.

Goldstein, A., Pryor, G.T., Otis, L.S. and Larsen, F. (1976) On the role of endogenous opioid peptides: failure of naloxone to influence shock escape threshold in the rat. *Life Sci.,* 18: 599–604.

Gouret, C., Mocquet, G. and Raynaud, G. (1976) Use of Freund's adjuvant arthritis test in anti-inflammatory drug screening in the rat: value of animal selection and preparation at the breeding center. *Lab. Anim. Sci.,* 26: 281–287.

Gracely, R.H., Dubner, R., Wolskee, P.J. and Deeter, W.R. (1983) Placebo and naloxone can alter postsurgical pain by separate mechanisms. *Nature (Lond.),* 306: 264–265.

Grevert, P. and Goldstein, A. (1977) Effects of naloxone on experimentally-induced ischaemic pain and on mood in human subjects. *Proc. Natl. Acad. Sci. USA* 74: 1291–1294.

Grevert, P. and Goldstein, A. (1978) Endorphins: naloxone fails to alter experimental pain or mood in humans. *Science,* 199: 1093–1095.

Grevert, P., Baizman, E.R. and Goldstein, A. (1978) Naloxone effects on a nociceptive response of hypophysectomized and adrenalectomized mice. *Life Sci.,* 23: 723–728.

Hagan, R.M. and Hughes, I.E. (1984) Opioid receptor subtypes involved in the control of transmitter release in cortex of the brain of the rat. *Neuropharmacology,* 23: 491–495.

Höllt, V., Haarmann, I., Millan, M.J. and Herz, A. (1987) Prodynorphin gene expression is enhanced in the spinal cord of chronic arthritic rats. *Neurosci. Lett.,* 73: 90–94.

Jacob, J.J. and Ramabadran, K. (1978) Enhancement of a nociceptive reaction by opioid antagonists in mice. *Br. J. Pharmacol.,* 64: 91–98.

Jacob, J.J., Tremblay, E.C. and Colombel, M.C. (1974) Facilitation de réactions nociceptives par la naloxone chez la souris et chez le rat. *Psychopharmacologia (Berl.),* 37: 217–223.

Kaplan, R. and Glick, S.D. (1979) Prior exposure to footshock induced naloxone hyperalgesia. *Life Sci.,* 24: 2309–2312.

Kayser, V. and Guilbaud, G. (1981) Dose-dependent analgesic and hyperalgesic effects of systemic naloxone in arthritic rats. *Brain Res.,* 226: 344–348.

Kayser, V. and Guilbaud, G. (1983) The analgesic effect of morphine, but not those of the enkephalinase inhibitor thiorphan, are enhanced in arthritic rats. *Brain Res.,* 267: 131–138.

Kayser, V. and Guilbaud, G. (1985) Can tolerance to morphine be induced in arthritic rats? *Brain Res.,* 334: 335–338.

Kayser, V. and Guilbaud, G. (1987a) Cross-tolerance between analgesic low doses of morphine and naloxone in arthritic rats. *Brain Res.,* 405: 123–129.

Kayser, V. and Guilbaud, G. (1987b) Local and remote modifications of nociceptive sensitivity during carrageenin-induced inflammation in the rat. *Pain,* 28–1: 99–108.

Kayser, V., Besson, J.M. and Guilbaud, G. (1986a) Analgesia

produced by low doses of the opiate antagonist naloxone in arthritic rats is reduced in morphine-tolerant animals. *Brain Res.,* 371: 37 – 41.

Kayser, V., Neil, A. and Guilbaud, G. (1986b) Repeated low doses of morphine induce a rapid tolerance in arthritic rats but a potentiation of opiate analgesia in normal animals. *Brain Res.,* 383: 392 – 396.

Kokka, N. and Fairhurst, A.S. (1977) Naloxone enhancement of acetic acid-induced writhing in rats. *Life Sci.,* 21: 975 – 980.

Kosterlitz, H.W. and Hughes, J. (1975) Some thoughts on the significance of enkephalin, the endogenous ligand. *Life Sci.,* 17: 91 – 96.

Langer, S.Z. (1981) Presynaptic regulation of the release of catecholamine. *Pharmacol. Rev.,* 32: 337 – 362.

Lasagna, L. (1965) Drug interaction in the field of analgesic drugs. *Proc. Roy. Soc. Med.,* 58: 978 – 983.

Levine, J.D. and Gordon, N.C. (1986) Method of administration determines the effects of naloxone on pain. *Brain Res.,* 365: 377 – 378;

Levine, J.D., Gordon, N.C., Jones, R.T., and Fields, H.L. (1978) The narcotic antagonist naloxone enhances clinical pain. *Nature (Lond.),* 272: 826 – 827.

Levine, J.D., Gordon, N.C. and Fields, H.L. (1979) Naloxone dose-dependently produces analgesia and hyperalgesia in post-operative pain. *Nature (Lond.),* 278: 740 – 741.

Lindblom, U. and Tegner, R. (1978) Are the endorphins active in clinical pain states? Narcotic antagonism in chronic pain patients. *Pain,* 7: 65 – 68.

Millan, M.J., Czlonkowski, A., Pilcher, C.W.T., Almeida, O.F.X., Millan, M.H., Colpaert, F.C. and Herz, A. (1987) A model of chronic pain in the rat: functional correlates of alterations in the activity of opioid systems. *J. Neurosci.,* 7: 77 – 87.

North, M.A. (1978) Naloxone reversal of morphine analgesia but failure to alter reactivity to pain in the formalin test. *Life Sci.,* 22: 295 – 302.

Pearson, C.M., Waksman, B.H. and Sharp, J.J. (1961) Studies of arthritis and other lesions induced in rats by injection of mycobacterial adjuvant. Changes affecting the skin and mucous membranes. Comparison of the experimental process with human disease, *J. Exp. Med.,* 113: 485 – 509.

Pert, A. and Walter, M. (1976) Comparison between naloxone reversal of morphine and electrical stimulation induced analgesia in the rat mesencephalon. *Life Sci.,* 19: 1023 – 1032.

Pinsky, C., Labella, F.S., Havlicek, V. and Dua, A.K. (1978) Apparent central agonist actions of naloxone in the unrestrained rat. In J.M. Van Ree and L. Terenius (Eds.), *Characteristics and Function of Opioids,* Elsevier/North-Holland Biomedical Press, Amsterdam, New York, Oxford, pp. 439 – 440.

Pircio, A.W., Fedele, C.T. and Bierwagen, M.E. (1975) A new method for the evaluation of analgesic activity using adjuvant induced arthritis in the rat. *Eur. J. Pharmacol.,* 31: 207 – 215.

Pomeranz, B. and Chiu, D. (1976) Naloxone blockade of acupuncture analgesia: endorphin implicated. *Life Sci.,* 19: 1757 – 1762.

Przewlocki, R., Przewlocka, B., Lason, W., Garzon, J., Stala, L. and Hertz, A. (1985) Opioid peptides, particularly dynorphin, and chronic pain. In J.M. Besson and Y. Lazorthes (Eds.), *Substances Opioides Medullaires et Analgésie,* INSERM, pp. 159 – 170.

Ramabadran, K. and Jacob, J.J. (1979) Stereospecific effects of opiate antagonists on superficial and deep nociception and on motor activity suggest involvement of endorphins on different opioid receptors. *Life Sci.,* 24: 1959 – 1970.

Rios, L. and Jacob, J.J. (1983) Local inhibition of inflammatory pain by naloxone and its N-methyl quaternary analogue. *Eur. J. Pharmacol.,* 96: 277 – 283.

Roch-Arveiller, M., Dunn, C.J. and Giroud, J.P. (1977) Comparaison des propriétés inflammatoires des fractions λ et de carrageenin. *J. Pharmacol. (Paris),* 8: 461 – 476.

Rosenfeld, J.P. and Rice, P.E. (1979) Effects of naloxone on aversive trigeminal and thalamic stimulation, and on peripheral nociception: a hypothesis of selective action and variability in naloxone testing. *Brain Res.,* 178: 609 – 612.

Satoh, M., Kawajiri, S.I., Yamamoto, M., Makino, H. and Takagi, H. (1979) Reversal by naloxone of adaptation of rats to noxious stimuli. *Life Sci.,* 24: 685 – 690.

Sewell, R.D.E. and Spencer, P.S.J. (1976) Antinociceptive activity of narcotic agonist and partial agonist analgesics and other agents in the tail-immersion test in mice and rats. *Neuropharmacology,* 15: 683 – 688.

Starke, K. (1981) Presynaptic receptors. *Annu. Rev. Pharmacol. Toxicol.,* 21: 7 – 30.

Tulunay, F.C., Sparber, S.B. and Takemori, A.E. (1975) The effect of dopaminergic stimulation and blockade on the nociceptive and antinociceptive responses of mice. *Eur. J. Pharmacol.,* 33: 65 – 70.

Ueda, H., Fukushima, N., Kitao, T., Ge, M. and Takagi, H. (1986) Low doses of naloxone produce analgesia in the mouse brain by blocking presynaptic autoinhibition of enkephalin release. *Neurosci. Lett.,* 65: 247 – 252.

Vinegar, R., Schreiber, W. and Hugo, R. (1969) Biphasic development of carrageenin edema in rats. *J. Pharmacol. Exp. Ther.,* 166: 96 – 103.

Walker, J.M., Berntson, G.G., Sadman, C.A., Coy, D.H., Schally, A.V. and Kastin, A.J. (1977) An analog of enkephalin having prolonged opiate-like effects in vivo. *Science,* 196: 85 – 87.

Winter, C.A., Risley, E.A. and Nuss, G.W. (1962) Carrageenin-induced edema in hind paw of the rat as an assay for anti-inflammatory drugs. *Proc. Soc. Exp. Biol. Med.,* 111: 544 – 547.

Woolf, C.J. (1980) Analgesia and hyperalgesia produced in the rat by intrathecal naloxone. *Brain Res.,* 189: 593 – 597.

Yaksh, T.L. Yeung, J.C. and Rudy, T.A. (1976) An inability to antagonise with naloxone the elevated threshold resulting from electrical stimulation of the mesencephalic central gray. *Life Sci.,* 18: 1193 – 1198.

H.L. Fields and J.-M. Besson (Eds.)
Progress in Brain Research, Vol. 77
© 1988 Elsevier Science Publishers B.V. (Biomedical Division)

CHAPTER 22

Intrathecal administration: methodological considerations

Donna L. Hammond

Department of Central Nervous System Diseases Research, G.D. Searle & Co., 4901 Searle Parkway, Skokie, IL 60077, USA

Introduction

In 1976, Yaksh and Rudy described a method for chronic catheterization of the spinal cord subarachnoid space. The introduction of this technique stimulated research in spinal cord function and its regulation by supraspinal nuclei, and demonstrated that the spinal cord is an important site of drug action. Fig. 1 depicts the rapid acceptance of this methodology, which has been cited 283 times since its introduction. The impact of this method can be attributed to two factors. First, it enables direct injection of drugs into the intrathecal space without need of restraint or anesthesia, and does not interfere with behavioral measures of action. Second, and more importantly, the site of action of the drug is restricted to the spinal cord. This chapter will review the methodological considerations of this technique.

Methodological considerations

Surgical technique

Although originally described for rats and rabbits, the technique has since been extended to cats, dogs and monkeys. Details of the procedure for various species are available in the literature and will only be cursorily described here (Yaksh and Rudy, 1976; LoPachin et al., 1981; Yaksh and Reddy, 1981; Martin et al., 1984). Under aseptic condi-

tions and after induction of anesthesia, a length of PE-10 polyethylene tubing is inserted through a slit in the atlanto-occipital membrane and threaded caudally for a specified distance in the subarachnoid space. To situate the catheter's tip at the junction of the thoracic and lumbar segments, this distance is 7.0 cm in 200-g rats (Tang and Schoenfeld, 1978), 8.5 cm in 350 – 400 g rats (LoPachin et al., 1981), and 30 cm in an adult cat or monkey (Yaksh, 1978; Yaksh and Reddy, 1981). Attention should be given to the selection of catheter length and segmental termination because the potency of

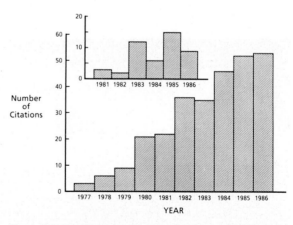

Fig. 1. Number of citations by year of the report by Yaksh and Rudy (1976) on chronic catheterization of the spinal cord subarachnoid space. Inset: number of citations by year of the report by Hylden and Wilcox (1980) on intrathecal injection in the mouse. Ordinates: number of citations. Abscissas: year of citation. (Data from Science Citation Index.)

an intrathecally administered drug is a function of its site of administration (see below). The catheter may be stretched before insertion to decrease dead volume and to facilitate its introduction into the spinal subarachnoid space (LoPachin et al., 1981).

Several methods have been devised to externalize and anchor the free end of the catheter through which the drug is injected (Yaksh and Rudy, 1976; LoPachin et al., 1981; Bahar et al., 1984; Dib, 1984; Martin et al., 1984). The most recent and easiest method for externalizing and securing the catheter in the rat is illustrated in Fig. 2. The catheter is prepared with a small knot loosely tied 9.5 – 10 cm from one end; the knot is secured by a drop of dental acrylic. After insertion of the catheter in the spinal subarachnoid space, the free end is threaded through a trocar that has been inserted through a skin incision on the dorsum of the head. The trocar is then removed and the catheter is gently pulled forward by its free end so that the knot is pulled under the skin and fascia overlying the skull; the catheter tip is situated 8.5 cm from the atlanto-occipital junction. The catheter is affixed to the skull by adhesions during the healing process. After flushing the catheter with several μl of saline, the free end may be occluded by a stylet, or more easily by heat-sealing. The catheter may

alternately be externalized at the lumbar or thoracic levels if compression of the spinal cord is a concern (Bahar et al., 1984; Dib, 1984; Martin et al., 1984).

Anesthetics as diverse as ether, ketamine and pentobarbital have been used for this procedure. Inhalation anesthetics such as halothane are preferable, as they have much shorter induction and recovery times (less than 5 min), thereby minimizing the animal's stress, and are more easily controlled to assure adequate anesthesia. Rapid recovery from anesthetic also permits immediate identification and disposal of animals with neurologic deficits. Animals apparently free of neurologic deficits on the day of surgery should be reexamined the following day. The animals are housed individually with free access to food and water during the 1-week postoperative care period.

Hylden and Wilcox (1980) have devised a method for injection of drugs into the spinal cord subarachnoid space of mice. The inset of Fig. 1 illustrates the rapid adoption of this method since its introduction. The drug is injected into the intrathecal space by percutaneous lumbar puncture in unanesthetized mice using a 30 ga 1/2-inch needle. Entry into the intrathecal space is indicated by a flick of the tail. This method obviates the need for

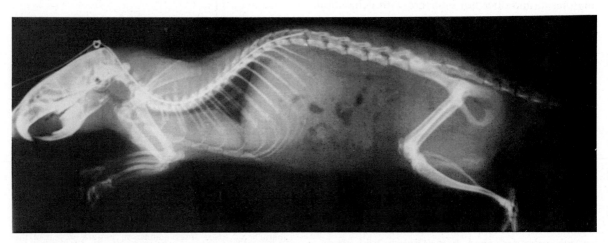

Fig. 2. Radiogram of a rat depicting the current technique for externalization of an intrathecal catheter. The catheter is filled with a radioopaque dye. Note the knot, secured by a drop of dental acrylic, that is situated under the fascia on the dorsum of the skull and affixed by adhesion. The tip of the catheter lies at the T12 – L1 segmental level. (Radiogram, courtesy of Dr. Tony Yaksh.)

preparative surgery and has the added advantages of being faster, cheaper and easier to perform. Because this method probably involves some distress, it should only be performed in unanesthetized mice by individuals who are proficient in the method as first determined by administration of dye in anesthetized mice.

Drug administration

In determining the volume of drug to be administered three factors must be considered: (1) dead volume of the catheter, (2) volume of the spinal subarachnoid space and (3) area over which the drug is to be distributed. The typical dead volume of an intrathecal catheter as depicted in Fig. 2 is 7 μl. The volume of drug solution and saline flush must be calculated so that there is no residual drug in the catheter. Investigators typically inject 10 μl of drug solution followed by 10 μl saline. The drug and saline flush are usually injected using a manually operated gear-driven syringe or by infusion pump over a 30 – 60 s period. In a number of studies, drug has been injected in 5 μl, a volume that dye studies indicate spreads about 0.5 – 1.5 cm from the tip of the catheter. However, volumes $\leqslant$ 5 μl should be avoided because circumferential staining of the spinal cord may be spotty (Yaksh and Rudy, 1976). This fact becomes important when one considers that the majority of catheters are not situated on the dorsal surface of the spinal cord, but rather lie on one side or the other of the spinal cord, under the spinal roots (Weisenfeld and Gustafsson, 1982; unpublished observations). Finally, scar tissue does form, enveloping the tip of the catheter and eventually the entire catheter. Although this tissue does not impede drug administration, it can alter the pattern of distribution. For these reasons, drug solutions should probably be administered in a 10-μl volume followed by a saline flush.

In the rat, 8 – 10 μl of Evans blue, trypan blue or bromophenol blue dye spreads 2.5 – 3.5 cm above and below the catheter tip. The spread of dye is volume dependent with larger volumes

spreading further rostrally (Martin et al., 1984; Tseng and Fujimoto, 1985; Tseng et al., 1983; Bryant et al., 1983). When examined 10 – 15 min after injection, the dye is primarily restricted to thoracic and lumbar segments of the spinal cord. Some staining of cervical segments may be apparent in a limited number of animals. In the mouse, 5 μl of methylene blue is restricted to lumbar and thoracic segments 10 min after injection (Hylden and Wilcox, 1980). In the cat, 300 μl does not stain the brain stem (Yaksh, 1978). The typical injection volume in the adult primate is 500 μl.

Estimates of the volume of spinal CSF are difficult to obtain, particularly for the rat. By measuring the concentration of radiolabelled tracers, several investigators estimate total CSF in the adult rat to be approximately 250 μl (Bass and Lundborg, 1973; Burns et al., 1976). Between 10 and 16 ml of CSF, depending on body weight, can be obtained from adult monkeys (Rieselbach et al., 1962). If the volume of intrathecal injection exceeds 1/4 the total CSF volume, the injectate will access basal cisterns and ventricles. If the volume is 10% of total CSF volume, the injectate may reach the basal cisterns. In order to restrict the injectate to the spinal cord, the volume of injection should probably be less than 10% of total CSF volume (Rieselbach et al., 1962). Total volumes of injection should therefore be less than 25 μl in the rat, 1.0 ml in the monkey and 400 μl in the cat.

Physicochemical properties of the drug

The relative potency, onset and duration of action of a compound are functions of its physicochemical properties. The two parameters of greatest interest are the equilibrium constant and the apparent partition coefficient. The equilibrium constant of a drug is usually expressed as its negative logarithm, or pK and corresponds to the pH at which 50% of the drug exists as the ionized form. The relative proportion of unionized to ionized drug is a function of the pH of the environment and can be calculated using the Henderson-

Hasselbach equation (Tallarida and Murray, 1987). The unionized form of drug is more lipid-soluble and membrane-permeable than the ionized form. In studies in which the relative potency of a series of structurally or pharmacologically related compounds is examined, the compounds are likely to differ with respect to pK and, consequently, the relative proportion of unionized to ionized drug. Although conclusions of efficacy will not be affected, these differences may confound conclusions concerning the relative potencies of the different compounds.

The apparent partition coefficient (P') of a compound is the ratio of its concentration in a lipid phase to its concentration in an aqueous phase after partitioning. An octanol/buffer system is frequently used for this determination. The apparent partition coefficient is usually expressed as its logarithm (log P') and is a function of the compound's lipid solubility. Calculations of the 'true' log P additionally consider the proportion of drug existing in the ionized and presumably non-partitionable form at the pH being studied, and will more closely reflect the true lipophilicity of a compound under the conditions of study (Timmermans et al., 1977). The larger the log P, the more lipophilic the compound and the more readily it will pass cell membranes and distribute into lipid soluble sites such as the spinal cord and brain. The lipid solubility of a compound is an important determinant of the onset and duration of its action, but not of its potency (Herz and Teschemacher, 1971; see below).

Despite their importance, these factors are not routinely discussed in studies of the efficacy of intrathecally administered drugs. This fact may be attributed to the paucity of structure-activity studies of series of chemically or pharmacologically related compounds. The influences exerted by the physicochemical properties of a drug are much more apparent when several, rather than one or two, compounds are examined. The most extensive examination of structure-activity relationships to date has been performed with adrenergic and opioid agonists. Unfortunately, the adrenergic agonists differ greatly in their sensitivity to uptake and oxidation. This fact severely hampers correlations of activity with physicochemical property as differences in metabolism will also affect potency, onset and duration of action. The situation is more favorable with the opioid alkaloids. Yaksh (1983) noted that opioid alkaloids with a large log P (lipophilic), such as lofentanyl, had a very rapid onset of action, but a relatively short duration of action. This observation is consistent with rapid uptake of lipophilic substances into tissue, followed by redistribution to other sites. In contrast, agents with lower log P values (hydrophilic), such as morphine, had a slower onset of action and a relatively long duration of action. This observation is consistent with their hydrophilic nature, slow uptake into tissue and slower redistribution. Similar observations have been made by Herz and Teschemacher (1971) after intraventricular administration of these compounds.

Site(s) of action

Spinal versus supraspinal

One of the observations cited to support a spinal site of action of intrathecally administered drugs is that only thoracic and lumbar segments of the spinal cord are stained after injection of the same volume of dye (see above). However, these studies only indicate how far the dye itself will spread. Unless the physicochemical properties of the dye duplicate those of the drug, no conclusions about the site(s) of action can, strictly speaking, be drawn. Furthermore, because the concentration of dye is arbitrary and the density of tissue staining is a subjective measure, the results are neither conclusive nor quantitative.

Another observation cited to support a spinal site of action is the finding that the apparent potency of a drug frequently differs as a function of the segmental level at which it is injected. Larson (1985) reported that the hyperalgesic activity of tryptamine and the analgesic activity of serotonin were highly and differentially dependent on the segmental level at which they were injected.

Tryptamine was more potent when administered to thoracic levels whereas serotonin was more potent when administered to lumbar levels of the spinal cord. Tang and Schoenfeld (1978) noted that morphine was more potent when injected at caudal levels of the spinal cord. Segmental differences in potency would not be expected if a drug distributed homogeneously in the spinal cord subarachnoid space or if its effect was mediated by redistribution to supraspinal structures. These data are consistent with the results obtained after intrathecal administration of dye suggesting that the action of the drug is limited to the spinal cord. In view of the differential segmental distribution of neurotransmitters and neurotransmitter binding sites, however, the segmental distribution of a drug may be an important factor in determinations of its apparent efficacy and relative potency.

A more quantitative definition of the site(s) of action is obtained after intrathecal administration of the drug in radiolabelled form. The physico-chemical properties of the radiolabelled drug are more likely to approximate those of the unlabelled drug and the label permits measures of concentration in tissue, plasma and CSF. Unfortunately, only a few such studies have been performed and the majority of these have examined the distribution of morphine and naloxone (Yaksh and Rudy, 1976, 1977; Hylden and Wilcox, 1980; Tang and Schoenfeld, 1978; Schmauss et al., 1983; Wolf and Mohrland, 1984; Tseng and Fujimoto, 1985). These two compounds differ appreciably in lipophilicity (Kaufman et al., 1975) and their distribution is predictive for other compounds of similar lipophilicities. However, little comparative data is available for compounds with lipophilicities that differ from morphine and naloxone.

The levels of radioactivity measured in the brain of rats 10 minutes after intrathecal injection of ^{14}C-urea, which distributes as body water, never exceed 0.25% of that injected in the spinal cord (Yaksh and Rudy, 1976). Ten minutes after intrathecal injection of ^{3}H-naloxone, the total amount of radioactivity recovered in brain is approximately 0.5% of that injected intrathecally

(Yaksh and Rudy 1976, 1977; Tang and Schoenfeld, 1978; Tseng and Fujimoto, 1985). This amount falls rapidly over the subsequent 50 min. With both ^{14}C-urea and ^{3}H-naloxone, the distribution of radioactivity within the spinal cord is restricted to the lumbar and thoracic segments, indicating that label found in the brain does not arrive by transit (bulk flow) in the CSF, but rather by uptake into blood and subsequent redistribution to supraspinal sites (Yaksh and Rudy, 1976). The amount of ^{3}H-morphine present in the brain 10 min after intrathecal injection in rats, however, is less than that observed for either urea or the more lipophilic naloxone. It does not exceed 0.1% of the amount delivered to the spinal cord (Yaksh and Rudy, 1977). Unlike either urea or naloxone, appreciable label is recovered from cervical segments 60 min after intrathecal administration of morphine in the rat, suggesting that a portion of the compound reaches supraspinal sites by rostral diffusion in the subarachnoid space. A similar study in sheep demonstrated that morphine appeared in cisternal CSF simultaneously with ^{14}C-sucrose, a marker of CSF bulk flow, and averaged 0.3% of the administered dose. This finding suggests that hydrophilic substances appear in the cisternal CSF and supraspinal structures as a consequence of bulk flow (Payne and Inturrisi, 1985). Lipophilic substances, in contrast, appear to reach supraspinal sites by uptake into the peripheral circulation and redistribution. These findings are consistent with observations that hydrophilic substances are restricted to the spinal cord subarachnoid space while lipophilic substances redistribute elsewhere. Tseng and Fujimoto (1985) demonstrated that only about 9% of intrathecally administered naloxone is recoverable in the spinal cord 15 min after injection. This observation contrasts with the results of studies with morphine in which greater than 90% is recoverable in the spinal cord up to 60 min after intrathecal injection (Yaksh and Rudy, 1977; Hylden and Wilcox, 1980).

The distribution of radiolabel has also been examined after intrathecal injection of radiolabelled morphine in the mouse (Hylden and Wilcox,

1980). Five minutes after a 5 μl injection, 98.8% of the radiolabel is present in the spinal cord. Twenty minutes after injection, this amount diminishes to 94.6%. Conversely, 0.4 and 0.8% of the radiolabel is present in forebrain and brain stem structures, respectively, 5 min after injection. The amount in forebrain and brain stem structures increases to 1.8% and 3.6%, respectively, 20 min after injection. These data suggest that in the mouse more drug reaches supraspinal structures than in the rat after intrathecal injection. Moreover, it is likely that an even greater percentage of drug may reach supraspinal structures after injection of lipophilic compounds such as naloxone or lofentanyl. This observation may indicate that the relative volume of injection (expressed as a percentage of total CSF) in the mouse is greater than in the rat. Other potential contributing factors are that the distance between the injection site and the brain (length of spinal cord) is shorter in the mouse, and that the transient increase in the spinal cord CSF pressure produced by the injection is greater in the mouse than in the rat (Bass and Lungborg, 1973). Given these factors and to exclude a potential supraspinal site of action, studies of intrathecally administered drugs in the mouse should demonstrate that intraventricular administration of the intrathecal dose does not mimic the effects observed after intrathecal administration. This additional control will also be required in the rat, if the peak effect of the compound is substantially delayed beyond 30 min (e.g. 45 min) at a time when supraspinal concentrations of the drug are increasing (Hylden and Wilcox, 1980; Schmauss et al., 1984).

Distribution to the peripheral circulation

As discussed above, absorption into the peripheral circulation from the spinal cord subarachnoid space is an important route of clearance for lipophilic substances, and less importantly, for hydrophilic substances as well. Yet, relatively little attention has been paid to quantitation of this phenomenon for species other than man. This may be partly attributed to the difficulty in obtaining sequential blood samples from small animals and in 'clearing' the blood sufficiently to reduce sample quenching for liquid scintillation counting. Nonetheless, the potential exists for rapid and efficient absorption of an intrathecally administered drug into the circulation with subsequent redistribution to supraspinal sites. Although the amount of compound in the circulation may be a fraction of that administered intrathecally, the concentration in brain may be several times greater than the plasma concentration as shown by Herz and Teschemacher with lipophilic substances such as etorphine. In the absence of quantitative data, it is imperative to demonstrate that intravenous administration of the intrathecal dose is without effect in order to substantiate claims that the site of drug action is restricted to the spinal cord. Several studies have attempted to address this issue by s.c. or i.p. administration of the intrathecal dose. These routes are not satisfactory as only a portion of the dose enters the peripheral circulation. The i.p. route is particularly inappropriate as what drug is absorbed enters the hepatic circulation and is subject to first-pass metabolism before distribution to the brain.

Effects on spinal cord blood flow

A factor that must be considered in intrathecal studies is that the observed effect is secondary to drug-induced alterations in spinal cord blood flow. With respect to antinociception, the possibility has been raised that the antinociceptive actions of epinephrine, norepinephrine and serotonin reflect vasoconstriction of the spinal cord. However, as noted by Reddy et al. (1980), the antinociceptive potency of these compounds does not parallel their potency as vasoconstrictors of cerebral vasculature. Thus, serotonin is a more potent vasoconstrictor than norepinephrine (Toda and Fujita, 1973), yet it is substantially less potent than norepinephrine as an analgesic after intrathecal administration (Yaksh and Wilson, 1979; Reddy et al., 1980) Angiotensin-II, another potent vasoconstrictor (Wei et al., 1978), does not alter the nociceptive threshold after intrathecal administration (Reddy et al., 1980). In the dog and cat, intrathecal injection of epinephrine or of phenylephrine does not alter spinal cord blood flow as measured by radioactive microspheres (Kozody et al., 1984; Porter et al., 1985), yet both compounds produce antinociception after intrathecal injection. These observations suggest that antinociceptive activity is not mediated by vasoconstriction. However, these observations do not indicate that the effects of intrathecally administered drugs are independent of spinal cord blood flow. Increases or decreases in spinal cord or dural blood flow may diminish or prolong, respectively, the duration of action of a compound. Interestingly, a decrease in dural blood flow is observed after intrathecal injection of epinephrine and phenylephrine (Kozody et al., 1984). This decrease in dural blood flow may explain the ability of epinephrine and phenylephrine to prolong the duration of action of spinally administered lipophilic local anesthetics such as tetracaine (see discussion in Kozody et al., 1984).

Conclusion

The conclusions of studies utilizing the intrathecal route of administration are based on the premise that the drug's site of action is restricted to the spinal cord. Although the studies discussed in this review suggest that this is likely the case, the most quantitative data to support this contention is provided by studies of the distribution of radiolabelled compounds in tissue and plasma after intrathecal administration. Unfortunately, not enough studies of this type have been performed with drugs of different physicochemical properties to support generalizations to the wide array of substances now being administered intrathecally. In the absence of such data and in order to conclude that a drug's action is exerted at a pharmacologically relevant receptor in the spinal cord, the following should be demonstrated:

1. The action of the drug is dose-dependent and stereospecific.

2. The onset and duration of action are consistent with its known physicochemical properties.

3. The effect is mimicked by other, structurally dissimilar compounds of similar pharmacological specificity.

4. The effect is antagonized by appropriate pharmacological antagonists.

5. Intravenous administration of the intrathecal dose does not mimic the effect observed after intrathecal administration.

6. Intraventricular administration of the intrathecal dose does not mimic the effect observed after intrathecal administration. This is particularly important for studies in the mouse and for compounds in which the peak effect is substantially delayed.

Acknowledgements

I would like to acknowledge the expert secretarial assistance of Grace Koek.

References

Bahar, M., Rosen, M. and Vickers, M.D. (1984) Chronic cannulation of the intradural or extradural space in the rat. *Br. J. Anaesth.,* 56: 405 – 410.

Bass, N.H. and Lundborg, P. (1973) Postnatal development of bulk flow in the cerebrospinal fluid system of the albino rat: clearance of carboxyl-[^{14}C]inulin after intrathecal infusion. *Brain Res.,* 52: 323 – 332.

Bryant, R.M., Olley, J.E. and Tyers, M.B. (1983) Antinociceptive actions of morphine and buprenorphine given intrathecally in the conscious rats. *Br. J. Pharmacol.,* 78: 659 – 663.

Burns, D., London, J., Brunswick, D.J., Pring, M., Garfinkel, D., Rabinowitz, J.L. and Mendels, J. (1976) A kinetic analysis of 5-hydroxyindoleacetic acid excretion from rat brain and CSF. *Biol. Psychiat.,* 11: 125 – 157.

Dib, B. (1984) Intrathecal chronic catheterization in the rat *Pharmacol. Biochem. Behav.,* 20: 45 – 48.

Herz, A. and Teschemacher, H.-J. (1971) Activities and sites of antinociceptive action of morphine-like analgesics and kinetics of distribution following intravenous, intracerebral and intraventricular application. *Adv. Drug Res.,* 6: 79 – 119.

Hylden, J.L. and Wilcox, G.L. (1980) Intrathecal morphine in mice: a new technique. *Eur. J. Pharmacol.,* 67: 313 – 316.

Kaufman, J.J., Semo, N.M. and Koski, W.S. (1975) Microelectrometric titration measurement of the pK$_a$'s and partition

320

and drug distribution coefficients of narcotics and narcotic antagonists and their pH and temperature dependence. *J. Med. Chem.,* 18: 647 – 655.

Kozody, R., Palahniuk, R.J., Wade, J.G. and Cumming, M.O. (1984) The effect of subarachnoid epinephrine and phenylephrine on spinal cord blood flow. *Can. Anaesth. Soc. J.,* 31: 503 – 508.

Larson, A.A. (1985) Distribution of CNS sites sensitive to tryptamine and serotonin in pain processing. In A.A. Boulton, L. Maitre, P.R. Bieck and P. Reiderer (Eds.), *Neuropsychopharmacology of the Trace Amines,* Humana, Clifton, NJ, pp. 241 – 249.

LoPachin, R.M., Rudy, T.A. and Yaksh, T.L. (1981) An improved method for chronic catheterization of the rat spinal subarachnoid space. *Physiol. Behav.,* 27: 559 – 561.

Martin, H., Kocher, L. and Chery-Croze, S. (1984) Chronic lumbar intrathecal catheterization in the rat with reduced-length spinal compression. *Physiol. Behav.,* 33: 159 – 161.

Payne, R. and Inturrisi, C.E. (1985) CSF distribution of morphine, methadone and sucrose after intrathecal injection. *Life Sci.,* 37: 1137 – 1144.

Porter, S.S., Albin, M.S., Watson, W.A., Bunegin, L. and Pantoja, G. (1985) Spinal cord and cerebral blood flow responses to subarachnoid injection of local anesthetics with and without epinephrine. *Acta Anaesthesiol. Scand.,* 29: 330 – 338.

Reddy, S.V.R., Maderdrut, J.L. and Yaksh, T.L. (1980) Spinal cord pharmacology of adrenergic agonist-mediated antinociception. *J. Pharmacol. Exp. Ther.,* 213: 525 – 533.

Rieselbach, R.E., DiChiro, G., Freireich, E.J., and Rall, D.P. (1962) Subarachnoid distribution of drugs after lumbar injection. *N. Engl. J. Med.,* 267: 1273 – 1278.

Schmauss, C., Hammond, D.L., Ochi, J.W. and Yaksh, T.L. (1983) Pharmacological antagonism of the antinociceptive effects of serotonin in the rat spinal cord. *Eur. J. Pharmacol.,* 90: 349 – 357.

Tallarida, R.J. and Murray, R.B. (1987) *Manual of Pharmacologic Calculations with Computer Programs,* 2nd edn., Springer-Verlag, New York, pp. 74 – 75.

Tang, A.H. and Schoenfeld, M.J. (1978) Comparison of subcutaneous and spinal subarachnoid injections of morphine and naloxone on analgesic tests in the rat. *Eur. J. Pharmacol.,* 52: 215 – 223.

Timmermans, P.B.M.W.M., Brands, A. and Van Zwieten, P.A. (1977) Lipophilicity and brain disposition of clonidine and structurally related imidazolidines. *Naunyn-Schmied. Arch. Pharmacol.,* 300: 217 – 226.

Toda, N. and Fujita, Y. (1973) Responsiveness of isolated cerebral and peripheral arteries to serotonin, norepinephrine, and transmural electrical stimulation. *Circulation Res.,* 33: 98 – 104.

Tseng, L.-F. and Fujimoto, J.M. (1985) Differential actions of intrathecal naloxone on blocking the tail-flick inhibition induced by intraventricular β-endorphin and morphine in rats. *J. Pharmacol. Exp. Ther.,* 232: 74 – 79.

Tseng, L.-F., Cheng, S.S. and Fujimoto, J.M. (1983) Inhibition of tail flick and shaking responses by intrathecal and intraventricular D-Ala^2-D-Leu^5-enkephalin and β-endorphin in anesthetized rats. *J. Pharmacol. Exp. Ther.,* 224: 51 – 54.

Wei, E.P., Kontos, H.A. and Patterson, J.L. (1978) Vasoconstrictor effect of angiotensin on pial arteries. *Stroke,* 9: 487 – 489.

Wiesenfeld, Z. and Gustafsson, L.L. (1982) Continuous intrathecal administration of morphine via an osmotic minipump in the rat. *Brain Res.,* 247: 195 – 197.

Wolf, D.L. and Mohrland, J.S. (1984) Alteration of shock titration thresholds in the cat following intrathecal substance P administration. *Peptides,* 5: 477 – 479.

Yaksh, T.L. (1978) Analgetic actions of intrathecal opiates in cat and primate. *Brain Res.,* 153: 205 – 210.

Yaksh, T.L. (1983) In vivo studies on spinal opiate receptor systems mediating antinociception. I. Mu and delta receptor profiles in the primate. *J. Pharmacol. Exp. Ther.,* 226: 303 – 316.

Yaksh, T.L. and Reddy, S.V.R. (1981) Studies in the primate on the analgetic effects associated with intrathecal actions of opiates, α-adrenergic agonists and baclofen. *Anesthesiology,* 54: 451 – 467.

Yaksh, T.L. and Rudy, T.A. (1976) Chronic catheterization of the spinal subarachnoid space. *Physiol. Behav.,* 17: 1031 – 1036.

Yaksh, T.L. and Rudy, T.A. (1977) Studies on the direct spinal action of narcotics in the production of analgesia in the rat. *J. Pharmacol. Exp. Ther.,* 202: 411 – 428.

Yaksh, T.L. and Wilson, P.R. (1979) Spinal serotonin terminal system mediates antinociception. *J. Pharmacol. Exp. Ther.,* 208: 446 – 453.

H.L. Fields and J.-M. Besson (Eds.)
Progress in Brain Research, Vol. 77
© 1988 Elsevier Science Publishers B.V. (Biomedical Division)

CHAPTER 23

Neuronal effects of controlled superfusion of the spinal cord with monoaminergic receptor antagonists in the cat

Jürgen Sandkühler and Manfred Zimmermann

II. Physiologisches Institut, Universität Heidelberg, Im Neuenheimer Feld 326, D-6900 Heidelberg, FRG

Introduction

Parallel and partially independent multiple descending inhibitory systems may be activated by electrical stimulation of the periaqueductal gray (PAG) or nucleus raphe magnus (NRM), respectively (Gebhart et al., 1983; Sandkühler et al., 1987). The descending inhibitory effects are possibly mediated by different neurotransmitters such as serotonin, noradrenaline (Davies and Quinlan, 1985; Hammond et al., 1985) or endogenous opioids (Duggan et al., 1976; Zorman et al., 1982), which may be released simultaneously in the spinal cord (Bowker et al., 1982; Hammond et al., 1985).

To identify the spinal neurotransmitters involved in the descending inhibition of spinal nociceptive neurons, the efficacy of stimulation-produced descending inhibition from the PAG or NRM was evaluated before and during superfusion of the spinal cord dorsum at the recording segment with selective receptor antagonists.

Material and techniques

Extracellular recordings were made through glass microelectrodes in the lumbar dorsal horn of cats which were deeply anesthetized with pentobarbital (initially 40 mg/kg i.p. and subsequently 6 – 12 mg/kg i.v., as required) and artificially ventilated with a gaseous mixture of N_2O/O_2 and halothane. Conventional animal preparation and recording techniques have been described in detail elsewhere (Sandkühler et al., 1987).

All neurons studied responded to noxious radiant heating applied to the glabrous skin of the ipsilateral hindpaw (50 or 52°C for 10 s) as well as to innocuous mechanical skin stimuli. Heat-evoked activity, analyzed as the total number of impulses in 25 s (corrected for spontaneous activity), was readily depressed during electrical stimulation in the PAG or in the NRM (0.1 ms pulse width, 200 – 800 µA, 100 ms trains at 100 Hz, repeated at 3 Hz). At the end of each experiment, brain stimulation sites were electrolytically marked and later verified histologically to be within the boundaries of the PAG or NRM, respectively.

Superfusion of the lumbar spinal cord dorsum

The spinal cord dorsum was superfused at the recording segments L5 – L7 by means of a small plexiglass chamber as illustrated in Fig. 1. The content of the pool ($\leqslant$ 200 µl) could be exchanged completely during extracellular single neuron recordings through polyethylene tubing connected to the chamber. All drugs used were dissolved in normal saline (methysergide 0.96 or 9.6 mM, phentol-

322

amine 4.8 or 9.6 mM or a mixture with methysergide 0.96 mM, phentolamine 9.6 mM plus naloxone 2.7 mM. In some experiments morphine was applied at 0.3 mM).

Means ± SEM are given and compared with the two-tailed Student's *t* test for paired or unpaired data, $p \leqslant 0.05$ was considered significant.

Results

Results are derived from a total of 23 nociceptive neurons located in laminae I – VI of the lumbar dorsal horn of 20 cats. Electrical stimulation of cutaneus nerves supplying the ipsilateral hindlimb at a strength supramaximal for the activation of A fibers was used as a search stimulus. All neurons included in this study responded to noxious radiant skin heating and to innocuous mechanical skin stimuli.

Superfusion of the spinal cord dorsum

In an attempt to identify the spinal receptors of the putative neurotransmitters which mediate the descending inhibition from the PAG or the NRM, we superfused the spinal cord at the recording segment with selective receptor antagonists (Fig. 1). To test whether drugs applied topically to the cord may influence the neuronal activity underneath, the pool was filled in four experiments with morphine at 0.3 mM and heat-evoked activity was depressed to 42.1 ± 9.6% of control 9 – 15 min after the beginning of the superfusion. This depression was partially reversed by naloxone (1.0 mg/kg, i.v.) and fully reversed by spinal naloxone (2.7 mM, Sandkühler, Fu and Zimmermann, unpublished observations, see also Fig. 1).

Methysergide. During superfusion of the spinal cord dorsum with methysergide at 0.96 mM, noxious heat-evoked responses were *not* significantly altered (reduction to 74.9 ± 18.1% of control); methysergide at the greater concentration (9.6 mM), however, depressed responses to 19.6 ± 6.9% of control ($t = 11.74, p \leqslant 0.0001, n = 7$),

see Fig. 2 for an example. The efficacy of stimulation-produced descending inhibition from the PAG or NRM was not, however, significantly affected by either concentration of methysergide (see Fig. 3).

Phentolamine. Noxious heat-evoked activity was depressed dose-dependently during superfusion of the spinal cord with phentolamine at 4.8 mM (to 70.2 ± 8.8% of control; $t = 3.36, p \leqslant 0.02, n = 8$) and at 9.6 mM (to 50.1 ± 11.0% of control; t

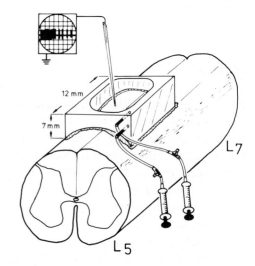

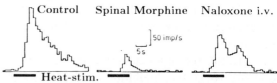

Fig. 1. Controlled superfusion of the spinal cord dorsum during extracellular recording in vivo. A small plexiglass chamber was fitted to the dorsal surface of the spinal cord at the recording segments (L5 – L7). The content of the pool (≤ 200 µl) could be exchanged completely and rapidly through polyethylene tubing during extracellular single neuron recordings. The dura mater was reflected and the pia mater was left intact except at the places for the electrode penetrations. To evaluate possible diffusion barriers, morphine was applied at 0.3 mM topically to the cord. The depression of noxious heat-evoked responses (50°C, 10 s) occurred 9 – 12 min after beginning of the superfusion and was partially reversible by intravenous naloxone (1.0 mg/kg), see peristimulus time histograms (bin width 1 s) at the bottom.

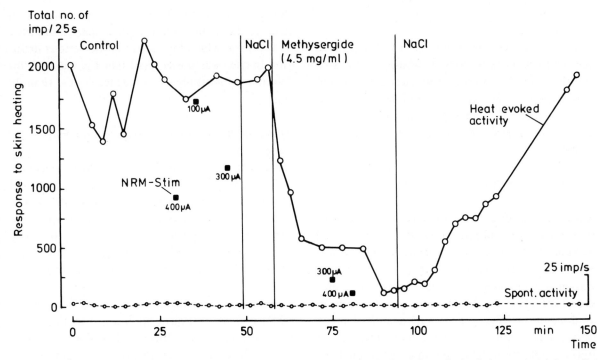

Fig. 2. Effect of spinal methysergide (4.5 mg/ml, 9.6 mM) on noxious heat-evoked activity and stimulation-produced descending inhibition from the NRM of a spinal dorsal horn neuron. Heat-evoked responses are expressed as total number of impulses (○) and plotted on the ordinate versus time course of the experiment. Responses during NRM stimulation at the indicated intensities are plotted as filled squares, spontaneous activity (○) is plotted at the bottom (right hand scale). Vertical lines indicate exchange of spinal pool content.

= 4.53, $p \leqslant 0.01$, $n = 7$). Stimulation-produced descending inhibition was, however, not affected significantly during superfusion with phentolamine (see Fig. 3).

In four experiments, the spinal cord dorsum was superfused with a solution containing methysergide (0.96 mM), phentolamine (9.6 mM) and naloxone (2.7 mM). Heat-evoked activity was depressed to 53.0 ± 10.8% of control ($t = 4.34$, $p \leqslant 0.05$) while the efficacy of stimulation-produced descending inhibition from the PAG or the NRM was not affected significantly (see Fig. 3).

The depression of noxious heat-evoked responses by these receptor antagonists was fully reversible within 1 – 2 h. Responses to non-noxious stimuli such as brushing of the skin or electrical stimulation of cutaneous nerves (n. tibialis posterior or n. peroneus superficialis) at intensities which activated only A fibers were not or much less affected by these receptor antagonists.

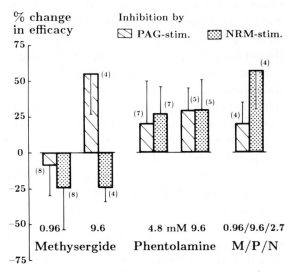

Fig. 3. Summary of the effect of spinal receptor antagonists on the efficacy of stimulation-produced descending inhibition. Percentages of changes in efficacy of descending inhibition are given as means ± SEM. M/P/N indicates a superfusate containing methysergide, phentolamine and naloxone. The concentrations of the receptor antagonists in the superfusate are expressed as mM at the bottom.

Discussion

The tonic descending inhibition of dorsal horn neuronal responses to noxious heating of the skin and the inhibition produced by electrical stimulation in the PAG or NRM was completely resistant to serotonergic, α-adrenergic and opiate receptor antagonists superfused topically at the recording segment.

Controlled superfusion of the cord dorsum

Selective receptor antagonists were applied topically, with known concentrations, to the spinal cord dorsum at the recording segment, by means of a small plexiglass chamber. This approach was chosen to avoid those very steep concentration gradients produced by the iontophoretic application of drugs not covering the dendritic area of many dorsal horn neurons studied; and further, the topical application should minimize extraspinal effects which are frequently observed after systemic application of receptor-antagonists (e.g. Foong et al., 1985). The method used here resembles to some extent the intrathecal application of drugs (Yaksh and Rudy, 1976). However, drugs in the present experiments were not diluted by the cerebrospinal fluid, and the area of spinal cord and the duration of exposure should be better defined.

None of the receptor antagonists tested reduced the efficacy of stimulation-produced descending inhibition of nociceptive dorsal horn cells. Insufficient drug concentrations, exposure area or exposure duration, or a diffusion barrier might be implicated to explain the lack of effect. None of these possibilities, however, seems likely, since the highest concentrations used here are comparable to those shown to be effective in awake animals after intrathecal application and the exposed area at the cord dorsum ($\sim$ 50 mm^2) should be large enough to cover all dendritic contacts of the neurons studied. At least 20 min elapsed between the beginning of the superfusion and the evaluation of the efficacy of descending inhibition. Finally, the rather water-soluble compound morphine affected dorsal horn neuronal responses to noxious skin heating via opiate receptors when applied topically to the cord, which indicated that no serious diffusion barrier was present and that the maximal inhibition by morphine was reached in less than 20 min.

Spinal administration of receptor antagonists

Both methysergide and phentolamine selectively and reversibly depressed dorsal horn neuronal responses to noxious radiant heating of the skin in a dose-dependent manner. These depressions were not antagonized by spinal naloxone and thus they are probably not mediated through an opiate link. A depression of nociceptive responses of some dorsal horn cells was also observed after i.v. administration of methysergide in cats (Foong et al., 1985) and after topical application to the spinal cord surface of rats (Jones and Gebhart, personal communication). Interestingly, the incidence of heat-responsive dorsal horn neurons in cats was reduced following depletion of serotonin (5HT) by pretreatment of the animals with p-chlorophenylalanine (Carstens et al., 1981).

The mechanism of the attenuation of heat-evoked responses by the serotonin receptor antagonist methysergide is not known, but it might be due to a partial agonistic activity, or due to the removal of tonic excitatory influences, since methysergide was found to readily antagonize the *excitatory* effect of iontophoretic 5HT or the *excitation* of some dorsal horn cells produced by NRM-stimulation (Belcher et al., 1978; Todd and Millar, 1984). Intraveneous or iontophoretic methysergide also antagonizes the *inhibition* of dorsal horn cells by serotonin or by PAG or NRM stimulation in some studies (Griersmith and Duggan, 1980; Yezierski et al., 1982) but not in others (Belcher et al., 1978; Mokha et al., 1986). The failure of methysergide to antagonize the inhibition produced by 5HT in some preparations is consistent with its ineffectiveness against NRM-induced descending inhibition. Alternatively, the lack of effect could also indicate that 5HT is *not* the primary neurotransmitter mediating the descending inhibition from the NRM of nociceptive dorsal horn cells (see discussions by Belcher et al., 1978; Mokha et al., 1986; Yezierski et al., 1982). This latter conclusion is consistent with reports showing that 5HT is exclusively present in unmyelinated (slowly conducting) descending fibers (Zahs et al., 1985), while descending inhibition from the NRM is, at least in part, mediated through fibers with faster conduction velocities (Light et al., 1986; Willis et al., 1977).

A depression of dorsal horn cell responses to noxious heat by topical phentolamine was also observed in rats (Jones and Gebhart, unpublished observations). In the dorsal horn, iontophoretic phentolamine was shown to 'often reduce spike amplitude and depress neuronal responses to all cutaneous stimuli' (Davies and Quinlan, 1985).

Although a selective depression of heat-evoked activity of dorsal horn cells by iontophoretic noradrenaline acting on α_2-receptors was described (Davies and Quinlan, 1985), and a non-selective depression of all responses by noradrenaline was reported by Howe and Ziegelgänsberger (1987), iontophoretic phentolamine failed to antagonize inhibition produced by iontophoretic noradrenaline in some reports (Belcher et al., 1978; Engberg and Ryall, 1966; Howe and Ziegelgänsberger, 1987) but not in all (Fleetwood-Walker et al., 1985). Phentolamine also antagonized the hyperpolarisation of lamina II cells by noradrenaline in a spinal cord slice preparation (North and Yoshimura, 1984).

Noradrenaline may also exite some spinal neurons (North and Yoshimura, 1984), specially those located at the base of the dorsal horn (Howe and Ziegelgänsberger, 1987). It has been discussed that the rare excitation of some spinal neurons by noradrenaline may be mediated through α_1-adrenoceptors (North and Yoshimura, 1984), while the depression may employ α_2-adrenoceptors (see discussion by Howe and Ziegelgänsberger, 1987). Here, the overall depression by phentolamine would then indicate a predominant antagonism at α_1-adrenoceptors.

It has been suggested that this unreliable antagonism of phentolamine of the depression by noradrenaline may explain its ineffectiveness against stimulation-produced descending inhibition of dorsal horn cells (Belcher et al., 1978).

To account for the possibility that serotonin, noradrenaline and endogenous opioids are released simultaneously in the spinal cord when stimulating electrically in the PAG or in the NRM, we have superfused the cord with a solution containing receptor antagonists against all three putative neurotransmitters. However, stimulation-produced descending inhibition was *not* affected, indicating that a possible *redundancy* of these inhibitory neurotransmitter systems may not have been the reason for the lack of effect by a single receptor antagonist.

Our results do not rule out the possibility that the synaptic release of serotonin or noradrenaline in the spinal cord plays a role in mediating stimulation-produced inhibition of nociceptive information in the dorsal horn. However, the present data do not support the view that the inhibition is mediated through $5HT_{1/2}$ or $\alpha_{1/2}$-adrenoceptors in the cord, respectively.

Descending inhibition of nocifensive motor reflexes. It was hypothetized that the depression of nociceptive dorsal horn cells may account for stimulation-produced descending inhibition of spinally mediated, nocifensive motor reflexes such as the rat tail-flick reflex (see Besson and Chaouch, 1987 for a recent review). The pharmacology in the spinal cord underlying the depression of single dorsal horn neurons or the depression of motor responses may in part be different.

Intrathecal methysergide, phentolamine (Hammond and Yaksh, 1984) or naloxone (Zorman et al., 1982) reduced or abolished stimulation-produced descending inhibition of the tail-flick reflex, whereas the depression of dorsal horn cells appears to be much more resistant against these receptor antagonists when applied to the *spinal cord* as shown in this and other reports (Belcher et al., 1978; Davies and Quinlan, 1985; Foong et al.,

1985; Griersmith et al., 1981).

Apart from obvious differences in species, state of the animals, noxious stimuli employed and route of drug administration, divergent results obtained from single cell recordings versus motor-reflex measurements may suggest that the underlying descending inhibitory mechanisms in the spinal cord may, at least in in part, be different.

Acknowledgements

We gratefully acknowledge the assistance of Q.-G. Fu during the experiments and the valuable comments of G.F. Gebhart on an earlier version of the manuscript. Supported by the Deutsche Forschungsgemeinschaft, Grant Zi 110.

References

Belcher, G., Ryall, R.W. and Schaffner, R. (1978) The differential effects of 5-hydroxytryptamine, noradrenaline and raphe stimulation on nociceptive and non-nociceptive dorsal horn interneurones in the cat. Brain Res., 151: 307 – 321.

Besson, J.-M. and Chaouch, A. (1987) Peripheral and spinal mechanisms of nociception. Physiol. Rev., 67: 67 – 186.

Bowker, R.M., Westlund, K.N., Sullivan, M.C., Wilber, J.F. and Coulter, J.D. (1982) Transmitters of the raphe-spinal complex: immunocytochemical studies. Peptides, 3: 291 – 298.

Carstens, E., Fraunhoffer, M. and Zimmermann, M. (1981) Serotonergic mediation of descending inhibition from midbrain periaqueductal gray, but not reticular formation, of spinal nociceptive transmission in the cat. Pain, 10: 149 – 167.

Davies, J. and Quinlan, J.E. (1985) Selective inhibition of responses of feline dorsal horn neurones to noxious cutaneous stimuli by tizanidine (DS103 – 282) and noradrenaline: involvement of α_2-adrenoceptors. Neuroscience, 16: 673 – 682.

Duggan, A.W., Hall, J.G. and Headly, P.M. (1976) Morphine, enkephalin and the substantia gelatinosa. Nature, 264: 456 – 458.

Engberg, I. and Ryall, R.W. (1966) The inhibitory action of noradrenaline and other monoamines on spinal neurones. J. Physiol. (London), 185: 298 – 322.

Fleetwood-Walker, S.M., Mitchell, R., Hope, P.J., Molony, V. and Iggo, A. (1985) An α_2-receptor mediates the selective inhibition by noradrenaline of nociceptive responses of identified dorsal horn neurones. Brain Res., 334: 243 – 254.

Foong, F.W., Terman, G. and Duggan, A.W. (1985)

Methysergide and spinal inhibition from electrical stimulation in the periaqueductal grey. Eur. J. Pharmacol., 116: 239 – 248.

Gebhart, G.F., Sandkühler, J., Thalhammer, J.G. and Zimmermann, M. (1983) Inhibition of spinal nociceptive information by stimulation in midbrain of the cat is blocked by lidocaine microinjected in nucleus raphe magnus and medullary reticular formation. J. Neurophysiol., 50: 1446 – 1459.

Griersmith, B.T. and Duggan, A.W. (1980) Prolonged depression of spinal transmission of nociceptive information by 5-HT administered in the substantia gelatinosa: antagonism by methysergide. Brain Res., 187: 231 – 236.

Griersmith, B.T., Duggan, A.W. and North, R.A. (1981) Methysergide and supraspinal inhibition of the spinal transmission of nociceptive information in the anaesthetized cat. Brain Res., 204: 147 – 158.

Hammond, D.L. and Yaksh, T.L. (1984) Antagonism of stimulation-produced antinociception by intrathecal administration of methysergide or phentolamine. Brain Res., 298: 329 – 337.

Hammond, D.L., Tyce, G.M. and Yaksh, T.L. (1985) Efflux of 5-hydroxytryptamine and noradrenaline into spinal cord superfusates during stimulation of the rat medulla. J. Physiol. (Lond.), 359: 151 – 162.

Howe, J.R. and Zieglgänsberger, W. (1987) Responses of rat dorsal horn neurons to natural stimulation and to iontophoretically applied norepinephrine. J. Comp. Neurol., 255: 1 – 17.

Light, A.R., Casale, E.J. and Ménétrey, D.M. (1986) The effects of focal stimulation in nucleus raphe magnus and periaqueductal gray on intracellularly recorded neurons in spinal laminae I and II. J. Neurophysiol., 56: 555 – 571.

Mokha, S.S., McMillan, J.A. and Iggo, A. (1986) Pathways mediating descending control of spinal nociceptive transmission from the nuclei locus coeruleus (LC) and raphe magnus (NRM) in the cat. Exp. Brain Res., 61: 597 – 606.

North, R.A. and Yoshimura, M. (1984) The actions of noradrenaline on neurones of the rat substantia gelatinosa in vitro. J. Physiol. (Lond.), 349: 43 – 55.

Sandkühler, J., Fu, Q.G. and Zimmermann, M. (1987) Spinal pathways mediating tonic or stimulation-produced descending inhibition from the periaqueductal gray or nucleus raphe magnus are separate in the cat. J. Neurophysiol., 58: 327 – 341.

Todd, A.J. and Millar, J. (1984) Antagonism of 5-hydroxytryptamine-evoked excitation in the superficial dorsal horn of the cat spinal cord by methysergide. Neurosci. Lett., 48: 167 – 170.

Willis, W.D., Haber, L.H. and Martin, R.F. (1977) Inhibition of spinothalamic tract cells and interneurons by brain stem stimulation in the monkey. J. Neurophysiol., 40: 968 – 981.

Yaksh, T.L. and Rudy, T.A. (1976) Chronic catheterization of the spinal subarachnoid space. *Physiol. Behav.,* 17: 1031–1036.

Yezierski, R.P., Wilcox, T.K. and Willis, W.D. (1982) The effects of serotonin antagonists on the inhibition of primate spinothalamic tract cells produced by stimulation in nucleus raphe magnus or periaqueductal gray. *J. Pharmacol. Exp. Ther.,* 220: 266–277.

Zahs, K.S., Lakos, S. and Basbaum, A.I. (1985) Immunoreactive serotonergic axons in the dorsolateral funiculus of the cat and rat. *Soc. Neurosci. Abstr.,* 11: 125.

Zorman, G., Belcher, G., Adams, J.E. and Fields, H.L. (1982) Lumbar intrathecal naloxone blocks analgesia produced by microstimulation of the ventromedial medulla in the rat. *Brain Res.,* 236: 77–84.

H.L. Fields and J.-M. Besson (Eds.)
Progress in Brain Research, Vol. 77
© 1988 Elsevier Science Publishers B.V. (Biomedical Division)

CHAPTER 24

Pharmacology of putative neurotransmitters and receptors: 5-hydroxytryptamine

M.H.T. Roberts

Department of Physiology, University College Cardiff, Cardiff CF1 1XL, UK

This volume contains many references to the data showing that systems which contain 5-hydroxytryptamine (5HT) alter the responses of many species to high-threshold cutaneous stimuli. As these data have also been reviewed many times (Roberts and Llewelyn, 1982; Roberts, 1984; Fields and Basbaum, 1984), they will not be discussed again in detail. Briefly, if neurons in the brain which contain 5HT are destroyed with the selectively neurotoxic compound 5,7-dihydroxytryptamine, the antinociceptive effects of morphine are strongly attenuated (Morland and Gebhart, 1980). Similarly, depletion of 5HT from central neurons with parachlorophenylalanine will also reduce the antinociceptive effects of (a) systemic morphine (Fennesy and Lee, 1970; Gorlitz and Frey, 1972; Le Bars et al., 1979), (b) periaqueductal gray (PAG) stimulation (Carstens et al., 1981) and (c) nucleus raphe magnus (NRM) stimulation (Oliveras et al., 1978). It is believed that the serotonergic raphe-spinal neurons are important because: lesions of the NRM reduce the antinociceptive effects of systemic morphine (Proudfit and Anderson, 1975), excitation of NRM cells causes antinociception (Fields and Basbaum, 1978), intrathecal administration of 5HT causes antinociception (Wang, 1977; Yaksh and Wilson, 1979), and microiontophoretic application of 5HT mimics the antinociceptive effects of NRM stimulation (Belcher et al., 1978; Davies and Roberts, 1981). It has further been shown that

antinociceptive PAG stimulation causes the release of 5HT from the spinal cord (Yaksh and Tyce, 1980) and that potentiating 5HT transmission with precursors or uptake inhibitors, potentiates the effects of morphine (Johansson and Von Knorring, 1979; Uzan et al., 1980) and is useful in the treatment of pain in man (Noel et al., 1978; Hosobuchi, 1978). These data and those from many electrophysiological experiments have given rise to the theoretical postulate (Fields and Basbaum, 1984) that raphe-spinal neurons which release 5HT into the dorsal horn of the spinal cord, inhibit the responses of spinal sensory cells to noxious stimuli.

The above very brief summary fails to reveal the rather fundamental difficulties that exist concerning the detail of the way in which 5HT functions to inhibit nociceptive responses. Ruda and Gobel (1980) reported the ultrastructural characteristics of spinal axonal endings which take up 5HT. [^{3}H]5HT was applied topically to the medulla and only the superficial laminae were studied by them. This may be because only the superficial laminae were subjected to a sufficient concentration of the topically applied 5HT or because terminals taking up 5HT occur only in substantia gelatinosa. It is likely to be the former, because the original publication of 5HT distribution (Fuxe, 1965) reported a higher concentration of 5HT terminals deeper in the dorsal horn than more superficially. Thus, it may follow that topical (or intrathecal?) application of 5HT or other compounds may influence only the most superficial layers of the cord and may fail to diffuse very far into the deeper layers. If physiological function of superficial and deep 5HT synapses is different, then intrathecally, intraspinally and systemically applied drugs may have confusingly different effects. Inhibition of deep, but not superficial cells, has been reported following stimulation of some sites in the brain (Rees and Roberts, 1987). The 5HT terminals in laminae I and II do seem to be relevant to the antinociceptive effects of brain stimulation, as Miletic et al. (1984) report that stimulation of NRM suppresses the responses of lamina-I- and lamina-II-stalked cells to a range of intense cutaneous stimuli. These same cell types possessed particularly dense synaptic contacts from 5HT terminals. It is not certain, however, that topically applied 5HT will mimic the effects of 5HT released from these axon terminals. This is because the release of 5HT from synaptic terminals may be inhibited by autoreceptors. Many of the confusing effects of 5HT agonists and antagonists may be due to them having a significant action upon the autoreceptor. As pointed out by Monroe and Smith (1985), the release of 5HT from spinal synaptosomes is inhibited by 5HT agonists and potentiated by 5HT antagonists. This may give rise to the opposite of the expected result if only postsynaptic actions of the drugs are considered. This would be particularly the case if 5HT systems are tonically active, which they seem to be as indicated by electrode recordings from NRM cells (Davies et al., 1988a,b) but seem not to be when effects of drugs are considered (Soja and Sinclair, 1980).

Another source of the immense variability in the effects of drugs on 5HT systems could stem from the considerable evidence for not only an antinociceptive role of descending noradrenergic and 5HT fibres (Jensen and Yaksh, 1986) but also for a strong interaction between the two systems. Archer et al. (1985) report that following selective destruction of noradrenaline cells in rats, intrathecal 5HT was no longer antinociceptive in tail flick, hot plate and shock titration tests. The im-

plications of this interaction to the design of pharmacological experiments are fairly clear, and it must be remembered that it is not possible to activate 5HT systems without involving noradrenergic fibres simply by stimulating in the region of NRM. Barbaro et al. (1985) have shown that the antinociceptive effects of NRM microstimulation on the tail flick are blocked by either intrathecal yohimbine or methysergide. It seems that NRM stimulation may well evoke activity in α_2-adrenoceptors, perhaps via a relay in the brain stem between NRM and the noradrenergic cells which project to the spinal cord. The paper by Barbaro et al. (1985) reveals another source of variability between experiments. The antagonistic effects of methysergide were not seen when the paw pressure test was used. This may be interpreted as being either because different tests are more or less sensitive to the effects of drugs generally, or because different neuronal systems may suppress responses to the different types of noxious cutaneous stimuli applied in these tests. Furthermore, it is fairly clear that tests which have a coordinated emotional response as the end point differ significantly from those which evoke a purely spinal reflex (Schmauss et al., 1983). Thus, Jensen and Yaksh (1985) report that intrathecal methysergide blocks inhibition of the tail flick by activation of PAG but fails to block the same inhibition of the hot plate response. Bjorkum and Berge (1986), also using the hot plate test, observed that neurotoxic lesion of ascending 5HT neurons in the brain potently reduced the antinociceptive effects of 5HT release by parachloramphetamine. Similar neurotoxic lesions of spinal 5HT pathways were much less effective. Even when spinal reflexes are studied, drugs may act on supraspinal sites, and an excellent example of this has been reported by Zemlan et al. (1983). 5HT agonists, which normally inhibit nociceptive spinal reflexes, were found to be hyperalgesic in spinal animals. A partial explanation of the loss of the antinociceptive effect may be that ascending 5HT systems in the brain inhibit the nociceptive responses of thalamic neurons (Anderson and Dafny, 1982) and, while the responses of these cells are obviously important for the mediation of the integrated response of the whole animal, they may well also activate descending inhibition in the spinal cord.

It is very noticeable that most of the studies referred to above have used methysergide as the intrathecally administered 5HT antagonist. Earlier studies had used antagonists such as cinanserin and found it to be effective (Yaksh et al., 1976; Chitour et al., 1982) but much less potent than methysergide. None of the 5HT antagonists seem to be able to block dependably the descending inhibition of spinal neurons. Griersmith and Duggan (1980) observed that iontophoretically applied methysergide was able to block the antinociceptive effects of 5HT applied iontophoretically into the vicinity of spinal laminae IV or V neurons. They noted, however, that very large ejecting currents were necessary and that the antagonist had to be applied for some time before the agonist. It was probably the failure to use such high currents that led Belcher et al. (1978) and Davies and Roberts (1981) to conclude that iontophoretically applied methysergide was ineffective on the depressant effects of 5HT in the spinal cord. Griersmith et al. (1981) subsequently reported, however, that methysergide, even when applied with high iontophoretic currents, was unable to block descending inhibition of multireceptive spinal neurons. The methysergide was also applied iontophoretically into the substantia gelatinosa and topically to the cord, but without effect. When given intravenously, however, methysergide effectively blocked the descending inhibition. The authors concluded that methysergide caused 'a depression of the firing of the cells of origin' of the descending inhibition. Yesierski et al. (1982) came to an essentially similar conclusion because the antagonists methysergide, metergoline, cinanserin and cyproheptadine were only weakly effective on spinal inhibition evoked by NRM stimulation but much more potent on inhibition evoked from PAG. These implications that antagonists were potent on a supraspinal site were investigated by Llewelyn et al. (1983, 1984). Using the spinal reflex tail flick to noxious heat in unanaesthetised rats it was observed that microinjection of 5 μg of 5HT into NRM was potently antinociceptive. The effect of 5HT was blocked by cinanserin (5 μg i.p.) and microinjection of methysergide into NRM blocked the effects of PAG stimulation. Cells containing 5HT have been reported to project from ventrolateral PAG to NRM (Beitz, 1982) and these may mediate the antinociceptive effects of PAG stimulation. Microinjections of the 5HT uptake blocker zimelidine, or the 5HT releasing agent fenfluramine, into NRM also potently inhibited the tail flick reflex (Llewelyn et al., 1984). Microiontophoretic applications of 5HT onto cells in NRM were potently excitatory, and these responses were abolished by very low currents of the 5HT antagonist cinanserin (Llewelyn et al., 1983). It would seem likely that the PAG to NRM relay, as well as the NRM to spinal cord pathway uses 5HT as a neurotransmitter.

5HT transmission onto NRM cells also seems likely from the data of Dickenson et al. (1986) who report that a 5HT depleting agent and a 5HT antagonist reduce both the excitatory and inhibitory responses of NRM cells to noxious peripheral stimuli. At about the same time as the above studies, Willcockson et al. (1983) reported a very detailed study of the responses of identified projection neurons in NRM to iontophoretically applied 5HT. They observed only depressant effects of 5HT. As the authors point out, the absence of excitory effects may be because they used pentobarbitone anaesthesia and it has been known since 1969 that in the cat neocortex the excitatory effects of 5HT are seen in unanaesthetised (encephale isole) and fluothane-anaesthetised cats but excitation is practically abolished by barbiturates (Johnson et al., 1969). Of course, it is also possible that because in the study by Llewelyn et al. (1983) the neurons were not physiologically identified, they may have all been interneurons. Perhaps NRM interneurons and NRM projection neurons possess different receptors to 5HT.

It is most likely that the existence of different receptor types to 5HT on central neurons is the factor which will eventually explain the many puzzling inconsistencies in the literature concerning the role of 5HT in sensory perception. It has been clear since the original observations of Gaddum and Picarelli (1957) that subgroups of the 5HT receptor must exist. The first demonstration of functional differences in the response of central neurons to 5HT was the study of Roberts and Straughan (1967), who reported that in the unanaesthetised cat cortex iontophoretically applied 5HT excited many cells and depressed others. Only the excitatory responses could be blocked by lysergic acid diethylamide or cinanserin and, therefore, only these responses could be related to an action of 5HT at a specific receptor. No antagonist could be found which influenced the depressant effects of 5HT. Many cells responded biphasically to 5HT (an initial depression followed by a subsequent excitation), and increasing the amount of 5HT ejected from the electrode increased the size of the excitatory phase at the expense of the inhibition. This suggested that the excitatory receptor was less sensitive to 5HT than the depressant receptor. The absence of selective agonists and antagonists which discriminated between these responses to 5HT prevented very much further investigation of the phenomenon. Further progress had to wait for the binding studies of Peroutka and Snyder (1979). These studies showed that the brain contained specific very high affinity (nanomolar) recognition sites for 5HT called $5HT_1$ sites and also specific low affinity (micromolar) sites called $5HT_2$ sites. These sites were distributed differently throughout the brain but there were many overlapping areas where both could be found. In general terms, agonists of 5HT showed high affinity for $5HT_1$ sites and antagonists high affinity for $5HT_2$ sites but, apart from this degree of discrimination, useful selective agonists and antagonists were not available. Subsequently, selective binding ligands were discovered and it became clear that a further subdivision of 5HT sites into $5HT_{1A}$ and $5HT_{1B}$ was necessary (Pedigo et al., 1981).

Following closely behind these binding studies were attempts to relate functional responses to activation of these binding sites. Without such studies, of course, only the affinity of a compound for a site is known, and it may or may not have efficacy. Without knowledge of efficacy a binding site should not be called a pharmacological receptor. Greatest progress has been made using functional responses to 5HT and its selective agonists and antagonists in behavioural, peripheral neuron and vascular studies. These studies have been summarised by Bradley et al. (1986) and a classification of functional receptors is proposed using terminology which is clearly derived from, but importantly not identical to, the classification of binding sites. They define the $5HT_3$ receptor which is not found in CNS (although this has recently been questioned by Brittain et al., 1987 and Jones et al., 1987), and it is unlikely, therefore, to mediate the central actions of 5HT in descending inhibitory pathways*. The $5HT_3$ receptor has clearly been shown, however, to mediate the provocation of pain from the blister base and the intradermal flare, so it will probably be involved with inflammatory pain (Richardson et al., 1985).

The $5HT_2$ receptor closely resembles the $5HT_2$ binding site. 5HT has a low potency and responses are antagonised very potently by ketanserin, methysergide and many other antagonists. The $5HT_1$-like receptor is so named because of profound differences from the $5HT_1$ binding sites. 5HT has a high potency and ketanserin does not block these functional receptors even at high doses. Methysergide, however, has some antagonistic potency at $5HT_1$ receptors, but only at much higher doses than required at $5HT_2$ receptors. There are several agonists which selectively bind to $5HT_1$ sites and also have functional efficacy (see below), but the selectively binding antagonist cyanopindolol does not have clear antagonistic actions at several of the $5HT_1$ functional receptors, e.g. the inhibitory receptor for 5HT on postganglionic sympathetic neurons (Charlton et al., 1986).

---

* See 'Footnote added in proof' on p. 338.

Recently, Davies et al. (1988a,b) have examined the effects of these new and selective ligands on the responses of randomly encountered central neurons recorded from the hindbrain raphe nuclei and sites up to 0.5 mm lateral. The high proportion of excitatory effects of 5HT in the fluothane-anaesthetised rat reported by Llewelyn et al. (1983) were confirmed. These excitatory responses were readily blocked by iontophoretic or intravenous administration of the highly $5HT_2$ selective antagonist ketanserin (200 μg/kg i.v.). This was not due to the α_1 blocking action of ketanserin. Methysergide (1 mg/kg) or metergoline (100 μg/kg) given intravenously or iontophoretically were also very effective and selective antagonists of excitation. Two agonists of 5HT, which have been shown to have greater affinity for $5HT_1$ binding sites than 5HT, and also to be relatively selective functional agonists at peripheral $5HT_1$ receptors were studied. 8-Hydroxy-2-(di-*n*-propylamino)tetralin (8-OH-DPAT) and 5-carboxamidotryptamine (5CT) were only rarely weak agonists of excitation. It seems clear that the excitatory receptor and the $5HT_2$ receptor are very similar or identical (Davies et al., 1988a).

A smaller but significant number of cells in, or close to, NRM were depressed by iontophoretically applied 5HT. These responses were of shorter latency than the excitatory responses and lasted for a shorter time. The $5HT_1$-like agonists, 8-OH-DPAT and 5CT, evoked very strong and long-lasting depressant responses which were much larger than those to 5HT. The transport numbers of these agonists were calculated and they did not differ significantly from the transport number for 5HT and it is unlikely, therefore, that their greater potency was due to greater release from the electrode by the iontophoretic current. Ketanserin given for long periods with high iontophoretic currents, or given intravenously with high doses (2 mg/kg i.v.), did not reduce these depressant responses. Methysergide at the $5HT_2$-effective dose of 1 mg/kg i.v. was also ineffective, but with very much higher doses of 30 mg/kg i.v. it reduced the depressant responses without affecting depres-

sant responses of the same cell to GABA. Methysergide in binding and functional studies affects $5HT_2$ sites preferentially but also has antagonistic actions on $5HT_1$-like receptors. It is very likely, therefore, that the depressant responses reflect the action of 5HT at a $5HT_1$-like receptor. This receptor may have some similarity to the $5HT_{1A}$ binding site, as 8-OH-DPAT is a potent agonist. The effects of cyanopindolol at this site are unresolved at present.

This description of $5HT_1$ and $5HT_2$ functional receptors in the central nervous system had long been predicted (Peroutka et al., 1981) but has not been clearly demonstrated previously. It is very likely from these data that the excitatory action of 5HT on NRM cells and the antinociceptive effects of 5HT microinjected into NRM, reported by Llewelyn et al. (1983), are due to the action of 5HT on $5HT_2$ receptors. 5HT antagonists potently block these actions of 5HT (Llewelyn et al., 1983). It seems less likely that the depressant and/or antinociceptive actions of 5HT in the spinal cord are mediated by a $5HT_2$ receptor. Intrathecally applied cinanserin is much less effective than methysergide (Yaksh et al., 1976) and, although intrathecal methysergide is clearly effective (Yaksh et al., 1979; Barbaro, 1985; Jensen and Yaksh, 1985a,b), the intrathecal dose which differentiates between spinal $5HT_1$ and $5HT_2$ receptors is not clearly known. Of course, if antagonists are administered intravenously, descending inhibitory influences may be altered by an action of the drug on brain stem cell bodies, and the nature of spinal receptors cannot be deduced (Post et al., 1986).

When methysergide is applied to spinal nociceptive neurons by iontophoresis, it does not block descending inhibitory influences (Belcher et al., 1978; Griersmith and Duggan, 1981), even though it does block the antinociceptive effects of 5HT if applied for a long time (Griersmith and Duggan, 1980). It does seem to be a sensible conclusion that methysergide is able to block the antinociceptive actions of 5HT in the spinal cord but that high concentrations of the drug are required. This is exactly to be expected if the antinociceptive 5HT receptors in the cord are of the $5HT_1$ type.

Many recent papers have addressed the pharmacological nature of the spinal 5HT receptor and binding site. Pazos et al. (1985a,b) have studied the nature of 5HT binding in the spinal cord and report a low to very low density of both $5HT_1$ and $5HT_2$ binding sites in the spinal cord. Mitchell and Riley (1985) confirm this observation and correctly stress that, although $5HT_1$ sites are more dense in the cord, $5HT_2$ sites are clearly present. Although $5HT_2$ sites are at low levels, an important physiological function for them cannot be discounted. Schmauss et al. (1983) investigated the nature of the functional antinociceptive 5HT receptor in the spinal cord. Intrathecal 5HT caused antinociception in the tail flick and hot plate tests. Co-administration, intrathecally, of methysergide, bromolysergic acid and ketanserin antagonised the effects of 5HT on tail flick and, as ketanserin was less effective than methysergide, they suggest that a spinal $5HT_1$ receptor mediates the antinociception detected with the tail flick test. It is necessary to remember, however, that according to the binding affinities of ketanserin at $5HT_1$ and $5HT_2$ sites ($>10\,000$-fold less affinity for the $5HT_1$ site), ketanserin should have practically no blocking effect at a $5HT_1$ site whereas it had an IC_{50} of 34.5 nmol. This is the equivalent of about 80 μg/kg which is just about the correct ED_{50} for 50% antagonism of $5HT_2$ receptors by systematically administered ketanserin. Either $5HT_2$ receptors are important in the spinal cord or ketanserin entered the blood stream to act at supraspinal $5HT_2$ sites. It is also possible that the α-adrenoceptor blocking action of ketanserin (Fozard, 1982) was responsible (Archer et al., 1985; Post et al., 1986).

Under very different experimental conditions, Ogren and Berge (1985) also concluded that $5HT_1$ receptors were involved in the antinociception evoked by parachloramphetamine-induced release of 5HT. They conclude this from the lack of antagonistic action of systemically administered ketanserin. The hot plate test was used, and this supraspinally organised response is affected by ascending 5HT systems as discussed previously. It

was also observed that, when given alone, ketanserin caused a marked hyperalgesia, and this seems to imply some complex, possibly supraspinal, role for $5HT_2$ receptors in tonic suppression of responsiveness to noxious stimuli.

The importance of precise measurement of dose and the need for information on which dose of a drug will discriminate between different receptor types is apparent from studies of 5HT agonists. Although 5-methoxy- and other tryptamines are described as $5HT_1$ agonists and may have antinociceptive effects due to an action on $5HT_1$ binding sites (Zemlan, 1983; Danysz et al., 1986; Post et al., 1986), the established binding affinities of these compounds for $5HT_{1A}$, $5HT_{1B}$ and $5HT_2$ sites show that their affinity for both of the $5HT_1$ sites is less than that of 5HT, and their affinity for $5HT_2$ sites is equal to or greater than that of 5HT (Engel et al., 1986). It is true that they bind to $5HT_1$ sites with greater affinity than to $5HT_2$ sites, but then, so does 5HT. These compounds discriminate less well between $5HT_1$ and $5HT_2$ sites than does 5HT itself. There is no justification for believing that they act preferentially at $5HT_1$ receptors and, in fact, their effects may well be mediated by $5HT_2$ receptors. This point has been clearly demonstrated by Green (1984) who showed that 5-methoxydimethyltryptamine and quipazine both evoked a behavioural response which was blocked by modest doses of $5HT_2$ antagonists. There are more selective ligands than these compounds. 8-OH-DPAT and 5CT both bind to $5HT_{1A}$ sites with slightly greater affinity than 5HT, and to $5HT_2$ sites with a slightly lower affinity than 5HT (Engel et al., 1986). Even these have quite reasonable affinity for $5HT_2$ sites, however, and a failure to block the effects of these compounds with known doses of the very selective $5HT_2$ antagonists (Leysen et al., 1984) is an essential part of identifying a functional role for $5HT_1$ receptors.

Berge et al. (1985) have studied the effects of 8-OH-DPAT on the tail flick response of mice to radiant heat. 8-OH-DPAT failed to change the response latency when given alone ($0.06 - 1$ mg/kg i.p.) but potently blocked the analgesic effects of morphine. It follows that it is far from proven that $5HT_1$ receptors mediate the antinociceptive effects of 5HT in the spinal cord. The major difficulty of course is the lack of a selective $5HT_1$ antagonist.

The work of Monroe, Smith and colleagues (1983, 1985, 1986) adds yet another dimension of complexity which cannot be ignored if sense is to be made of the role of 5HT in descending spinal inhibition. They studied the release of 5HT from synaptosomes prepared from the spinal cord. They observed that some agonists of 5HT reduce the release of 5HT and that the antagonists quipazine and methiothepin block this autoreceptor-mediated inhibition of release – i.e. antagonists may potentiate release. This means that antagonists with a preferential affinity for presynaptic autoreceptors may enhance transmission at 5HT synapses. These autoreceptors are likely to be $5HT_1$-like receptors but Monroe et al. (1985) observed that, although ketanserin does not change the release of 5HT evoked by potassium, it increased the basal release of 5HT. Even ketanserin, therefore, may have some presynaptic actions in vivo.

In conclusion, it is clear that synaptic transmission mediated by $5HT_2$ receptors has an important role in the inhibition of responses to noxious stimuli. It is likely that antinociceptive $5HT_2$ receptors are supraspinal but they seem to influence descending inhibitory systems as well as supraspinally organised behavioural responses. It is unlikely that functionally antinociceptive $5HT_2$ synapses are located in the spinal cord, even though $5HT_2$ binding sites exist there. The antinociceptive spinal 5HT synapses probably contain $5HT_1$ receptors, but proof requires a selective $5HT_1$ antagonist and this is presently not available. Full recognition of distinctive pharmacological differences between the receptor subtypes will go a long way towards unravelling these complex antinociceptive mechanisms.

Acknowledgements

The ideas and concepts in this review have been developed in the course of long discussions with Michael Davies and Huw Rees. Their contribution is gratefully acknowledged. The laboratory is supported by the Wellcome Trust.

References

Anderson, E. and Dafny, N. (1982) Microiontophoretically applied 5HT reduces responses to noxious stimulation in the thalamus. Brain Res., 241: 176 – 178.

Archer, T., Arwestrom, E., Jonsson, G. and Post, C. (1985) Complete blockade and attenuation of 5-hydroxytryptamine induced analgesia following Na depletion in rats and mice. Acta Pharmacol. Toxicol., 57: 255 – 261.

Barbaro, N.M., Hammond, D.L. and Fields, H.L. (1985) Effects of intrathecally administered methysergide and yohimbine on microstimulation-produced antinociception in the rat. Brain Res., 343: 223 – 229.

Beitz, A.J. (1982) The sites of origin of brain stem neurotensin and serotonin projections to the rodent nucleus raphe magnus. J. Neurosci., 2: 829 – 842.

Belcher, G., Ryall, R.W. and Schaffner, R. (1978) The differential effects of 5-hydroxytryptamine, noradrenaline, and raphe stimulation on nociceptive and non-nociceptive dorsal horn interneurones in the cat. Brain Res., 151: 307 – 321.

Berge. O.-G., Fasmer, O.B., Ogren, S.O. and Hole, K. (1985) The putative serotonin receptor agonist 8-hydroxy-2-(di-n-propylamino) tetralin antagonises the antinociceptive effect of morphine. Neurosci. Lett., 54: 71 – 75.

Bjorkum, A.A. and Berge, O.-G. (1986) The relative importance of ascending and descending serotonergic pathways in PCA induced analgesia. Acta Physiol. Scand., 128: 19.

Bradley, P.B., Engel, G., Feniuk, W., Fozard, J., Humphrey, P.P.A., Middlemiss, D.N., Mylecharane, E.J., Richardson, B.P. and Saxena, P.R. (1986) Proposals for the classification and nomenclature of functional receptors for 5-hydroxytryptamine. Neuropharmacology, 25: 563 – 576.

Brittain, R.T., Butler, A., Coates, I.H., Fortune, D.H., Hagan, R., Hill, J.M., Humber, D.C., Humphrey, P.P.A., Ireland, S.J. Jack, D., Jordan, C.C., Oxford, A., Straughan, D.W. and Tyers, M.B. (1987) GR 38032F, a novel selective $5HT_3$ receptor antagonist. Br. J. Pharmacol., 90: 87P.

Carstens, E., Fraunhoffer, M. and Zimmermann, M. (1981) Serotonergic mediation of descending inhibition from midbrain periaqueductal gray, but not reticular formation, of spinal nociceptive transmission in the rat. *Pain,* 10: 149 – 167.

Charlton, K.G., Bond, R.A. and Clarke, D.E. (1986) An inhibitory prejunctional $5HT_1$-like receptor in the isolated perfused rat kidney: apparent distinction from the $5HT_{1A}$, $5HT_{1B}$ and $5HT_{1C}$ subtypes. *Naunyn-Schmiedeb. Arch. Pharmacol.,* 332: 8 – 15.

Chitour, D., Dickenson, A.H. and Le Bars, D. (1982) Pharmacological evidence for the involvement of serotonergic mechanisms in diffuse noxious inhibitory controls (DNIC). *Brain Res.,* 236: 329 – 337.

Danysz, W., Minor, B.G., Post, C. and Archer, T. (1986) Chronic treatment with antidepressant drugs and the analgesia induced by 5-methoxy-*n,n*-dimethyltryptamine: attenuation by desipramine. *Acta Pharmacol. Toxicol.,* 59: 103 – 112.

Davies, J.E. and Roberts, M.H.T. (1981) 5-Hydroxytryptamine reduces substance P responses on dorsal horn interneurons: a possible interaction of neurotransmitters. *Brain Res.,* 217: 399 – 404.

Davies, M., Wilkinson, L.S. and Roberts, M.H.T. (1988a) Evidence for excitatory $5-HT_2$ receptors on rat brain stem neurons. *Br. J. Pharmacol.,* in press.

Davies, M., Wilkinson, L.S. and Roberts, M.H.T. (1988b) Evidence for depressant $5HT_1$-like receptors on rat brain stem neurons. *Br. J. Pharmacol.,* in press.

Dickenson, A.H. and Goldsmith, G. (1986) Evidence for a role of 5-hydroxytryptamine in the responses of rat raphe magnus neurones to peripheral noxious stimuli. *Neuropharmacology,* 25: 863 – 868.

Engel, G., Gothert, M., Hoyer, D., Schlicker, E. and Hillenbrand, K. (1986) Identity of inhibitory presynaptic 5-hydroxytryptamine (5HT) autoreceptors in the rat brain cortex with $5HT_{1B}$ binding sites. *Naunyn-Schmiedeb. Arch. Pharmacol.,* 332: 1 – 7.

Fennessy, M.R. and Lee, J.R. (1970) Modification of morphine analgesia by drugs affecting adrenergic and tryptaminergic mechanisms. *J. Pharm. Pharmacol.,* 22: 930 – 935.

Fields, H.L. and Basbaum, A.I. (1978) Brainstem control of spinal transmission neurons *Annu. Rev. Physiol.,* 40: 193 – 221.

Fields, H.L. and Basbaum, A.I. (1984) Endogenous pain control mechanisms. In P.D. Wall and R. Melzack (Eds.), *Textbook of Pain.* Churchill Livingston, pp. 142 – 152.

Fozard, J.R. (1982) Mechanisms of the hypotensive effect of ketanserin. *J. Cardiovasc. Pharmacol.,* 4: 829 – 838.

Fuxe, K. (1965) Evidence for the existence of monoamine neurons in the central nervous system. IV. Distribution of monoamine terminals in the central nervous system. *Acta Physiol. Scand.,* 64, Suppl. 247: 41 – 85.

Gaddum, J.H. and Picarelli, Z.P. (1957) Two kinds of tryptamine receptor. *Br. J. Pharmacol. Chemother.,* 12: 323 – 328.

Gorlitz, B.D. and Frey, H.H. (1972) Central monoamines and antinociceptive drug action. *Eur. J. Pharmacol.,* 20: 171 – 180.

Green, A.R. (1984) 5-HT-mediated behaviour: animal studies. *Neuropharmacology,* 23: 1521 – 1528.

Griersmith, B.T. and Duggan, A.W. (1980) Prolonged depression of spinal transmission of nociceptive information by 5-HT administered in the substantia gelatinosa: antagonism by methysergide. *Brain Res.,* 187: 231 – 236.

Griersmith, B.T., Duggan, A.W. and North, R.A. (1981) Methysergide and supraspinal inhibition of the spinal transmission of nociceptive information in the anaesthetised cat. *Brain Res.,* 204: 147 – 158.

Hosobuchi, Y. (1978) Dietary supplementation with L-tryptophan reverses tolerance to analgesia induced by periaqueductal gray stimulation in humans. In Leong-Way (Ed.), *Endogenous and Exogenous Opiate Agonists and Antagonists.* Pergamon Press, Toronto, pp. 375 – 378.

Jensen, T.S. and Yaksh, T.L. (1985a) Spinal monoamine and opiate systems partly mediate the antinociceptive effects produced by glutamate at brain stem sites. *Brain Res.,* 321: 287 – 297.

Jensen, T.S. and Yaksh, T.L. (1985b) Glutamate induced analgesia: effects of spinal serotonin, norepinephrine and opioid antagonists. In H. Fields et al. (Eds.), *Advances in Pain Research and Therapy, Vol 9.* Raven Press, New York.

Jensen, T.S. and Yaksh, T.L. (1986) II. Examination of spinal monoamine receptors through which brain stem opiate-sensitive systems act in the rat. *Brain Res.,* 363: 114 – 127.

Johansson, F. and Von Knorring, L. (1979) A double blind controlled study of a serotonin uptake inhibitor (zimelidine) versus placebo in chronic pain patients. *Pain,* 7: 69 – 78.

Johnson, E.S., Roberts, M.H.T. and Straughan, D.W. (1969) The responses of cortical neurons to monoamines under differing anaesthetic conditions. *J. Physiol. (Lond.),* 203: 261 – 280.

Jones, B.J., Oakley, N.R. and Tyers, M.B. (1987) The anxiolytic activity of GR 38032F, a $5HT_3$ receptor antagonist, in the rat and cynomolgus monkey. *Br. J. Pharmacol.,* 90: 88 p.

Le Bars, D., Rivot, J.P., Guilbaud, G., Menetrey, D. and Besson, J.-M. (1979) The depressive effect of morphine on the C fibre response of dorsal horn neurones in the spinal rat pretreated or not by pCPA. *Brain Res.,* 176: 337 – 353.

Leysen, J.E., de Chaffoy de Courcelles, D., de Clerck, F., Niemegeers, C.J.E. and van Nueten, J.M. (1984) Serotonin-S_2 receptor binding sites and functional correlates. *Neuropharmacology,* 23: 1493 – 1501.

Llewelyn, M.B., Azami, J. and Roberts, M.H.T. (1983) Effects of 5-hydroxytryptamine applied into nucleus raphe magnus on nociceptive thresholds and neuronal firing rate. *Brain Res.,* 258: 59 – 68.

Llewelyn, M.B., Azami, J. and Roberts, M.H.T. (1984) The effect of modification of 5-hydroxytryptamine function in nucleus raphe magnus on nociceptive threshold. *Brain Res.,* 306: 165 – 170.

Miletic, V., Hoffert, M.A., Ruda, M.A. Dubner, R. and Shinegaga, Y. (1984) Serotoninergic contacts on identified cat spinal dorsal horn neurons and their correlation with nucleus raphe magnus stimulation. *J. Comp. Neurol.,* 228: 129 – 141.

Mitchell, R. and Riley, S. (1985) Characterisation of receptors for 5-hydroxytryptamine in spinal cord. *Trans. Biochem. Soc.,* 13: 955.

Mohrland, J.S. and Gebhart, G.F. (1980) Effect of selective destruction of serotonergic neurons in nucleus raphe magnus on morphine-induced antinociception. *Life Sci.,* 27: 2627 – 2632.

Monroe, P.J. and Smith, D.J. (1983) Characterisation of multiple [^{3}H]5-hydroxytryptamine binding sites in rat spinal cord tissue. *J. Neurochem.,* 41: 349 – 355.

Monroe, P.J. and Smith, D.J. (1985) Demonstration of an autoreceptor modulating the release of [^{3}H]5-hydroxytryptamine from a synaptosomal-rich spinal cord tissue preparation. *J. Neurochem.,* 45: 1886 – 1894.

Monroe, P.J., Michaux, K. and Smith, D.J. (1986) Evaluation of the direct actions of drugs with a serotonergic link in spinal analgesia on the release of [^{3}H]serotonin from spinal cord synaptosomes. *Neuropharmacology,* 25: 261 – 265.

Noel, M.A., Mays, K.S. and Byrne, W.L. (1978) Oral tryptophan as a potential adjunctive therapy in chronic pain patients. In Leong-Way (Ed.), *Endogenous and Exogenous Opiate Agonists and Antagonists.* Pergamon Press, Toronto. pp. 371 – 374.

Ogren, S.O. and Berge, O.G. (1985) Evidence for selective serotonergic receptor involvement in parachloramphetamine induced antinociception. *Naunyn-Schmiedeb. Arch. Pharmacol.,* 329: 135 – 140.

Oliveras, J.L., Hosobuchi, Y., Guilbaud, G. and Besson, J.M. (1978) Analgesic electrical stimulation of the feline nucleus raphe magnus: development of tolerance and its reversal by 5-HTP. *Brain Res.,* 146: 404 – 409.

Pazos, A., Cortes, R. and Palacios, J.M. (1985a) Quantitative autoradiographic mapping of serotonin receptors in the rat brain II. Serotonin-2 receptors. *Brain Res.,* 346: 231 – 249.

Pazos, A. and Palacios, J.M. (1985b) Qualitative autoradiographic mapping of serotonin receptors in the rat brain. I. Serotonin-1 receptors. *Brain Res.,* 346: 205 – 230.

Pedigo, N.W., Yamamura, H.I. and Nelson, D.L. (1981) Discrimination of multiple [^{3}H]5-hydroxytryptamine binding sites by the neuroleptic spiperone in rat brain. *J. Neurochem.,* 36: 220 – 226.

Peroutka, S.J. and Snyder, S.H. (1979) Multiple serotonin receptors: differential binding of [^{3}H]5-hydroxytryptamine, [^{3}H]lysergic acid diethylamide and [^{3}H]spiroperidol. *Molec. Pharmacol.,* 16: 687 – 699.

Peroutka, S.J., Lebovitz, R.M. and Snyder, S. (1981) Two distinct central serotonin receptors with different physiological functions. *Science,* 212: 827 – 829.

Post, C., Minor, B.G., Davies, M. and Archer, T. (1986) Analgesia induced by 5-hydroxytryptamine receptor agonists is blocked or reserved by noradrenaline-depletion in rats. *Brain Res.,* 363: 18 – 27.

Proudfit, H.K. and Anderson, E.G. (1975) Morphine analgesia: blockade by raphe magnus lesions. *Brain Res.,* 98: 612 – 618.

Rees, H. and Roberts, M.H.T. (1987) Anterior pretectal stimulation alters the responses of spinal dorsal horn neurones to cutaneous stimulation in the rat. *J. Physiol. (Lond.),* 385: 415 – 436.

Richardson, B.P., Engel, G., Donatsch, P. and Stadler, P.A. (1985) Identification of serotonin M-receptor subtypes and their specific blockade by a new class of drugs. *Nature,* 316: 126 – 131.

Roberts M.H.T. (1984) 5-Hydroxytryptamine and antinociception. *Neuropharmacology,* 23: 1529 – 1536.

Roberts, M.H.T. and Llewelyn, M.B. (1982) The supraspinal control of pain. *Bioscience,* 32: 587 – 594.

Roberts, M.H.T. and Straughan, D.W. (1967) Excitation and depression of cortical neurons by 5-hydroxytryptamine. *J. Physiol. (Lond.).,* 193: 269 – 294.

Ruda, M.A. and Gobel, S. (1980) Ultrastructural characterisation of axonal endings in the substantia gelatinosa which take up [^{3}H]serotonin. *Brain Res.,* 184: 57 – 83.

Schmauss, C, Hammond, D.L., Ochi, J.W. and Yaksh, T.L. (1983) Pharmacological antagonism of the antinociceptive effects of serotonin in the spinal cord. *Eur. J. Pharmacol.* 90: 349 – 357.

Soja, P.J. and Sinclair, J.G. (1980) Evidence against a serotonin involvement in the tonic descending inhibition of nociceptor-driven neurones in the cat spinal cord. *Brain Res.,* 199: 225 – 230.

Uzan, A., Kabouche, M., Rataud, J. and Le Fur, G. (1980) Pharmacological evidence of a possible tryptaminergic regulation of opiate receptors by using indalpine, a selective 5-HT uptake inhibitor. *Neuropharmacology,* 19: 1075 – 1079.

Wang, J.K. (1977) Antinociceptive effect of intrathecally administered serotonin. *Anesthesiology,* 271: 269 – 271.

Willcockson, W.S., Gerhart, K.D., Cargill, C.L. and Willis, W.D. (1983) Effects of biogenic amines on raphe spinal tract cells. *J. Pharmacol. Exp. Ther.,* 225: 637 – 645.

Yaksh, T.L. and Tyce, G.M. (1980) Resting and K$^+$-evoked release of serotonin and norephinephrine in vivo from the rat and cat spinal cord. *Brain Res.,* 192: 133 – 146.

Yaksh, T.L. and Wilson, P.R. (1979) Spinal serotonin terminal system mediates antinociception. *J. Pharmacol. Exp. Ther.* 208: 446 – 453.

Yaksh, T.L., Du Chateau, J.C. and Rudy, R.A. (1976) Antagonism by methysergide and cinanserin of the antinociceptive action of morphine administered in the periaqueductal gray. *Brain Res.,* 104: 367 – 372.

Yezierski, R.P., Wilcox, T.K. and Willis, W.D. (1982) The effects of serotonin antagonists on the inhibition of primate spinothalamic tract cells produced by stimulation in nucleus raphe magnus or periaqueductal gray. *J. Pharmacol. Exp. Ther.,* 220: 266 – 277.

Zemlan, F.P., Kow, L.-M. and Pfaff, D.W. (1983) Spinal serotonin (5HT) receptor subtypes and nociception. *J. Pharmacol. Exp. Ther.,* 226: 477 – 485.

* Footnote added in proof

The publication by Kilpatric et al. in December 1987 of the distribution of $5HT_3$ binding sites in the brain, significantly alters this suggestion. However, the behavioural effects of the very potent antagonists at $5HT_3$ receptors are not known to include marked hyperalgesia.

Reference

Kilpatrick, G.J., Jones, B.J. and Tyers, M.B. (1987) Identification and distribution of $5HT_3$ receptors in rat brain using radioligand binding. *Nature,* 330: 746 – 748.

H.L. Fields and J.-M. Besson (Eds.)
Progress in Brain Research, Vol. 77
© 1988 Elsevier Science Publishers B.V. (Biomedical Division)

CHAPTER 25

The use of microiontophoresis in the study of the descending control of nociceptive transmission

R.G. Hill

Parke-Davis Research Unit, Addenbrooke's Hospital Site, Cambridge CB2 2QB, UK

Introduction

A major problem in the study of descending control mechanisms is presented by the need to iden-the mechanism and locus of action of both endogenous neural messengers and of exogenously administered drugs used as tools. One way of simplifying this problem is to use micro-methods to apply drugs to discrete areas of the central nervous system. The use of microiontophoresis (or alternatively micropressure) application from a glass micropipette is the technique of choice, particularly when combined with the extra or intracellular recording of neuronal activity from the same pipette assembly. This technique, like all others, has drawbacks as well as advantages, and this review attempts to point out the more obvious pitfalls for the unwary. Specific examples are given of instances in which micro-methods of drug application have proved helpful in the context of the subject of this volume.

The methodological detail of the microiontophoresis and micropressure has been dealt with at length elsewhere, thus this review makes no attempt to be exhaustive. For a complete account of all aspects of the subject, the books by Purves (1981) and Stone (1985) are recommended. Earlier reviews by Curtis (1964), Kelly (1975) Krnjevic (1971) and a relevant symposium (Bradley et al., 1974) may also be found helpful.

Theoretical basis of microiontophoresis

The terms microiontophoresis, microionophoresis and microelectrophoresis are now used interchangeably. All describe the movements of charged drug out of glass micropipettes by the application of an electric current of appropriate polarity and include contributions from the phenomena of electro-osmosis and bulk flow without attribution. It has been generally assumed that release of drug from a solution within a micropipette is directly related to the charge applied to that pipette, i.e. it obeys Faraday's (or more correctly Hittorf's) Law − see Purves (1981). The first well-controlled studies that supported this view were performed by Krnjevic et al. (1963), who showed that microiontophoretic release of acetylcholine was proportional to the amount of charge passed down to a charge of 2.5 coulombs. However, in the investigation of the time course of the response of single neurons in the cat cerebral cortex to microiontophoretic application of γ-aminobutyric acid (GABA), Hill and Simmonds (1973) obtained results suggesting that the rate of microiontophoretic release of GABA at ejecting currents below 40 nA is not constant but, in fact, increases with time during the first minute of application. In a subsequent study using ^{24}Na as a model radiolabelled cation (as labelled drugs were not sufficiently radioactive), Clarke et al. (1973) showed that there was, indeed, a progressive increase in the rate of release over the first 30 to 40 s of ejection. This effect could be minimized by reducing the retaining current (q.v. later) and was, therefore, explained as being due to dilution of the solution in the tip of the pipette. That is to say, during the passage of a retaining current ions would be drawn in from the solution surrounding the pipette tip and then, during a reversal of the current in order to expel the drug, a substantial part of the current would be carried initially by those ions previously drawn in from the surrounding medium. This phenomenon is independent of the ionic species involved, and will apply to drug solutions as much as to ^{24}Na. Measurements of labelled drug release by other workers have generally failed to see the initial rise in rate of release (see Clarke et al., 1973; Kelly, 1975, for references) as the radioligands used were insufficiently active to allow the study of release occurring over periods of less than 1 min.

The practical importance of the above discussion is in relation to the microiontophoresis of highly potent drugs that can diffuse from a micropipette in sufficient quantities to exert an effect. A retaining current (Del Castillo and Katz, 1957) of opposite polarity to the drug is, therefore, passed through the pipette between periods of active ejection in order to prevent diffusional release, thereby leading to the dilution referred to above. The expelling current 'per se' may therefore not be a good index of the dose of drug applied. In pipettes with large tip apertures, when there is a significant component of diffusional release (Clarke et al., 1973), this may be most apparent as diffusion only depends upon the concentration of drug in the pipette and not on the applied current.

The practical consequence is that the effect of the microiontophoretic drug application cannot be relied upon to be reproducible unless the current applied is kept constant together with the duration of each current application and (most easily forgotten) the time between each application (i.e. the duration of the retaining current). Bradshaw and Szabadi (1974) expand on these considerations. The combination of a consistent retaining current

with a regular cycle of drug application can allow very reproducible responses to a drug which can be shown to be proportional to the applied current (see Fig. 1, taken from Hill and Simmonds, 1973). It is noteworthy that published transport numbers (i.e. that proportion of the current carried by the drug molecules) are an approximate guide only to the amount of drug that is likely to be released in a given experimental situation. Considerable variability can be seen, even down to differences between the amounts of drug released by adjacent barrels of the same pipette. It should always be remembered that a current can be carried equally well by a drug cation leaving the micropipette or by a physiological anion entering it.

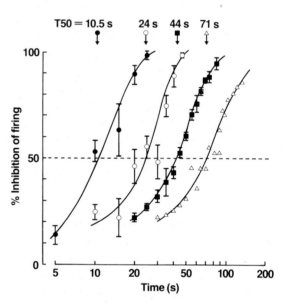

Fig. 1. Time-courses of inhibition of neuronal firing rate produced by micro-iontophoretic application of γ-aminobutyric acid (GABA) with four different currents: 20 nA (●), 10 nA (○), 5 nA (■) and 2 nA (△). Each curve was obtained from the same neuron located in the middle suprasylvian cortical gyrus of a cat anaesthetized with halothane. The neuron was driven by continuous microiontophoretic application of 20 nA L-glutamate. Each of the points for the 20 nA, 10 nA and 5 nA applications of GABA is the mean ± SEM of three values obtained from three separate applications of the same current of GABA. The values of T_{50} shown are the times taken to achieve 50% inhibition of neuron firing. (Redrawn from Hill and Simmonds, 1973.)

It is sometimes possible to expel unionized or zwitterionic substances such as peptides from micropipettes by exploitation of the phenomenon of electro-osmosis. This occurs because glass/aqueous medium interfaces tend to accumulate a net positive charge. This means that application of a positive potential to a pipette results in bulk flow of the aqueous medium, carrying drug molecules along with it. It is probably reasonable to assume that all current-induced release of drugs from micropipettes is, in fact, a combination of microiontophoresis and electro-osmosis. It is, however, likely that the relative contribution of the two processes varies with the concentration of the drug solution such that electro-osmosis will be more important in dilute solutions.

It has become common practice in some laboratories to make up solutions of potent and/or poorly soluble drugs in 150 mM sodium chloride solution rather than in water. Sometimes this is argued to carry more current than the drug solution alone (which may, in any case, have an infinite electrical resistance!) or to actually allow dilution of a potent drug solution such that a fraction of the applied current will be carried by drug ions and the remainder by sodium or chloride. In practice, the effects are unpredictable, and its use is best justified in terms of trial and error. It is true, however, that a positive current applied to sodium chloride solutions will produce bulk flow of the solution, as the water of hydration associated with the sodium ions moves, and thus drug ejection can be increased. These factors are considered in detail in Stone (1985), but is is worth stressing that microiontophoresis is an empirical technique.

Micropressure ejection of drug

As an alternative to microiontophoresis, pressure can be applied to the top of a barrel containing drug solutions in order to expel small amounts (pico- to nano-litres). Release appears to be related to the pressure applied, but tip size of the pipette can be critical in determining the amount released (whereas it seems to have little significance when microiontophoresis is used). It is important to note that, in most cases, neither a retaining current nor negative pressure are applied to pressure pipettes between applications and, thus, diffusional release is uncontrolled when this technique is employed. In the author's experience this method can work well in in vitro brain slices where relatively large tipped pipettes can be used but in vivo it has proved to be disappointing.

Construction of micropipettes

There is no doubt that the most trouble-free and reproducible results with either microiontophoresis or with micropressure are obtained when a single barrelled glass micropipette is used. Most experiments in vivo, however, require that multibarrelled assemblies are used, in order to apply a selection of drugs to the neuron under study. The author's experience has been that best results are obtained with micropipette blanks constructed from individual 100-mm lengths of 2-mm borosilicate glass tubing, but commercial blanks are now available from a number of sources. Pulling the micropipette should be a multistage process, taking care initially to ensure that the barrels are fused together by twisting through 45° when the glass is softened. The finished micropipette should be checked under a microscope for cracks between individual barrels (pipettes with 5 to 10 barrels have been found to work satisfactorily) and discarded if any are found. The filling of the micropipette with drug solutions is facilitated by using glass with an integral glass fibre so that drug is carried into the tip by capillarity, and by breaking back the tip to between 5 and 7 μm in diameter prior to filling. Detailed descriptions of micropipette preparation are given in Stone (1985), Chapter 2.

Marking of electrode position

The simplest use of microiontophoresis or micropressure in the investigation of descending inhibitory processes is its use to mark recording positions within the CNS. This can be achieved simply with extracellular dye deposition or, in a more elegant way, by filling the neuron being recorded from with dye or HRP injected from an intracellular pipette. The latter technique allows details of the morphology of an individual neuron to be determined. The extracellular marker that works best, and which can also be used (in a sodium chloride or acetate solution) in a recording or current balancing barrel, is pontamine sky blue (2.5% w/v) (Hellon, 1971). It provides an easily visible mark when negative currents of approximately 2 μA are passed for 10 min. It is best used, if the experimental protocol allows, to make a single mark at the end of an electrode track rather than to attempt to mark individual neurons, as repeated use sometimes leads to failure of dye ejection even though current is still being passed by the pipette. The subject of intracellular marking of neurons is comprehensively covered in Brown and Fyffe (1984), and those contemplating using this technique would be well advised to consult that monograph, as there are many pitfalls to overcome. The author's laboratory is currently using lucifer yellow to locate neurons from which intracellular recordings have been made, and we find that a 3% solution of Lucifer Yellow CH (Sigma) in 0.5 M KCl allows acceptable recordings to be made and provides good filling of the neurons (30 to 50 ms pulses at 1 nA, 25 Hz for approximately 10 min).

Microiontophoresis of drugs

In the context of descending control there are two main areas where microiontophoresis (and possibly micropressure) drug application can be of particular use. These are firstly the application of an agonist to determine whether a particular population of neurons is sensitive or not, and to characterize the response and its time course. Secondly, pharmacological antagonists can be used to block synaptic excitation or inhibition in order to identify the transmitter utilized by a particular pathway. There are obviously common problems associated with these two experimental situations, which have been touched on in the discussion of

the underlying principles, but there are also clear differences, so these two topics will be dealt with separately.

Microiontophoresis of agonists

A variety of endogenous substances are candidates for investigation as transmitters in descending control. Endogenous opioids, first implicated by the observation of naloxone-reversible inhibition after PAG stimulation (Akil et al., 1976), are found within the dorsal horn of the spinal cord (Hökfelt et al., 1977), probably as a result of the presence of both intrinsic interneurons and descending inhibitory pathways. Monoamines, including noradrenaline (NA), dopamine (DA), 5-hydroxytryptamine (5HT) and adrenaline are located in spinal cord (Carlsson et al., 1964). Most, if not all, are present in descending pathways with 5HT terminals originating from medullary raphe nuclei, NA primarily from locus coeruleus, medial and lateral parabrachial nuclei and associated areas, DA from hypothalamus and A11 and adrenaline from rostral ventrolateral medulla. Depletion of monoamines changes the antinociceptive effect of PAG stimulation (Akil and Liebeskind, 1975) and intrathecal administration of NA, 5HT or the DA receptor agonist, apomorphine, have all been shown shown to be antinociceptive (Reddy et al., 1980; Schmauss et al., 1983; Jensen and Smith, 1982). GABA and glycine are ubiquitous inhibitory substances, and must be considered for a role in any synaptic inhibitory process.

Microiontophoresis has been used in a number of attempts to characterize the actions of these substances on dorsal horn neurons. Opioid peptides, when applied close to the cell bodies of dorsal horn neurons, inhibit spontaneous firing and neuronal responses to both noxious and nonnoxious stimuli (Duggan et al., 1976). Subsequent in vitro studies have shown that this is likely to be a consequence of an increase in outward potassium conductance and hyperpolarization of the neuronal soma (Allerton et al., 1987), although an in vivo intracellular study failed to see this action (Zieglgänsberger and Tulloch, 1979). Microiontophoretic application of opioid peptides into the substantia gelatinosa whilst recording neuronal activity deeper within the dorsal horn with a second micropipette, gave a rather different picture (Duggan et al., 1977); there was little reduction in the response to non-noxious stimuli, whilst that to a noxious stimulus was reduced. The physiological consequences of this difference have been discussed elsewhere, but in terms of the microiontophoretic method it is an important reminder that the site of application of a drug can alter its effect on the pattern of neuronal responses. When glutamate was applied at various sites on the motoneuron dendritic tree using a 'staggered' micropipette assembly, Zieglgänsberger and Champagnat (1979) found that the latency of glutamate responses was less when the application site was dendritic rather than somatic, which suggests that the primary site of action for this substance is distal to the soma.

Monoamines, when applied microiontophoretically, have a variety of actions on spinal neurons, but the predominant effect is one of depression of neuronal activity (Headley et al., 1978). Noradrenaline has been shown to have a selective effect on the responses to noxious as compared with nonnoxious stimuli (Headley et al., 1978) and to have a time course of effect similar to that of neuronal inhibition evoked by stimulation of descending pathways (see Fig. 2). The microiontophoretic application of catecholamines can be monitored 'in situ', using the technique of cyclic voltametry (Armstrong-James et al., 1981) in which a carbon fibre filled barrel of the pipette assembly functions alternately as an extracellular recording electrode or electrochemical electrode, allowing a direct correlation of transport number with pharmacological effect. It is also relevant to note that fluorescence histochemistry has been used to estimate the spread of α-methylnoradrenaline and of noradrenaline following microiontophoretic application (Candy et al., 1974), leading to the conclusion that after 2-min application with a current of 50 nA the drug had spread approximately 0.5 mm from the electrode tip.

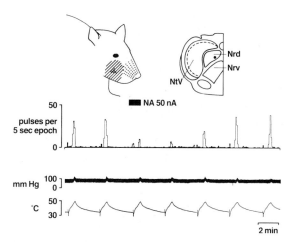

Fig. 2. Ratemeter record illustrating the depressant effect of noradrenaline (NA) (solid bar, 50 nA) on responses evoked by noxious heat of a noci-multireceptive neuron in the caudal trigeminal nucleus of a urethane-anaesthetized rat. The thermal stimulus consisted of heated water which was applied as a thermal ramp (see bottom trace for monitored stimulus temperature) to the whole receptive field (shaded region on face outline responsive only to noxious stimuli, and cross-hatched region additionally responsive to low threshold mechanical stimuli). NA depressed the evoked response, elevating the threshold by 47.5%, and the effect was particularly marked in the succeeding trial, the effect lasting some 6 min. Thermal responses of this neuron were also inhibited by periventricular grey stimulation (98% inhibitory effect), which lasted 9 min (the animal had previously displayed 70% behavioural antinociception to brain stimulation). Note the deflections of blood pressure (middle trace) which indicated that the thermal stimulus was noxious. The neuron was recorded from laminae V–VI of the medullary dorsal horn (filled circle on diagram of transverse section of medulla). (Redrawn from Cahusac, 1984.)

One common problem in the interpretation of responses to the microiontophoretic application of monoamines is that the naturally occurring amines are mixed agonists. When applied to the vicinity of a neuron they may gain access to more than one receptor subtype and, thus, produce a biphasic effect. This is illustrated in Fig. 3, and can to some extent be avoided by using substances which are receptor subtype selective rather than the natural ligands. For example, it is possible to produce consistent depression of medullary neurons if the α_2 agonist clonidine is used rather than noradrenaline (Cahusac and Hill, 1983), whereas the α_1 agonist

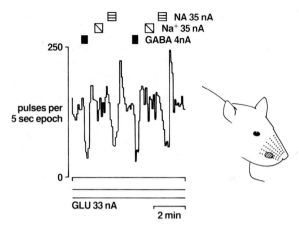

Fig. 3. Ratemeter record of a biphasic response of a low threshold caudal trigeminal mechanoreceptive neuron driven with glutamate (open bar, 33 nA) to iontophoretic noradrenaline (NA) (striped bars, 35 nA). NA produced a clear depression of firing during application and an excitation following the application. By contrast, iontophoretic GABA (solid bars, 4 nA) caused a monophasic depression of firing, whilst 35 nA passed through a NaCl solution filled barrel (crossed bars) had no effect. The neuron's receptive field is shown as the shaded area on the face outline. (Redrawn from Cahusac, 1984.)

phenylephrine is more consistently found to excite neurons (Cahusac, 1984).

A detailed account of the actions of 5HT- and receptor-selective analogues and which illustrates the above point very well, is given in Chapter 24 in this volume, by Roberts.

In summary, when agonists are applied by microiontophoresis, consideration should be given to the observation that the location of drug application can influence the effects recorded, and that drugs can spread further in the tissues following micropipette application, than might be supposed. Additionally, as natural ligands are mixed agonists that in nature are rendered selective by physiological release in the vicinity of the appropriate receptor subtype, it can be more practicable to characterize responses using synthetic, receptor subtype selective agonists.

Microiontophoresis of antagonists

It is frequently observed that when agonist and an-

tagonist applications are made from the same micropipette then clear and appropriate pharmacology can be recorded (e.g. see Fig. 4), but that when a microiontophoretically applied antagonist is used to challenge a physiological event, then results are less consistent. The reasons for this are discussed in detail by Curtis (1976) and are illustrated in Fig. 5, which is taken from his review. Briefly, when agonist and antagonist are administered from the same pipette assembly, they are likely to 'see' the same population of receptors and, thus, the fact that the overall distribution of drug around the neuron is asymmetric is of little consequence. However, when a synaptic process such as postsynaptic inhibition is being studied, then synapses close to the micropipette will receive a high (possi-

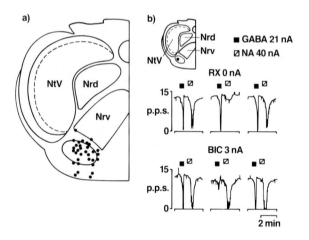

Fig. 4. (a) Diagram of a transverse section of the medulla at a level 1 mm caudal to the obex. The filled circles represent recording positions which are shown in and around the lateral reticular nucleus (unlabelled and in outline) ventrolateral to nucleus reticularis ventralis (Nrv). Other abbreviations: Nrd, nucleus reticularis dorsalis; NtV, nucleus of the tract of the Vth nerve. (b) Discontinuous, sequential ratemeter records showing the differential antagonist actions of microioonotophoretic RX781094 (RX) (top set of records) and bicuculline (BIC) (bottom set of records) on depression of spontaneous firing by cycled iontophoretic applications of GABA (21 nA) and noradrenaline (NA) (40 nA). The sets of records in temporal sequence from left to right represent control, during antagonist application, and recovery. RX781094 selectively reduced the depression induced by noradrenaline, and bicuculline selectively reduced the GABA depression. The filled circle in the diagram at the top of the Fig. represents the recording site for this neuron. (Redrawn from Cahusac and Hill, 1983.)

bly unspecific) concentration of antagonist whereas those distant from it may receive little if any. It may, therefore, be appropriate to apply agonists by microiontophoresis but to give antagonists systemically (provided that they cross the blood-brain barrier). Some antagonists are difficult to use microiontophoretically, and naloxone, for example (see Hill, 1981), is released in large amounts (compared with morphine in adjacent barrels) when used as a simple aqueous solution, but its re-

lease is unpredictable when sodium chloride solutions are used (Pepper, 1978). Additionally, it is sometimes possible to produce blockade of GABA receptors as well as of opioid receptors with microiontophoretic naloxone (see Fig. 6), and appropriate controls should therefore always be performed. Flupenthixol has been found to block both DA and 5HT excitations and inhibitions of nigral neurons (Dray et al., 1976), and bicuculline has been reported to block 5HT inhibitions on hypothalamic and cortical neurons (Mayer and Straughan, 1981) when these substances were applied by microiontophoresis.

In summary, antagonists may be more appropriately given systemically than by microiontophoresis, and specificity of effect should never be assumed without appropriate supporting results.

Future prospects

Micromethods of drug application have proved very useful in the past and will continue to do so in the future. The commercial availability of equipment for microiontophoresis and micropressure drug application has made it possible for those who do not adequately grasp the underlying principles (and therefore could not have constructed their own equipment) to use the technique. Elementary considerations, such as making sure that passing current through the drug barrel has more effect than passing current through an adjacent barrel filled with sodium chloride solution, can thus sometimes be neglected. A skeptical attitude to the results obtained will always be required.

The combination of microiontophoresis with electrochemical detection (Armstrong-James et al., 1981) or with antibody microprobes (Duggan and Morton, this volume) will allow measurement of endogenous transmitter release and monitoring of microiontophoretic ejection, thus increasing the level of quality control. Increasing use of in vitro techniques is likely, as preparations of mammalian spinal cord can now be kept viable for long periods and have been used for the investigation of descending control systems (Bagust et al., 1985).

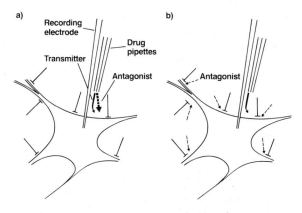

Fig. 5. Diagram illustrating the differences in distribution of agonist and antagonist drugs around a single neuron when administered from a micropipette or when injected systemically. In (a) the situation of release of both antagonist and agonist from adjacent barrels of the same pipette is illustrated. The situation of attempted antagonism of synaptic transmitter by microiontophoretic antagonist is also shown here. In (b) the likely distribution of systemically administered antagonist is illustrated. See text for further explanation. (Redrawn from Curtis, 1976.)

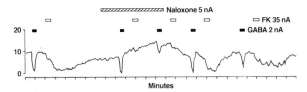

Fig. 6. A continuous chart recorder trace of the firing rate of a caudal reticular neurone in the medulla of a urethane anaesthetized rat. During the periods indicated by the bars the opioid peptide FK 33-824 (open bars) and GABA (solid bars) were applied microiontophoretically. Naloxone, applied during the period indicated by the hatched bar, blocked the long inhibition of firing produced by FK 33-824 and partially reduced the response to GABA. (Redrawn from Morris et al., 1984.)

346

Acknowledgements

I would like to thank my colleagues, particularly my graduate students for their contributions.

References

Akil, H. and Liebeskind, J.C. (1975) Monoaminergic mechanisms of stimulation produced analgesia. *Brain Res.,* 94: 279 – 296.

Akil, H., Mayer, D.J. and Liebeskind, J.C. (1976) Antagonism of stimulation-produced analgesia by naloxone, a narcotic antagonist. *Science,* 191: 961 – 962.

Allerton, C.A., Boden, P. and Hill, R.G. (1987) Actions of mu- and kappa-opioids on deep dorsal horn neurones in rat transverse spinal cord slices 'in vitro'. J. Physiol. (Lond.), 396: 153.

Armstrong-James, M., Fox, K., Kruk, Z.L. and Millar, J. (1981) Quantitative iontophoresis of catecholamines using multibarrel carbon fibre microelectrodes. *J. Neurosci. Meth.,* 4: 385 – 406.

Bagust, J., Kelly, M.E.M. and Kerkut, G.A. (1985) An isolated mammalian brainstem-spinal cord preparation suitable for the investigation of descending control of motor activitiy. *Brain Res.,* 327: 370 – 374.

Bradley, P.B., Roberts, M.H.T. and Straughan, D.W. (1974) Recent advances in methods for studying the pharmacology of single cortical neurons. *Neuropharmacology,* 13: 401 – 573.

Bradshaw, C.M. and Szabadi, E. (1974) The measurement of dose in microelectrophoretic experiments. *Neuropharmacology,* 13: 407 – 416.

Brown, A.G. and Fyffe, R.E.W. (1984) *Intracellular Staining of Mammalian Neurones.* Academic Press, London, 115 pp.

Cahusac, P.M.B. (1984) *A Behavioural and Neuropharmacological Study of the Modulation of Trigeminal Nociception in the Rat.* PhD Thesis, University of Bristol, UK.

Cahusac, P.M.B. and Hill, R.G. (1983) Alpha-2 adrenergic receptors on neurones in the region of the lateral reticular nucleus in the rat. *Neurosci. Lett.,* 42: 270 – 284.

Candy, J.M., Boakes, R.J., Key, B.J. and Worton, E. (1974) Correlation of release of amines and antagonists with their effects. *Neuropharmacology,* 13: 423 – 430.

Carlsson, A., Falck, B., Fuxe, K. and Hillarp, N.A. (1964) Cellular localization of monoamines in the spinal cord. *Acta Physiol. Scand.,* 60: 112 – 119.

Clarke, G., Hill, R.G. and Simmonds, M.A. (1973) Microiontophoretic release of drugs from micropipettes: use of ^{24}Na as a model. *Br. J. Pharmacol.,* 48: 156 – 161.

Curtis, D.R. (1964) Microelectrophoresis. In W.L. Nastuk (Ed.), *Physical Techniques in Biological Research, Vol. V, Electrophysiological Methods, Part A.* Academic Press, New York, pp. 144 – 190.

Curtis, D.R. (1976) The use of transmitter antagonists in microelectrophoretic investigations of central synaptic transmission. In P.B. Bradley and B.N. Dhawan (Eds.), *Drugs and Central Synaptic Transmission.* Macmillan, London, pp. 7 – 35.

Del Castillo, J. and Katz, B. (1957) A study of curare action with an electrical micromethod. *Proc. Roy. Soc. B.,* 146: 339 – 356.

Dray, A., Gonye, T.J. and Oakley, N.R. (1976) Effects of α-flupenthixol on dopamine and 5-hydroxytryptamine responses of substantia nigra neurones. *Neuropharmacology,* 15: 793 – 796.

Duggan, A.W., Hall, J.G. and Headley, P.M. (1976) Morphine, enkephalin and the substantia gelatinosa. *Nature (Lond.),* 264: 456 – 458.

Duggan, A.W., Hall, J.G. and Headley, P.M. (1977) Enkephalins and dorsal horn neurones of the cat: effects on responses to noxious and innocuous skin stimuli. *Br. J. Pharmacol.,* 61: 399 – 408.

Headley, P.M., Duggan, A.W. and Griersmith, B.T. (1978) Selective reduction by noradrenaline and 5-hydroxytryptamine of nociceptive responses of cat dorsal horn neurones. *Brain Res.,* 145: 185 – 189.

Hellon, R.F. (1971) The marking of electrode tip positions in nervous tissue. *J. Physiol. (Lond.),* 214: 12.

Hill, R.G. (1981) The status of naloxone in the identification of pain control mechanism operated by endogenous opioids. *Neurosci. Lett.,* 21: 217 – 222.

Hill, R.G. and Simmonds, M.A. (1973) A method for comparing the potencies of γ-aminobutyric acid antagonists on single cortical neurones using microiontophoretic techniques. *Br. J. Pharmacol.,* 48: 1 – 11.

Hökfelt, T., Ljungdahl, A., Terenius, L., Elde, R. and Nilsson, G. (1977) Immunohistochemical analysis of peptide pathways possibly related to pain and analgesia: enkephalin and substance P. *Proc. Natl. Acad. Sci. USA,* 74: 3081 – 3085.

Jensen, T.S. and Smith, D.F. (1982) Dopaminergic effects on tailflick responses in spinal rats. *Eur. J. Pharmacol.,* 79: 129 – 133.

Kelly, J.S. (1975) Microiontophoretic application of drugs onto single neurones. In L.L. Iversen, S.D. Iversen and S.H. Snyder (Eds.), *Handbook of Psychopharmacology, Vol. 2, Principles of Receptor Research.* Plenum Press, New York, pp. 29 – 67.

Krnjevic, K. (1971) Microiontophoresis. In R. Fried (Ed.), *Methods of Neurochemistry.* Marcel Dekker, New York. pp. 129 – 172.

Krnjevic, K., Mitchell, J.F. and Szerb, J.C. (1963) Determination of iontophoretic release of acetylcholine from micropipettes. *J. Physiol. (Lond.),* 165: 421 – 436.

Mayer, M.L. and Straughan, D.W. (1981) Effects of 5-hydroxytryptamine on central neurones antagonized by bicuculline and picrotoxin. *Neuropharmacology,* 20: 347 – 350.

Morris, R., Cahusac, P.M.B. and Hill, R.G. (1984) The effects of microiontophoretically-applied opioids and opiate antagonists on nociceptive responses of neurones of the caudal reticular formation of the rat. *Neuropharmacology,* 23: 497 – 504.

Pepper, C.M. (1978) *The Effects of Opiates and Opioid Peptides on Thalamic Neurones in the Rat.* PhD. Thesis. Bristol University, UK.

Purves, R.D. (1981) *Microelectrode Methods for Intracellular Recording and Iontophoresis.* Academic Press, London, pp. 146.

Reddy, S.V.R., Maderdrut, J.L. and Yaksh, T.L. (1980) Spinal cord pharmacology of adrenergic agonist-mediated antinociception. *J. Pharmacol. Exp. Ther.,* 213: 525 – 533.

Schmauss, C., Hammond, D.L., Ochi, J.W. and Yaksh, T.L. (1983) Pharmacological antagonism of the antinociceptive effects of serotonin in the rat spinal cord. *Eur. J. Pharmacol.,* 90: 349 – 357.

Stone, T.W. (1985) Microiontophoresis and pressure ejection. In *IBRO Handbook Series – Methods in the Neurosciences, Vol. 8.* John Wiley and Sons, Chichester, pp. 214.

Zieglgänsberger, W. and Champagnat, J. (1979) Cat spinal motoneurones exhibit topographic sensitivity to glutamate and glycine. *Brain Res.,* 160: 95 – 104.

Zieglgänsberger, W. and Tulloch, I.F. (1979) The effects of methionine and leucine enkephalin on spinal neurones of the cat. *Brain Res.,* 167: 53 – 64.

H.L. Fields and J.-M. Besson (Eds.)
Progress in Brain Research, Vol. 77
© 1988 Elsevier Science Publishers B.V. (Biomedical Division)

CHAPTER 26

Serotonin receptor subtypes and the modulation of pain transmission

Frank P. Zemlan, Michael M. Behbehani and R. Maureen Murphy

Division of Geriatrics, Office of the Dean, University of Cincinnati College of Medicine, Cincinnati, OH 45267-0555, USA

5-HT receptor pharmacology

Recent pharmacologic data has identified three major subtypes of the serotonin (5HT) receptor (Bradley et al., 1986). These three receptor subtypes, $5HT_1$, $5HT_2$ and $5HT_3$ have different anatomical distributions which are important for understanding the unique effect each receptor subtype has on primary afferent and central pain transmission. The purpose of the present paper is to review data on all three major 5HT receptor subtypes focusing primarily on $5HT_1$ receptors.

The antecedent for the present classification system of 5HT receptors is the original data of Gaddum and Picarelli (1957), where the ability of 5HT to induce contraction of the guinea pig ileum was related to two distinct mechanisms. First, 5HT resulted in muscle contractions by a direct action on 5HT receptors located on smooth muscle, an action preferentially antagonized by phenoxybenzamine (dibenzyline) and therefore refered to as the D-receptor. Second, 5HT produces muscle contraction by an indirect effect on cholinergic ganglionic neurons innervating the guinea pig ileum; an effect of 5HT preferentially antagonized by morphine (M-receptors). Recent synthesis of compounds having higher affinity and selectivity for D- and M-receptors has led to the present terminology (Bradley et al., 1986). D-receptors demonstrate high affinity for the $5HT_2$ antagonists ketanserin and LY53857 (Leysen et al., 1981) while

M-receptors demonstrate high affinity for the $5HT_3$ antagonists ICS 205-930 and MDL 72 222 and the $5HT_3$ agonist 2-methyl-5HT (Richardson et al., 1985; Fozard, 1984). For the present, $5HT_1$ receptors are identified as receptors having a high affinity for 5HT but not demonstrating a pharmacology similar to $5HT_2$ or $5HT_3$ receptors. As would be expected, $5HT_1$ receptors are a heterogeneous group. In spinal cord, two major subgroups of the $5HT_1$ receptor may be pharmacologically and functionally distinguished. These data on the pharmacology and function of 5HT receptor subtypes is summarized in Fig. 1 and discussed below.

Spinal 5HT receptors and pain

Several lines of evidence indicate that the descending bulbospinal serotonin system mediates pain transmission by suppressing incoming noxious input to the spinal cord (Basbaum et al., 1976; Fields et al., 1977). Although these early studies support the inhibitory role of 5HT on incoming noxious stimulation, several studies indicate that the serotonergic system may also facilitate pain transmission especially at the spinal level. Anatomically, the locations of both 5HT inhibitory and excitatory synapses have been identified in the dorsal horn of the spinal cord (Ruda and Gobel, 1980). Approximately 20 to 30% of dorsal horn nociceptive neurons demonstrate increased unit activity following stimulation of nucleus raphe magnus (NRM) or 5HT iontophoresis (Belcher et al., 1978; Behbehani and Zemlan, unpublished). Using several behavioral endpoints, studies indicate that serotonin may differentially affect complex (supraspinal) and reflex (spinal) responses to noxious stimulation. Specifically, 5HT increases hot plate (supraspinal) thresholds (Schmauss et al., 1983), while the effects of 5HT at the spinal level are more variable resulting in moderate and biphasic alterations on tail flick thresholds (Ogren and Berge, 1984), and decreased spinal reflex thresholds (Zemlan et al., 1983). With the recent discovery of multiple $5HT_1$ binding sites in the spinal cord (Zemlan et al., 1985; Monroe and Smith, 1983) similar to multiple $5HT_1$ binding sites previously identified in cortex (Sills et al., 1984a), it is possible that the opposing effects of 5HT at the spinal level may be mediated by particular $5HT_1$ receptor subtypes.

Currently available data suggest that the primary type of 5HT receptor in rat spinal cord is the $5HT_1$ receptor. There do not appear to be significant numbers of $5HT_2$ receptors in spinal cord as no measurable specific binding of the $5HT_2$-selective antagonist, ^3H-ketanserin, has been reported (Leysen et al., 1982; Monroe and Smith, 1983). We are currently exploring the possibility that measurable $5HT_3$ receptors may exist in spinal cord. In this regard, we have found that spinal cord 5HT receptors are guanine-nucleotide sensitive (Zemlan and Murphy, 1987). As $5HT_1$ receptors are guanine-nucleotide sensitive (Sills et al., 1984b) while $5HT_3$ receptors appear to be guanine-nucleotide insensitive (Robaut et al., 1985); these data suggest that the number of $5HT_3$ receptors in spinal cord would be expected to be small.

Our present receptor-binding and functional data indicate the presence in spinal cord of two distinct $5HT_1$ receptor subtypes which have opposite effects on spinal pain transmission. Spinal cord $5HT_{1A}$ receptors were directly labeled with ^3H-8-OH-DPAT (Zemlan and Murphy, 1987).

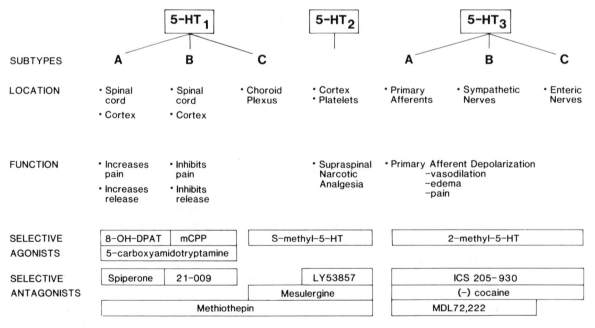

Fig. 1. Serotonin (5HT) receptor subtypes. The pharmacology of spinal cord $5HT_{1A}$ and $5HT_{1B}$ receptors is presented in the text of the present article along with electrophysiologic and behavioral data illustrating the role of these receptors in pain transmission. Similarly, the pharmacology of peripheral $5HT_{3A}$ receptors is discussed in the text along with their role in the organisms response to injury.

Comparison of B_{max} values generated from saturation isotherms indicated that ^3H-8-OH-DPAT labeled about 25% as many total binding sites as ^3H-5HT in the presence of divalent cations (^3H-8-OH-DPAT B_{max} = 83.1 ± 6.3 fmol/mg; ^3H-5HT B_{max} = 335.7 ± 63.0 fmol/mg). Competition studies employing the $5HT_{1A}$-selective compounds 8-OH-DPAT, buspirone and 5-MeODMT identified high affinity binding of these compounds in the nanomolar range which labeled between 23% to 29% of the ^3H-5HT binding sites suggesting that $5HT_{1A}$ receptors represent about 25% of 5HT receptors in spinal cord (Table I). This estimate of $5HT_{1A}$ sites in spinal cord based on radioligand binding data is similar to that reported for cervical enlargement employing quantitative autoradiography, where approximately 35% of the specific ^3H-5HT binding was displaced by 10 nM 8-OH-DPAT (Pazos and Palacios, 1985). In spinal cord, 5-MeODMT, 8-OH-DPAT and buspirone demonstrated low nanomolar affinity for the $5HT_{1A}$ receptors (Table I) which is similar to reported K_D and K_i values for these compounds in frontal cortex, hippocampus and striatum (Peroutka, 1986; Gozlan et al., 1983; Hall et al., 1985; Pazos et al., 1985). In spinal cord, 8-OH-DPAT and buspirone demonstrated over 1000-fold selectivity for the $5HT_{1A}$ binding site which is similar to the selectivity reported for these compounds in frontal cortex. 5-MeODMT demonstrated about 500-fold selectivity in spinal cord which is somewhat higher than the 100-fold selectivity reported for cortical $5HT_{1A}$ receptors (Peroutka, 1986). In spinal cord, ^3H-8-OH-DPAT binding was monophasic, indicating binding to a single population of receptors similar to other CNS regions; however, addition of guanine nucleotides decreased the total number of ^3H-8-OH-DPAT binding sites by about 60% (Zemlan and Murphy, 1987). In this regard, spinal cord $5HT_{1A}$ receptors resemble cortical $5HT_{1A}$ receptors, which also demonstrate sensitivity to guanine nucleotides; this contrasts with hippocampal and striatal $5HT_{1A}$ binding sites which are not affected by GTP (Nor-

TABLE I

Computer-derived kinetic parameter estimates for high and low affinity competition of 5HT agonists and antagonists against ^3H-5HT-labeled binding sites in spinal cord

	1A sites		1B sites	
	%	K_i (nM)	%	K_i (nM)
8-OH-DPAT	29 ± 4	5 ± 3	31 ± 3	31 491 ± 19 179
Buspirone	23 ± 7	30 ± 11	35 ± 6	29 470 ± 9 788
5-MeODMT	25 ± 4	81 ± 15	33 ± 4	41 226 ± 10 951
mCPP	23 ± 1	20 867 ± 4 790	35 ± 2	0.4 ± 0.06
Quipazine	24 ± 1	2 639 ± 714	34 ± 3	26 ± 16
TFMPP	27 ± 6	14 183 ± 4 171	33 ± 4	98 ± 4
5-HT	–	6 ± 1	–	6 ± 1
5-MT	–	43 ± 8	–	43 ± 8
Metergoline	–	151 ± 19	–	151 ± 19
Cyproheptadine	–	803 ± 55	–	803 ± 55

Reported values are the mean and asymptotic SEM K_i and percentage bound for the high and low affinity competitor binding sites. Assignment to 1A and 1B receptor subtypes was made on the basis of 100 nM masking experiments employing either the 1A-selective compound 8-OH-DPAT or the 1B-selective compound mCPP. Computer estimates from competition studies performed in triplicate at four ligand concentrations (0.3 nM to 5 nM).

man et al., 1985; Hall et al., 1985).

In spinal cord, the $5HT_{1B}$-selective compounds mCPP and quipazine demonstrated high affinity competition for about 35% of the ^{3}H-5HT-labeled spinal cord binding sites (Table I). This high affinity mCPP and quipazine binding was insensitive to addition of 100 nM 8-OH-DPAT, indicating that these high affinity binding sites are independent of the $5HT_{1A}$ site; these are predominantly $5HT_{1B}$ sites as the selective $5HT_{1C}$ compound, mesulergine (Pazos et al., 1985) demonstrated high affinity competition for spinal cord ^{3}H-5HT binding. This relative paucity of $5HT_{1C}$ binding sites in spinal cord observed in the present study is consistent with autoradiographic data indicating that $5HT_{1C}$ sites in cervical enlargement are limited to lamina I and represent only about 1% to 2% of the total number of ^{3}H-5HT binding sites (Pazos and Palacios, 1985). In comparison, TFMPP demonstrated high affinity displacement for only 38% of the spinal cord ^{3}H-5HT-labeled sites and the high affinity TFMPP binding was insensitive to 8-OH-DPAT (Table I).

In summary, $5HT_{1A}$ receptors represent about 25% while $5HT_{1B}$ receptors represent about 33% of spinal cord 5HT receptors. The remaining 42% of spinal cord 5HT receptors represent a new subtype of $5HT_1$ receptor with a unique pharmacology currently being explored.

The selective $5HT_{1A}$ and $5HT_{1B}$ agonists identified in the receptor-binding studies were employed to examine the involvement of $5HT_{1A}$ and $5HT_{1B}$ receptors in spinal nociceptive reflexes. Administration of the selective $5HT_{1B}$ agonists mCPP and TFMPP produced a dose-response related decrease in sensitivity to noxious stimulation for the ventroflexion withdrawal reflex in spinal rats (Table II). These $5HT_{1B}$ receptors are associated with spinal neurons which are innervated by descending 5HT fibers originating in the ventral medulla (Zemlan et al., 1983; Bowker et al., 1983). Electrical stimulation of these 5HT cells of origin produce behavioral analgesia (Fields and Anderson, 1978; Basbaum et al., 1976) and inhibition of dorsal horn nociceptive neurons (Belcher et

al., 1978; Headley et al., 1978). We have recently reported that dorsal horn nociceptive neurons inhibited by both ventral medullary stimulation and iontophoretic application of 5HT, are also inhibited by iontophoretic application of the selective $5HT_{1B}$ agonist mCPP (Harris et al., 1986). In these experiments (Fig. 2), ejection currents for mCPP necessary to inhibit glutamate-induced firing of lamina V type nociceptive neurons were 1/5 that required for 5HT, consistent with the presently reported K_i values of these two compounds for spinal cord $5HT_{1B}$ receptors (Table I). While $5HT_{1B}$ agonists inhibited the response of dorsal horn nociceptive neurons, no effect of iontophoretic application of the selective $5HT_{1A}$ agonists 8-OH-DPAT or 5-MeODMT was observed across the entire range of ejection currents

TABLE II

Effect of the 1A-selective agonists 8-OH-DPAT and buspirone, and the 1B-selective agonists mCPP and TFMPP on the nociceptive withdrawal reflex in the spinal rat

Drug	n	Percentage change			
		0.1 mg/kg	0.4 mg/kg	2.0 mg/kg	13.0 mg/kg
mCPP	11	−22	−22	−76[b]	−50[a]
		(20)	(21)	(17)	(22)
TFMPP	9	+23	−47[a]	−58[b]	−79[b]
		(31)	(10)	(12)	(8)
Buspirone	9	+59	+86[a]	+119[b]	+138[b]
		(35)	(37)	(36)	(34)
8-OH-DPAT	13	+69[b]	+67[a]	+51[b]	+262[b]
		(17)	(17)	(18)	(35)

Drugs were administered systemically (i.p.) at increasing doses and the sensitivity to noxious stimulation quantified as percentage change from mean predrug response levels. Values are means ± SEM. Pretreatment with the 1A antagonist, spiperone (1 mg/kg) blocked the ability of 2 mg/kg buspirone to increase the sensitivity of the reflex to noxious stimulation. Values greater than zero represent increased sensitivity to noxious stimulation of the reflex receptive field area while values less than zero represent decreased sensitivity (analgesia).
[a] $p < 0.05$, [b] $p < 0.01$ when compared to mean predrug response levels.

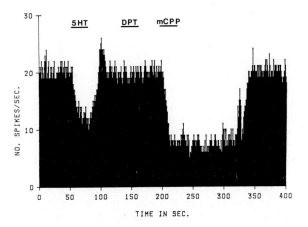

Fig. 2. The effect of the non-selective serotonin agonist 5HT, the $5HT_{1A}$ selective agonist, 8-OH-DPAT (DPT) and the $5HT_{1B}$ selective agonist mCPP on a wide-dynamic-range dorsal horn neuron in the rat. All units employed in the study were silent and demonstrated an inhibition of glutamate-induced activity following both electrical stimulation of nucleus raphe magnus and iontophoresis of 5HT. As illustrated in the initial portion of the spike histogram, iontophoresis of 80 nA 5HT for 20 s resulted in a significant decrease in glutamate-induced activity. Iontophoresis of 60 nA 8-OH-DPAT for 20 s was without effect on glutamate-induced activity, while application of 60 nA mCPP for 20 s produced a long-lasting inhibition.

published). These data suggest that the excitatory effect of 5HT on dorsal horn neurons may be mediated by spinal cord $5HT_{1A}$ receptors. The opposing effects of $5HT_{1A}$ and $5HT_{1B}$ receptors on spinal pain transmission may help explain contradictory studies regarding the role of the descending 5HT system in the control of spinal pain.

Primary afferent 5HT receptors and pain

It has been known for several decades that intradermal administration of 5HT mimics the effects of mechanical or chemical insult in man including vasodilation (flare response), edema formation and the perception of pain. For example, application of 5HT results in vasodilation and the perception of pain when applied to a blister base on the human forearm (Sicuteri et al., 1965). The ability of 5HT to induce pain is mimicked in a dose-dependent manner by the selective $5HT_3$ agonist 2-methyl-5HT, while the dose response curve is shifted over two log units to the left for the

employed. The present reflex data and the above iontophoresis data suggest that the analgesia associated with the descending 5HT system may be mediated by dorsal horn $5HT_{1B}$ receptors.

As seen in Table II, administration of the $5HT_{1A}$-selective agonists 8-OH-DPAT and buspirone produced a dose response related increase in sensitivity of spinal nociceptive reflexes to noxious stimulation which was blocked by treatment with the $5HT_{1A}$-selective antagonist spiperone. In the above described single unit studies, only dorsal horn nociceptive neurons which were inhibited by ventral medullary stimulation and 5HT iontophoresis were studied. Considering the entire population of dorsal horn nociceptive neurons, about 20% to 30% demonstrate increased unit activity following ventral medullary stimulation or 5HT iontophoresis (Belcher et al., 1978; Behbehani and Zemlan, un-

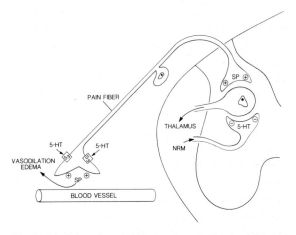

Fig. 3. Administration of $5HT_3$ agonists results in both vascular responses similar to those observed in peripheral injury, and perceived pain in man. The underlying mechanism of these effects appears related to depolarization of primary afferent substance P containing C fibers as described in the text. The increased release of substance P induces central pain via increased activity in dorsal horn nociceptive neurons which in turn are inhibited by descending 5HT fibers originating in nucleus raphe magnus (NRM).

354

5HT$_2$ agonist S-methyl-5HT (Richardson et al., 1985). Conversely, the pain-inducing effect of 5HT is blocked by the selective 5HT$_3$ antagonist ICS 205-930 but not by methysergide which is an antagonist at 5HT$_1$ and 5HT$_2$ receptors. Similarly, the dose-dependent vasodilation seen after intradermal administration of 5HT is blocked by the selective 5HT$_3$ antagonist, MDL 72 222 but not by classical 5HT antagonists (Orwin and Fozard, 1986).

The ability of 5HT$_3$ agonists to mimic some of the effects of peripheral injury, including vasodilation and pain induction may be explained by the ability of 5HT$_3$ agonists to produce depolarization of primary afferents associated with pain transmission, particularly substance P containing primary afferents. Studies with ICS 205-930 indicate that 5HT$_3$ receptors are located on sensory nerve endings (Fig. 1). In the isolated vagus nerve, both the non-selective 5HT agonist, 5HT as well as the 5HT$_3$ agonist 2-methyl-5HT produce a significant depolarization of non-myelinated C fibers, while the 5HT$_2$-selective compound S-methyl-5HT was without effect (Richardson et al., 1985). This depolarizing effect was predominantly on small diameter C fibers preferentially associated with pain transmission, and not on larger diameter fibers. Conversely, the depolarizing effect of 5HT could be blocked by the selective 5HT$_3$ antagonists ICS 205-930 and cocaine while 5HT$_1$ and 5HT$_2$ antagonists were without effect. The primary effect of depolarization appears to be increased release of transmitter from C fibers, particularly substance P in the presence of a noxious stimulus (Orwin and Fozard, 1986). Increased substance P release would result in the perception of pain in the presence of a subthreshold sensory stimulus, as observed in the case of a blister base. Second, as arterial infusion of substance P results in a dose-dependent vasodilation and plasma extravasation, these two aspects of peripheral injury also appear modulated by 5HT$_3$ receptors (Lembeck and Holzer, 1979).

References

Asarch, K.B., Ransom, R.W. and Shih, J.C. (1985) 5-HT-1a and 5-HT-1b selectivity of two phenylpiperazine derivatives: evidence for 5-HT-1b heterogeneity. Life Sci., 36: 1265.

Basbaum, A.I., Clanton, C.H. and Fields, H.L. (1976) Opiate and stimulus-produced analgesia: functional anatomy of a medullo-spinal pathway. Proc. Natl. Acad. Sci. USA, 73: 4685.

Belcher, G., Ryall, R.W. and Schaffer, R. (1978) The differential effects of 5-hydroxytryptamine, noradrenaline and raphe stimulation on nociceptive and non-nociceptive dorsal horn interneurons in the cat. Brain Res., 151: 307.

Bowker, R.M., Westlund, K.N., Sullivan, M.C., Wilber, J.F. and Coulter, J.D. (1983) Descending serotonergic, peptidergic and cholinergic pathways from the raphe nuclei: a multiple transmitter complex. Brain Res., 288: 33.

Bradley, P.B., Engle, G., Feniuk, W., Fozard, J.R., Humphrey, P.P.A., Middlemiss, D.N., Mylecharane, E.J., Richardson, B.P. and Saxena, P.R. (1986) Proposals for the classification and nomenclature of functional receptors for 5-hydroxytryptamine. Neuropharmacology, 25: 563.

Fields, H.L. and Anderson, S.D. (1978) Evidence that raphe spinal neurons mediate opiate and midbrain stimulation-produced analgesia. Pain, 5: 333.

Fields, H.L., Basbaum, A.I., Clanton, C.H. and Anderson, S.D. (1977) Nucleus raphe magnus inhibition of spinal cord dorsal horn neurones. Brain Res., 126: 441.

Fozard, J.R. (1984) Neuronal 5-HT receptors in the periphery. Neuropharmacology, 23: 1473.

Gaddum, J.H. and Picarelli, Z.P. (1957) Two kinds of tryptamine receptor. Br. J. Pharmacol. Chemother., 12: 323.

Gozlan, H., El Mestikawy, S., Pichat, L., Glowinski, J. and Hamon, M. (1983) Identification of presynaptic autoreceptors using a new ligand: 3H-PAT. Nature, 305: 140.

Hall, M., El Mestikawy, S., Emerit, M., Pichat, L., Hamon, M. and Gozlan, H. (1985) [^{3}H]8-Hydroxy-2-(di-n-propylamino)-tetralin binding to pre- and postsynaptic 5-hydroxytryptamine site in various regions of the rat brain. J. Neurochem., 44: 1686.

Harris, G.D., Zemlan, F.P., Murphy, R.M. and Behbehani, M.M. (1986) Spinal cord 5-HT 5-HT$_{1A}$ and 5-HT$_{1B}$ receptor subtypes: relation to pain transmission. Neurosci. Abstr., 12: 1015.

Headley, P.M., Duggan, A.W. and Griersmith, B.T. (1978) Selective reduction by noradrenaline and 5-hydroxytryptamine of nociceptive responses of cat dorsal horn neurons. Brain Res., 145: 185.

Lembeck, M. and Holzer, P. (1979) Substance P as neurogenic mediator of antidromic vasodilation and neurogenic plasma extravasation. *Naunyn-Schmiedeb. Arch. Pharmacol.,* 310: 175.

Leysen, J.E., Awouters, F., Kennis, L., Laduron, P.M., Vandenberk, J. and Janssen, P.A.J. (1981) Receptor binding profile of R 41 468, a novel antagonist at 5-HT$_2$ receptors. *Life Sci.,* 28: 1015.

Leysen, J.E., Niemegeers, C.J.E., Van Nueten, J.M. and Laduron, P.M. (1982) [^{3}H]Ketanserin (R 41 468), a selective ^{3}H-ligand for serotonin$_2$ receptor binding sites. *Molec. Pharmacol.,* 21: 301.

Monroe, P.J. and Smith, D.J. (1983) Characterization of multiple [^{3}H]5-hydroxytryptamine binding sites in rat spinal cord tissue. *J. Neurochem.,* 41: 349.

Norman, A.B., Battaglia, G. and Creese, I. (1985) [^{3}H]WB4101 labels the 5-HT$_{1A}$ receptor subtype in rat brain: guanine nucleotide and divalent cation sensitivity. *Mol. Pharmacol.,* 28: 487.

Ogren, S.-O. and Berge, O.-G. (1984) Test dependent variations in the antinociceptive effects of *p*-chloroamphetamine-induced release of 5-hydroxytryptamine. *Neuropharmacology,* 23: 915.

Orwin, J.M. and Fozard, J.R. (1986) Blockade of the flare response to intradermal 5-hydroxytryptamine in man by MDL 72.222, a selective antagonist at neuronal 5-hydroxytryptamine receptors. *Eur. J. Clin. Pharmacol.,* 30: 209.

Pazos, A. and Palacios, M. (1985) Quantitative autoradiographic mapping of serotonin receptors in rat brain. I. Serotonin-1 receptors. *Brain Res.,* 364: 205.

Pazos, A., Hoyer, D. and Palacios, J.M. (1985) The binding of serotonergic ligands to the porcine choroid plexus: characterization of a new type of serotonin recognition site. *Eur. J. Pharmacol.,* 106: 539.

Peroutka, S.J. (1986) Pharmacological differentiation and characterization of 5-HT$_{1a}$, 5-HT$_{1b}$, and 5-HT$_{1c}$ binding sites in rat frontal cortex. *J. Neurochem.,* 47: 529.

Richardson, B.P., Engel, G., Donatsch, P. and Stadler, P.A.

(1985) Identification of serotonin M-receptor subtypes and their specific blockade by a new class of drugs. *Nature,* 316: 126.

Roubat, C., Fillion, M.P., Dufois, S., Fayolle-Bauguen, C., Rousselle, J.-C., Gillet, G., Benkirane, S. and Fillion, G. (1985) Multiple high affinity binding sites for 5-hydroxytryptamine: a new class of sites distinct from 5-HT$_1$ and S$_2$. *Brain Res.,* 346: 250.

Ruda, M.A. and Gobel, S. (1980) Ultrastructural characterization of axonal endings in the substantia gelatinosa which take up [^{3}H]serotonin. *Brain Res.,* 184: 57.

Schmauss, C., Hammond, D.L., Ochi, J.W. and Yaksh, T.L. (1983) Pharmacological antagonism of the antinociceptive effects of serotonin in the rat spinal cord. *Eur. J. Pharmacol.,* 90: 349.

Sicuteri, E., Faniciullaci, M., Franchi, G. and Del Bianco, P.L. (1965) Serotonin-bradykinin potentiation on the pain receptors in man. *Life Sci.,* 4: 309.

Sills, M.A., Wolfe, B.B. and Frazer, A. (1984a) Determination of selective and nonselective compounds for the 5-HT$_{1A}$ and 5-HT$_{1B}$ receptor subtypes in rat frontal cortex. *J. Pharmacol. Exp. Ther.,* 231: 480.

Sills, M.A., Wolfe, B.B. and Frazer, A. (1984b) Multiple states of the 5-hydroxytryptamine receptor as indicated by the effects of GTP on [^{3}H]5-hydroxytryptamine binding in rat frontal cortex. *Mol. Pharmacol.,* 26: 10.

Zemlan, F.P., Kow, L.-M. and Pfaff, D.W. (1983) Spinal serotonin (5-HT) receptor subtypes and nociception. *J. Pharmacol. Exp. Ther.,* 226: 477.

Zemlan, F.P., Murphy, R.M. and Behbehani, M.M. (1985) Conformational states of 5-HT$_1$ receptors modulating spinal cord pain transmission: GTP sensitivity. *Neurosci. Abstr.,* 11: 125.

Zemlan, F.P. and Murphy, R.M. (1987) Pharmacologic characterization of spinal cord 5-HT$_1$ receptor subtypes and their role in the modulation of pain transmission. *Brain Res.,* in press.

H.L. Fields and J.-M. Besson (Eds.)
Progress in Brain Research, Vol. 77
© 1988 Elsevier Science Publishers B.V. (Biomedical Division)

CHAPTER 27

Pharmacologic evidence for the modulation of nociception by noradrenergic neurons

Herbert K. Proudfit

Department of Pharmacology, University of Illinois College of Medicine at Chicago, P.O. Box 6998, Chicago, IL 60680, USA

Introduction

The discovery of neuronal systems in the brain stem and spinal cord which modulate nociception has stimulated a large research effort which has provided a wealth of information regarding the characteristics of these neuronal systems. These systems have a widespread distribution in the CNS including the forebrain, midbrain, brain stem, and spinal cord. Furthermore, a large number of neurotransmitters appears to be involved in modulating nociception including norepinephrine, serotonin, acetylcholine, enkephalins, neurotensin, bombesin, and many other peptides and amino acids. The participation of monoaminergic neurons in the modulation of nociception has been more fully characterized than that of the other transmitters, which is largely due to the availability of pharmacologic agents which produce relatively selective alterations in metabolism, synthesis, uptake, release, and receptor binding. This review will be primarily concerned with noradrenergic (NA) neurons and pharmacologic evidence that these neurons constitute a major neuronal system which serves to alter the responsiveness of organisms to noxious stimuli.

General evidence for modulation of nociception by bulbospinal noradrenergic neurons

Anatomical evidence

The vast majority of studies examining the participation of NA neurons in pain modulation have focused on the spinal cord since numerous fluorescence histochemical and immunocytochemical studies have demonstrated a dense plexus of NA terminals and varicosities in the superficial dorsal horn (Carlsson et al., 1964; Fuxe, 1965; Nygren and Olson, 1977; Westlund et al., 1980, 1982, 1983, 1984). In addition, several autoradiographic studies have demonstrated a relatively dense concentration of α_2-NA receptors in the substantia gelatinosa of the spinal cord dorsal horn (Young and Kuhar, 1979; Seybold and Elde, 1984; Unnerstall et al., 1984; Dashwood et al., 1985). The existence of NA terminals and receptors in the region of the dorsal horn where small-diameter nociceptive afferents terminate (Light and Perl, 1979; Ralston and Ralston, 1979) suggests that NA systems may modulate the transmission of nociceptive information from primary afferents to ascending pain transmission neurons. A large body of experimental evidence has accumulated during the past decade to substantiate this proposal and to document the modulation of nociceptive processes by spinally-projecting NA neurons located in the brain stem.

Numerous studies have attempted to determine the origins of the NA neurons which terminate in the spinal cord, using a variety of tract tracing methods and combinations of lesions and histochemical methods (Ross and Reis, 1974; Nygren and Olson, 1977; Satoh et al., 1977; Commissiong et al., 1978; Karoum et al., 1980; Commissiong, 1981; Westlund et al., 1981, 1982, 1983, 1984; Stevens et al., 1982). The results of these studies have demonstrated NA projections to the spinal cord from the nucleus locus coeruleus (LC), medial and lateral parabrachial nuclei, nucleus subcoeruleus, A5 nucleus, and the A7 nucleus. Although several reports have indicated that NA neurons in the A1 and A2 catecholamine nuclei also project to the spinal cord (Dahlström and Fuxe, 1965; Satoh et al., 1977; Fleetwood-Walker and Coote, 1981), recent more definitive experiments have not been able to demonstrate NA projections from these nuclei (Westlund et al., 1981, 1983, 1984; McKellar and Loewy, 1982).

The terminations of spinally projecting NA neurons have been examined using a variety of tract tracing and lesioning methods (Nygren and Olson, 1977; Commissiong et al., 1978; Westlund and Coulter, 1980). The findings of these reports indicate that spinally projecting NA neurons which innervate the dorsal horn are located in the ventral LC, nucleus subcoeruleus, and probably the A5 and A7 catecholamine nuclei.

Electrophysiological evidence

The functional significance of bulbospinal NA terminals in the spinal cord dorsal horn has been demonstrated by a large number of reports. For example, iontophoretically applied norepinephrine (NE) inhibits the activation of dorsal horn neurons by noxious peripheral stimuli (Engberg and Ryall, 1966; Headley et al., 1978; Belcher et al., 1978;

Willcockson et al., 1984; Fleetwood-Walker et al., 1985; Howe and Zieglgänsberger, 1987). Several lines of evidence indicate that the inhibitory action of NE is mediated by α_2-NA receptors: (1) the α_2 agonist clonidine also produces inhibition, (2) the inhibition produced by NE is blocked by α_2 antagonists, and (3) α_1 agonists do not produce inhibition (Fleetwood-Walker et al., 1985). In addition, in vitro studies have demonstrated that NE inhibits dorsal horn neurons by an α_2 receptor-mediated hyperpolarization resulting from increased potassium conductance (North and Yoshimura, 1985). Some studies have also demonstrated an excitatory effect of iontophoretically applied NE on identified dorsal neurons responsive to noxious stimuli (Todd and Millar, 1983; Howe and Zieglgänsberger, 1987). Similar studies using in vitro spinal cord preparations have also reported that NE excites unidentified neurons recorded in the superficial dorsal horn; an action mediated by α_1-NA receptors (North and Yoshimura, 1985). These findings suggest that spinally projecting NA neurons modulate the activity of nociceptive dorsal horn neurons to produce either antinociception or augment nociception.

Descending NA neurons may also modulate nociception by altering the release of neurotransmitters from the terminals of small diameter primary afferents. For example, NE blocks the release of substance P from minced spinal cord (Pang and Vasko, 1986), cultured chick dorsal root ganglion cells (Fischbach et al., 1981; Holz et al., 1985), and superfused spinal cord (Kuraishi et al., 1985; Yaksh and Go, 1985). Additional evidence that NE can reduce transmitter release from nociceptive afferent terminals is the demonstration that intravenous administration of the α_2 agonist clonidine increases the excitability of C fiber primary afferent terminals in spinally transected cats (Calvillo and Ghignone, 1986). Increases in terminal excitability may reflect primary afferent depolarization which has been associated with decreased transmitter release (Schmidt, 1971). Although other conflicting evidence has shown that iontophoretically applied NE reduces the excitability of C fiber terminals, the significance of these results is not certain since the effects of NE could not be antagonized by either phentolamine or yohimbine (Jeftinija et al., 1981, 1983). The balance of the evidence supports the suggestion that activation of spinally projecting NA neurons produces antinociception, at least in part, by reducing transmitter release from small-diameter nociceptive afferents in the spinal cord dorsal horn.

Behavioral evidence

The actions of NE on primary afferent transmitter release and nociceptive neurons in the dorsal horn appear to be related to nociception since behavioral studies have repeatedly demonstrated that potent antinociceptive effects can be induced by intrathecal administration of various NA agonists. For example, numerous authors have demonstrated that intrathecal injection of NE produces dose-dependent antinociception (Kuraishi et al., 1979, 1985; Reddy and Yaksh, 1980; Reddy et al., 1980; Howe and Yaksh, 1982; Howe et al., 1983; Hylden and Wilcox, 1983). The antinociceptive actions of adrenergic agonists appear to be mediated by α_2-NA receptors (Howe et al., 1983; see review by Yaksh, 1985); a conclusion based on the relative potencies of α_1- and α_2-NA agonists for inducing antinociception.

Additional evidence suggesting that α_2 receptors in the spinal cord modulate nociception, has been provided by the effects of intrathecally administered NA antagonists which are selective for either α_1 or α_2 receptor subtypes. These studies demonstrated that compounds selective for α_2 receptors such as yohimbine produce hyperalgesia at lower doses than compounds which are selective for α_1 receptors such as prazosin and WB4101 (Sagen and Proudfit, 1984). These observations also suggest that the α_2 receptors in the spinal cord have a postsynaptic location. Thus, if α_2 receptors were located presynaptically and regulated NE release, then α_2 antagonists such as yohimbine should block these receptors, increase the release

of NE, and produce antinociception as does intrathecal injection of NE. Therefore, the observation that intrathecal injection of α_2 antagonists enhances nociception (produce hyperalgesia) argues against the existence of presynaptic α_2 receptors (Sagen and Proudfit, 1984). These results also indicate that descending NA neurons tonically inhibit the activation of nociceptive dorsal horn neurons, an action mediated by α_2-NA receptors. Additional evidence supporting this conclusion is the observation that depletion of spinal cord NE by intrathecal injection of 6-hydroxydopamine also enhances nociception (Reddy et al., 1980; Howe and Yaksh, 1982; Howe et al., 1983; Sagen et al., 1983).

Evidence for modulation of nociception by specific bulbospinal noradrenergic neurons

The origins of spinally projecting NA neurons which terminate in the spinal cord dorsal horn have not been clearly defined. However, the available anatomical evidence indicates that these neurons originate in the ventral LC, nucleus subcoeruleus, A5, and A7 catecholamine nuclei (see previous discussion). Recently, a number of electrophysiological and behavioral studies have provided additional evidence that NA neurons in these nuclei terminate in the dorsal horn, and furthermore, that these neurons are involved in modulating nociception.

Nucleus locus coeruleus/subcoeruleus

The role of LC NA neurons in modulating nociception has been demonstrated by several studies using electrical stimulation to activate LC neurons (Segal and Sandberg, 1977; Sandberg and Segal, 1978; Margalit and Segal, 1979; Jones and Gebhart, 1986; Janss et al., 1987b). Furthermore, the stimulation-induced antinociception is reduced by intrathecal injection of the non-selective NA antagonist phentolamine and the selective α_2 antagonist yohimbine, but not by prazosin, a selective α_1 antagonist (Jones and Gebhart, 1986).

These results support the notion that activation of spinally projecting NA neurons in the LC induces antinociception which is mediated by α_2-NA receptors in the spinal cord dorsal horn.

Electrophysiological studies, demonstrating that electrical stimulation of LC neurons inhibits nociceptive dorsal horn neurons, provides additional evidence that bulbospinal NA neurons modulate nociception (Hodge et al., 1981, 1983a, b; Iggo et al., 1981; Mokha et al., 1983, 1985, 1986; Jones and Gebhart, 1986, 1987). Microinjection of glutamic acid into the LC also inhibits nociceptive dorsal horn neurons (Jones and Gebhart, 1986) which confirms the assumption that electrical stimulation activates LC neurons and not fibers passing through the LC. Although inhibition of nociceptive dorsal horn neurons is the most common effect of LC stimulation, several reports indicate that LC stimulation also excites dorsal horn neurons (Iggo et al., 1981; Mokha et al., 1983). These observations are consistent with iontophoretic studies which demonstrate that some nociceptive dorsal horn neurons are activated by NE (Todd and Millar, 1983; Howe and Zieglgänsberger, 1987).

The role of NE in mediating the inhibitory actions produced by LC stimulation has been questioned, since depletion of NE in the spinal cord by 6-hydroxydopamine treatment or by reserpine did not alter the effects of LC stimulation (Hodge et al., 1983). Janss and coworkers (1987b) have similarly demonstrated that depletion of spinal cord NE by 6-hydroxydopamine does not attenuate the antinociceptive effects of LC stimulation, although intrathecal injection of α_2-NA antagonists does decrease the effects of LC stimulation (Jones and Gebhart, 1986). These authors have further demonstrated that supersensitivity develops following intrathecal injection of 6-hydroxydopamine, and is accompanied by an increase in the number of α_2-NA binding sites in the spinal cord. These authors suggest that the failure of 6-hydroxydopamine to block LC-induced antinociception is due to receptor supersensitivity which compensates for the loss of NA terminals in the spinal cord (Janss et al., 1987b). Thus, the failure of spinal cord NE depletion to attenuate the LC-induced inhibition of nociceptive dorsal horn neurons may be due to compensatory up-regulation of NA receptors in the spinal cord dorsal horn.

A1 catecholamine nucleus

Although there is convincing evidence that the A1 catecholamine nucleus does not project to the spinal cord dorsal horn (see previous discussion), electrical stimulation of neurons in the area of the A1 nucleus produces antinociception (Janss et al., 1987a,b; Gebhart and Ossipov, 1986) which is blocked by intrathecal injection of yohimbine (α_2 adrenoceptor antagonist) (Gebhart and Ossipov, 1986; Janss et al., 1987b). In addition, the antinociception induced by A1 stimulation can be blocked by intrathecal injection of methysergide (Gebhart and Ossipov, 1986). These data suggest that stimulation of neurons in the A1 nucleus produces antinociception which is mediated by spinally projecting NE and 5HT neurons. Since the NA neurons in the A1 nucleus do not appear to project to the spinal cord, the antinociception induced by A1 stimulation may be mediated by an indirect pathway involving other areas of the brain stem. Since the nucleus raphe magnus receives axonal projections from the A1 nucleus (Takagi et al., 1981; Dong and Shen, 1986) and the lateral reticular nucleus (Abols and Basbaum, 1981), it is possible that the antinociceptive actions of A1 stimulation are mediated by activation of NRM neurons. This suggestion is supported by evidence demonstrating that electrical- (Hammond and Yaksh, 1984; Barbaro et al., 1985) or glutamate-induced (Jensen and Yaksh, 1984) stimulation of the NRM produces antinociception which is mediated by spinally projecting serotonergic and NA neurons. Furthermore, electrical stimulation of the NRM, using current parameters known to produce antinociception, increases the release of endogenous NE and 5HT into spinal cord superfusates (Hammond et al., 1985).

Stimulation of neurons in the A1 catecholamine nucleus appears to induce antinociception by inhibiting nociceptive dorsal horn neurons (Morton et al., 1983; Janss and Gebhart, 1987). These studies demonstrated that either electrical or glutamate-induced stimulation of the lateral reticular nucleus, near the A1 nucleus, reduced both spontaneous and noxious-evoked activity of nociceptive dorsal horn neurons (Morton et al., 1983) or identified spinothalamic tract cells (Janss and Gebhart, 1987).

Rostral A5 catecholamine nuclei

Although there is not a great deal of evidence implicating A5 NA neurons in the modulation of nociceptive processes, several recent studies have provided suggestive evidence that electrical stimulation of these neurons can induce antinociception. For example, electrical stimulation of the rostral part of the A5 catecholamine nucleus produces antinociception (Miller and Proudfit, 1985, 1986, 1987). These effects appear to be directly mediated by spinally projecting NA neurons since the antinociception can be blocked by intrathecal injection of the α_2-NA antagonist yohimbine and the mixed antagonist phentolamine (Miller and Proudfit, 1987). α_1 and β adrenoceptors do not appear to be involved since neither WB4101, an α_1 antagonist, nor propranolol, a β antagonist, had any effect on the magnitude or duration of A5 stimulation-induced antinociception. The descending pathway from the A5 nucleus to the spinal cord does not appear to involve a relay in the raphe magnus, since intrathecal injection of the 5HT antagonist methysergide was without effect (Miller and Proudfit, 1985). In addition, reversible inactivation of NRM neurons produced by microinjection of tetracaine into the NRM did not alter the antinociception induced by electrical stimulation of A5 neurons (Miller and Proudfit, 1985). The active stimulation sites were near NA neurons located in the rostral part of the A5 nucleus near the exit of the trigeminal nerve in the ventrolateral pons. It should be noted that stimulation at some sites produced aversive reactions which precluded analgesiometric testing (Miller and Proudfit, 1984).

In addition, electrical stimulation of the rostral part of the A5 catecholamine nucleus inhibits nociceptive dorsal horn neurons (Clark et al., 1987). Stimulation sites were located in the ventrolateral pontine tegmentum (VLPT) just medial to the rubrospinal tract. Of the 44 cells tested, the response to noxious stimulation was increased in 18 cells, inhibited in 17 cells, and 9 cells were not affected. Excitation and inhibition were elicited from similar locations in the VLPT. These results indicate that simulation in the VLPT produces both excitation and inhibition of nociceptive dorsal horn neurons. These findings are consistent with behavioral studies which indicate that both antinociceptive and aversive effects can be elicited by electrical stimulation of various sites in the VLPT.

Evidence for modulation of nociception by intrabulbar noradrenergic neurons

In addition to the large body evidence supporting the modulation of nociception by bulbospinal NA neurons, there is also evidence that bulbar NA neurons which project to areas within the brain stem also modulate nociception. This evidence indicates that NA neurons in the ventrolateral pontine tegmentum modulate the excitability of neurons located in the ventromedial medulla, such as those in the nucleus raphe magnus and the adjacent nucleus reticularis paragigantocellularis, which are involved in regulating nociception.

Anatomical studies

Biochemical studies (Saavedra et al., 1976; Versteeg et al., 1976; Hammond and Proudfit, 1980) have demonstrated a relatively high concentration of NE in the medial medulla and fluorescence histochemical studies (Dahlström and Fuxe, 1964; Fuxe, 1965; Palkovits and Jacobowitz, 1974; Swanson and Hartman, 1975; Levitt and Moore,

362

1979; Hammond et al., 1980b; Westlund et al., 1980, 1984; Takagi et al., 1981; Jones and Friedman, 1983; Dong and Shen, 1986) have demonstrated that the NRM contains a dense concentration of NA terminals and varicosities. In addition, immunocytochemical studies have demonstrated dopamine-β-hydroxylase immunoreactive varicosities which appear to make contact with the somata and proximal dendrites of serotonergic neurons in the NRM (Pretel and Ruda, 1985). Studies of the fine structure of NA synapses on NRM neurons using permanganate fixation have demonstrated that NA axon terminals primarily form axodendritic contacts on NRM neurons (Takagi et al., 1981). The existence of both α_1- and α_2-NA receptors in the NRM region (Young and Kuhar, 1980; Unnerstall et al., 1984) further supports the presence of functional NA synapses on NRM neurons.

The origin of the NA neurons, which project to the medial medulla, has been studied by several laboratories. Most reports agree that the NA terminals in the NRM do not originate in the LC (Levitt and Moore, 1979; Hammond and Proudfit, 1980; Sagen and Proudfit, 1981; Takagi et al., 1981), although Dong and Shen (1986) did demonstrate some NA neurons in LC and subcoeruleus which project to the NRM region. Several regions of the ventrolateral medulla, the A1 and A3 catecholamine groups, appear to contain some NA neurons which project to the NRM region (Sagen and Proudfit, 1981; Takagi et al., 1981; Dong and Shen, 1986). However, others have not demonstrated such projections (McKellar and Loewy, 1982). The A5 nucleus was reported to contain the largest number of NA neurons projecting to the NRM region (Sagen and Proudfit, 1981), but other reports (Takagi et al., 1981; Dong and Shen, 1986) did not observe projection neurons from this nucleus. The reasons for these conflicting results are not clear, although evidence from other experimental approaches, such as the effects of lesioning various catecholamine cell groups on nociception, suggest that the A5 catecholamine neurons may be the major projec-

tion to the NRM (Sagen and Proudfit, 1986). This evidence is discussed in a later section.

Electrophysiological studies

The NA projection to neurons in the medial medulla appears to be inhibitory, since iontophoretically applied NE depresses the firing rate of most identified raphe-spinal NRM neurons (Wessendorf and Anderson, 1983; Willcockson et al., 1983). In contrast to these reports, NE excited most NRM neurons not identified as projecting to the spinal cord (Behbehani et al., 1981). In addition, preliminary evidence has indicated that NE also excites NRM neurons which were identified as 'on' cells (Heinricher et al., 1987). Since the neurons examined in these reports were not identified as having raphe-spinal projections, the differences in responses to NE may be due to differences in the populations of neurons examined. That is, NE may inhibit most raphe-spinal NRM neurons, but may excite most other NRM neurons.

Pharmacological studies

The functional significance of the NA innervation of neurons located in the NRM has been addressed in a series of experiments designed to examine the effects of various NA agonists and antagonists microinjected into the NRM region on nociception. Microinjection of adrenergic antagonists such as phentolamine into the NRM produces antinociception (Hammond et al., 1980a,b; Sagen and Proudfit, 1981, 1985; Sagen et al., 1983). These results have been interpreted to indicate that raphe-spinal neurons located in the NRM region are tonically inhibited by NA neurons and the blockade of these NA receptors by microinjection of phentolamine disinhibits (activates) these raphe-spinal neurons.

Effect of drugs selective for noradrenergic receptor subtypes

The existence of both α_1- and α_2-NA receptors in the NRM region (Young and Kuhar, 1980; Unnerstall et al., 1984) suggests that the interpretation of the neurotransmitter actions of NE on raphe-spinal neurons may be complex, since these two receptor subtypes may serve different functions. The classical model of NA receptor subtypes derived from studies of the peripheral nervous system postulates postsynaptic α_1 receptors located on effector organs and presynaptic α_2 receptors involved in the feedback regulation of NE release (Langer, 1977, 1981; Starke, 1977). Recent studies designed to investigate the nature of the α-NA receptor subtypes in the NRM have demonstrated that both α_1- and α_2-NA receptors in the NRM are involved in modulating nociception (Sagen and Proudfit, 1985). These studies involved microinjection of α_1- and α_2-NA agonists and antagonists into brain stem sites corresponding to the NRM and the region lateral to the NRM and dorsal to the pyramidal tracts. The results demonstrated that such injections produce alterations in nociception that are consistent with the classical model of adrenergic receptor subtypes in which α_1 receptors are located postsynaptically and α_2 receptors are located on NA terminals and regulate NE release. The evidence in support of this conclusion is as follows. Since the NA projection to raphe-spinal neurons in the NRM is inhibitory (Wessendorf and Anderson, 1983; Wessendorf et al., 1981; Willcockson et al., 1983), blockade of this action by an α_1 antagonist should disinhibit (activate) NRM neurons and produce antinociception. Injection of the selective α_1 antagonist prazosin (Greengrass and Bremner, 1979; Hornung et al., 1979) produces antinociception which is consistent with the proposed interpretation. An α_2 agonist should also produce antinociception by decreasing the amount of NE release from the presynaptic terminals. The α_2 agonist, clonidine, decreases NE release from NA terminals peripheral tissues (Langer, 1977, 1981; Starke, 1977) and cerebral cortex (Taube et al., 1977), and binds selectively to α_2-NA receptors in the brain (Greenberg et al., 1976). Microinjection of clonidine into the NRM region produced antinociception, a finding which

is consistent with the existence of presynaptic α_2 receptors that inhibit NE release (Sagen and Proudfit, 1985). Thus, the antinociception induced by these two drugs appears to result from a decrease in the inhibitory actions of endogenously released NE. Prazosin appears to produce antinociception by a direct blockade of postsynaptic α_1 receptors while clonidine appears to act indirectly by presynaptic inhibition of NE release, an effect mediated by α_2 receptors.

In contrast, both the α_1 agonist, phenylephrine, and the α_2 antagonist, yohimbine, produce an increase in nociception (hyperalgesia). The enhancement of nociception is most likely due to inhibition of raphe-spinal NRM neurons, since lesions of the NRM (Proudfit, 1980b, 1981; Proudfit and Anderson, 1975) or injection of local anesthetic solutions into this region (Proudfit, 1980a) also produce hyperalgesia. Since NE inhibits NRM neurons, other agonists which act at postsynaptic NA receptors would be expected to have inhibitory actions and enhance nociception. Thus, the hyperalgesia produced by microinjecting phenylephrine into the NRM probably results from inhibition of raphe-spinal neurons, an action mediated by postsynaptic α_1 receptors. Microinjection of the α_2 antagonist, yohimbine, into the NRM also produces hyperalgesia. It has been well documented that α_2 antagonists such as yohimbine increase the release of endogenous NE from presynaptic terminals by binding to presynaptic α_2 receptors (see review by Berthelsen and Pettinger, 1977). Therefore, α_2 antagonists such as yohimbine may induce hyperalgesia by increasing the amount of NE released and enhancing the inhibition of raphe-spinal NRM neurons. Thus, the hyperalgesia induced by these two drugs appears to result from an increase in the inhibition of raphe-spinal NRM neurons. Phenylephrine appears to produce hyperalgesia by directly inhibiting NRM neurons, an action mediated by activation of postsynaptic α_1 receptors. Yohimbine appears to indirectly inhibit NRM neurons by acting on presynaptic α_2 receptors to enhance NE release.

In summary, these results support the proposal

that NA neurons modulate the activity of NRM neurons involved in the control of nociceptive processes. Furthermore, these results are consistent with the model which postulates a postsynaptic α_1 receptor and a presynaptic α_2 receptor which modulates the release of NE. Thus, both postsynaptic α_1 receptors and presynaptic α_2 receptors which regulate NE release appear to be involved in the brain stem control of nociception.

The antinociception resulting from blockade of postsynaptic NA receptors located on NRM neurons, appears to be mediated by the release of 5HT in the spinal cord, since it can be blocked by intrathecal injection of methysergide (Hammond et al., 1980b). In addition, the activation of raphe-spinal neurons may also be accompanied by a subsequent activation of bulbospinal NA neurons and release of NE in the spinal cord. This conclusion is supported by several lines of evidence. For example, the antinociception produced by the injection of phentolamine into the NRM can be reversed by phentolamine injected into the spinal cord subarachnoid space (Sagen and Proudfit, 1981). In addition, depletion of spinal cord 5HT, NE, or both, also blocks the antinociception produced by microinjection of phentolamine into the NRM region (Sagen et al., 1983). Finally, microinjection of phentolamine into the NRM significantly increases the release of endogenous 5HT and NE into spinal cord superfusates (Sagen and Proudfit, 1987). These results suggest that the antinociception induced by blockade of NA receptors on raphe-spinal neurons is mediated by activation of both raphe-spinal serotonergic neurons and bulbospinal NA neurons. The activation of descending serotonergic and NA neurons by electrical (Hammond and Yaksh, 1985; Hammond et al., 1985; Barbaro et al., 1985) and chemical stimulation (Jensen and Yaksh, 1984) of raphe-spinal NRM neurons supports the conclusion that microinjection of phentolamine into the NRM region produces antinociception by activating bulbo-spinal monoaminergic neurons.

Location of bulbospinal noradrenergic neurons activated by NRM stimulation

The involvement of spinally projecting serotonergic neurons in the antinociception produced by NRM stimulation is not surprising, since the NRM is a primary source of descending serotonergic neurons (see review by Bowker et al., 1982). However, since there are no NE-containing neurons in the NRM, stimulation of NRM neurons must activate spinally projecting NA neurons in other brain regions which inhibit nociceptive neural processes in the spinal cord.

Evidence discussed earlier in this review indicates that spinally projecting NA neurons appear to be located in the ventral LC, nucleus subcoeruleus, A5, and A7 catecholamine nuclei. Recent evidence indicates that NA neurons located in the rostral portion of the A5 nucleus may be involved in mediating the antinociception induced by stimulation of neurons in the NRM (Sagen and Proudfit, 1983; Miller and Proudfit, 1987; Clark et al., 1987). For example, electrical stimulation of neurons in the A5 nucleus induced antinociception which was antagonized by intrathecal injection of the NA antagonists phentolamine and yohimbine (Miller and Proudfit, 1987). In addition, such stimulation also inhibited the activity of spinal cord dorsal horn neurons evoked by noxious thermal or mechanical stimuli (Clark et al., 1987). Preliminary evidence indicates that the inhibition of dorsal horn neurons can be reversed by phentolamine topically applied to the dorsal surface of the spinal cord (Clark and Proudfit, unpublished). More direct evidence indicates that large electrolytic lesions which included both A7 and rostral A5 neurons produced hyperalgesia and blocked the antinociception induced by microinjection of NA antagonists into the NRM region (Sagen and Proudfit, 1983). Recent studies have demonstrated that selective lesions of the A5 nucleus (at the level of Vth nerve exit) also produced hyperalgesia and blocked the antinociceptive actions of NA antagonists microinjected into the NRM (Sagen, Miller and Proudfit, unpublished). These results provide suggestive evidence that chemical or electrical stimulation of neurons in the NRM region produces antinociception which is mediated, at least in part, by activating bulbospinal NA neurons located in the rostral portion of the A5 catecholamine nucleus.

Origin of noradrenergic projections to NRM

Although some of the anatomical evidence for the origin of the NA projection to the NRM suggests a projection from the A1 nucleus (Dong and Shen, 1986; Takagi et al., 1981), there are numerous behavioral and electrophysiological studies which argue against the existence of a projection from the A1 nucleus. Since blockade of NA receptors located on neurons in the NRM produces antinociception, lesions of the NA neurons that project to, and inhibit NRM neurons should also produce antinociception. However, lesions of the A1 catecholamine nucleus either do not alter nociception (Bragin and Durinyan, 1983), or enhance nociception (Morton et al., 1983, 1984). These authors demonstrated that lesions of the lateral reticular nucleus, which appear to include the A1 nucleus, increase the response of dorsal horn neurons to electrical stimulation of unmyelinated C fibers (Hall et al., 1982; Morton et al., 1983, 1984). These results indicate that A1 lesions enhance rather than reduce nociception, thus, these data are not consistent with an inhibitory NA projection from the A1 group to neurons in the NRM region. Furthermore, the effects of A1 stimulation on nociception and the responses of nociceptive dorsal horn neurons are not consistent with a projection from the A1 group to neurons in the NRM. Since the available evidence indicates that NE inhibits raphe-spinal neurons (see previous discussion), one would predict that stimulation of the NA neurons which project to the NRM would enhance nociception and increase the responsiveness of nociceptive dorsal horn neurons to noxious stimuli. However, recent reports have

demonstrated that electrical and chemical stimulation near A1 neurons produces antinociception (Janss et al., 1987a,b; Gebhart and Ossipov, 1986) which is mediated in part by spinally projecting NA neurons (Janss et al., 1987b; Gebhart and Ossipov, 1986). In addition, stimulation of neurons in the lateral reticular nucleus, near A1 neurons, inhibits the activation of dorsal horn neurons by noxious thermal stimuli (Janss and Gebhart, 1987) and stimulation of C fiber afferents (Morton et al., 1983). Thus, the vast majority of behavioral and electrophysiological evidence argues against an inhibitory NA projection from A1 neurons to raphe-spinal neurons located in the NRM.

Although NA neurons in the A1 group do not appear to innervate NRM neurons, there is some indirect evidence which supports the existence of a NA projection from the A5 catecholamine group to raphe-spinal neurons in the NRM (Sagen and Proudfit, 1986). These studies demonstrated that bilateral electrolytic lesions of the A5 nuclei (at the level of the VIIth nerve exit) produced antinociception which persisted for longer than 3 weeks. This observation is consistent with previous studies which demonstrated that blockade of NA receptors on NRM neurons produced by microinjection of NA antagonists also produces antinociception (Hammond et al., 1980a,b; Sagen and Proudfit, 1981, 1985; Sagen et al., 1983). Furthermore, the antinociception observed following A5 lesions was significantly attenuated by intrathecal injections of either NA or serotonergic antagonists. Similarly, previous studies have shown that the antinociception produced by microinjecting NA antagonists in the NRM is also attenuated by intrathecal injections of these antagonists (Sagen and Proudfit, 1981; Hammond et al., 1980b). Finally, preliminary results indicate that A5 lesions (at the level of the VIIth nerve exit) significantly attenuate the antinociceptive effects of microinjecting phentolamine into the NRM (Miller and Proudfit, unpublished results). These observations lead to the suggestion that the NA neurons located in the caudal part of the A5 catecholamine nucleus modulate nociception by tonically inhibiting raphe-spinal neurons located in the NRM.

Summary

Four major systems of NA neurons which modulate nociception have been described. Three of these systems appear to be involved in producing antinociception, while the fourth appears to enhance nociception.

One system of bulbospinal NA neurons which modulates nociception is located in the LC and subcoeruleus regions of the dorsolateral medulla. Stimulation of these neurons has been demonstrated to produce antinociception and inhibition of spinal cord dorsal horn neurons activated by noxious cutaneous stimulation.

The NA neurons located in the A1 nucleus, part of the lateral reticular nucleus of the ventrolateral medulla, constitute a second NA pain modulation system. Electrical or chemical stimulation of the neurons in the A1 region produces antinociception and inhibition of spinal cord dorsal horn neurons. Although these neurons do not appear to project to the spinal cord, the antinociception produced by electrical stimulation of these neurons can be blocked by intrathecal NA antagonists. Thus, the antinociception induced by stimulating this area may be mediated by activation of spinally projecting NA neurons located elsewhere in the brain stem.

A third bulbospinal NA system originates in the rostral part of the A5 nucleus and may include the A7 nucleus. Electrical stimulation of neurons in these regions produces antinociception which can be blocked by intrathecal injection of NA antagonists. Stimulation at some sites near the A5 nucleus not only inhibits some nociceptive dorsal horn neurons, but also increases the responses of a significant number of dorsal horn neurons to noxious stimuli.

The fourth system of NA neurons, located in the caudal A5 nucleus, projects to and tonically inhibits spinally projecting neurons located in the ventromedial medulla (VMM). Local injection of NA antagonists in the VMM activates (disinhibits) VMM neurons and produces antinociception. The antinociception induced by such injections is mediated by spinally projecting serotonergic and NA neurons. Similar injections of agonists produce hyperalgesia, presumably by inhibiting spinally projecting VMM neurons. Activation of this system appears to enhance nociception, in contrast to the antinociceptive actions of the other three NA pain modulation systems.

References

Abols, I.A. and Basbaum, A.I. (1981) Afferent connections of the rostral medulla of the cat. *J. Comp. Neurol.,* 201: 285 – 297.

Barbaro, N.M., Hammond, D.L. and Fields, H.L. (1985) Effects of intrathecally administered methysergide and yohimbine on microstimulation-produced antinociception in the rat. *Brain Res.,* 343: 223 – 229.

Behbehani, M.N., Pomeroy, S.L. and Mack, C.E. (1981) Interaction between central gray and nucleus raphe magnus: role of norepinephrine. *Brain Res. Bull.,* 6: 361 – 364.

Belcher, G., Ryall, R.W. and Schaffner, R. (1978) The differential effects of 5-hydroxytryptamine, noradrenaline, and raphe stimulation of nociceptive and non-nociceptive dorsal horn interneurons in the cat. *Brain Res.,* 151: 307 – 332.

Berthelsen, S. and Pettinger, W.A. (1977) A functional basis for classification of α-adrenergic receptors. *Life Sci.,* 21: 595 – 606.

Bowker, R.M., Westlund, K.N., Sullivan, M.C., Wilber, J.F. and Coulter, J.D. (1983) Descending serotonergic, peptidergic and cholinergic pathways from the raphe nuclei: a multiple transmitter complex. *Brain Res.,* 288: 33 – 48.

Bragin, E.O. and Durinyan, R.A. (1983) A study of the catecholamine systems of the lateral reticular nucleus and the serotonergic systems of the raphe magnus in various types of analgesia. *Pain,* 17: 225 – 234.

Calvillo, O. and Ghignone, M. (1986) Presynaptic effect of clonidine on unmyelinated afferent fibers in the spinal cord of the cat. *Neurosci. Lett.,* 64: 335 – 339.

Carlsson, A., Falck, B., Fuxe, K. and Hillarp, N.A. (1964) Cellular localization of monoamines in the spinal cord. *Acta Physiol. Scand.,* 60: 112 – 119.

Clarke, F.M., Fitzgerald, L.F. and Proudfit, H.K. (1987) Alterations in the activity of dorsal horn neurons produced by electrical stimulation of neurons in the ventrolateral pontine tegmentum. *Soc. Neurosci. Abstr.,* 13: 303.

Commissiong, J.W. (1981) Evidence that the noradrenergic projection decussates at the spinal level. *Brain Res.,* 212: 145 – 151.

Commissiong, J.W., Hellström, S.O. and Neff, N.H. (1978) A new projection from locus coeruleus to the spinal ventral columns: histochemical and biochemical evidence. *Brain Res.,* 148: 207–213.

Dahlström, A. and Fuxe, K. (1965) Evidence for the existence of monoamine-containing neurons in the central nervous system. I. Demonstration of monoamines in the cell bodies of brain stem neurons. *Acta Physiol. Scand.,* Suppl. 232: 1–55.

Dashwood, M.R., Gilbey, M.P. and Spyer, K.M. (1985) The localization of adrenoceptors and opiate receptors in regions of the cat central nervous system involved in cardiovascular control. *Neuroscience,* 15: 537–551.

Dong, X. and Shen, E. (1986) Origin of monoaminergic innervation of the nucleus raphe magnus – a combined monoamine histochemistry and fluorescent retrograde tracing study in the rat. *Scientia Sinica,* 6: 599–608.

Engberg, I. and Ryall, R.W. (1966) The inhibitory actions of noradrenaline and other monoamines on spinal neurons. *J. Physiol. (Lond.),* 185: 298–322.

Fleetwood-Walker, S.M. and Coote, J.H. (1981) The contribution of brain stem catecholamine cell groups to the innervation of the sympathetic lateral cell column. *Brain Res.,* 205: 141–155.

Fleetwood-Walker, S.M., Mitchell, R., Hope, P.J., Molony, V. and Iggo, A. (1985) An α_2 receptor mediates the selective inhibition by noradrenaline of nociceptive responses of identified dorsal horn neurones. *Brain Res.,* 334: 243–254.

Fischbach, G.D., Dunlap, K., Mudge, A. and Leeman, S. (1981) Peptide and amine transmitter effect on embryonic chick sensory neurons in vitro. *Adv. Biochem. Psychopharmacol.,* 28: 175–188.

Fuxe, K. (1965) Evidence for the existence of monoamine neurons in the central nervous system. *Acta Physiol. Scand.,* Suppl. 247: 37–84.

Gebhart, G.F. and Ossipov, M.H. (1986) Characterization of inhibition of the spinal nociceptive tail-flick reflex in the rat from the medullary lateral reticular nucleus. *Neuroscience,* 6: 701–713.

Greenberg, D.A., U'Prichard, D.C. and Snyder, S.H. (1976) Alpha-noradrenergic receptor binding in mammalian brain: differential labeling of agonists and antagonist states. *Life Sci.,* 19: 69–76.

Greengrass, P. and Bremner, R. (1979) Binding characteristics of ^{3}H-prazosin to brain α-adrenergic receptors. *Eur. J. Pharmacol.,* 55: 323–326.

Hall, J.G., Duggan, A.W., Morton, C.R. and Johnson, S.M. (1982) The location of brainstem neurones tonically inhibiting dorsal horn neurones of the cat. *Brain Res.,* 215: 215–222.

Hammond, D.L. and Proudfit, H.K. (1980) Effects of locus coeruleus lesions on morphine-induced antinociception. *Brain Res.,* 188: 79–91.

Hammond, D.L. and Yaksh, T.L. (1984) Antagonism of stimulation-produced antinociception by intrathecal administration of methysergide or phentolamine. *Brain Res.,* 298: 329–337.

Hammond, D.L., Levy, R.A. and Proudfit, H.K. (1980a) Hypalgesia following microinjection of noradrenergic antagonists in the nucleus raphe magnus. *Pain,* 9: 85–101.

Hammond, D.L., Levy, R.A. and Proudfit, H.K. (1980b) Hypoalgesia induced by microinjection of a norepinephrine antagonist in the raphe magnus: reversal by intrathecal administration of a serotonin antagonist. *Brain Res.,* 201: 475–479.

Hammond, D.L., Tyce, G.M. and Yaksh, T.L. (1985) Efflux of 5-hydroxytryptamine and noradrenaline into spinal cord superfusates during stimulation of the rat medulla. *J. Physiol. (Lond.),* 359: 151–162.

Headley, P.M., Duggan, A.W. and Griersmith, B.T. (1978) Selective reduction by noradrenaline and 5-hydroxytryptamine of nociceptive responses of cat dorsal horn neurones. *Brain Res.,* 145: 185–189.

Heinricher, M.M., Haws, C.M. and Fields, H.L. (1987) Opposing actions of norepinephrine and clonidine on single pain-modulating neurons in rostral ventromedial medulla. *Pain,* Suppl. 4: S28.

Hodge, C.J., Jr., Apkarian, A.V., Stevens, R., Vogelsang, G. and Wisnicki, H.J. (1981) Locus coeruleus modulation of dorsal horn unit responses to cutaneous stimulation. *Brain Res.,* 204: 415–420.

Hodge, C.J., Jr., Apkarian, A.V., Owen, M.P. and Hanson, B.S. (1983a) Changes in the effects of stimulation of locus coeruleus and nucleus raphe magnus following dorsal rhizotomy. *Brain Res.,* 288: 325–329.

Hodge, C.J., Jr., Apkarian, A.V., Stevens, R.T., Vogelsang, G.D., Brown, O. and Franck, J.I. (1983b) Dorsolateral pontine inhibition of dorsal horn cell responses to cutaneous stimulation: lack of dependence on catecholaminergic systems in cat. *J. Neurophysiol.,* 50: 1220–1235.

Holz, G.G., Kream, R.M. and Dunlap, K. (1985) Norepinephrine inhibits field stimulation-evoked release of substance P from chick dorsal root ganglion cells in culture. *Soc. Neurosci. Abstr.,* 11: 126.

Hornung, R., Presek, P. and Glossmann, H. (1979) Alpha-adrenoceptors in rat brain: direct identification with prazosin. *Naunyn-Schmiedeb. Arch. Pharmacol.,* 308: 223–230.

Howe, J.R. and Yaksh, T.L. (1982) Changes in sensitivity to intrathecal norepinephrine and serotonin after 6-hydroxydopamine (6-OHDA), and 5,6-dihydroxytryptamine (5,6-DHT) or repeated monoamine administration. *J. Pharmacol. Exp. Ther.,* 220: 311–321.

Howe, J.R. and Zieglgänsberger, W. (1987) Responses of rat dorsal horn neurons to natural stimulation and to iontophoretically applied norepinephrine. *J. Comp. Neurol.,* 255: 1–17.

Howe, J.R., Wang, J.-Y. and Yaksh, T.L. (1983) Selective antagonism of the antinociceptive effect of intrathecally applied alpha-adrenergic agonists by intrathecal prazosin and intrathecal yohimbine. *J. Pharmacol. Exp. Ther.*, 224: 552–558.

Hylden, J.L.K. and Wilcox, G.L. (1983) Pharmacological characterization of substance P-induced nociception in mice. Modulation by opioid and noradrenergic agonists at the spinal cord level. *J. Pharmacol. Exp. Ther.*, 226: 398–404.

Iggo, A., McMillan, J.A. and Mokha, S.S. (1981) Modulation of spinal cord multireceptive neurones from locus coeruleus and nucleus raphe magnus in the cat. *J. Physiol.*, 319: 107–108P.

Janss, A.J. and Gebhart, G.F. (1987) Quantitative characterization and spinal pathway mediating inhibition of spinal nociceptive transmission from the lateral reticular nucleus in the rat. *J. Neurophysiol.*, 59: 226–247.

Janss, A.J., Cox, B.F., Brody, M.J. and Gebhart, G.F. (1987a) Dissociation of antinociceptive from cardiovascular effects of stimulation in the lateral reticular nucleus in the rat. *Brain Res.*, 405: 140–149.

Janss, A.J., Jones, S.L. and Gebhart, G.F. (1987b) Effect of spinal norepinephrine depletion on descending inhibition of the tail flick reflex from the locus coeruleus and lateral reticular nucleus in the rat. *Brain Res.*, 400: 40–52.

Jeftinija, S., Semba, K. and Randic, M. (1981) Norepinephrine reduces excitability of single cutaneous afferent C-fibers in the cat spinal cord. *Brain Res.*, 219: 456–463.

Jeftinija, S., Semba, K. and Randic, M. (1983) Norepinephrine reduces excitability of single cutaneous primary afferent C and A fibers in the cat spinal cord. *Adv. Pain Res. Ther.*, 5: 271–276.

Jensen, T.S. and Yaksh, T.L. (1984) Spinal monoamine and opiate systems partly mediate the antinociceptive effects produced by glutamate at brainstem sites. *Brain Res.*, 321: 287–298.

Jones, B.E. and Friedman, L. (1983) Atlas of catecholamine perikarya, varicosities and pathways in the brainstem of the cat. *J. Comp. Neurol.*, 215: 382–396.

Jones, S.L. and Gebhart, G.F. (1986a) Characterization of coeruleospinal inhibition of the nociceptive tail-flick reflex in the rat: mediation by spinal α_2-adrenoceptors. *Brain Res.*, 364: 315–330.

Jones, S.L. and Gebhart, G.F. (1986b) Quantitative characterization of ceruleospinal inhibition of nociceptive transmission in the rat. *J. Neurophysiol.*, 56: 1397–1410.

Jones, S.L. and Gebhart, G.F. (1987) Spinal pathways mediating tonic, coeruleospinal, and raphespinal descending inhibition in the rat. *J. Neurophysiol.*, 58: 138–159.

Karoum, F., Commissiong, J.W., Neff, N.H. and Wyatt, R.J. (1980) Biochemical evidence for uncrossed locus coeruleus projections to the spinal cord. *Brain Res.*, 196: 237–241.

Kuraishi, T., Harada, T. and Takagi, H. (1979) Noradrenaline regulation of pain-transmission in the spinal cord mediated by α-adrenoceptors. *Brain Res.*, 174: 333–336.

Kuraishi, Y., Hirota, N., Sato, Y., Kaneko, S., Satoh, M. and

Takagi, H. (1985) Noradrenergic inhibition of the release of substance P from the primary afferents in the rabbit spinal dorsal horn. *Brain Res.*, 359: 177–182.

Langer, S.Z. (1977) Presynaptic receptors and their role in the regulation of transmitter release. *Br. J. Pharmacol.*, 60: 481–497.

Langer, S.Z. (1981) Presynaptic regulation of the release of catecholamines. *Pharmacol. Rev.*, 32: 337–362.

Levitt, P. and Moore, R.J. (1979) Origin and organization of brainstem catecholamine innervation in the rat. *J. Comp. Neurol.*, 186: 505–528.

Light, A.R. and Perl, E.R. (1979) Reexamination of the dorsal root projection to the spinal dorsal horn including observations on the differential termination of coarse and fine fibers. *J. Comp. Neurol.*, 186: 1171–32.

Margalit, D. and Segal, M. (1979) A pharmacologic study of analgesia produced by stimulation of the nucleus locus coeruleus. *Psychopharmacology*, 62: 169–173.

McKellar, S. and Loewy, A.D. (1982) Efferent projections of the A1 catecholamine cell group in the rat: an autoradiographic study. *Brain Res.*, 241: 11–29.

Miller, J.F. and Proudfit, H.K. (1984) Stimulation-produced analgesia from pontine ventrolateral tegmentum. *Soc. Neurosci. Abstr.*, 10: 102.

Miller, J.F. and Proudfit, H.K. (1985) Stimulation-produced analgesia from ventrolateral pontine tegmentum is not mediated through the nucleus raphe magnus. *Soc. Neurosci. Abstr.*, 11: 638.

Miller, J.F. and Proudfit, H.K. (1987) Stimulation-produced analgesia from sites in the ventrolateral pons is mediated by a spinal alpha-2 adrenergic system. *Soc. Neurosci. Abstr.*, 13: 303.

Mokha, S.S., McMillan, J.A. and Iggo, A. (1983) Descending influences on spinal nociceptive neurons from locus coeruleus: actions, pathway, neurotransmitters, and mechanisms. *Adv. Pain Res. Ther.*, 5: 387–392.

Mokha, S.S., McMillan, J.A. and Iggo, A. (1985) Descending control of spinal nociceptive transmission. Actions produced on spinal multireceptive neurones from the nuclei locus coeruleus (LC) and raphe magnus. *Exp. Brain Res.*, 58: 213–226.

Mokha, S.S., McMillan, J.A. and Iggo, A. (1986) Pathways mediating descending control of spinal nociceptive transmission from the nuclei locus coeruleus (LC) and raphe magnus (NRM) in the cat. *Exp. Brain Res.*, 61: 597–606.

Morton, C.R., Johnson, S.M. and Duggan, A.W. (1983) Lateral reticular regions and the descending control of dorsal horn neurones of the cat: selective inhibition by electrical stimulation. *Brain Res.*, 275: 13–21.

Morton, C.R., Duggan, A.W. and Zhao, Z.Q. (1984) The effects of lesions of medullary midline and lateral reticular areas on inhibition in the dorsal horn produced by periaqueductal grey stimulation in the cat. *Brain Res.*, 301: 121–130.

North, R.A. and Yoshimura, M. (1984) The actions of

noradrenaline on neurones of the rat substantia gelatinosa in vitro. *J. Physiol. (Lond.)*, 349: 43 – 55.

Nygren, L.-G. and Olson, L. (1977) A new major projection from locus coeruleus: the main source of noradrenergic nerve terminals in the ventral and dorsal columns of the spinal cord. *Brain Res.*, 132: 85 – 93.

Palkovits, M. and Jacobowitz, D.M. (1974) Topographical atlas of catecholamine and acetylcholinesterase-containing neurons of the rat brain. II. Hindbrain (mesencephalon, rhombencephalon). *J. Comp. Neurol.*, 157: 29 – 42.

Pang, I.H. and Vasko, M.R. (1986) Morphine and norepinephrine but not 5-hydroxytryptamine and gamma-amino butyric acid inhibit the potassium-stimulated release of substance P from rat spinal cord slices. *Brain Res.*, 6: 268 – 279.

Pretel, S. and Ruda, M.A. (1985) Immunocytochemical investigation of monoaminergic interaction in brain stem raphe nuclei of the cat. *Soc. Neurosci. Abstr.*, 11: 579.

Proudfit, H.K. (1980a) Effects of raphe magnus and raphe pallidus lesions on morphine-induced analgesia and spinal cord monoamines. *Pharmacol. Biochem. Behav.*, 13: 705 – 714.

Proudfit, H.K. (1980b) Reversible inactivation of raphe magnus neurons: effects on nociceptive threshold and morphine-induced antinociception. *Brain Res.*, 201: 459 – 464.

Proudfit, H.K. (1981) Time-course of alterations in morphine-induced analgesia and nociceptive threshold following medullary raphe lesions. *Neuroscience*, 6: 945 – 951.

Proudfit, H.K. and Anderson, E.G. (1975) Morphine analgesia: blockade by raphe magnus lesions. *Brain Res.*, 98: 612 – 618.

Ralston, H.J., III, and Ralston, D.D. (1979) The distribution of dorsal root axons in laminae I, II and III of the macaque spinal cord: a quantitative electron microscope study. *J. Comp. Neurol.*, 184: 643 – 684.

Reddy, S.V.R. and Yaksh, T.L. (1980) Spinal noradrenergic terminal system mediates antinociception. *Brain Res.*, 189: 391 – 401.

Reddy, S.V.R., Maderdrut, J.L. and Yaksh, T.L. (1980) Spinal cord pharmacology of adrenergic agonist-mediated antinociception. *J. Pharmacol. Exp. Ther.*, 213: 525 – 533.

Ross, R.A. and Reis, D.J. (1974) Effects of lesions of locus coeruleus on regional distribution of dopamine-β-hydroxylase activity in rat brain. *Brain Res.*, 73: 161 – 166.

Saavedra, J.M., Grobecker, H. and Zivin, J. (1976) Catecholamines in the raphe nuclei of the rat. *Brain Res.*, 114: 339 – 345.

Sagen, J. and Proudfit, H.K. (1981) Hypoalgesia induced by blockade of noradrenergic projections to the raphe magnus: reversal by blockade of noradrenergic projections to the spinal cord. *Brain Res.*, 223: 391 – 396.

Sagen, J. and Proudfit, H.K. (1983) The role of the A7 catecholamine group in the modulation of pain perception. *Soc. Neurosci. Abstr.*, 9: 785.

Sagen, J. and Proudfit, H.K. (1984) Effect of intrathecally administered noradrenergic antagonists on nociception in the rat. *Brain Res.*, 310: 295 – 301.

Sagen, J. and Proudfit, H.K. (1985) Evidence for pain modulation by pre- and postsynaptic noradrenergic receptors in the medulla oblongata. *Brain Res.*, 331: 285 – 293.

Sagen, J. and Proudfit, H.K. (1986) Alterations in nociception following lesions of the A5 catecholamine nucleus. *Brain Res.*, 370: 93 – 101.

Sagen, J. and Proudfit, H.K. (1987) Release of endogenous monoamines into spinal cord superfusates following the microinjection of phentolamine into the nucleus raphe magnus. *Brain Res.*, 406: 246 – 254.

Sagen, J., Winker, M.A. and Proudfit, H.K. (1983) Hypoalgesia induced by the local injection of phentolamine in the nucleus raphe magnus: blockade by depletion of spinal cord monoamines. *Pain*, 16: 253 – 263.

Sandberg, D.E. and Segal, M. (1978) Pharmacological analysis of analgesia and self-stimulation elicited by electrical stimulation of catecholamine nuclei in the rat brain. *Brain Res.*, 152: 529 – 542.

Satoh, K., Tohyama, K., Yamamoto, K., Sakumoto, T. and Shimizu, N. (1977) Noradrenaline innervation of the spinal cord studied by the horseradish peroxidase method combined with monoamine oxidase staining. *Exp. Brain Res.*, 30: 175 – 186.

Schmidt, R.F. (1971) Presynaptic inhibition in the vertebrate central nervous system. *Ergebn. Physiol.*, 63: 20 – 101.

Segal, M. and Sandberg, D. (1977) Analgesia produced by electrical stimulation of catecholamine nuclei in the rat brain. *Brain Res.*, 123: 369 – 372.

Seybold, V.S. and Elde, R.P. (1984) Receptor autoradiography in thoracic spinal cord: correlation of neurotransmitter binding sites with sympathoadrenal neurons. *J. Neurosci.*, 4: 2533 – 2542.

Starke, K. (1977) Regulation of noradrenaline release by presynaptic receptor systems. *Rev. Physiol. Biochem. Pharmacol.*, 77: 1 – 124.

Stevens, R.T., Hodge, C.J. and Apkarian, A.V. (1982) Kölliker-Fuse nucleus: the principal source of pontine catecholaminergic cells projecting to the lumbar spinal cord of cat. *Brain Res.*, 239: 589 – 594.

Swanson, L.W. and Hartman, B.K. (1975) The central adrenergic system. An immunofluorescence study of the location of cell bodies and their efferent connections in the rat utilizing dopamine-β-hydroxylase as a marker. *J. Comp. Neurol.*, 163: 467 – 506.

Takagi, H., Yamamoto, K., Shiosaka, S., Senba, E., Takutsuki, K., Inagaki, S., Sakanaka, M. and Toyama, M. (1981) Morphological study of noradrenaline innervation in the caudal raphe nuclei with special reference to fine structure. *J. Comp. Neurol.*, 203: 15 – 22.

Taube, H.D., Starke, K. and Borowski, E. (1977) Presynaptic

receptor systems on the noradrenergic neurones of rat brain. *Naunyn-Schmiedeb. Arch. Pharmacol.,* 299: 123 – 141.

Todd, A.J. and Millar, J. (1983) Receptive fields and responses to iontophoretically applied noradrenaline and 5-hydroxytryptamine of units recorded in laminae I-III of cat dorsal horn. *Brain Res.,* 288: 159 – 167.

Unnerstall, J.R., Kopajtic, T.A. and Kuhar, M.J. (1984) Distribution of α_2 agonist binding sites in the rat and human central nervous system: analysis of some functional, anatomic correlates of the pharmacologic effects of clonidine and related adrenergic agents. *Brain Res. Rev.,* 7: 69 – 101.

Versteeg, D.H.G., Van der Gugten, J., De Jong, W. and Palkovits, M. (1976) Regional concentrations of noradrenaline and dopamine in rat brain. *Brain Res.,* 113: 563 – 574.

Wessendorf, M.W. and Anderson, E.G. (1983) Single unit studies of identified bulbospinal serotonergic units. *Brain Res.,* 279: 93 – 103.

Wessendorf, M.W., Proudfit, H.K. and Anderson, E.G. (1981) The identification of serotonergic neurons in the nucleus raphe magnus by conduction velocity. *Brain Res.,* 214: 168 – 173.

Westlund, K.N. and Coulter, J.D. (1980) Descending projections of the locus coeruleus and subcoeruleus/medial parabrachial nuclei in monkey: axonal transport studies and dopamine-β-hydroxylase. *Brain Res. Rev.,* 2: 235 – 264.

Westlund, K.N., Bowker, R.M., Ziegler, M.G. and Coulter, J.D. (1981) Origins of spinal noradrenergic pathways demonstrated by retrograde transport of antibody to dopamine-β-hydroxylase. *Neurosci. Lett.,* 25: 243 – 249.

Westlund, K.N., Bowker, R.M., Ziegler, M.G. and Coulter, J.D. (1982) Descending noradrenergic projections and their spinal terminations. In H.G.J.M. Kuypers and G.F. Martin (Eds.), *Descending Pathways to the Spinal Cord, Progress in Brain Research, Vol. 57.* Elsevier, Amsterdam, pp. 219 – 238.

Westlund, K.N., Bowker, R.M., Ziegler, M.G. and Coulter, J.D. (1983) Noradrenergic projections to the spinal cord in the rat. *Brain Res.,* 263: 15 – 31.

Westlund, K.N., Bowker, R.M., Ziegler, M.G. and Coulter, J.D. (1984) Origins and terminations of descending noradrenergic projections to the spinal cord of monkey. *Brain Res.,* 292: 1 – 16.

Willcockson, W.S., Gerhart, K.D., Cargill, C.L. and Willis, W.D. (1983) Effects of biogenic amines on raphe-spinal tract cells. *J. Pharmacol. Exp. Ther.,* 225: 637 – 645.

Willcockson, W.S., Chung, J.M., Hori, Y., Lee, K.H. and Willis, W.D. (1984) Effects of iontophoretically released amino acids and amines on primate spinothalamic tract cells. *J. Neurosci.,* 4: 732 – 740.

Yaksh, T.L. (1985) Pharmacology of spinal adrenergic systems which modulate spinal nociceptive processing. *Pharmacol. Biochem. Behav.,* 22: 845 – 858.

Yaksh, T.L. and Go, V.L.W. (1985) Physiology and pharmacology of the release of substance P from spinal primary afferents. *Soc. Neurosci. Abstr.,* 11: 121.

Young, W.S., III, and Kuhar, M.J. (1980) Noradrenergic α_1 and α_2 receptors: light microscopic and autoradiographic localization. *Proc. Natl. Acad. Sci. USA,* 77: 1696 – 1700.

H.L. Fields and J.-M. Besson (Eds.)
Progress in Brain Research, Vol. 77
© 1988 Elsevier Science Publishers B.V. (Biomedical Division)

CHAPTER 28

Sites of action of opiates in production of analgesia

T.L. Yaksh, N.R.F. Al-Rodhan and T.S. Jensen[a]

Department of Neurologic Surgery, Mayo Clinic, Rochester, MN 55905, USA and [a] Department of Neurology, University of Copenhagen, KAS, Gentofte, 2900 Hellerup, Denmark

Introduction

Certain unconditioned thermal, mechanical or chemical stimuli can evoke activity in small primary afferents and evoke an organized escape response in the unanesthetized animal. Opiates given systemically can powerfully and selectively alter that response in a fashion which suggests that the encoding of the physical stimulus has been altered. This effect appears to be mediated by specific classes of receptors as characterized by their pharmacological profile (ordering of the structure-activity relationship, and reversal by agents with affinity for, but no efficacy at the opiate site, i.e. antagonists). As regards the localization of these receptors, opiates may exert a direct effect on the peripheral terminals of primary afferent nociceptors and alter thereby peripheral sensitivity (Russell et al., 1987). However, the ability to induce the effects by central administration of the agonists at doses which are not systemically active and to antagonize the effects of systemically administered agonists with antagonists given into the central nervous system (see Herz and Teschemacher, 1971; Yaksh and Rudy, 1978), clearly emphasizes a central action. The issues to be considered here are (1) with which CNS structures are these opioid receptors associated; (2) given the existence of several classes of opioid receptors (μ/μ_1, δ and $\varkappa$) which of the receptors are relevant to the observed modulation of pain behavior produced by the locally acting agents; and (3) by what

mechanisms do these opioid receptors alter pain processing?

Technical issues

If it is presumed that a drug exerts an action within the neuraxis on discrete populations of opioid receptors to alter 'pain' behavior, three considerations present themselves: (1) administration of the agent, (2) assessment of the role and identity of the receptor mediating any observed drug effects, and (3) assessment of pain behavior.

Drug administration

A direct assessment of the locus of action of a drug may be achieved by the administration of the agent specifically into discrete regions using chronically implanted catheters. The broad range of investigations described herein involves consideration of both supraspinal and spinal elements.

Elucidation of the supraspinal action of a drug by local administration may be accomplished by stereotaxically directed, chronically implanted stainless steel guide cannulae (typically 23 to 24 gauge tw). Such guides are permanently affixed to the skull with screws and dental acrylic. These may then be used to insert smaller (typically 28 – 32 gauge) injection cannulae to varying depths into the parenchyma of the unanesthetized animal. Agents may then be delivered in volumes of up to 0.5 μl and the effects of the agents on a circumscribed tissue volume assessed. The ability to define the locus of drug effect is critically dependent upon variables such as volume of injection, drug concentration and characteristics of drug diffusion. These variables have been discussed elsewhere (Herz and Teschemacher, 1971; Yaksh and Rudy, 1978). The consequence of such variables is that time of onset for a given agent will be dependent upon the physical proximity to the relevant receptors, the volume of tissue which must be affected, and the concentration gradient of the drug and the rate of diffusion. A principal physical factor defining the rate of diffusion in brain is the tortuosity of the extracellular space (rate of straightline diffusion in tissue $\div$ rate of diffusion in water: Fenstermacher and Patlak (1975). Lipophobic molecules (such as morphine) or larger molecules (such as peptides) diffuse relatively slowly. In contrast, the diffusion of lipophilic molecules in tissue is rapid, but surprisingly limited since they are rapidly cleared into the capillary net as they diffuse from the point of injection. If their blood levels remain low, the anatomical distribution of microinjected lipophilic drugs can be very limited. Practically, actual measurement of diffusion gradients in tissue rarely provides convincing evidence for or against anatomical localization of the effect, as the actual concentration of drug at the receptor which exists, the concentration necessary, and the fraction of relevant receptor population affected are never known. More direct evidence has been achieved by assessing (1) the minimum time of onset of effect and (2) the maximum distance a given drug may be injected from an 'active' region to obtain a measured physiological effect. These measures indicate for that concentration of drug and microinjection volume employed that a pharmacologically adequate concentration of drug has been achieved at a particular site. Thus, as will be discussed below, in the rat, with the injection of 5 μg of morphine in 0.5 μl, prominent differences in activity may be observed following injection at sites separated by 1 mm.

The probable action of drugs at spinal sites has been assessed using catheters chronically placed in the intrathecal space. Such catheterization procedures have been described for a variety of species including dogs (Atchison et al., 1986), rat and rabbit (Yaksh and Rudy, 1976, 1977), cats and primates (Yaksh, 1978a). The issues of localization of drug effect are similar to those noted for intracranial application. To the extent that a drug must penetrate the spinal cord, factors of lipophilicity and concentration gradients are relevant. Issues relating to diffusion from the CSF into neural tissue have been previously discussed (Herz and Teschemacher, 1971; Yaksh, 1981). The likelihood of the supraspinal redistribution of a pharmacologically relevant concentration of spinally administered drug rises with the volume and dose injected and the time after administration. Hydrophilic agents diffuse into tissue more slowly and are cleared more slowly — they thus tend to show slower onset of effect and lower blood levels than equivalent doses of lipophilic agents after intrathecal injection (see Yaksh et al., 1986; Cousins and Mather, 1984).

Characterization of the receptor

As the action of systemically administered opiates is characterized by the nature of their pharmacological profile, so too is that of the intracerebrally administered drug. Because of the high concentrations of agents normally involved (e.g. a solution of 5 μg/0.5 μl of morphine is approximately 30 mM), it cannot be assumed that a receptor-selective agonist is indeed acting upon a particular receptor. Conversely, such concentrations do not provide a priori evidence that the drug effects are 'non-selective'. As minimum criteria, if a given receptor is proposed to mediate a particular physiological effect (1) the relative ordering of potency of other agonists for that receptor given into that region should parallel their activity in other bioassay systems having the same receptor; (2) the effect should be antagonized by the appropriate antagonists given into the same site. Absence of such information (or lack of the relevant agents) makes interpretation of receptor selectivity difficult, if not highly speculative.

Assessment of pain behavior

Given that the aim is to determine the presence and role of different opioid receptors in different CNS structures viz the 'analgesic' actions of an opioid, the bioassay is the behavioral response of the unanesthetized animal to a strong, unconditioned, physical stimulus which would otherwise evoke escape behavior. Chronically placed catheters permit drug administration to be made without significant restraint in the unanesthetized animal. Behaviors most frequently measured are broadly defined as spinal and supraspinally mediated, e.g. thermally evoked tail flick (D'Amour and Smith, 1941) or skin twitch (Martin et al., 1976) for the former; and hot plate induced paw licking (Woolfe and MacDonald, 1944), shock- or pinch-evoked vocalization/withdrawal (Randall and Selitto, 1957), writhing in response to peritoneal irritants, distention of the viscus (Hendershot and Forsaith, 1959; Ness and Gebhart, 1987) or shock titration threshold (Yaksh and Reddy, 1981), favoring of the hindpaw following local injection of irritants (Dubuisson and Dennis, 1977), for the latter.

Three points should be emphasized as minimum criteria for assessing the effects of a manipulation in terms of the theoretical construct of 'analgesia'. First, the blockade of the response must not occur because the motor output of the CNS to the response system was blocked (e.g. an inhibition of motor neurons; co-excitation of extensors and flexors resulting in rigidity, etc.). Secondly, analgesia implies a selective obtundation of the response otherwise evoked by a noxious stimulus without alterations in the response to non-noxious stimuli (e.g. anesthesia). Such specificity is difficult to ascertain in the animal model and is rarely determined. The continued ability, however, to evoke simple tactile driven reflexes such as placing and stepping or tendon reflexes, can provide evidence that transmission by at least some large diameter primary afferents is intact. Thirdly, the

criteria of specificity relate to changes in the content of the message which is evoked by a strong stimulus and which reaches the sensorium where the complex escape response is organized. Absolute dependence by the investigator on a spinal circuit precludes direct assessment of a change in rostrad transmission. Thus, while animal studies may usefully assess the effects of drugs on spinal nociceptive reflexes, the determination of analgesia should ideally use a response which is ultimately organized at the supraspinal level. In short, the occurrence of an effect on the organized behavior evoked by an unconditioned stimulus without changes in the ability of the animal to otherwise respond or a general suppression of behavior, is a minimal criterion necessary to imply analgesia.

Localization of supraspinal opioid receptors related to analgesia

Given the above considerations, the brains of several species have been mapped using stereotaxically implanted guides for regional sensitivity to the effects of opioid drugs with respect to a variety of pain behaviors.

Intracerebral mapping in rodents

Fig. 1 displays a composite summary of 521 histologically identified brain sites in the sagittal plane in which the effect of a unilateral microinjection of morphine (5 μg/0.5 μl) was examined on the hot plate response in several studies (Yaksh et al., 1976; Yeung et al., 1977; Walker and Yaksh, 1986; Jensen and Jaksh, 1986a,b,c; Yaksh and Camarata, unpublished observations). Several points are evident. First, over 78% of the sites examined in these whole brain mapping studies showed no responsiveness to this injection. Second, increases in hot plate response latencies were observed following the unilateral administration into several discrete regions. These include the mesencephalic periaqueductal gray and the region in and around the medial and paramedial medulla. In addition to the above sites, it was observed that similar

374

microinjections, made bilaterally into the corticomedial amygdala and mesencephalic reticular formation also yield effects on supraspinally organized measures. Table I summarizes the relative activity of morphine, given into several brain regions of the rat, measured by the effects on nociceptive (tail flick, hot plate) and non-nociceptive measures (catalepsy, seizures). The effects of morphine (5 µg/0.5 µl) on hot plate and tail flick response latency in histologically identified sites in the coronal planes of greatest activity from recent studies in this laboratory (Jensen and

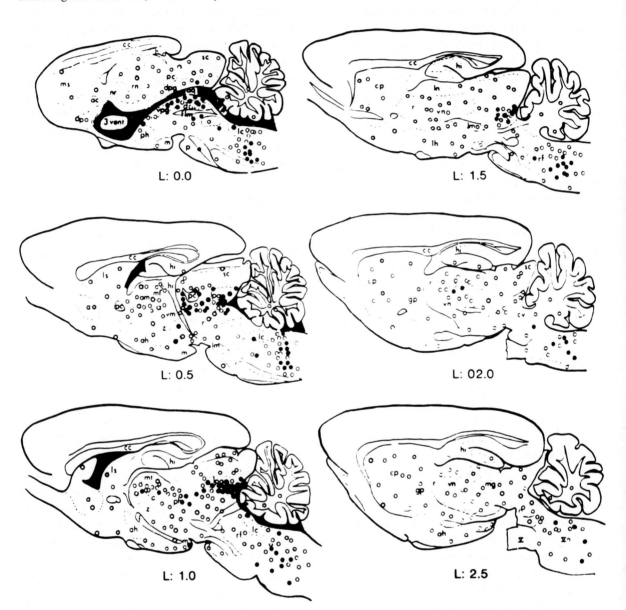

Fig. 1. Schematic of sagittal sections through rat brain showing individual histologically identified microinjection sites where the local application through stereotaxically implanted cannulae of 5 µg/0.5 µl of morphine sulfate produced a block of the hot plate or tail flick response in the rat. (Data are a composite of work by Yaksh et al., 1976; Yeung et al., 1977; Jensen and Yaksh, 1986a,b,c; Yaksh and Camarata, unpublished observations.)

Yaksh, 1986a; unpublished data) are presented in Fig. 2. As indicated, in spite of the likely location of activity in a given brain region such as the PAG, all microinjections do not produce the same magnitude of effect. This variability likely reflects upon possible technical failures of the microinjection system, misjudged histological placement or local heterogeneities in sensitivity (see below).

Mesencephalic periaqueductal/periventricular gray

The earliest studies pointing to a discrete localization of opiate action in brain using modern microinjection techniques were those of Tsou and Jiang (1964). Those studies, sophisticated even by today's standards, revealed that microinjections into the periventricular gray modify the thermally evoked hindlimb flexor reflex in a nalorphine-reversible fashion. Subsequent investigations in the rat (Jacquet and Lajtha, 1976; Sharpe et al., 1974; Yaksh et al., 1976; Lewis and Gebhart, 1977; Jensen and Yaksh, 1986c), mouse (Criswell, 1976), cat (Ossipov et al., 1984), dog (Wettstein et al., 1982) and primate (Pert and Yaksh, 1974, 1975; see below), repeatedly emphasized the sensitivity of the mesencephalic periaqueductal system and confirmed the species generality of this action. Fig. 3 presents the effects of morphine microinjected into the mesencephalic PAG on tail flick and hot plate response latencies. As indicated, this effect is characterized by a rapid increase in response latencies and in the intensity of the tail shock required to evoke a response in the shock

TABLE I

Effects of intracerebrally administered morphine on nociceptive and non-nociceptive aspects of behavior in the rat

	Antinociception		Catalepsy	Seizures	References
	spinal reflex (tail flick)	supraspinal (hot plate)			
Diencephalon					
medial thalamus	$(-)^a$	$(-)$	II	II	1, 3
lateral thalamus	$(-)$	$(-)$	II	II	1, 3
amygdala (corticomedial)	$(-)$	II	$(-)$	$(-)$	2
Mesencephalon					
periaqueductal gray	I	I	II	$(-)$	3, 7, 8, 9, 10
mesencephalic reticular function	III	III	II	$(-)$	4
Medulla					
medial medulla (raphe magnus)	III	1 – 2	$(-)$	$(-)$	6, 10
lateral medulla (nucl. giganto-cellularis)	III	1 – 2	$(-)$	$(-)$	5, 10
Spinal cord	I	I	$(-)$	$(-)$	11, 12

^{a} Dose range of morphine sulfate required to produce a maximum effect in the rat: I = 1 – 5 μg; II = 5 – 15 μg; III = > 15 μg; (–), inactive or for antinociceptive measures, prominent side effects occur at comparable doses.

References:
1, Walker and Yaksh, 1986
2, Rodgers, 1977
3, Yaksh et al., 1976
4, Haighler and Spring, 1978
5, Takagi et al., 1977; Kuraishi et al., 1978; Ossipov et al., 1984
6, Takagi et al., 1976; Dickenson et al., 1979

7, Jacquet and Lajtha, 1976
8, Sharpe et al., 1974
9, Lewis and Gebhart, 1977
10, Jensen and Yaksh, 1986a
11, Yaksh and Rudy, 1977
12, Yaksh and Rudy, 1976.

titration paradigm. This effect of PAG morphine on those measures can uniformly be antagonized by the systemic administration of naloxone. As indicated in the shock titration, those sites lying caudal in the PAG typically displayed the greatest sensitivity and shortest latency of onset (see below). Fig. 3 A displays the rapid increase in hot plate and tail flick response latency observed after the injection of 5 µg/0.5 µl into the mesencephalic PAG. The increase in the response latencies was

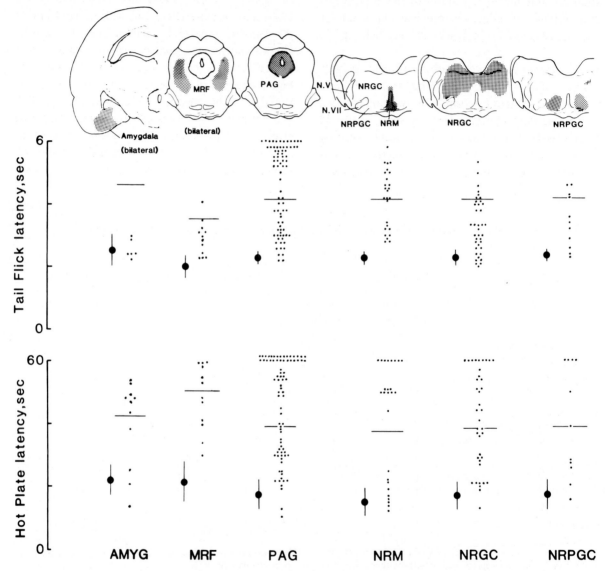

Fig. 2. Plot showing the maximum tail flick (upper) and hot plate (lower) response latency observed within 15 min after an intracerebral injection of morphine sulfate (5 µg/0.5 µl) in the sites within the medial amygdala (bilateral), mesencephalic reticular formation (MRF: bilateral), periaqueductal gray (PAG), nucleus raphe magnus (NRM), nucleus reticularis gigantocellularis (NRGC) and the nucleus reticularis paragigantocellularis (NRPGC). Each point represents a specific site (unilateral) or pair of sites (bilateral). The general distribution of the microinjection sites is indicated by the shaded area in the schematic at top. The mean ± SEM of the baseline response latency of each group is presented at left of each plot. (Adapted from Jensen and Yaksh, 1986a; and unpublished observations.)

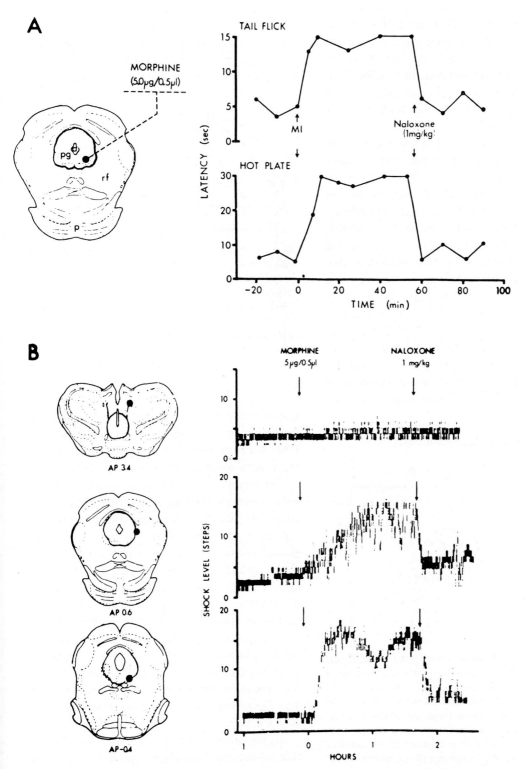

Fig. 3. (A) Effect of morphine (5 μg/0.5 μl) given into the periaqueductal gray at the site indicated in the schematic (left) on the tail flick and hot plate response latency in a single rat (right) at the time indicated, naloxone (1 mg/kg) was administered i.p. (B) Effect of microinjections of morphine (5 μg/0.5 μl) given into three sites (location indicated by the schematics on the left) on the tail shock titration. At the time indicated, naloxone (1 mg/kg) was administered i.p. (Adapted from Yaksh et al., 1976.)

378

not due to a motor blockade as the action of drug was to increase the intensity of stimulus required to evoke the effect. As shown in Fig. 3 B, the microinjection of morphine into the caudal PAG resulted in a progressive rise in the level of shock required to evoke the response in a discrete trial shock titration paradigm.

As shown in Fig. 4, systematic mapping of the distribution of activity within the PAG revealed that the most prominent action was found in or near the caudal, ventrolateral aspects of the region. As shown in Fig. 5, sequential microinjection at sites 1 to 3 mm below guide tip resulted in a maximum effect in the ventrolateral aspect of the PAG. Sites more shallow or deep showed a comparatively lesser effect. Similarly, assessing the latency of onset after microinjection (Fig. 4), or the dose-dependent sensitivity as a function of distance from midline (Fig. 5) indicated that those sites which lay in the ventrolateral quadrant displayed the shortest latency and greatest sensitivity. That the drug effect observed did not derive from a movement into the ventricular lumen was sug-

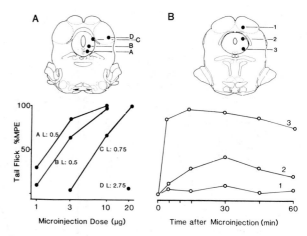

Fig. 5. (A) Dose response curves plotting the percentage of the maximal possible effect (MPE) versus the log dose of morphine sulfate given in 0.5 μl into four brain sites (A, B, C, D) which correspond to the sites indicated in the schematic. (Adapted from Yaksh et al., 1976.) (B) Time response curve for the tail flick following the microinjection of morphine (5 μg/0.5 μl) at progressively deeper sites through the same guide cannula. The respective three sites are indicated in the schematic. Each injection was separated by a 5-day period from the previous one.

gested by the observation that for sites equidistant to the lumen, those in the dorsal quadrant of the PAG were routinely less active than sites laying in the ventral quadrant (Yaksh et al., 1976).

The effects of morphine given into the PAG have been demonstrated on a variety of nociceptive endpoints including those mediated by spinal (e.g. tail flick) and supraspinal (hot plate, paw pinch, evoked vocalization and withdrawal, writhing and shock titration) (see above references). As shown in Fig. 2, not all sites judged in or near the PAG were active. Importantly, however, sites at which morphine evoked an increase in the tail flick response, a corresponding increase in the hot plate response latency was also noted. Fig. 6 displays the corresponding response latency for hot plate and tail flick following microinjection into a given site. The linear regression line associating these data shows a slope of −1.

An important issue, not typically considered, is that of whether the antinociceptive effects produced by unilateral microinjections of morphine into

Stereotaxic Coordinate (mm)

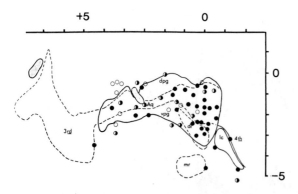

Fig. 4. Sagittal section shows the profile of the mesencephalic periaqueductal gray 0.5 mm off midline in the rat. The abscissa and ordinate of the sagittal section are the anterior-posterior and horizontal. Vertical stereotaxic coordinates in mm. The areas outlined by broken lines are projections of midline structures. Schematic shows sites where the microinjection of morphine (5 μg/0.5 μl) resulted in a blockade of the tail flick response within 5 min (●), 5 to 20 min (◗) or greater than 20 min (○) after the microinjection.

the periaqueductal gray are somatotopically organized. Systematic examination of the pinch response revealed no systematic laterality of the antinociception. Yaksh and colleagues (1976) reported a rostrocaudal distribution such that those sites in the caudal PAG tended towards a whole body effect, while those rostrally tended towards an effect on forepaw, face and pinch (see also Kasman and Rosenfeld, 1986).

Mesencephalic reticular formation

Haigler and Spring (1978) reported that microinjections of 10 μg, bilaterally could elevate tail flick and hot plate latencies. As shown in the data on Fig. 2, the apparent potency is greater in the supraspinally mediated hot plate response. Significantly, unilateral injections have only a minor effect on the nociceptive response. The question of somatotopic organization of the antinociceptive effects has not been addressed.

Medulla

Two principal distributions of sites have been reported. Those lying lateral in the paramedial medulla, a region anatomically defined as the nucleus reticularis gigantocellularis and the medial medulla where the caudal raphe nuclei (e.g. raphe magnus) are located. Early studies by Takagi and colleagues first emphasized the probable importance of the paramedial medulla, notably the region anatomically described as the nucleus reticularis gigantocellularis and this action has been subsequently confirmed (Takagi et al., 1978; Akaike et al., 1978; Azami et al., 1982; Satoh et al., 1983; Jensen et al., 1986a).

Subsequently, others have also emphasized the effects of morphine administered in the medial medulla, notably the nucleus raphe magnus and paramedial medulla (Levy and Proudfit, 1979; Dickenson et al., 1979; Jensen et al., 1986a; Prado and Roberts, 1984). It should be stressed that, in spite of what appears to be extensive mapping in the caudal brain stem, the extent of this region and the distribution of sensitivity has not been satisfactorily assessed at this time. Thus, the possible role

of more caudal raphe nuclei such as raphe pallidus and obscurus, has not been determined systematically.

To date, microinjections of morphine into the medulla have been shown to significantly increase the response latencies on thermal spinal and supraspinally mediated measures as well as paw pinch and writhing (see above references). In spite of this, it should be noted that unlike the PAG sites, morphine's action in the medulla is clearly

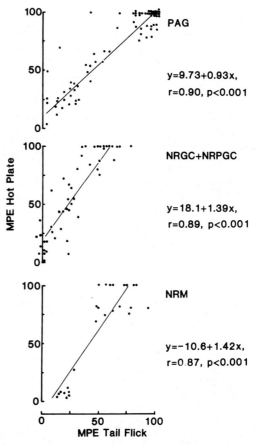

Fig. 6. Scatter plot diagram with maximal possible effect (MPE) of the tail flick (abscissa) plotted vs. the MPE of hot plate (ordinate) values shown in Fig. 1. Each dot represents the MPE tail flick and hot plate values within 15 min after an intracerebral injection of morphine sulfate (5 μg/0.5 μl) into a site within the periaqueductal gray (top), nucleus raphe magnus (middle) or nucleus reticularis gigantocellularis and nucleus reticularis paragigantocellularis (bottom). The straight lines represent the calculated regression lines for which the equation is shown in each figure. (From Jensen and Yaksh, 1986a.)

380

distinguishable. As indicated in Fig. 6, doses of morphine which block the 52.5°C hot plate rarely, if ever, result in a complete block of the spinally mediated tail flick. Even injections of doses of 20 μg bilaterally fail to completely block the tail flick response (in contrast to the PAG). It should be stressed that the distinction between PAG and medullary sites, as regards the effect on spinal reflexes, is not absolute. It is probable that milder stimuli might evoke a response which is subject to complete blockade by medullary microinjections of morphine. The important issue is that in parallel tests, the ability of opiates given into the PAG, results in a proportional effect on hot plate and tail flick response, while in the medulla this relative activity is different.

The issues of somatotopic organization of the analgesia elicited by microinjections of opiates in this region have not been assessed.

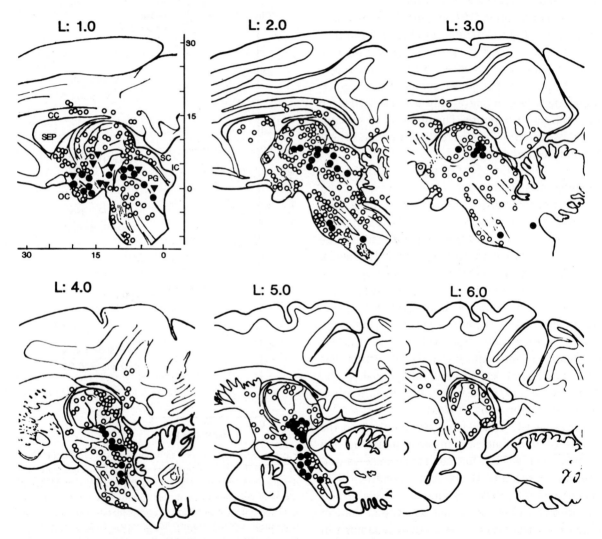

Fig. 7. Schematic drawings taken from sagittal histology (1 – 6 mm from midline) of the rhesus monkey. Each dot displays the effects of a single injection of morphine sulfate (2 μl) given through chronically implanted guide cannulae. ○, < 50% increase in baseline shock titration threshold with 40 μg/2 μl; ●, > 50% increase in the baseline shock titration threshold with 40 μg/2 μl; ▼, > 50% increase above baseline with 10 – 20 μg/2 μl. The stereotaxic axes are given for the most medial (L: 1.0) section. (Adapted from Pert and Yaksh, 1974; Yaksh, unpublished observations.)

Amygdala

Bilateral microinjections of morphine into the corticomedial region of the amygdala were reported by Rodgers (1977) to have prominent effects on supraspinal responses such as the jump portion of the flinch jump task. In our own work, unilateral injections given into a variety of amygdalar sites (Yaksh et al., 1976) failed to have any effect on either hot plate or tail flick. However, subsequent examination confirmed the observation of Rodgers, with significant increases in hot plate, but not tail flick response latencies being observed after bilateral injections (see Fig. 2).

Intracerebral mapping in primate

Early systematic studies in the primate revealed a distribution of sites which lay along the mesencephalic periaqueductal gray. Like in the rat, distributions of these sites were observed to extend rostrally into the periventricular gray of the diencephalon. Fig. 7 presents a summary of 420 histologically identified sites showing the effects of intracerebral morphine on the shock titration threshold in the rhesus monkey. The most active sites were those which lay in the caudal aspects of the PAG. Rostrally, unlike in the rat, a number of sites were found in the caudal ventral aspect of the medial thalamus. Pert and Yaksh (1974, 1975) also noted a second distribution of less active sites located more laterally. These sites extended caudally from the mesencephalic reticular formation. Because of the stereotaxic angle of insertion, unlike in the rat, the deeper the microinjection sites, the more 'caudal' were the areas studied. Thus, as the strategy of these experiments was to map deeper sites until an active locus was observed, medial sites (ventral to the PAG) were not explored. These results thus provide support for the probable role of paramedial medullary sites in the antinociceptive actions of morphine, but the role of medial sites in the primate pons and medulla remain unaddressed. Oliveras and colleagues (1986a,b) have examined the effect of morphine microinjected into the trigeminal nucleus (see below).

Intracerebral opiates in man

Though intraparenchymal studies have not been attempted in man, the intraventricular administration of several opioids including morphine (Lazorthes et al., 1985, and see his chapter in this volume; Lenzi et al., 1985; Leavens et al., 1982; Lobato et al., 1983) and β-endorphin (Foley et al., 1979) in terminal cancer patients have been shown to produce analgesia. Latency of onset to the reported analgesia has varied but has usually been on the order of 30 min or less.

Spinal opioid receptors associated with analgesia

The spinal administration of opioids and the effect on pain behavior have been carried out in a wide variety of species including mouse (Hylden and Wilcox, 1983), rabbit (Yaksh and Rudy, 1976), cat (Yaksh, 1978b; Yaksh et al., 1986), sheep (Eisenach, 1987) and primate (Yaksh, 1978a; Yaksh and Reddy, 1981; Yaksh, 1983), and a powerful analgesia has been routinely reported. As shown in Fig. 8, intrathecal morphine will yield a potent and long-lasting elevation in the tail flick and hot plate response latencies, and a caudal block of the animal's response to pinch. Similarly, intrathecal morphine yields an increase in the intensity of tail shock required to evoke a response. Similarly, spinal (intrathecal or epidural) administration has been shown to increase the nociceptive threshold and to diminish the pain report in a variety of human studies (see Yaksh and Noueihed, 1985; Cousins and Mather, 1984). Intraparenchymal injections of opioids into spinal cord in unanesthetized animals have not been routinely accomplished. Oliveras and colleagues (1986a,b) have observed that microinjections of morphine in the medullary trigeminal nucleus will result in significant increases in the thermal nociceptive threshold. Microinjection into the dorsal horn of the cat lumbar spinal cord has been shown to suppress C fiber ventral root reflexes (Bell et al., 1980). The time of onset of intrathecally (topically) applied opiates varies directly with their lipid partition coefficient (see for example

Yaksh et al., 1986), and this timing corresponds with the observed depression of dorsal horn neurons assessed after the topical application of the respective agents (Suzukawa et al., 1983; Homma et al., 1983). These results suggesting the delay in onset after intrathecal injection reflect upon the need for the drug to reach the site of action in the dorsal horn.

Pharmacology of supraspinal and spinal opioid receptors associated with analgesia

With regard to the general question of the role of opioid receptors, the antinociceptive effects produced by intracerebral morphine in the several brain regions have in general been shown to be dose dependent, mimicked by other opioid alkaloids (such as methadone, levorphanol, sufentanil), uniformly antagonized by intracerebral and systemically administered naloxone and, where examined, stereospecific (see above and Yaksh, 1984b, for references). In spinal cord, comparable studies have similarly revealed over a wide range of doses that the antinociceptive effects of intrathecal opioid alkaloids possess a characteristically opioid receptor pharmacology (see Yaksh and Noueihed, 1985). These minimal criteria, thus, early established that the focal action of opiates on these brain regions and in spinal cord were exerting their effects by a local opioid receptor.

There is evidence for several subclasses of opioid receptors. The focal injection procedures allow us to consider whether the receptors in the several regions which alter nociceptive processing are the same. Assessment of this issue hinges upon the establishment of the pharmacological profile associated with the observed effects produced by the intracerebrally administered agents, and comparison of this profile to that known to describe currently proposed subpopulations of opioid receptors. An abbreviated listing of the several putative receptor-defining agonists and antagonists is presented in Table II. Specific assessment of these pharmacological criteria has not been uniformly carried out for all regions, and different receptors may mediate effects observed in the different brain regions.

Table III presents a summary of experiments examining the agonist pharmacology of sites in the mesencephalic periaqueductal gray and the

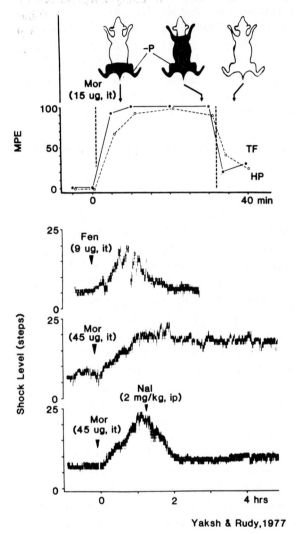

Fig. 8. (Top) Effect of the intrathecal administration of morphine (45 μg/5 μl) in the rat on the hot plate and tail flick response latency as a function of time after injection. At the time indicated, naloxone (1 mg/kg, i.p.) was administered. The figures above the response latency indicate in black the regions which were rendered non-responsive to forelimb pinch at that time point. (Bottom) Effects of intrathecal fetanyl or morphine in the rat on the shock titration paradigm. At the time indicated in the bottom panel, naloxone (1 mg/kg, i.p.) was administered. (Adapted from Yaksh and Rudy, 1977.)

TABLE II

Pharmacological profile of several proposed subclasses of opioid receptors

	Agonists	Antagonists
μ	Sufentanil, morphine, DAGO	β-FNA[a], naloxone
μ_1	Meptazinol	Naloxonazine[a], naloxone
δ	DADL, DSTLE, DPLPE	ICI-178,864, naloxone[b]
$\varkappa$	U50488H	(?)[c], Naloxone[b]
ϵ	β-Endorphin	(?), Naloxone

[a] Non-equilibrium, non-competitive antagonists. See Ward et al. (1982); Ling et al. (1986).
[b] Naloxone has approximately 0.1 × the affinity for the δ and $\varkappa$ sites as compared to the μ site.
[c] (?), a well-defined selective antagonist is not available.

β-FNA, β-funalnaltrexamine
DADL, D-Ala^2-D-Leu^5-enkephalin
DAGO, D-Ala^2-MePhe^4, Gly-ol^5-enkephalin
DPLPE, D-penicillamine^2-L-penicillamine^5-enkephalin
DSTLE, D-Ser^2-Thr^6-leucine enkephalin
U50488H, (trans-3,4-dichloro-N-methyl-N-[2-1(1-pyrrolindinyl)cyclohexyl]) benzeneacetamide
ICI-178,864, N,N-diallyl-Tyr-Aib-Aib-Phe-Leu-OH.

paramedial medulla, and after spinal intrathecal injection. In all cases where agents are listed as active, the drug has been shown to produce a monotonic dose-dependent increase in the hot plate response latency.

Periaqueductal gray

Though considerably more work remains, the first order analysis of the results in Table III suggests that within the PAG, sites exist with affinity for μ type agents (morphine, sufentanil, DAGO). Significantly, the ligand DSLET is active but DPDPE at the highest concentration which can be delivered in 1 μl is not. Though both peptides are thought to have high affinity for the δ receptor (Clark et al., 1986; Itzhak and Pasternak, 1986), they differ in that DSLET, in contrast to DPDPE, also has high affinity for μ sites (Clark et al., 1986; Itzhak and Pasternak, 1986). The purported μ_1

receptor agonist, meptazinol (Dray et al., 1986), is weakly active as is the $\varkappa$ agonist, U50488H. Though this may suggest that the μ_1 and $\varkappa$ type sites may be relevant, it should be stressed that these drugs are active only at concentrations above those at which DPDPE can be tested, and the likelihood of non-specific effects must be considered.

With regard to antagonists, Jensen and Yaksh (1986a) observed that the intracerebral administration of naloxone resulted in a dose-dependent depression of the effects of PAG morphine and DADL. Significantly, these effects of PAG DADL have been reported not to be antagonized by the putative δ- receptor antagonist, ICI-174,846 (Al-Rodhan and Yaksh, unpublished observations). In recent studies we have observed that the effect of μ agonists (sufentanil, DAGO, morphine) as well as DSLET, meptazinol and U50488H are uniformly antagonized by the μ-specific, non-equilibrium

TABLE III

Effect in the rat on the hot plate response latency of selected receptor preferring opioid ligands administered into the periaqueductal gray, medulla and spinal cord

Site	Ordering of activity on the hot plate test (relative to morphine)
Periaqueductal gray[a]:	sufentanil (0.01) > β-endorphin (0.06) ≥ DADL (0.2) > DSLET (0.3) > morphine (1) ≥ DAGO (1.1) >> meptazinol (26) > U50488H (33) >> DPDPE = 0
Medial medulla[a]:	sufentanil (0.06) > DSLET (0.35) ≥ DADL (0.03) > morphine (1)
Spinal cord[b]:	DAGO (0.02) ≥ sufentanil (0.02) > β-endorphin (0.25) ≥ DSLET (0.5) > morphine (1) ≥ DPDPE (2.0) >> meptazinol (> 100) = U50488H (> 100) = 0

[a] Data from Jensen and Yaksh (1986c); Al-Rodhan and Yaksh, in preparation. All drugs delivered in volumes of 0.5 μl.
[b] Data from Yaksh and Henry (1978); Yaksh et al. (1986); Schmauss and Yaksh (1983); Mjanger and Yaksh, unpublished. All drugs delivered in volumes of 10 μl.

antagonist, β-FNA (Al-Rodhan and Yaksh, unpublished observations). This supports a probable role of a common μ receptor site for these agents in the PAG. Systematic studies in mice, with intraventricular injections, arrive at a similar conclusion (Fang et al., 1986). Though the precise locus of action of the intraventricular opiates in the mouse is unknown, early studies by Criswell have shown morphine-sensitive sites in the PAG (Criswell, 1976).

Medulla

Current studies on the action of opioids in the medulla have shown that the rank ordering of potency in the medulla differs from that in the PAG with DADL and DSLET becoming more potent. Naloxone administered at the site also produced prominent antagonism of the effects of morphine and less so DADL. Further evidence that these agents are acting at discriminable sites is that in the PAG all agents (e.g. DADL and morphine) result in a 1:1 relationship between the blockade of the hot plate and tail flick. Whereas in the medulla, μ agonists (morphine and sufentanil) show a diminished efficacy on the hot plate. In contrast, DADL is able to yield a complete block. Thus, based on relative sensitivity to naloxone antagonism and a differential structure-activity series in the PAG and medulla, we speculate that there are μ sites in the PAG and μ and δ sites in the medulla. Indeed, early reports by Takagi et al. (1978) emphasized the potency in the medulla of met-enkephalin, a relatively selective δ receptor agonist. Systematic examination of the antagonist pharmacology is necessary to address these issues.

Spinal cord

As summarized in Table III, the ordering of activity in the cord is consistent with the presence of three classes of receptors: μ, δ, and $\varkappa$. Examination of the effects of these agents on the writing response also supports this separation. Thus, in contrast to the structure activity relationship noted on the thermal measures, the ordering of activity or the writing suggests the presence of μ and $\varkappa$, but a lesser effect of δ receptor agonists. Similar results have been recently reported by Millan and colleagues (personal communication, Munich, 1987).

With regard to antagonists, naloxone has been shown to produce a dose-dependent shift to the right of the intrathecal morphine dose-response curve (Yaksh and Rudy, 1977). Calculation of the pA_2 values of naloxone against a variety of agonists indicates significant differences between μ, δ and $\varkappa$ agonists (see Yaksh and Noueihed, 1985), suggesting distinguishable sites. β-FNA has been shown to readily block the effect of intrathecal μ (DAGO and morphine), but at comparable doses had no effect on the actions of δ (DPLPE) specific agonists (Russell et al., 1987; Mjanger and Yaksh, in preparation).

Pharmacology of intracerebral/intrathecal opioids in man

Regarding intracerebroventricular injection of opioids in man, there is no data concerning their pharmacology. Thus far, morphine (see above) and β-endorphin (Foley et al., 1979) have been administered. Systematic examination of the ability to reverse the analgesia with naloxone has not to our knowledge been reported (see Lazorthes this symposium).

In contrast, considerable data exists regarding the actions of these agents in the human spinal cord. Table III presents the approximate ordering of activity of a variety of agents given by the epidural route with the estimated endpoint being the approximate dose which gives 'adequate' analgesia. As indicated, DADL, a δ-preferring ligand has been shown to be active. Agents with probable $\varkappa$ properties such as nalbuphine (Wang et al., 1985) and butorphanol (Chu et al., 1987) have been reported to have mild analgesic actions. These limited observations, though supportive, do not prove the presence of either δ or $\varkappa$ receptors.

With regard to antagonism, Rawal and colleagues have demonstrated that naloxone in the range of 10 $\mu g \cdot kg^{-1} \cdot h^{-1}$, i.v. will produce an approximate 50% reduction in the analgesic effects produced by epidural morphine. This dose falls within a factor of 3 of the dose known to double the ED_{50} of intrathecal μ receptor agonists in rats and primates (see Yaksh and Noueihed, 1985). Together, the comparability of the relative ordering of the SAR for spinally administered agonists in rats and man, along with the sensitivity to systemically administered opiates, argues for a similarity in the spinal receptors which mediates analgesia in man and animals.

Neural mechanisms whereby opioids acting in the several brain regions modulate nociceptive transmission

In view of the anatomical diversity of substrates where opiates may act to modulate the nociceptive response, it appears unlikely that the mechanisms underlying the effects observed following injection into the several brain regions, could be the same. We will briefly consider several probable circuits involving the brain and spinal cord.

Brain stem

Currently, we believe that there are four likely mechanisms whereby opiates acting in the PAG may alter nociceptive transmission: indirect bulbospinal inhibition, indirect brain stem/brain stem inhibition, direct inhibition of brain stem transmission, and forebrain projections.

Bulbospinal projections

Early studies in intact and spinal transected animals with systemic opiates pointed to the probable bulbospinal pathways on the inhibition of spinal cord reflexes (Takagi et al., 1955). Subsequently, discrete lesions of the dorsolateral quadrant of the spinal cord were observed to diminish the antinociceptive effects of systemic morphine (Barton et al., 1980; Basbaum et al., 1977). This supraspinal effect on spinal function has been con-

firmed in a large number of periaqueductal/periventricular microinjection studies (Tsou and Jang, 1964; see also Yaksh and Rudy, 1978). Mesencephalic and raphe (Bennett and Mayer, 1979; Du et al., 1984; Gebhart et al., 1984) microinjection of opiates have been shown to inhibit activity in dorsal horn nociceptors, though excitation has also been observed (Dickenson and LeBars, 1986). These effects coincide with the work by early Swedish investigators indicating that bulbospinal monoamine pathways, when activated, could prominently modulate activity in flexor reflex afferents (Anden et al., 1966). Several direct lines of evidence support the likelihood that PAG and medullary opioid receptor linked systems do activate such bulbospinal pathways and thereby directly regulate spinal cord nociceptive processing.

(a) Opiates acting supraspinally result in an increase in spinal cord turnover or release of serotonin and noradrenaline (Yaksh and Tyce, 1979; Takagi et al., 1979).

(b) The effects of PAG morphine on nociceptive responses are closely mimicked by the local spinal administration of serotonergic or adrenergic agonists. Thus, locally applied noradrenaline and 5HT will block activity in dorsal horn nociceptors (Headley et al., 1978), and the intrathecal administration of these amines will result in a powerful and functionally specific analgesia in several species (Yaksh and Wilson, 1979; Reddy et al., 1980; Kuraishi et al., 1979). Intrathecal clonidine has been shown to produce analgesia in man (Tamsen and Gordh, 1984). The analgesic effects of the spinal noradrenergic agonists appear, by virtue of their agonist and antagonist pharmacology, to act via an α_2 receptor (see Yaksh, 1985).

(c) The effects on spinal reflexes of opioids injected into the mesencephalon and medulla are antagonized, as shown in Fig. 9 by the spinal administration of adrenergic and serotonergic receptor antagonists (Yaksh, 1979; Jensen and Yaksh, 1986b). Importantly, the pharmacology of the spinal adrenergic receptor sites occupied after the supraspinal administration of morphine is indistinguishable from that assessed with the intrathecally administered adrenergic agonist (e.g. an α_2 but not an α_1 or β receptor: Camarata and Yaksh, 1985).

(d) Finally, that the antinociceptive effects of PAG opiates reflect the net 'activation' of a bulbospinal system is emphasized by the fact that the effects are mimicked by the intracerebral administration of excitatory amino acids (glutamate) or by electrical stimulation, and the spinal pharmacology of this stimulation as assessed by intrathecally administered antagonists in blocking these supraspinally evoked efferents cannot be distinguished from that of the intracerebrally administered opiates (Jensen and Yaksh, 1984; Satoh et al., 1983; Hammond and Yaksh, 1984).

The mechanism whereby opiates produce this net bulbospinal activation, when they appear to result locally in an inhibition of the activity of single units (see Gebhart, 1982; Duggan and North, 1984), is not known. Yaksh and colleagues (1976) suggested the obvious alternative that the PAG effects of morphine reflected the inhibition of a tonic inhibition on PAG outflow, though they had no direct evidence to support their hypothesis. Demonstration of GABAergic neurons in the PAG (Otterson and Storm-Mathisen, 1984) and the antinociceptive effects of GABA antagonists on PAG outflow (Moreau and Fields, 1987) suggest the viability of this proposal.

Given that PAG projections to the spinal cord are sparse and are not monoaminergic, early studies emphasized the probability that functionally excitatory projections from PAG to the cells of origin and monoaminergic bulbospinal pathways

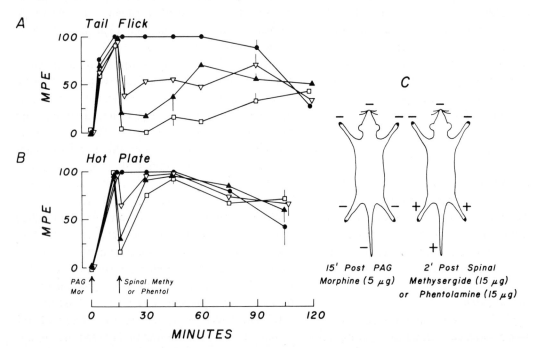

Fig. 9. The effect expressed as the mean and SE of the maximum percent effect (MPE) on the tail flick (A) and hot plate (B) of rats receiving an injection of morphine sulfate (5 μg/0.5 μl) into the PAG at time 0 (first arrow). At the second arrow, each animal received in different experiments an intrathecal injection (15 μl) of either saline (●———●), methysergide bimaleate (15 μg; ▽———▽), phentolamine-HCl (15 μg; ▲———▲) or both methysergide and phentolamine (15 μg each; □———□). SE are presented on every other data point to preserve figure clarity. C (left) shows that the response to forceps pinch applied to all four limbs was blocked by 15 min after the injection of morphine. This blockade was observed in all animals. Two minutes after the injection of methysergide or phentolamine, all animals showed a return of the withdrawal response to the hindquarters only. See text for further details and discussion.

in the pons and medulla were an important intermediary link (Behbehani and Fields, 1979).

While there is persuasive evidence for the significance of bulbospinal pathways in modulating spinal nociceptive processing, these pathways appear not to be the only mechanism by which supraspinal opiates act to regulate the organized behavioral response to noxious stimuli. Thus, perhaps most interesting is that, while the spinal administration of monoamine antagonists can completely reverse the inhibition of spinal reflexes produced by PAG opiates (see Fig. 9), spinal monoamine receptor antagonism has a relatively transient effect on the supraspinally organized response to the nociceptive stimulus (e.g. as measured on the hot plate response and behavior, evoked by forceps pinch). While these observations could mean that bulbospinal inhibition plays little role in modulating spino-bulbar transmission (e.g. that it only affects spinal motor reflexes), we consider it more likely that these results emphasize the presence of additional supraspinal mechanisms which modulate the response of the animal to aversive stimuli independently of powerful descending modulatory influences. Thus, in their absence, other possible systems are revealed.

Brainstem-brainstem inhibition

The role of spino-reticulo-thalamic networks in pain transmission has been long postulated (Bowsher et al., 1968). Mohrland and Gebhart (1980) have shown that stimulation in the PAG will result in an inhibition in nucleus reticularis gigantocellularis neurons. Thus, it is conceivable that a 'local' descending inhibition may be relevant.

Direct inhibition of brain stem afferent transmission

It is clear that many of the regions in which opiates act in rat and primate (e.g. the medulla or the PAG) receive input from spinobulbar fibers or collaterals from spinodiencephalic fibers (Bowsher et al., 1968). Though indirect, the fact that spinobulbar cell bodies possess opioid receptors

(see below), and given the probability that receptors are transported to distal cell terminals (Atweh et al., 1978), it is likely that spinobulbar fibers also have opioid receptors on their bulbar terminals. In early studies, it was noted that a crude rostrocaudal somatotopy existed for microinjection of morphine into the PAG, with rostral sites blocking the response to mechanical stimuli applied to the rostral body, and caudal injections blocking pinches applied at rostral and caudal body sites (Yaksh et al., 1976). This corresponds with reports of somatotopically organized evoked activity in this structure (Liebeskind and Mayer, 1971). We speculate that local opioids may block afferent activity into the bulbar core. If true, local lesions or local anesthetics should yield antinociception. Though neither manipulation has been reported to be effective in the PAG (see Yaksh and Rudy, 1978 for references), lesions of the medullary reticular formation have been shown to be effective (Halpern and Halverson, 1974).

Forebrain projections

While there is little direct evidence supporting the hypothesis that rostral projections are affected by a bulbar action of opiates or that such rostral projections may be relevant to pain transmission, early studies examining the effect of various lesions on morphine analgesia focussed on raphe dorsalis, a serotonin-containing nucleus which projects rostrally (see Messing and Lytle, 1977), and the possibility exists that opiates may activate systems relevant to the emotionality context of the pain message and may employ these systems as a substrate (Xuan et al., 1986). More recently, Han and colleagues, in an extremely interesting series of experiments, have shown the probable role of the nucleus accumbens, the amygdala and the habenula in a circuit where rostrofugal projections partially involving serotonergic fibers alter withdrawal responses in the rabbit (see Xuan et al., 1986).

Forebrain sites

Though the mechanisms of opiate analgesia in the

brain stem are only incompletely understood, forebrain systems are even less appreciated. The effects of opioids in the amygdala reflect upon this. As noted in Table I amygdalar injections do not alter spinal reflex function. Thus, the mechanism probably does not relate to any spinopetal interactions. Alternatively, the amygdala has long been associated with various aspects of emotionality and the well-appreciated efforts of systemic morphine in the emotional-affective component of pain may be related to an effect on such systems. Similarly, it should be stressed that other portions of the limbic forebrain systems related to emotionality may be involved, and the failure to detect their relevance to pain, particularly as in chronic circumstances, may be the result of insensitive experimental test paradigms. It should also be stressed that a bilateral action of the drug may be necessary for the opioid effect on pain behavior to be manifested. This may be the case for such systems which modulate the affective aspects of the behavioral response (e.g. compare Rodgers, 1977 to Yaksh et al., 1976). More recently, Han and colleagues have presented evidence that the forebrain effects of morphine in the rabbit also require bilateral injections (Han, this volume).

Spinal cord

The application of opiates to the spinal surface or directly into tissue by local microtechniques, yields a powerful, pharmacologically specific and functionally selective inhibition of activity evoked in wide dynamic range or nociceptive specific neurons evoked by $A\delta/C$ fiber stimulation (see Yaksh and Noueihed, 1985). Within the spinal cord, there is evidence that opioids act to alter nociceptive transmission selectively by an action both presynaptic on or postsynaptic to the primary afferent.

Evidence for a presynaptic action is based on: (a) the observation that opioid binding in the dorsal horn is largely within the substantia gelatinosa, and is significantly, but subtotally, diminished by rhizotomy or by treatment with a small primary af-

ferent neurotoxin capsaicin (LaMotte et al., 1976; Gamse et al., 1979); (b) that opiates will diminish terminal excitability (Carstens et al., 1979); and (c) that opiates will reduce the stimulation-evoked secretion of substance P, a small primary afferent peptide neurotransmitter (Yaksh et al., 1980; Go and Yaksh, 1987; Pang and Vasko, 1986).

That spinal opiates may also act postsynaptically on primary afferents is emphasized (a) by the partial effects of rhizotomy in opioid binding, and (b) by the ability of opiates to diminish the response evoked by iontophoretically applied glutamate (Zieglgänsberger and Bayerl, 1976).

Though opiate binding is found in the dorsal roots (Fields et al., 1980), it does not appear that such axonal sites play a role in the actions of intrathecal opiates in the adult animals. Thus, recording in situ from adult DRG cells revealed no effect of opiates (Williams and Zieglgänsberger, 1981), though significant μ, δ and $\varkappa$ efferents or ion currents have been identified in cultured spinal ganglion cells (Werz and MacDonald, 1983, 1985).

Interaction between brain and spinal opioid receptor-linked systems

Given the multiple sites of potential action revealed by microinjection studies, we may consider how they interact. When an opiate is given systemically, all of the systems are concurrently affected. Several lines of evidence may be considered.

Intracerebral agonist studies

As outlined above, an action of morphine in either spinal or intracerebroventricular sites can produce a monotonic, dose-dependent increase in the response to noxious stimuli. Though the distribution may be limited, the concentration of agents required to produce these effects is clearly higher than would be anticipated following a systemic injection.

Antagonist studies

When opioids are given systemically, it is possible to produce a dose-dependent rightward shift in the morphine dose response curve by administering an opioid antagonist either into the cerebral ventricles or into the spinal cord (see Yaksh and Rudy, 1978, for references). At high concentrations of systemic opiates, further shifts in the dose response curves by either intracerebral or intrathecal antagonists are not observed. Given that opiates acting only in circumscribed brain regions (e.g. brain stem vs. spinal cord) can produce analgesia, the inability to produce continued shifts in the systemic dose response curves with local naloxone appears contradictory.

Synergy studies

Yaksh and Rudy (1978) proposed that the several phenomena might be explained by presuming a synergistic interaction between brain stem and spinal cord opioid sensitive systems. Such a synergistic interaction would theoretically be revealed by the results of the above cited opioid antagonist experiments, and by studies in which the dose response interaction between intraventricular and intrathecal morphine was examined. In such studies, it was indeed confirmed that there is a synergistic interaction between brain stem and spinal opioid sensitive systems (Yeung and Rudy, 1980). A corollary of this hypothesis is that, if the bulbospinal pathway mediates the effects of brain stem morphine on spinal processing, then there should also be a synergistic interaction between spinal morphine and spinal α_2 agonists. This has indeed been demonstrated (Monasky and Yaksh, 1986; Yaksh and Reddy, 1981; Wigdor and Wilcox, 1987). We believe that the substrate for this interaction is revealed by the observation that the slope of the stimulus intensity/cell response curve of spinal neurons is reduced both by bulbospinal stimulation (Gebhart et al., 1984) and by spinal opiates (Yaksh, 1978a). Such an interaction between manipulations which alter the gain of the system would indeed be expected to show a non-linear (non-additive) functional interaction.

Future directions

The methodology of applying opiates to very circumscribed brain regions in the unanesthetized animal and assessing the effects of pharmacologically manipulating distant terminals (as with the intrathecal injection of monoamine antagonists), provides a powerful tool to assess the hodology of these systems relevant to the organization of pain behavior. In spite of the numerous studies, discrete examination of the sites of action of opioids in brain has not sufficiently defined the distribution of the relevant receptor systems. At present, the analysis has focussed rather specifically on mesencephalic and medullary sites. We might further query the role of regions within the pontine reticular formation. Caudally, we actually do not know how far the distribution of medial medullary sites extends. Given the prominent role of the thalamus in pain transmission, and the likely presence of opioid receptors on these terminals, why is the role of the thalamus in this regard so obscure and controversial? Does the forebrain projection circuit relate to an alteration in the 'perception' of the stimulus message and if so, is this change in response limited to pain or is it a generalized reorganization of motivational aspects of behavior affecting global behavioral constructs? These latter questions bring the issue back to the hands of the psychophysicists who query whether opioids change the perceived intensity of the applied stimulus or its affective impact or, more likely, both. Finally, the effects of opiates at moderate systemic doses produce changes which are the 'gold standard' of analgesia. As such, understanding the effects of opiates on sensory responses may tell us a great deal about the syntax of the communication which occurs between the spinal cord and the brain.

Acknowledgements

This work was funded in part by NIH Grant NS-

16541 (TLY), the King Faisal Specialist Hospital and Research Center, Riyadh, Saudi Arabia (NRFA), and the Danish Medical Research Council and the Knud Hojgaard's Foundation (TSJ). Travel funds to TLY were provided in part by Astra Pharmaceuticals.

References

Akaike, A., Shibata, T., Satoh, M. and Takagi, H. (1978) Analgesia induced by microinjection of morphine into, and electrical stimulation of, the nucleus reticularis paragigantocellularis of rat medulla oblongata. *Neuropharmacology,* 17: 775 – 778.

Anden, N.-E., Jukes, M.G.M., Lundberg, A. and Vyklicky, L. (1966) The effect of DOPA on the spinal cord. *Acta Physiol. Scand.,* 67: 373 – 386.

Atchison, S.R., Durant, P.A.C. and Yaksh, T.L. (1986) Cardiorespiratory effects and kinetics of intrathecally injected D-Ala^2-D-Leu^5-enkephalin and morphine in unanesthetized dogs. *Anesthesiology,* 65: 609 – 616.

Atweh, S.F., Murrin, L.C. and Kuhar, M.J. (1978) Presynaptic localization of opiate receptors in the vagal and accessory optic systems: an autoradiographic study. *Neuropharmacology,* 17: 65 – 71.

Azami, J., Llewelyn, M.B. and Roberts, M.H.T. (1982) The contribution of nucleus reticularis paragigantocellularis and nucleus raphe magnus to the analgesia produced by systemically administered morphine, investigated with the microinjection technique. *Pain,* 12: 229 – 246.

Barton, C., Basbaum, A.I. and Fields, H.L. (1980) Dissociation of supraspinal and spinal actions of morphine: a quantitative evaluation. *Brain Res.,* 188: 487 – 498.

Basbaum, A.I., Marley, N.J.E., O'Keefe, J. and Clanton, C.H. (1977) Reversal of morphine and stimulus produced analgesia by subtotal spinal cord lesions. *Pain,* 3: 43 – 56.

Behbehani, M.M. and Fields, H.L. (1979) Evidence that an excitatory connection between the periaqueductal gray and the nucleus raphe magnus mediates stimulation produced analgesia. *Brain Res.,* 170: 85 – 93.

Bell, J.A., Sharpe, L.G. and Berry, J.N. (1980) Depressant and excitant effects of intraspinal microinjections of morphine and methionine-enkephalin in the cat. *Brain Res.,* 196: 455 – 465.

Bennett, G.J. and Mayer, D.J. (1979) Inhibition of spinal cord interneurons by narcotic microinjection and focal electrical stimulation in the periaqueductal gray matter. *Brain Res.,* 172: 243 – 257.

Bowsher, D., Mallart, A., Petit, D. and Albe-Fessard, D. (1968) A bulbar relay to the centre median. *J. Neurophysiol.,* 31: 288 – 300.

Camarata, P.J. and Yaksh, T.L. (1985) Characterization of the spinal adrenergic receptors mediating the spinal effects produced by the microinjection of morphine into the periaqueductal gray. *Brain Res.,* 336: 133 – 142.

Carstens, E., Tulloch, I., Zieglgänsberger, W. and Zimmermann, M. (1979) Presynaptic excitability changes induced by morphine in single cutaneous afferent C- and A-fibers. *Pflügers Arch.,* 379: 143 – 147.

Chu, G., Cool, M. and Kurtz, N. (1987) Comparison of epidural butorphanol and morphine for control of post-caesarean section pain. *Anaesthesist,* 36: 377 – 391.

Clark, J.A., Itzhak, Y., Hruby, V.J., Yamamura, H.I. and Pasternak, G.W. (1986) [D-Pen^2,D-Pen^5]enkephalin (DPDPE): a δ-selective enkephalin with low affinity for μ_1 opiate binding sites. *Eur. J. Pharmacol.,* 128: 303 – 304.

Cousins, M.J. and Mather, L.E. (1984) Intrathecal and epidural administration of opioids. *Anesthesiology,* 61: 276 – 310.

Criswell, H.D. (1976) Analgesia and hyperreactivity following morphine microinjection into mouse brain. *Pharmacol. Biochem. Behav.,* 4: 23 – 26.

D'Amour, F.E. and Smith, D.L. (1941) A method for determining loss of pain sensation. *J. Pharmacol. Exp. Ther.,* 72: 74 – 79.

Dickenson, A.H. and Le Bars, D. (1987) Supraspinal morphine and descending inhibitions acting on the dorsal horn of the rat. *J. Physiol.,* 384: 81 – 107.

Dickenson, A.H., Oliveras, J.-L. and Besson, J.-M. (1979) Role of the nucleus raphe magnus in opiate analgesia as studied by the microinjection technique in the rat. *Brain Res.,* 170: 95 – 111.

Dray, A., Nunan, L. and Wire, W. (1986) Meptazinol: unusual in vivo opioid receptor activity at supraspinal and spinal sites. *Neuropharmacology,* 25: 343 – 349.

Du, H.-J., Kitahata, L.M., Thalhammer, J.G. and Zimmermann, M. (1984) Inhibition of nociceptive neuronal responses in the cat's spinal dorsal horn by electrical stimulation and morphine microinjection in nucleus raphe magnus. *Pain,* 19: 249 – 257.

Dubuisson, D. and Dennis, G. (1977) The formalin test: a quantitative study of the analgesic effects of morphine, meperidine, and brain stem stimulation in rats and cats. *Pain,* 4: 161 – 174.

Duggan, A.W. and North, R.A. (1984) Electrophysiology of opioids. *Pharmacol. Rev.,* 35: 219 – 281.

Eisenach, J.C., Dewan, D.M., Rose, J.C. and Angelo, J.M. (1987) Epidural clonidine produces antinociception, but not hypotension in sheep. *Anesthesiology,* 66: 496 – 501.

Fang, F.G., Fields, H.L. and Lee, N.M. (1986) Action at the mu receptor is sufficient to explain the supraspinal analgesic effect of opiates. *J. Pharmacol. Exp. Ther.,* 238: 1039 – 1044.

Fenstermacher, J.D. and Patlak, C.S. (1975) The exchange of material between cerebrospinal fluid and brain. In *Fluid Environment of the Brain,* Academic Press, New York, pp.

201 – 214.

Fields, H.L., Emson, P.C., Leigh, B.K., Gilbert, R.F.T. and Iversen, L.L. (1980) Multiple opiate receptor sites on primary afferent fibres. *Nature*, 284: 351 – 353.

Foley, K.M., Kourides, I.A., Inturrisi, C.E., Kaiko, R.F., Zaroulis, C.G., Posner, J.B., Houde, R.W. and Li, C.H. (1979) β-Endorphin: analgesic and hormonal effects in humans. *Proc. Natl. Acad. Sci. USA*, 76: 5377 – 5381.

Gamse, R., Holzer, P. and Lembeck, F. (1979) Indirect evidence for presynaptic location of opiate receptors in chemosensitive primary sensory neurones. *Naunyn-Schmiedeb. Arch. Pharmacol.*, 308: 281 – 285.

Gebhart, G.F. (1982) Opiate and opioid peptide effects on brain stem neurons: relevance to nociception and antinociceptive mechanisms. *Pain*, 12: 93 – 140.

Gebhart, G.F., Sandkühler, J., Thalhammer, J. and Zimmerman, M. (1984) Inhibition in spinal cord of nociceptive information by electrical stimulation and morphine microinjections at identical sites in midbrain of the cat. *J. Neurophysiol.*, 51: 75 – 89.

Go, V.L.W. and Yaksh, T.L. (1987) Release of substance P from the cat spinal cord. *J. Physiol.*, 383, 391: 141 – 167.

Haigler, H.J. and Spring, D.D. (1978) A comparison of the analgesic and behavioral effects of [D-Ala²]met-enkephalinamide and morphine in the mesencephalic reticular formation of rats. *Life Sci.*, 23: 1229 – 1240.

Halpern, B.P. and Halverson, J.D. (1974) Modification of escape from noxious stimuli after bulbar reticular formation lesions. *Behav. Biol.*, 11: 215 – 229.

Hammond, D.L. and Yaksh, T.L. (1984) Antagonism of stimulation-produced antinociception by intrathecal administration of methysergide or phentolamine. *Brain Res.*, 298: 329 – 337.

Headley, P.M., Duggan, A.W. and Griersmith, B.T. (1978) Selective reduction by noradrenaline and 5-hydroxytryptamine of nociceptive responses of cat dorsal horn neurones. *Brain Res.*, 145: 185 – 189.

Hendershot, L.C. and Forsaith, J. (1959) Antagonism of the frequency of phenylquinone-induced writhing in the mouse by weak analgesics and non-analgesics. *J. Pharmacol. Exp. Ther.*, 125: 237 – 240.

Herz, A. and Teschemacher, H. (1971) Activities and sites of antinociceptive action of morphine-like analgesics and kinetics of distribution following intravenous, intracerebral and intraventricular application. *Adv. Drug Res.*, 6: 79 – 119.

Homma, E., Collins, J.G., Kitahata, L.M. and Kawahara, M. (1983) Suppression of noxiously evoked WDR dorsal horn neuronal activity by spinally administered morphine. *Anesthesiology*, 58: 232 – 236.

Hylden, J.L.K. and Wilcox, G.L. (1983) Pharmacological characterization of substance P-induced nociception in mice: modulation by opioid and noradrenergic agonists at the spinal level. *J. Pharmacol. Exp. Ther.*, 226: 398 – 404.

Itzhak, Y. and Pasternak, G.W. (1986) Interaction of [D-Ser²,Leu⁵]enkephalin-Thr⁶ (DSLET), a relatively selective delta ligand, with mu₁ opioid binding sites. *Life Sci.*, 40: 307 – 311.

Jacquet, Y.F. and Lajtha, A. (1976) The periaqueductal gray: site of morphine analgesia and tolerance as shown by 2-way cross-tolerance between systemic and intracerebral injections. *Brain Res.*, 103: 501 – 513.

Jensen, T.S. and Yaksh, T.L. (1984) Spinal monoamine and opiate system pathways mediate the antinociceptive effects produced by glutamate at brainstem sites. *Brain Res.*, 321: 287 – 297.

Jensen, T.S. and Yaksh, T.L. (1986a) I. Comparison of antinociceptive action of morphine in the periaqueductal gray, medial and paramedial medulla in rat. *Brain Res.*, 363: 99 – 113.

Jensen, T.S. and Yaksh, T.L. (1986b) II. Examination of spinal monoamine receptors through which brain stem opiate-sensitive systems act in the rat. *Brain Res.*, 363: 114 – 127.

Jensen, T.S. and Yaksh, T.L. (1986c) III. Comparison of the antinociceptive action of mu and delta opioid receptor ligands in the periaqueductal gray matter, medial and paramedial ventral medulla in the rat as studied by the microinjection technique. *Brain Res.*, 372: 301 – 312.

Kasman, G.S. and Rosenfeld, J.P. (1986) Opiate microinjections into midbrain do not affect the aversiveness of caudal trigeminal stimulation but produce somatotopically organized peripheral hypoalgesia. *Brain Res.*, 383: 271 – 278.

Kuraishi, Y., Fukui, K., Shiomi, H., Akaike, A. and Takagi, H. (1978) Microinjection of opioids into the nucleus reticularis gigantocellularis of the rat: analgesia and increase in the normetanephrine level in the spinal cord. *Biochem. Pharmacol.*, 27: 2756 – 2758.

Kuraishi, Y., Harada, Y. and Takagi, H. (1979) Noradrenaline regulation of pain-transmission in the spinal cord mediated by α-adrenoceptors. *Brain Res.*, 174: 333 – 336.

LaMotte, C., Pert, C.B. and Snyder, S.H. (1976) Opiate receptor binding in primate spinal cord: distribution and changes after dorsal root section. *Brain Res.*, 112: 407 – 412.

Lazorthes, Y., Verdie, J.C., Bastide, R., Lavados, A. and Descouens, D. (1985) Spinal versus intraventricular chronic opiate administration with implantable drug delivery devices for cancer pain. *Appl. Neurophysiol.*, 48: 234 – 241.

Leavens, M.E., Hill, C.S., Jr., Cech, D.A., Weyland, J.B. and Weston, J.S. (1982) Intrathecal and intraventricular morphine for pain in cancer patients: initial study. *J. Neurosurg.*, 56: 241 – 245.

Lenzi, A., Galli, G., Gandolfini, M. and Marini, G. (1985) Intraventricular morphine in paraneoplastic painful syndrome of the cervicofacial region: experience in thirty-eight cases. *Neurosurgery*, 17: 6 – 11.

Levy, R.A. and Proudfit, H.K. (1979) Analgesia produced by microinjection of baclofen and morphine at brainstem sites. *Eur. J. Pharmacol.*, 57: 43 – 55.

Lewis, V.A. and Gebhart, G.F. (1977) Evaluation of the periaqueductal central gray (PAG) as a morphine specific locus of action and examination of morphine-induced and stimulation-produced analgesia at coincident PAG loci. *Brain Res.*, 124: 283–303.

Liebeskind, J.C. and Mayer, D.J. (1971) Somatosensory evoked responses in the mesencephalic central gray matter of the rat. *Brain Res.*, 27: 135–151.

Ling, G.S.F., Simantov, R., Clark, J.A. and Pasternak, G.W. (1986) Naloxonazine actions in vivo. *Eur. J. Pharmacol.*, 129: 33–38.

Lobato, R.D., Madrid, J.L., Fatela, L.V., Rivas, J.J., Reig, E. and Lamas, E. (1983) Intraventricular morphine for control of pain in terminal cancer patients. *J. Neurosurg.*, 59: 627–633.

Martin, W.R., Eades, C.G., Thompson, J.A., Huppler, R.E. and Gilbert, P.E. (1976) The effects of morphine- and nalorphine-like drugs in the nondependent and morphine-dependent chronic spinal dog. *J. Pharmacol. Exp. Ther.*, 197: 517–532.

Messing, R.B. and Lytle, L.D. (1977) Serotonin containing neurons: their possible role in pain and analgesia. *Pain*, 4: 1–21.

Mohrland, S. and Gebhart, G. (1980) Effects of focal electrical stimulation and morphine microinjection in the periaqueductal gray of the rat mesencephalon on neuronal activity in the medullary reticular formation. *Brain Res.*, 201: 23–37.

Monasky, M.S. and Yaksh, T.L. (1986) Synergistic interaction of intrathecal morphine and an α_2-agonist (ST-91) on antinociception in the rat. *Soc. Neurosci. Abst.*, 12: 1016.

Moreau, J.-L. and Fields, H.L. (1987) Evidence for GABA involvement in midbrain control of medullary neurons that modulate nociceptive transmission. *Brain Res.*, 397: 37–46.

Ness, T.J. and Gebhart, G.F. (1987) Quantitative comparison of morphine and clonidine effects upon visceral and cutaneous spinal nociceptive transmission in the rat. *Pain*, Suppl. 4: S409.

Oliveras, J.-L., Maixner, W., Dubner, R., Bushnell, M.C., Duncan, G., Thomas, D.A. and Bates, R. (1986a) Dorsal horn opiate administration attenuates the perceived intensity of noxious heat stimulation in behaving monkey. *Brain Res.*, 371: 368–371.

Oliveras, J.-L., Maixner, W., Dubner, R., Bushnell, M.C., Kenshalo, D.R., Jr., Duncan, G.H., Thomas, D.A. and Bates, R. (1986b) The medullary dorsal horn: a target for the expression of opiate effects on the perceived intensity of noxious heat. *J. Neurosci.*, 6: 3086–3093.

Ossipov, M.H. and Gebhart, G.F. (1986) Opioid, cholinergic and α-adrenergic influences on the modulation of nociception from the lateral reticular nucleus of the rat. *Brain Res.*, 384: 282–293.

Ossipov, M.H., Goldstein, F.J. and Malseed, R.T. (1984) Feline analgesia following central administration of opioids. *Neuropharmacology*, 23: 925–929.

Ottersen, O.P. and Storm-Mathisen, J. (1984) Glutamate- and GABA-containing neurons in the mouse and rat brain, as demonstrated with a new immunocytochemical technique. *J. Comp. Neurol.*, 229: 374–392.

Pang, I.H. and Vasko, M.R. (1986) Morphine and norepinephrine, but not 5-hydroxytryptamine and γ-aminobutyric acid inhibit the potassium stimulated release of substance P from rat spinal cord slices. *Brain Res.*, 376: 268–279.

Pert, A. and Yaksh, T.L. (1974) Sites of morphine induced analgesia in the primate brain: relation to pain pathways. *Brain Res.*, 80: 135–140.

Pert, A. and Yaksh, T.L. (1975) Localization of the antinociceptive action of morphine in primate brain. *Pharmacol. Biochem. Behav.*, 3: 133–138.

Prado, W.A. and Roberts, M.H.T. (1984) Antinociception from a stereospecific action of morphine microinjected into the brainstem: a local or distant site of action. *Br. J. Pharmacol.*, 82: 877–882.

Randall, L.O. and Selitto, J.J. (1957) A method for measurement of analgesic activity on inflamed tissue. *Arch. Int. Pharmacodyn. Ther.*, 111: 409–419.

Reddy, S.V.R., Maderdrut, J.L. and Yaksh, T.L. (1980) Spinal cord pharmacology of adrenergic agonist-mediated antinociception. *J. Pharmacol. Exp. Ther.*, 213: 525–533.

Rodgers, R.J. (1977) Elevation of aversive threshold in rats by intraamygdaloid injection of morphine sulfate. *Pharmacol. Biochem. Behav.*, 6: 385–390.

Russell, N.J.W., Schaible, H.-G. and Schmidt, R.F. (1987) Opiates inhibit the discharges of fine afferent units from inflamed knee joint of the cat. *Neurosci. Lett.*, 76: 107–112.

Russell, R.D., Leslie, J.B., Su, Y.-F., Watkins, W.D. and Chang, K.-J. (1987) Continuous intrathecal opioid analgesia: tolerance and cross-tolerance of mu and delta spinal opioid receptors. *J. Pharmacol. Exp. Ther.*, 240: 150–158.

Satoh, M., Oku, R. and Akaike, A. (1983) Analgesia produced by microinjection of L-glutamate into the rostral ventromedial bulbar nuclei of the rat and its inhibition by intrathecal α-adrenergic blocking agents. *Brain Res.*, 261: 361–364.

Schmauss, C. and Yaksh, T.L. (1983) In vivo studies on spinal opiate receptor systems mediating antinociception. II. Pharmacological profiles suggesting a differential association of mu, delta and kappa receptors with visceral chemical and cutaneous thermal stimuli in the rat. *J. Pharmacol. Exp. Ther.*, 228: 1–12.

Schmauss, C., Shimohigashi, Y., Jensen, T.S., Rodbard, D. and Yaksh, T.L. (1985) Studies on spinal opiate receptor pharmacology. III. Analgetic effects of enkephalin dimers as measured by cutaneous thermal and visceral chemical evoked responses. *Brain Res.*, 337: 209–215.

Sharpe, L.G., Garnett, J.E. and Cicero, T.J. (1974) Analgesia and hyperreactivity produced by intracranial microinjections of morphine into the periaqueductal gray matter of the rat. *Behav. Biol.*, 11: 303–313.

Suzukawa, M., Matsumoto, M., Collins, J.G., Kitahata, L.M. and Yuge, O. (1983) Dose-response suppression of noxiously evoked activity of WDR neurons by spinally administered fentanyl. *Anesthesiology, 58:* 510 – 513.

Takagi, H., Matsumura, M., Yanai, A. and Ogiu, K. (1955) The effect of analgesics on the spinal reflex activity of the cat. *Jpn. J. Pharmacol., 4:* 176 – 187.

Takagi, H., Doi, T. and Akaike, A. (1976) Microinjection of morphine into the medial part of the bulbar reticular formation in rabbit and rat: inhibitory effects on lamina V cells of spinal dorsal horn and behavioral analgesia. In H. W. Kosterlitz (Ed.), *Opiates and Endogenous Opioid Peptides,* pp. 191 – 198. Elsevier/North-Holland Biomedical Press, Amsterdam.

Takagi, H., Satoh, M., Akaike, A., Shibata, T. and Kuraishi, Y. (1977) The nucleus reticularis gigantocellularis of the medulla oblongata is a highly sensitive site in the production of morphine analgesia in the rat. *Eur. J. Pharmacol., 45:* 91 – 92.

Takagi, H., Satoh, M., Akaike, A., Shibata, T., Yajima, H. and Ogawa, H. (1978) Analgesia by enkephalins injected into the nucleus reticularis gigantocellularis of rat medulla oblongata. *Eur. J. Pharmacol., 49:* 113 – 116.

Takagi, H., Shiomi, H., Kuraishi, Y., Fukui, K. and Ueda, H. (1979) Pain and the bulbospinal noradrenergic system: Pain-induced increase in normetanephrine content in the spinal cord and its modification by morphine. *Eur. J. Pharmacol., 54:* 99 – 107.

Tamsen, A. and Gordh, T. (1984) Epidural clonidine produces analgesia. *Lancet, 1:* 231 – 232.

Tsou, K. and Jang, C.S. (1964) Studies on the site of analgesic action of morphine by intracerebral microinjection. *Scient. Sin., 13:* 1099 – 1109.

Walker, G.E. and Yaksh, T.L. (1986) Studies on the effects of intrathalamically injected DADL and morphine on nociceptive thresholds and electroencephalographic activity: A thalamic δ receptor syndrome. *Brain Res., 383:* 1 – 14.

Wang, J.J., Chan, K.H., Lee, T.Y. and Mok, M.S. (1985) Epidural nalbuphine hydrochloride in painless labor. *Ma Tsui Hsueh Tsa Chi, 23:* 3 – 11.

Ward, S.J., Portoghese, P.S. and Takemori, A.E. (1982) Pharmacological characterization *in vivo* of the novel opiate, β-funaltrexamine. *J. Pharmacol. Exp. Ther., 220:* 494 – 498.

Werz, M.A. and MacDonald, R.L. (1983) Opioid peptides with differential affinity for mu and delta receptors decrease sensory neuron calcium-dependent action potentials. *J. Pharmacol. Exp. Ther., 227:* 394 – 402.

Werz, M.A. and MacDonald, R.L. (1985) Dynorphin and neoendorphin peptides decrease dorsal root ganglion neuron calcium-dependent action potential duration. *J. Pharmacol. Exp. Ther., 234:* 49 – 56.

Wettstein, J.G., Kamerling, S.G. and Martin, W.R. (1982) Effects of microinjections of opioids into and electrical stimulation (ES) of the canine periaqueductal gray (PAG) on EEG electrogenesis (EEG), heart rate (HR), pupil diameter (PD), behavior and analgesia. *Neurosci. Abstr., 8:* 229.

Wigdor, S. and Wilcox, G.L. (1987) Central and systemic morphine antinociception in the mouse: contribution of descending serotonergic and noradrenergic pathways. *J. Pharmacol. Exp. Ther.,* in press.

Williams, J. and Zieglgänsberger, W. (1981) Mature spinal ganglion cells are not sensitive to opiate receptor mediated actions. *Neurosci. Lett., 21:* 211 – 216.

Woolfe, G. and MacDonald, A.D. (1944) The evaluation of the analgesic action of pethidine hydrochloride (Demerol). *J. Pharmacol. Exp. Ther., 80:* 300 – 307.

Xuan, Y.T., Shi, Y.S., Zhou, Z.F. and Han, J.S. (1986) Studies on the mesolimbic loop of antinociception. II. A serotonin-enkephalin interaction in the nucleus accumbens. *Neuroscience, 19:* 403 – 409.

Yaksh, T.L. (1978a) Analgetic actions of intrathecal opiates in cat and primate. *Brain Res., 153:* 205 – 210.

Yaksh, T.L. (1978b) Inhibition by etorphine of the discharge of dorsal horn neurons: effects upon the neuronal response to both high- and low-threshold sensory input in the decerebrate spinal cat. *Exp. Neurol., 60:* 23 – 40.

Yaksh, T.L. (1979) Direct evidence that spinal serotonin and noradrenaline terminals mediate the spinal antinociceptive effects of morphine in the periaqueductal gray. *Brain Res., 160:* 180 – 185.

Yaksh, T.L. (1981) Spinal opiate analgesia: characteristics and principles of action. *Pain, 11:* 293 – 346.

Yaksh, T.L. (1983) In vivo studies on spinal opiate receptor systems mediating antinociception. I. Mu and delta receptor profiles in the primate. *J. Pharmacol. Exp. Ther., 226:* 303 – 316.

Yaksh, T.L. (1984a) Multiple opioid receptor systems in brain and spinal cord: Part 1. *Eur. J. Anaesthesiol., 1:* 171 – 199.

Yaksh, T.L. (1984b) Multiple opioid receptor systems in brain and spinal cord: Part 2. *Eur. J. Anaesthesiol., 1:* 201 – 243.

Yaksh, T.L. (1985) Pharmacology of spinal adrenergic systems which modulate spinal nociceptive processing. *Pharmacol. Biochem. Behav., 22:* 845 – 858.

Yaksh, T.L. and Henry, J.L. (1978) Antinociceptive effects of intrathecally administered human β-endorphin in the rat and cat. *Can. J. Physiol. Pharmacol., 56:* 754 – 760.

Yaksh, T.L. and Noueihed, R. (1985) The physiology and pharmacology of spinal opiates. *Annu. Rev. Pharmacol. Toxicol., 25:* 433 – 462.

Yaksh, T.L. and Reddy, S.V.R. (1981) Studies in the primate on the analgetic effects associated with intrathecal actions of opiate, α-adrenergic agonists and baclofen. *Anesthesiology, 54:* 451 – 467.

Yaksh, T.L. and Rudy, T.A. (1976) Analgesia mediated by a direct spinal action of narcotics. *Science, 192:* 1357 – 1358.

Yaksh, T.L. and Rudy, T.A. (1977) Studies on the direct spinal action of narcotics in the production of analgesia in the rat. *J. Pharmacol. Exp. Ther., 202:* 411 – 428.

394

Yaksh, T.L. and Rudy, T.A. (1978) Narcotic analgesics: CNS sites and mechanisms of action as revealed by intracerebral injection techniques. *Pain,* 4: 299 – 359.

Yaksh, T.L. and Tyce, G.M. (1979) Microinjection of morphine into the periaqueductal gray evokes the release of serotonin from spinal cord. *Brain Res.,* 171: 176 – 181.

Yaksh, T.L. and Wilson, P.R. (1979) Spinal serotonin terminal system mediates antinociception. *J. Pharmacol. Exp. Ther.,* 208: 446 – 453.

Yaksh, T.L., Yeung, J.C. and Rudy, T.A. (1976) Systemic examination in the rat of brain sites sensitive to the direct application of morphine: observation of differential effect within the periaqueductal gray. *Brain Res.,* 114: 83 – 103.

Yaksh, T.L., Jessell, T.M., Gamse, R., Mudge, A.W. and Leeman, S.E. (1980) Intrathecal morphine inhibits substance P release from mammalian spinal cord in vivo. *Nature,* 286: 155 – 156.

Yaksh, T.L., Noueihed, R.Y. and Durant, P.A.C. (1986) Studies of the pharmacology and pathology of intrathecally administered 4-anilinopiperidine analogues and morphine in rat and cat. *Anesthesiology,* 64: 54 – 66.

Yeung, J.C. and Rudy, T.A. (1980) Multiplicative interaction between narcotic agonisms expressed at spinal and supraspinal sites of antinociceptive action as revealed by concurrent intrathecal and intracerebroventricular injections of morphine. *J. Pharmacol. Exp. Ther.,* 215: 633 – 642.

Yeung, J.C., Yaksh, T.L. and Rudy, T.A. (1977) Concurrent mapping of brain sites for sensitivity to the direct application of morphine and focal electrical stimulation in the production of antinociception in the rat. *Pain,* 4: 23 – 40.

Zieglgänsberger, W. and Bayerl, H. (1976) The mechanisms of inhibition of neuronal activity by opiates in the spinal cord of the cat. *Brain Res.,* 115: 111 – 128.

H.L. Fields and J.-M. Besson (Eds.)
Progress in Brain Research, Vol. 77
© 1988 Elsevier Science Publishers B.V. (Biomedical Division)

CHAPTER 29

Intracerebroventricular morphinotherapy for control of chronic cancer pain

Yves Lazorthes[a], Jean-Claude Verdié[a], Brigitte Caute[b], Ricardo Maranhao[a] and Mathieu Tafani[c]

[a] *Clinique de Neurochirurgie, CHU Rangueil, Chemin du Vallon, 31054 Toulouse,* [b] *Laboratoire de Pharmacie Galénique, Faculté des Sciences Pharmaceutiques, Chemin des Maraîchers, et Laboratoire de Pharmacologie et Toxicologie Fondamentales, CNRS, 205 route de Narbonne, 31400 Toulouse and* [c] *Service de Médecine Nucléaire – Laboratoire des Radio-Isotopes, CHU Purpan, Place du Dr. Baylac, 31052 Toulouse, France*

Introduction

A series of recent reports concerning the direct action of morphine both on the spinal cord (Conseiller et al., 1972; Duggan et al., 1977) and on the brain (Akaike et al., 1978; Hayes et al., 1979; Le Bars et al., 1980a; Lewis and Gebhart, 1977; Tsou and Jang, 1964; Yaksh and Rudy, 1978) and also the discovery (Hughes, 1975; Pert and Snyder, 1973; Simon, 1982) and localization (Atweh and Kuhar, 1977a,b) of specific opiate binding sites and endogenous ligands have given rise to the rapid development of a new therapy for chronic pain. It is the direct administration of opiates, especially morphine, into the perispinal and intraventricular cerebrospinal fluid: intrathecal morphinotherapy.

Experimental studies (Yaksh and Rudy, 1977, 1978; Yaksh, 1981) have shown that morphine administered directly to the cerebrospinal fluid of the rat, cat and primate, brings about analgesia which is intense and durable, localized, dose-dependent, stereo specific and naloxone-reversible.

The considerable clinical interest in this new type of administration of morphine first led to the development of spinal intrathecal morphinotherapy (Lazorthes et al., 1980, 1985b; Muller et al., 1982; Onofrio et al., 1981; Penn et al., 1984; Saunders and Coombs, 1983; Tung et al., 1982; Wang, 1977). It is mainly indicated for intractable pain caused by cancer in the lower half of the body, since with spinal administration the analgesic effect is more limited and the risk of central respiratory depression higher when the pain to be treated by spinal administration is of diffuse or cervico-cephalic origin.

Thus, various authors, basing their work on the existence of intracerebral opiate receptors (Atweh and Kuhar, 1977b; Pert and Snyder, 1973; Simon, 1982), especially in the region of the walls of the third and fourth ventricles and on the analgesic action caused by intracerebral microinjections of morphine (Akaike et al., 1978; Dickenson et al., 1979; Tsou and Jang, 1964; Yaksh, 1978), have proposed and used direct intraventricular administration of morphine in human patients (Blond et al., 1985; Leavens et al., 1982; Lenzi et al., 1985; Lobato et al., 1983; Nurchi, 1984; Roquefeuil et al., 1983; Thiebaud et al., 1985).

Various clinical studies have compared the efficiency, the specificity and the risks of the two types of intrathecal opiate administration, spinal and intraventricular, in order to determine the appropriateness of each method (Lazorthes, 1986; Lazorthes et al., 1985c; Leavens et al., 1982; Nurchi, 1984).

Material and methods

Patient selection criteria

For intracerebroventricular morphinotherapy (ICVM) selection of patients is based on strict clinical criteria (Lazorthes et al., 1985c): (1) chronic pain secondary to inoperable malignant tumors; (2) pain not relieved by medical treatment and, in particular, tolerance of or significant side effects from using oral or parenteral morphine; (3) intractable bilateral, midline or diffuse pain beyond the possibilities of percutaneous or open surgical interruption of the nociceptive pathways; (4) subdiaphragmatic pain secondary to cervicothoracic cancers; (5) chronic pain of the lower half of the body (subdiaphragmatic), only after failure of spinal morphine analgesia; (6) absence of general risks of complications such as coagulation disturbances, cutaneous infection, septicemia, etc.; (7) informed consent from the patient and the family; (8) presence of a favorable domestic environment for ambulatory surveillance and ICVM treatment.

When the topography of pain involves a transitional area (lower thoracic, diaphragmatic or upper abdominal), ICVM is indicated after a negative trial of a lumbar intrathecal injection of a small dose of morphine (2.5 to 5 mg maximum).

The patients

From 1984 to April 1987, we selected just 51 patients for chronic ICVM via an implanted access port. The age range was from 40 – 80 yr (mean: 62). The duration of intractable pain before ICVM therapy ranged from 2 – 36 months (mean: 8 months). All were tolerant to oral or parenteral opiate agonists. The distribution of the primary malignant tumors and the topography of the chronic pain were: diffuse cancers, 5 (including 2 cases of Kahler's disease); diffuse bony or visceral metastases, 7 (including 2 cases with kidney cancer, 1 with melanoma, 1 with prostatic cancer, 1 with breast cancer, 1 with bladder cancer and 1

with vaginal cancer); cervicocephalic cancers, 13; thoracic or lung cancers, 20; abdominal or pelvic cancers, 6.

All six patients with abdominal or pelvic cancer had subdiaphragmatic pain, but there was a contraindication for a spinal intrathecal administration of opioids via a lumbar access port: three cases with upper abdominal tumors (1 pancreatic and 2 stomach cancers) with non-significant pain relief after lumbar intrathecal morphine trials (5 mg); one case with rectum cancer with pelvic and perineal pain with lumbosacral skin necrosis and suppuration; one case with uterus cancer with pelvic and sciatica pain presenting an intracranial hypertension due to a cerebellar metastasis. The sixth patient, a rectum cancer, had been treated before for 7 months with spinal administration until she developed tolerance (no analgesia after 20 mg of intrathecal morphine).

Implantation technique

The details concerning chronic administration, i.e. description of the drug administration devices and techniques of implantation under local anesthesia or neuroleptanalgesia, have been reported in previous publications (Lazorthes, 1986; Lazorthes et al., 1985a,c).

For chronic ventricular administration we have always used a subcutaneous access port connected to a ventricular catheter placed in the frontal horn of the lateral ventricle as close as possible to the foramen of Monro, or sometimes catheterized into the third ventricle.

The implanted access ports have different volumes: initially, we implanted a large reservoir (volume 2 ml) derived from the ventricular Ommaya reservoir. Currently we prefer to implant a smaller reservoir (1 ml) as proposed by Lenzi et al. (1985), or a pediatric miniport (0.2 ml).

Administration technique and morphine titration

The access port is percutaneously pricked, by a sterile technique, using a 25-gauge needle connected to a 2.5-ml syringe. First, to confirm that the system is functioning perfectly, 2 ml of cerebrospinal fluid (CSF) are withdrawn. This CSF sample is kept to flush the access port after morphine injection. In case of doubt, the permeability of the device can be checked by a contrast injection.

Slow administration of a preservative-free morphine sulfate solution (concentrations: 1 ml = 10 mg or 1 ml = 1 mg) was carried out with a 1-ml syringe. A 0.22 μm millipore filter can be inserted between the syringe and the needle in order to further ensure that the solution is free of bacteria. Serial CSF samples are drawn for chemical and bacteriological analyses.

In order to limit the risk of side effects and to test the efficiency, the first morphine dose is always 0.125 mg. Later, and according to the analgesia produced, the doses are progressively increased to 0.25, 0.5, 1.0 mg and so on! The patients are kept under close neurological observation and cardiorespiratory monitoring (apnea monitoring) throughout this titration period. Nurses must be ready to reverse a respiratory depression promptly with naloxone.

Kinetics of ^{123}I-labelled morphine

To study the diffusion of morphine into the ventricular system, and its correlation with the induced analgesia (latency, intensity, duration), we studied the isotopic transit of ^{123}I-morphine (Tafani et al., 1988) in six patients. Serial gamma camera images of the brain and spinal cord were performed after intraventricular injection of ^{123}I-morphine (0.5 to 1 mCi corresponding to 10 μg of morphine), diluted in 1 ml of saline, through an implanted access port of small volume (0.2 ml).

We compared the capacity of iodomorphine and morphine to bind to opiate receptors.

A classical 'in vitro' binding study was carried out on a tissue rich in μ-type opiate receptors: the membrane fraction of rabbit cerebellum. The affinity constant K_i was determined by the amount of specifically bound high-affinity ligand (^{3} hetor-

phine), $K_d = 0.1$ μM, at a concentration of 0.5 μM.

Finally absence of deiodation was checked 'in vitro' by maintaining iodomorphine at 37°C in 9% NaCl for 2 h. 'In vivo', the absence of label in the thyroid indicates absence of deiodation.

Results

Criteria of evaluation

Clinical evaluation of analgesia was based upon a multifactorial approach (Lazorthes et al., 1985b,c), using the estimation of three criteria related to pain: (1) pain relief graded using a subjective linear scale; (2) consequences concerning the patient's activity; (3) complementary consumption of analgesic drugs.

Analgesia was analyzed considering all three criteria together. This provides a comparative 'quantitative' evaluation in any given patient. Unexpected side effects due to direct chronic ICVM, such as central depression and tolerance, were monitored and noted as well as complications due to the implanted devices.

One of us (B.C.) had the responsibility to instruct the patient, the family members, and/or the nurses responsible for the ambulatory treatment. She was also in charge of keeping in contact with them and with the general physician during ambulatory surveillance at home.

Clinical results on analgesia

The mean follow-up for this series of 51 patients was 115 days (range 12 – 230). The initial daily doses of morphine were 0.30 mg (mean value), in a range from 0.10 – 1 mg. All the patients reported significant analgesia within 5 – 60 min (mean latency: 20 min), and pain relief lasting from 12 h to 7 days (mean: 36 h). During the course of treatment, the daily doses of morphine increased moderately; the terminal daily doses reached a mean value of 0.70 mg, over a range from 0.10 – 20 mg. Table I illustrates the progressive increase in morphine consumption with time. However, the increase remains very moderate, since the ratio between the initial and terminal doses is only from 1.26 to 3.41.

The final results (concerning 49 dead patients) are: 46 patients (94%) had 75% or more pain relief; functional activity was significantly improved in 29 patients (59%); drug intake was reduced in 47 patients (96%) and overall there were 43 cases

TABLE I

Changes in the initial and terminal daily doses of ICV morphine (mg/24 h)

Group	Days	n	Mean dose		Ratio TD/ID
			initial (ID)	terminal (TD)	
A	0 – 20	6	0.23	0.29	1.26
B	21 – 40	13	0.29	0.71	2.40
C	41 – 60	11	0.29	0.71	2.40
D	61 – 80	7	0.30	0.73	2.43
E	81 – 100	4	0.34	0.93	2.73
F	101 – 230	10	0.34	1.16	3.41
Mean	115	51	0.30	0.70	2.4

TABLE II

Morphine side effects after intracerebroventricular administration (n = 51)

	Titration period	Chronic administration	Total
Nausea, vomiting	24	5	29
Itching	4	–	4
Headache	2	–	2
Constipation	2	–	2
Urinary retention	1	–	1
Dizziness	5	–	5
Drowsiness	6	1	7
Miosis	3	–	3
Respiratory depression	2	–	2
Disorientation, euphoria	6	–	6
Hallucination, agitation	1	–	1

of good and excellent results (88%) with a mean follow-up of 3 months (115 days).

Until now, we have only observed two cases of tolerance. Progressive increases of the daily morphine doses up to 20 mg, without analgesia, were observed for one patient who was initially, 32 days before, totally pain-free with 1 mg a day. For another patient, it was necessary to increase the daily dose from 0.5 mg to 15 mg to produce sufficient analgesia.

Three other patients only required a moderate increase of daily morphine, without reaching doses more than four times the initial therapeutic doses. In the majority of cases (45 cases), the analgesia was stable during the total follow-up.

Side-effects of morphine

Table II summarizes the side effects observed during the total follow-up (initial trial, titration period and chronic administration).

Minor morphine side effects (nausea, vomiting, constipation, urinary retention, itching, dizziness, headache, disorientation, euphoria or drowsiness) were initially observed but always transiently, and some patients had multiple side effects.

During the trial and titration period, we observed three major central side effects. In two cases, after administration of 1 and 1.5 mg of morphine, respectively, the patients progressively developed drowsiness, miosis and respiratory depression. In a third case, after an injection of 1 mg, visual hallucination and behavioral disorders developed. These three central complications were immediately reversed by systemic naloxone administration with only small effects on the induced analgesia.

In this series (51 patients), we only had three complications due to local infection of the implant. In one case it was necessary to remove the implant. In the other two cases, with transient purulent meningitis, recovery occurred after direct intraventricular administration of antibiotics via the implanted reservoir. No patients presented CSF fistula. In one case, we had to replace the access port, due to catheter kinking.

Kinetics of ^{123}iodomorphine ICV

Iodomorphine binding was seen to be 10 times lower (K_i 50 nM) than that of morphine. In the rat, however, the analgesic activity was maintained (analgesia was evaluated by electrical stimulation of the tail after lumbar intrathecal injection, using the technique of Yaksh and Rudy, 1977), since the dose-effect response was identical to that obtained with morphine.

During the period following ICV injection of iodomorphine, photographs were taken with a gamma camera, on an average of 30 per h. Slow migration of the radioactivity was observed, but it never spread below the thoracic region. The migration was fairly constant and very slow, only about 5% of the injected radioactivity had left the cerebral ventricles after the first hour.

Discussion

In 51 patients suffering from intractable chronic cancer pain despite treatment with oral or parenteral opiates (up to 800 mg oral morphine per day) and also in one patient who had become tolerant to intrathecal lumbar morphinotherapy, we obtained significant analgesia with low doses of morphine (0.1 to 1 mg) using ICV administration.

The time-course of ICVM analgesia is only relatively reproducible: analgesia takes effect in 5 to 30 min (average: 15 min), maximum intensity is reached in 15 – 60 min, duration of analgesia lasts between 12 h and 7 days (average: 36 h). These values are in perfect agreement with those of other authors (Blond, 1988; Lenzi et al., 1985; Lobato et al., 1985; Nurchi, 1984; Roquefeuil et al., 1984; Thiebaud et al., 1985).

How can we explain the variability observed in the establishment of central morphine analgesia after ICV administration if it is related to the time required for morphine to reach its site of action at a concentration sufficient to produce a significant modification of pain perception? This variability is all the more surprising as the latency is often as long as that found with parenteral morphino-

therapy. The speed of diffusion into the ventricular CSF, the meningo-cerebral barrier (ependyma) and the cerebral parenchyma depends on the dose of morphine administered and on its lipid partition coefficient. But this does not fully explain the differences observed (Yaksh and Rudy, 1978). Another explanation may be the position of the distal end of the ventricular catheter (generally implanted in the lateral ventricle) with respect to the orifice (foramen of Monro) communicating with the third ventricle, and to the aqueduct of Sylvius in the walls of which the highest density of opiate receptors occurs (Atweh and Kuhar, 1977b). The exact position of the catheter was not always checked, but each time it was, a significant correlation was found. For example, in a patient who only felt effective analgesia very late (after an average of 60 min) from an ICV administration of 1 mg of morphine, the tip of the catheter was found to be situated at the central part of an abnormally dilated lateral ventricle. An opaque substance administered via the catheter with the patient lying on her back, diffused into the rear of the ventricle before spreading forwards to the foramen of Monro and then into the third ventricle. This diffusion was reversed and analgesia accelerated when the injection was carried out with the patient placed on her front and left side for 30 min. Similarly in another patient, where the tip of the catheter was just in front of the foramen of Monro, administration of 0.25 mg gave total analgesia in 15 min. In order to confirm these results, it would be necessary to verify the exact position of the catheter tip by peroperative ventriculography for each implantation and to establish correlations with the latency of ICVM analgesia.

The analgesia obtained spreads rapidly throughout the whole body, as is perfectly illustrated by the case of diffuse pain from widespread bone metastases. This effect has been reported by all authors and it agrees with experimental data from animals with regard to analgesia induced by intracerebral microinjections (Akaike et al., 1978; Dickenson and Le Bars, 1983; Le Bars et al.,

1980a) or ICV administration (Bouhassira et al., 1986; Bouhassira et al., 1988).

During the follow-up period (on average 115 days), repeated ICV administration required a steady increase in the daily doses of morphine (on average 0.30 mg at the start and 0.70 mg at the end of treatment) to maintain the analgesic effects.

In a recent series of five patients we also noted that implantation of intraventricular access ports of low volume (0.1 ml instead of 2.0 ml) and in addition, the use of less concentrated morphine solutions (1 mg/ml instead of 10 mg/ml) allow further reduction of the initially effective ICV morphine dose. Consequently, with regard to these five patients, the average effective daily dose was 0.20 mg, rising to just 0.40 mg at the end of treatment.

The average daily doses of morphine administered, as well as the range of doses used at the start and end of treatment, are comparable to those reported in the literature (see Table IV) for similar follow-ups. Only Obbens et al. (1987) report the use of much higher doses, between 3 and 60 mg/24 h for an average follow-up of 92 days, and the required doses are relative to the prior doses of systemic morphine: the greater the

systemic morphine dose, the greater the ICVM dose. They also report much more frequent gradual tolerance phenomena. These results conflict with ours (Table I) and those of larger clinical series (Blond, 1988; Lenzi et al., 1985; Lobato et al., 1985; Thiebaud et al., 1985) (Table IV).

As already published (Lobato et al., 1983; Roquefeuil et al., 1984, 1985; Thiebaud et al., 1985), and unlike our initial expectation, the risk of central respiratory depression on ICVM is low: we only observed it twice — during the initial titration period — over a running total follow-up of 4 500 patient days. Drowsiness is also rare (7 cases, 6 of which occurred in the initial period), in spite of the high doses sometimes used at the end of treatment.

Behavioural disturbances such as hallucination and nervousness, and dysphoria were noted more often using this site of administration ($n = 7$) than is reported after spinal intrathecal administration of morphine (Lazorthes et al., 1985c; Leavens et al., 1982; Nurchi, 1984; Thiebaud et al., 1985).

Apart from initial and transient nausea or vomiting, no digestive disturbances, in particular no constipation, were lasting, so ICVM never had to be interrupted. Moreover, in this series no cases

TABLE III

ICVM — literature data in chronological order; A: etiology and topography of pain of cancerous origin

	n	Diffuse metastases	Cervico-facial	Thoracic	Abdomino-pelvian
Leavens et al., 1982	4	–	–	–	4
Lobato et al., 1983, 1985	44	12	19	4	9
Roquefeuil et al., 1983, 1985, 1984	8	3	1	3	1
Nurchi, 1984	5	3	2	–	–
Thiebaud et al., 1985	32	6	16	2	8
Lenzi et al., 1985	38	5	29	4	–
Blond et al., 1985, 1988	79	19	58	2	–
Obbens et al., 1987	20	–	–	–	20
Lazorthes and Verdié	51	12	13	20	6
Total	281	60	138	35	48

of urinary retention were observed; this would appear to be a directly spinal effect (Lazorthes, 1986; Lazorthes et al., 1985b; Leavens et al., 1982; Muller et al., 1982; Penn et al., 1984; Saunders and Coombs, 1983; Tung et al., 1982; Wang, 1977; Yaksh, 1981).

The lasting effectiveness and the low incidence of side effects are in relatively good agreement with the data reported in the literature between 1982 and 1987 (Blond, 1988; Blond et al., 1985; Leavens et al., 1982; Lenzi et al., 1985; Lobato et al., 1983, 1985; Nurchi, 1984; Roquefeuil et al., 1983, 1984, 1985; Thiebaud et al., 1985) as summarized in Tables III and IV.

The analysis, in chronological order (from 1982 to 1987) of reports concerning ICVM shows that the overall clinical experience, including our own, is still very limited as not even 300 cases have been studied.

Our experience with PVG stimulation (Lazorthes et al., 1983) in eight patients suffering from chronic pain of neoplasic origin led us to drop this technique permanently in favor of ICVM. In fact,

in six cases with a significant follow-up (3 – 12 months), a rapid tolerance (3 – 7 weeks) to deep brain stimulation developed and was not satisfactorily reversed by simultaneous parenteral administration of drugs with a serotonergic action (L-tryptophan, 5-HTP and amitriptyline).

The choice between spinal intrathecal and intraventricular morphinotherapy depends, in our opinion and in that of most authors reciprocally and complementary (Lazorthes, 1986; Lazorthes et al., 1985c), mainly on the topography of the pain. Table III shows that all the authors, with the exception of Obbens et al. (1987), limit the use to pains situated in the upper half of the body subsequent to diffuse, cervicocephalic and thoracic cancers or to abdominopelvian cancers accompanied by pain in the upper body from metastases not responding to spinal intrathecal morphinotherapy. However, for chronic pain of cancerous origin in the lower half of the body we prefer, for ethical and clinical reasons, to start always with intrathecal morphinotherapy.

Even though the effectiveness of the analgesia

TABLE IV

ICVM – literature data; B: daily doses, follow-up and results

	n	Doses (mg) min.-max.	Follow-up (days) range	ave.	Analgesia (B + E) (%)	Tolerance	Side effects respir.	vigil.
Leavens et al., 1982	4	0.5 – 7	2 – 90	85	75	1	–	–
Lobato et al., 1983, 1985	44	0.25 – 16	6 – 150	55	97	–	3	5
Roquefeuil et al., 1983, 1985, 1984	8	0.4 – 7	8 – 120	73	80	1	–	2
Nurchi, 1984	5	2 – 4	8 – 48		100	–	1	–
Thiebaud et al., 1985	32	0.10 – 15	4 – 230	50	90	9	1	6
Lenzi et al., 1985	38	0.5 – 2	4 – 292	65	95	–	1	5
Blond, 1985, 1988	79	0.05 – 3	3 – 132	65	94	–	2	–
Obbens et al., 1987	20	3 – 60	7 – 510	98	> 50	+ + +	–	3
Lazorthes and Verdié	51	0.10 – 20	12 – 230	115	88	2	2	7

brought about by ICVM seems clear, the neurophysiological mechanism is still being debated. Is the effect purely supraspinal and, if so, what descending control systems are brought into play to modulate the input of the nociceptive messages to the spinal cord? The present hypotheses and theories are based on various neurophysiological data.

– Firstly, behavioural studies demonstrating the analogies which exist between the analgesia induced by microinjections of morphine (Akaike et al., 1978; Clark et al., 1983; Dickenson et al., 1979; Lewis and Gebhart, 1977; Tsou and Jang, 1964; Yaksh and Rudy, 1978) and the analgesia caused by electrical neurostimulation (Akaike et al., 1978; Fields and Basbaum, 1978; Hayes et al., 1979; Lewis and Gebhart, 1977; Penn et al., 1984) of the periventricular grey matter and of the nuclei of the brain stem, such as the nucleus raphe magnus, which are rich in morphine receptors (Atweh and Kuhar, 1977b), have suggested to some authors (Fields and Basbaum, 1978, 1984; Willis, 1984) that morphine acts via these structures strengthening the activity of the descending inhibitory control.

– Secondly, electrophysiological studies analysing the activity of the converging spinal neurons after cerebral microinjections of morphine (Clark et al., 1983; Dickenson and Le Bars, 1983, 1988; Le Bars et al., 1980a), or after intracerebroventricular (third ventricle) administration of increasing doses of morphine (0.6 – 40 μg) (Bouhassira et al., 1986; Bouhassira et al., 1988). The demonstration of an increasing activation of the neuronal responses to the C fibres has led to conclusions which are contrary to those accepted until now, i.e. morphine depresses the activity of the descending inhibitory controls (Duggan et al., 1980; Le Bars et al. 1980b) arising from the brain stem.

– Third, the apparent contradictions led Le Bars et al. (1980b) to propose an alternative hypothesis based on the fact that the ICV administration of low doses of morphine blocks, in a dose-dependent way, the diffuse noxious inhibitory controls (DNIC) induced by nociceptive stimulation. So, analgesia would be brought about by restoring the somesthetic background noise arising from DNIC depression (Bouhassira et al., 1986; Villanueva and Le Bars, 1986).

A common point in all these hypotheses is that ICV administered morphine acts directly and at low doses on central structures rich in opiate receptor sites and that the same structures are involved in the descending inhibition originating from the brain stem which exerts its action on the neurons of the dorsal horn.

We have attempted to bring together various arguments aiming at demonstrating that the intense and diffuse analgesia reported with ICVM is independent of any direct action of morphine having diffused to the spine.

(1) The time-course and the topography of the analgesia brought about by ICVM, as discussed previously, is different from that observed after spinal morphinotherapy (Lazorthes, 1986; Lazorthes et al., 1985c).

(2) HPLC assay of the morphine present in the lumbar CSF after ICV administration showed that perispinal diffusion occurs later than establishment of analgesia and that the diffusion is not sufficient to cause direct spinal analgesia (Caute et al., 1988). Thus, in a patient with two intrathecal access sites implanted (one in the lateral ventricle and the other lumbar), repeated ICV administration of 1.0 then 1.5 mg of morphine did not lead to significant concentrations of morphine being found at the spinal level 1 h after ICV injection. These preliminary results require confirmation.

(3) The study of the kinetics of iodomorphine administered ICV showed: (a) that the migration of radioactivity is very slow, (b) that after 1 h (i.e. after maximum latency of establishment of analgesia) only 5% of the injected dose had left the cerebral ventricles and (c) and that the diffusion did not go further than the thoracic region.

Conclusions

The use of morphinotherapy by intracerebroventricular (ICVM) administration in the treatment of chronic intractable pain of cancerous origin is based on recent fundamental data. This new method has drawn a very wide clinical interest not only because it is very effective, but also because it is relatively non-invasive and the drug effect is completely reversible. It takes part in the evolution of modern neurosurgical techniques based on activation of the neurophysiological control mechanisms.

Used in patients who have become tolerant to large doses of parenterally administered morphine, ICVM brings about fast and complete analgesia with very small doses (average dose = 0.30 mg/24 h). Tolerance with ICVM is reduced since the terminal average daily dose (for an average follow-up of 115 days) was 0.70 mg for the series analysed (*n* = 51). Although the site of administration is central, the side effects − notably central depression − are very moderate, mainly observed in the initial period and rapidly reversible. There is, however, always a potential risk, and close surveillance is necessary. This method of intraventricular administration is complementary to lumbar intrathecal administration: which technique is used depends mainly on the site of the pain − ICVM is particularly indicated for chronic neoplasic pain of cervicocephalic, thoracic or diffuse origin arising from widespread bone metastases.

References

Akaike, A., Shibata, T., Satoh, M. and Takagi, H. (1978) Analgesia induced by microinjection of morphine into and electrical stimulation of the nucleus reticularis paragigantocellularis of the rat medulla oblongata. *Neuropharmacology*, 17: 775 – 778.

Atweh, S.F. and Kuhar, M.J. (1977a) Autoradiographic localization of opiate receptors in rat brain. I. Spinal cord and lower medulla. *Brain Res.*, 124: 53 – 67.

Atweh, S.F. and Kuhar, M.J. (1977b) Autoradiographic localization of opiate receptors in rat brain. II. The brain stem. Brain Res., 129: 1 – 12.

Blond, S. (1988) Morphinothérapie intra-cérébro-ventriculaire. A propos de 79 cas. *Neurochirurgie*, in press.

Blond, S., Dubar, M., Meynadier, J., Combelles, Pruvot, M. and Vitrac, P. (1985) Cerebral intraventricular administration of morphine in cancer patients with intractable pain. *The Pain Clinic*, 1: 77 – 79.

Bouhassira, D., Villanueva, L. and Le Bars, D. (1986) Effects of intraventricular (i.c.v.) morphine upon diffuse noxious inhibitory controls (DNIC) in the rat. *Neurosci. Lett.*, 26: 5410.

Bouhassira, D., Villanueva, L. and Le Bars, D. (1988) Intracerebroventricular morphine restores the basic somesthetic activity of dorsal horn convergent neurones in the rat. *Eur. J. Pharmacol.*, 148: 273 – 277.

Caute, B., Monsarrat, B., Gouardères, Ch., Verdié, J.C., Lazorthes, Y., Cros, J. and Bastide, R. (1988) CSF morphine levels and analgesia after lumbar intrathecal administration of isobaric and hyperbaric solutions in humans. *Pain*, 32: 141 – 146.

Clark, S.L., Edeson, R.O. and Ryall, R.W. (1983) The relative significance of spinal and supraspinal actions in the antinociceptive effect of morphine in the dorsal horn: an evaluation of the microinjection technique. *Br. J. Pharmacol.*, 79: 807 – 818.

Conseiller, C., Menetrey, D., Le Bars, D. and Besson, J.M. (1972) Effet de la morphine sur les activités des interneurones de la couche V de Rexed de la corne dorsale chez le chat spinal. *J. Physiol.*, 65: 220.

Dickenson, A.H. and Le Bars, D. (1983) Morphine microinjections into periaqueductal grey matter of the rat: effect on dorsal horn neuronal responses to C fibre activity and diffuse noxious activity controls. *Life Sci.*, 33: 549 – 554.

Dickenson, A.H. and Le Bars, D. (1988) Lack of evidence for increased descending inhibition on the dorsal horn of the rat following periaqueductal grey morphine microinjections. *Br. J. Pharmacol.*, 92: 271 – 280.

Dickenson, A.H., Oliveras, J.L. and Besson, J.M. (1979) Role of the nucleus raphe magnus in opiate analgesia as studied by the microinjection technique in the rat. *Brain Res.*, 170: 95 – 111.

Duggan, A.W., Hall, J.G. and Headley, P.M. (1977) Suppression of transmission of nociceptive impulses by morphine: selective effects of morphine administered in the region of the substantia gelatinosa. *Br. J. Pharmacol.*, 61: 65 – 76.

Duggan, A.W., Griersmith, H.T. and North, R.A. (1980) Morphine and supraspinal inhibition of spinal neurones: evidence that morphine decreases tonic descending inhibition in the anaesthetized cat. *Br. J. Pharmacol.*, 69: 461 – 466.

Fields, H.L. and Basbaum, A.I. (1978) Brain stem control of spinal pain transmission neurons. *Annu. Rev. Physiol.*, 40: 193 – 221.

Fields, H.L. and Basbaum, A.I. (1984) Endogenous pain control mechanisms. In P.D. Wall and R. Melzack (Eds.), *Textbook of Pain*, Churchill Livingstone, Edinburgh, pp. 142 – 152.

Hayes, R.L., Price, D.D., Ruda, M. and Dubner, R. (1979) Suppression of nociceptive responses in the primate by electrical stimulation of the brain or morphine administration: behavioural and electrophysiological comparisons. *Brain Res.*, 167: 417 – 421.

Hughes, J. (1975) Isolation of an endogenous compound from

brain with pharmacological properties similar to morphine. *Brain Res.,* 88: 295 – 308.

Lazorthes, Y. (1986) Morphinothérapie intrathécale chez l'homme. *Rec. Méd. Vét.,* 162: 1409 – 1419.

Lazorthes, Y., Gouardères, Ch., Verdié, J.C., Montsarrat, B., Bastide, R., Campan, L. and Cros, J. (1980) Analgésie par injection intrathécale de morphine. Etude pharmacocinétique et application aux douleurs irréductibles. *Neurochirurgie,* 26A: 159 – 164.

Lazorthes, Y., Siegfried, J., Gouardères, Ch., Bastide, R., Cros, J. and Verdié, J.C. (1983) Periventricular grey matter stimulation versus chronic intrathecal morphine in cancer pain. In J.J. Bonica (Ed.), *Advances in Pain Research and Therapy., Vol. 5,* Raven Press, New York, pp. 467 – 475.

Lazorthes, Y., Verdié, J.C., Bastide, R., Caute, B. and Clemente, G. (1985a) Les systèmes implantables pour administration épidurale et intrathécale d'opioides. In J.M. Besson and Y. Lazorthes (Eds.), *Spinal Opioids and the Relief of Pain: Basic Mechanisms and Clinical Applications, Vol. 127,* INSERM Editions, Paris, pp. 391 – 415.

Lazorthes, Y., Verdié, J.C., Bastide, R., Clergue, M.L., Lavados, A., Caute, B. and Cros, J. (1985b) Chronic spinal administration of opiate: application in the treatment of intractable cancer pain. In J.M. Besson and Y. Lazorthes (Eds.), *Spinal Opioids and the Relief of Pain: Basic Mechanisms and Clinical Applications, Vol. 127,* INSERM Editions, Paris, pp. 437 – 463.

Lazorthes, Y., Verdié, J.C., Bastide, R., Lavados, A. and Descouens, D. (1985c) Spinal versus intraventricular chronic opiate administration with implantable drug delivery devices for cancer pain. *Appl. Neurophysiol.,* 48: 234 – 241.

Leavens, M.E., Hills, C.S. Jr., Cech, D.A., Weyland, J.B. and Weston, J.S. (1982) Intrathecal and intraventricular morphine for pain in cancer patients. Initial study. *J. Neurosurg.,* 56: 241 – 245.

Le Bars, D., Dickenson, A.H. and Besson, J.M. (1980a) Microinjection of morphine within nucleus raphe magnus and dorsal horn neurone activities related to nociception in the rat. *Brain Res.,* 189: 467 – 481.

Le Bars, D., Guilbaud, G., Chitour, D. and Besson, J.M. (1980b) Does systemic morphine increase descending inhibitory controls of dorsal horn neurones involved in nociception? *Brain Res.,* 202: 223 – 228.

Lenzi, A., Galli, G., Gandolfini, M. and Marini, G. (1985) Intraventricular morphine in paraneoplasic painful syndrome of the cervico-facial region: experience in thirty eight cases. *Neurosurgery,* 17: 6 – 11.

Lewis, V.A. and Gebhart, G.F. (1977) Evaluation of the periaqueductal central gray (PAG) as a morphine-specific locus of action and examination of morphine-induced and stimulation-produced analgesia at coincident PAG loci. *Brain Res.,* 124: 283 – 303.

Lobato, R.D., Madrid, J.L., Fatela, L.V., Rivas, J.J., Reig, E. and Lamas, E. (1983) Intraventricular morphine for control of pain in terminal cancer patients. *J. Neurosurg.,* 59: 627 – 633.

Lobato, R.D., Madrid, J.L., Fatela, L.V., Gozalo, A., Rivas, J.J. and Sarabia, R. (1985) Analgesia elicited by low-dose intraventricular morphine in terminal cancer patients. In H. Fields et al. (Eds.), *Advances in Pain Research and Therapy, Vol. 9,* Raven Press, New York, pp. 673 – 681.

Muller, H., Borner, U., Stoyanov, M. and Hempelmann, G. (1982) Theoretical aspects and practical considerations concerning selective opiate analgesia. *Spinal Opiate Analgesia,* 144: 9 – 17.

Nurchi, G. (1984) Use of intraventricular and intrathecal morphine in intractable pain associated with cancer. *Neurosurgery,* 15: 801 – 803.

Obbens, E.A.M.T., Hill, C.S., Leavens, M.E., Ruthenbeck, S.S. and Otis, F. (1987) Intraventricular morphine administration for control of chronic cancer pain. *Pain,* 28: 61 – 68.

Oliveras, J.L., Hosobuchi, Y., Redjemi, F., Guilbaud, G. and Besson, J.M. (1977) Opiate antagonist, naloxone, strongly reduces analgesia induced by stimulation of a raphe nucleus (centralis inferior). *Brain Res.,* 120: 221 – 229.

Onofrio, B., Yaksh, T.L. and Arnold, P.G. (1981) Continuous low-dose intrathecal morphine administration in the treatment of chronic pain of malignant origin. *Mayo Clin. Proc.,* 56: 516 – 520.

Penn, R.D., Paice, J.A., Gottschalk, W. and Ivankovich, A.D. (1984) Cancer pain relief using chronic morphine infusion: early experience with a programmable implanted drug pump. *J. Neurosurg.,* 61: 302 – 306.

Pert, C.B. and Snyder, S.M. (1973) Opiate receptor: demonstration in nervous tissue. *Science,* 179: 1011 – 1014.

Roquefeuil, B., Benezech, J., Batier, C., Blanchet, P., Gros, C. and Mathieu-Daude, J.C. (1983) Intérêt de l'analgésie morphinique par voie ventriculaire dans les algies rebelles néoplasiques. *Neurochirurgie,* 29: 135 – 141.

Roquefeuil, B., Benezech, J. and Batier, C. (1985) Intérêt de l'analgésie morphinique par voie ventriculaire dans les algies rebelles néoplasiques. In L. Simon, B. Roquefeuil and J. Pelissier (Eds.), *La Douleur Chronique,* Masson, Paris, pp. 212.

Roquefeuil, B., Benezech, J., Blanchet, P., Batier, C., Frerebeau, Ph. and Gros, C. (1984) Intraventricular administration of morphine in patients with neoplasic intractable pain. *Surg. Neurol.,* 21: 155 – 158.

Saunders, R.L. and Coombs, D.W. (1983) Dartmouth-Hitchcock Medical Center experience with continuous intraspinal narcotic analgesia. In H. Schmidek and W.E. Sweet (Eds.), *Operative Neurosurgical Techniques, Vol. 2,* Grune and Stratton, New York, pp. 1211 – 1212.

Simon, E.J. (1982) Opiate receptors and opioid peptides: an overview. *Ann. NY Acad. Sci.,* 327 – 339.

Tafani, M., Danet, B., Verdié, J.C. and Lazorthes, Y., Esquerré, J.P. and Simon, J. (1988) Human brain and spinal cord scan after intra-cerebroventricular administration of iodine 123 morphine. *Nucl. Med. Biol.,* in press.

Thiebaut, J.B., Blond, S., Farcot, J.M., Thurel, C., Matge, G., Schach, G., Meynadier, J. and Bucheit, F. (1985) La morphine par voie intraventriculaire dans le traitement des douleurs néoplasiques. *Méd. Hyg.,* 43: 636 – 646.

Tsou, K. and Jang, C.S. (1964) Studies on the site of analgesic action of morphine by intracerebral microinjection. *Scientia Sinica,* 13: 1099 – 1109.

Tung, A.S., Tenicela, R., Barr, G. and Winter, P. (1982) Intrathecal morphine in cancer patients tolerant to systemic opiates. *Spinal Opiate Analgesia,* 144: 138 – 140.

Villanueva, L. and Le Bars, D. (1986) Indirect effects of intrathecal morphine upon Diffuse Noxious Inhibitory Controls (DNICs) in the rat. *Pain,* 26: 233 – 243.

Wang, J.K. (1977) Analgesic effect of intrathecally administered morphine. *Reg. Anesth.,* 4: 2 – 3.

Willer, J.C., Roby, A. and Le Bars, D. (1984) Psychological and electrophysiological approaches to the pain-relieving effects of heterotopic nociceptive stimuli. *Brain,* 107: 1095 – 1112.

Willis, W.D. (1984) The raphe spinal system. In C.D. Barnes (Ed.), *Brainstem Control of Spinal Cord Function,* Academic Press, London, pp. 141 – 214.

Yaksh, T.L. (1978) Analgesic actions of intrathecal opiates in cat and primate. *Brain Res.,* 153: 205 – 210.

Yaksh, T.L. (1981) Spinal opiate analgesia: characteristic and principles of actions. *Pain,* 11: 293 – 346.

Yaksh, T.L. and Rudy, T.A. (1977) Studies on the direct spinal action of narcotics in the production of analgesia in the rat. *J. Pharmacol. Exp. Ther.,* 202: 411 – 428.

Yaksh, T.L. and Rudy, T.A. (1978) Narcotic analgetics: CNS sites and mechanisms of action as revealed by intracerebral injection techniques. *Pain,* 4: 299 – 359.

H.L. Fields and J.-M. Besson (Eds.)
Progress in Brain Research, Vol. 77
© 1988 Elsevier Science Publishers B.V. (Biomedical Division)

CHAPTER 30

Endogenous opioids and pain: status of human studies and new treatment concepts

Robert C.A. Frederickson and Richard E. Chipkin

Searle Research and Development, G.D. Searle and Co., Skokie, IL and Department of Pharmacology, Schering/Plough Corporation, Bloomfield, NJ, USA

Introduction

The tremendous cost, both financially and sociologically, of opioid addiction has spurred the search during the last century for non-abusable strong analgesics. Despite an intense and continuing effort, however, the goal has not yet been met. The discovery of the endogenous opioids fueled the latest spurt of enthusiasm and optimism. The evidence is now persuasive that these endogenous peptides play a role in nociceptive mechanisms, but the development of the ideal non-abusable analgesic based on this new knowledge has not yet come to fruition. Abuse potential or physical dependence liability is not the only area of potential improvement in analgesics. There is still a great need to develop potent centrally active analgesic drugs with less respiratory depression, psychotomimetic effects and gastrointestinal effects. There are also a host of specialty uses requiring certain particular properties. Analgesic drugs based on the endogenous opioids may yet fill some of these needs. The endogenous systems involved in pain perception and analgesia and the changes in endogenous opioids in various body fluids in different pain conditions are being reviewed elsewhere in this volume. Therefore, this chapter will concentrate on the status of efforts to develop new clinically effective analgesic agents based on the

endogenous opioid systems and will update a previous review of this topic (Frederickson, 1986).

Evidence for role of endogenous opioids in pain/analgesia

Support for the role of the endogenous opioids in the modulation of pain has come from several different lines of research including stimulation- and stress-induced analgesia, placebo and nitrous oxide induced analgesia and the effects of the antagonist naloxone and of inhibitors of opioid degradation such as thiorphan. This has been reviewed in detail previously (Frederickson, 1984).

Stimulation- and stress-induced analgesia are discussed elsewhere in this volume. Both stress and stimulation of appropriate brain areas can produce analgesia which can be at least partially reversed by naloxone, thus implicating endogenous opioids. It has been suggested that while levels of endogenous opioids in the cerebrospinal fluid (CSF) may reflect function in the modulation of pain, it is unlikely that plasma levels reflect any such role (e.g. Frederickson, 1984). The significance of endogenous opioids in the CSF is reviewed in the previous chapter.

Evidence has also derived from investigations of the ability of enzyme inhibitors to potentiate and of antagonists such as naloxone to block analgesia induced by acupuncture, nitrous oxide, brain stimulation or exposure to stress and from the ability of naloxone to produce hyperalgesia in the basal condition. The tonic activity of the endogenous systems, however, is apparently very low, and many factors appear to influence their likelihood of becoming activated. Thus, results have been negative in some studies, and this has led to some controversy. One confounding factor is the diurnal rhythm in the levels of the endogenous opioids and the receptors upon which they act. Further complications arise from the existence of both opioid and non-opioid mechanisms of analgesia. These factors have probably contributed to some of the negative results reported. Nevertheless, there is very strong positive evidence that endogenous opioids function in some manner to modulate nociception and this has been reviewed in some detail previously (Frederickson, 1984; Akil et al., 1984).

Concepts for new pain treatment based on endogenous opioids

The endogenous opioids themselves have no apparent clinical utility as analgesics. The actions of the enkephalins are too brief, due to rapid enzymatic degradation and β-endorphin does not cross the blood-brain barrier readily enough. Furthermore, another morphine-like μ-selective analgesic is hardly needed. Two fairly recent discoveries, however, have provided the basis for two new approaches to development of unique analgesics. The first is the demonstration that there are multiple receptors for the opioids (e.g. Goodman et al., 1980; Pasternak et al., 1983). The second is that there is no efficient neuronal uptake system for the endogenous opioids such that the predominant mode of inactivation must be enzymatic (Frederickson, 1984; Chipkin, 1986). This provides a rationale for the following drug development targets.

(1) δ-Receptor-selective opioid ligands

The three major opioid receptors defined to date are the μ, $\varkappa$ and δ receptors. At present, most strong analgesics act at the μ receptor and this is associated with physical dependence and abuse liability. The mixed agonist-antagonist analgesics presented a diminished abuse liability, presumably by providing analgesia via $\varkappa$ receptors in the spinal cord. Agents active on these receptors, however, tend to be psychotomimetic. There is now evidence for analgesia-producing δ receptors, both spinally and supraspinally, which may provide analgesia with diminished abuse liability and without psychotomimetic activity.

(2) Inhibitors of enzymatic degradation of endogenous opioids

If the critical pathway controlling the activity of the endogenous opioids is enzymatic, then enzyme inhibitors should have similar pharmacology to the endogenous ligands. Enkephalinase is the neutral metalloendopeptidase that cleaves methionine[5]- and leucine[5]-enkephalin at the glycinyl[3]-phenylalanine[4]-amide bond. It is proposed that inhibitors of this enzyme would have analgesic properties, and this has been demonstrated in animal models (Roques et al., 1980; Chipkin et al., 1983; Frederickson, 1984).

Some dogmas have been spreading which seem to prejudice the feasibility of developing useful new therapy based on the above concepts. These include the belief that analgesia is mediated via μ, but not δ receptors, that the opioid peptides produce physical dependence just as do the opiates, and that opioid peptides cannot cross the blood-brain barrier (B-B-B) adequately to produce analgesia. The next three sections will deal with these dogmas.

Evidence for δ-receptor-mediated analgesia

Earlier, the prevalent opinion was that analgesia is mediated by the μ receptor and not the δ receptor (e.g. Gacel et al., 1981). An early indication of the likely existence of δ receptor mediated analgesia came from a correlation of the in vitro and in vivo activities of morphine and metkephamid (Frederickson et al., 1980, 1981). This was corroborated by further observations (Table I) of the analgesic ED_{50}'s after intracerebroventricular administration of a series of opioids of widely differing μ-versus δ-receptor preference. The ED_{50}'s correlated very well with IC_{50} values on the mouse vas deferens and K_i values for inhibition of ^{3}H-DADL (D-Ala[2]-D-Leu[5]-enkephalin) binding (both measures of δ activity) but less well with measures of μ activity (guinea-pig ileum and ^{3}H-naloxone binding).

Other experimental means of evaluating comparative receptor types in pharmacologically induced behavioral changes include cross-tolerance studies and studies with selective antagonists. Cross-tolerance between metkephamid and morphine was assessed in the mouse writhing test for analgesia (Hynes and Frederickson, 1982). The results of these studies indicated the lack of cross-tolerance between metkephamid and morphine, supporting the concept that a non-μ-receptor-mediated mechanism contributes to the analgesia produced by metkephamid. A μ mechanism, however, may have contributed to the action of higher doses of metkephamid. Further support for the concept that metkephamid produces analgesia by an action on δ receptors was provided by studies with the antagonist naloxazone (Hynes and Frederickson, 1982). It was possible to determine a dose of this reputed irreversible antagonist which, given 20 h earlier, would selectively antagonize morphine-induced analgesia without effecting analgesia produced by metkephamid. These studies suggested that metkephamid produces analgesia by some mechanism or receptor-type not utilized by morphine under the conditions of the experiments described. This different mechanism is presumed to be δ-mediated because metkephamid does not recognize the $\varkappa$ receptor.

Considerable further evidence for δ-receptor-mediated analgesia, particularly at the spinal level, has been accumulating. Hylden and Wilcox (1983) reported evidence that antinociceptive activity induced in mice by intrathecal opioids was mediated by both μ and δ receptors but not by $\varkappa$ receptors. Tung and Yaksh (1982) reported identical findings for opioid-mediated antinociception in the rat spinal cord. Tseng (1982) utilized cross-tolerance studies to differentiate morphine and DADL and provided evidence for both μ and δ receptors mediating analgesia in the spinal cord.

Vaught and colleagues (1987) have provided some very interesting evidence supporting this concept of separate μ-mediated and δ-mediated analgesia. They have demonstrated that in the Jimpy mouse, which is deficient in cerebroside sulfate, morphine is inactive as an analgesic whereas δ-selective agents retain their analgesic activity. Similarily, in the CXBK mouse, which is deficient in the μ receptor, but retains a normal component of δ receptors, the analgesic response to morphine and DAGO, a μ-selective peptide, is diminished while no change is seen in the analgesia induced by DPLPE, a highly selective δ-receptor agent. This convincing data from animal studies, supporting the presence of δ-receptor-mediated analgesia, has been further corroborated by studies of intrathecal administration of opioids in humans, and this will be discussed in a later section.

TABLE I

Compound	Analgesic ED_{50}[a] (ng/mouse, ICV)	IC_{50} (nM)[b]	
		MVD (δ)	GPI (μ)
DSLET[c]	7.2	1.3	65
Metkephamid	2.2	10.0	21
Morphine	82.7	540.0	100
LY164929[d]	144.5	372.0	13

[a] ED_{50} (dose which provides an increase of greater than 2 standard deviations in latency to escape jump in 50% of mice tested) in hot-plate (52°C) test after intracerebroventricular (ICV) administration.
[b] Concentration which inhibits by 50% the amplitude of the electrically induced twitch of the mouse vas deferens (MVD) or guinea-pig ileum (GPI) strips in a muscle bath.
[c] [D-serine[2], threonine[6]]Leu-enkephalin, a relatively δ-selective peptide.
[d] A μ-selective analog of metenkephalin.

410

Physical dependence and the δ receptor

The above section provides evidence for δ-receptor-mediated analgesia and the question arises whether this might be associated with less physical dependence than μ-mediated analgesia. A number of investigators have reported the development of physical dependence consequent upon prolonged exposure to opioid peptide analogs and they have implied a close correlation, therefore, between analgesia and physical depedence, independent of receptor types (Miglecz et al., 1979; Wei, 1981; Wei and Loh, 1976). None of these studies focusses carefully, however, on correlating the production of physical dependence with receptor selectivity. Rather, they merely demonstrated that opioid peptides, like opioid alkaloids, can produce physical dependence. None of the peptides tested were devoid of μ activity and the protocol for such studies was to expose the organism to increasing levels of drug until dependence was produced. None of these studies, therefore, answers whether δ-receptor activation may be associated with similar or less physical dependence than μ-receptor

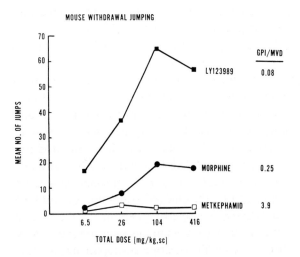

Fig. 1. Correlation of physical dependence with μ- versus δ-receptor selectivity. Mice were treated with each of the compounds at 6.5 mg/kg, s.c. twice daily, for 32 days. Mouse withdrawal jumping was precipitated and scored by injection of naloxone (10 mg/kg, s.c.). LY123989 is a μ-selective analog of metenkephalin.

activation. Some of the animal and human studies with metkephamid and DADL described herein suggest that δ-mediated analgesia may be associated with less physical dependence than μ-mediated analgesia. This concept is supported by the data shown in Fig. 1. Careful studies comparing in a quantitative dose-related fashion the analgesic versus physical dependence-producing properties after intraventricular administration of highly μ-selective and highly δ-selective enkephalin analogs (taking into account their relative bioavailabilities and enzymatic susceptibilities), will be required to better clarify this important question.

Opioid peptides and the blood-brain barrier

There is clearly a significant blood-brain barrier (B-B-B) to peptides and this includes the opioid peptides. The B-B-B to peptides has been the subject of several recent reviews (Meisenberg and Simmons, 1983; Pardridge, 1983). These peptides diffuse very slowly through these tight junctions and, furthermore, brain capillaries have a high aminopeptidase activity and therefore rapidly degrade enkephalins. Modification of the two-position of enkephalins, such as by replacement of Gly^2 by D-Ala^2, however, does improve penetration and there are brain structures, furthermore, with diminished barriers such as the circumventricular organs and the choroid plexus. Thus, enkephalin analogs can penetrate the B-B-B sufficiently after systemic administration to have behavioral effects. This is exemplified, for example, by metkephamid which is very potent indeed after intravenous administration (Frederickson et al., 1981).

Thus, while B-B-B passage of peptides is limited, this is not the limiting factor in the potential therapeutic use of enkephalin analogs. One major limitation to realization of the therapeutic potential of peptides, including enkephalin analogs, is the lack of sufficient oral bioavailability. These peptides suffer dramatic degradation in the gut, and the small proportion of a dose delivered to the gut which reaches the circulation suffers further substantial degradation in the first pass through the liver (e.g. Holland et al., 1986). A major focus of effort, therefore, should be on increasing peptide survival through the gut and liver or on finding ways to bypass the gut and liver.

Clinical studies

Opioid peptides

β-Endorphin has been considered the most potent of the opioid peptides, due most likely to its lesser susceptibility to enzymatic degradation than the smaller enkephalins. β-Endorphin does not readily cross the blood-brain barrier, however, and, therefore, none of the natural endogenous opioids produce analgesia after systemic administration in animal or man.

β-Endorphin is reported, however, to have profound analgesic effects in man after intrathecal administration. In one study, long-lasting analgesia was produced by intrathecal administration of 3 mg synthetic β-endorphin to patients with intractable cancer pain (Oyama et al., 1980a). In a subsequent study intrathecal administration of 1 mg β-endorphin, prior to delivery, provided rapid and prolonged analgesia in obstetric patients (Oyama et al., 1980b).

Onofrio and Yaksh (1983) reported that 1 mg DADL, given intrathecally, provided powerful long-lasting analgesia in a patient with intractable cancer pain who had become tolerant to intrathecal morphine. These authors suggested that δ-receptor ligands may be a pharmacological alternative to agents such as morphine and β-endorphin which appear to produce spinal analgesia through a common μ receptor.

The analgesic efficacy of intrathecal DADL was confirmed and extended in a subsequent study in a larger number of cancer patients with chronic pain (Moulin et al., 1985). In another study, 0.25 mg DADL intrathecally restored analgesia, without respiratory depression, in a morphine-tolerant patient. Importantly, DADL was reported to restore analgesia without preventing the morphine withdrawal syndrome which could, however, be treated with a small dose of morphine (Krames et al., 1986).

These data with DADL, while limited and needing expansion, nevertheless support the animal data suggesting the existence of a separate δ-mediated analgesia associated with less physical dependence than for μ-mediated analgesia. Thus, β-endorphin appears to use the same receptor as does morphine and shows cross-tolerance with morphine while DADL seems more potent than β-endorphin (true relative potencies in man have not yet been determined) and does not show cross-tolerance to morphine. This supports the suggestion that a δ-receptor ligand such as DADL be alternated with a μ-receptor ligand such as morphine to provide pain relief to chronic pain patients. Moulin et al. (1986) conducted a study of the comparative pharmacokinetics of morphine and DADL after intrathecal administration and concluded that the pharmacokinetics were very similar for both agents. DADL persists long enough in CSF to spread supraspinally, however, and thus it provides no advantage over morphine in this regard. A better drug for this purpose would have the same receptor profile as DADL but disappear more rapidly from the CSF, while sticking very tightly to the receptors once attached (K. Foley, personal communication).

A number of opioid peptides have been evaluated in man for antinociceptive activity after systemic administration. Dermorphin is an opiate-like heptapeptide (H-Tyr-D-Ala-Phe-Gly-Tyr-Pro-Ser-NH$_2$) isolated from frog skin (Broccardo et al., 1981). Intravenous infusion of 0.16 mg/kg dermorphin induced a long-lasting increase in the threshold of nociceptive flexion reflex in normal male subjects (Sandrini et al., 1986). Attempts at antagonism suggested that dermorphin acts at least partially on a non-μ receptor, possibly δ, and the authors speculate that this may explain its potent analgesic properties with only moderate tolerance and physical dependence in animal studies.

A modified enkephalin analog, D-Met^2,Pro^5-enkephalinamide, was also examined on pain tolerance and cognitive function in normal male volunteers (Székely et al., 1986). The investigators used the submaximum effort tourniquet technique and found that this peptide at 10 mg given s.c. decreased pain intensity rating similarly to a dose of 20 mg dihydrocodeine. They reported side effects including heaviness in the limbs, conjunctival injection, dry mouth and epigastric oppression.

Metkephamid (Fig. 2) is an analog of Met[5]-enkephalin, with several simple modifications. Since this compound was more extensively studied and progressed further in the clinic than any other modified opioid peptide, it will be dealt with in more detail.

Metkephamid competes with labeled opioid ligands for binding in brain homogenate and produces potent naloxone-reversible depression of the electrically induced twitch of both mouse vas deferens (MVD) and guinea pig ileum (GPI), with IC_{50} values in the nanomolar range (Frederickson et al., 1982). In the mouse vas deferens preparation, pA_2 values for naloxone versus metkephamid, normorphine and metenkephalin were determined to be 7.60, 8.32, and 7.4, respectively. These data suggested that metkephamid and metenkephalin share preference for a similar receptor, presumably the δ receptor. This differs from normorphine, which prefers the μ receptor. This was corroborated by the GPI/MVD ratios which were about 4.1 for metkephamid and 0.25 for morphine, indicating a 16-fold greater δ-receptor selectivity for metkephamid compared with morphine. This contrasted with the ratios for competing with [3H]naloxone versus [3H]DADL binding in brain homogenates, which were 0.6 and 0.1, respectively, for metkephamid and morphine. These latter data indicated that, although metkephamid had a 6-fold greater preference for the δ receptor than did morphine in the binding studies, it still had a slightly higher absolute affinity for the μ receptor than for the δ receptor. Metkephamid has little or no affinity for the х receptor.

Metkephamid has a definite antinociceptive effect when administered by systemic routes of administration, being anywhere from one-third to 10 times as potent as morphine, depending on the test system and the route of administration. When given by the intraventricular route, metkephamid was almost 100-fold more potent than morphine. The relative analgesic potencies of metkephamid and morphine by this route correlated much better with their relative potencies on the mouse vas deferens preparation than on the guinea-pig ileum preparation. This suggested that metkephamid was providing analgesia, at least partly, by an action at a δ receptor, as discussed earlier. This would imply a diminished dependence liability, and indeed metkephamid produced little stimulation of locomotor activity or naloxone-precipitated withdrawal jumping in mice compared with morphine. Chronic treatment of rats with metkephamid, furthermore, produced only slightly more physical dependence than did saline, unlike other drugs similarly tested such as morphine, meperidine, and pentazocine. Metkephamid was also reported to have a lesser depressant effect than morphine on respiration in a rodent model.

The ability of metkephamid to cross the placental barrier was assessed by measuring the maternal and fetal serum levels in rats and sheep at various times after intramuscular injection of metkephamid (Frederickson et al., 1982). In the rat, the fetal/maternal ratio of metkephamid in blood at 1 h after injection was about 1/60 compared with 1/1.8 for meperidine. In sheep, the fetal/maternal ratio for metkephamid was less than 1/200, compared with ratios of about 1/1 reported for meperidine. This finding has now been confirmed in human subjects (Henry, personal communication). It indicates a remarkable advantage of metkephamid over meperidine for use in obstetric analgesia.

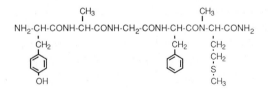

Fig. 2. Structure of metkephamid (LY127623, Lilly).

The preclinical profile of metkephamid described above demonstrated that metkephamid was different enough from standard analgesics and promised enough therapeutic advantage to warrant entering clinical trial. Metkephamid was administered to normal male volunteers in single intramuscular doses ranging from 0.5 to 150 mg in early safety studies (Frederickson et al., 1980). No clinically relevant effects were seen by routine clinical chemistry, electrolytes, urinalysis, hemograms, EKG, blood pressure, or heart rate. Serum prolactin was increased, but no change in serum growth hormone was observed after 75 mg.

Clinical tests in postoperative pain have demonstrated metkephamid to be efficacious as an analgesic in man. In one controlled double-blind clinical trial (Calimlim et al., 1982), metkephamid at a single parenteral dose of 70 mg was compared with meperidine at 100 mg and placebo in 30 patients with severe postoperative pain. All measures indicated that the analgesic activity of metkephamid 70 mg was significantly greater than placebo and not less than that of meperidine 100 mg. The duration of activity was about 4 h, and up to the 4-h point metkephamid 70 mg appeared more efficacious than did meperidine 100 mg (Fig. 3). The frequency of remedication with metkephamid was also less than with meperidine or placebo. In a second controlled double-blind study (Bloomfield et al., 1983), metkephamid at 70 mg and 140 mg intramuscularly was compared with meperidine at 100 mg and placebo in 60 post-partum women with severe pain after episiotomy. Using subjective reports as indices of response, patients rated pain intensity, pain relief, and side effects at periodic intervals for 6 h. Metkephamid at the 140-mg dose was rated most effective, followed in order by meperidine (100 mg), metkephamid (70 mg), and placebo. Only metkephamid at 140 mg and meperidine at 100 mg showed statistically significant superiority over placebo. Both treatments took effect within 1/2 h, peaked at 1 – 2 h and with 140 mg metkephamid, maximum analgesia was sustained for 6 h, i.e. 2 h longer than with meperidine.

There was a higher incidence of minor side effects with metkephamid than with the other treatments in these studies, but these effects were relatively transient and were not distressing to the patients. The side effects peculiar to metkephamid were a sensation of heavy limbs, dry mouth, eye redness, and nasal stuffiness. The spectrum of

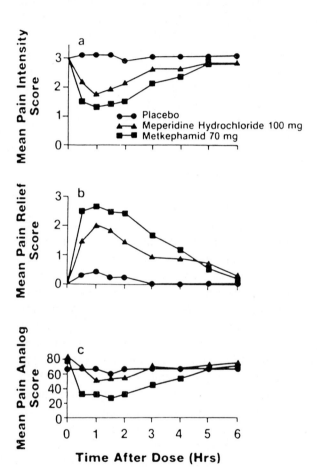

Fig. 3. Time-effect curves of analgesic activity of metkephamid (70 mg) compared to placebo and meperidine (100 mg). Pain was assessed subjectively at each interview by (a) a reported pain score on an ordinal scale of 0 (no pain) to 4 ('terrible' pain), (b) a reported score for pain relief compared to premedication pain level on an ordinal scale of 0 (no relief) to 4 (complete relief), and (c) an analog scale of pain consisting of 20-cm line marked 0 ('no pain') at one end and 100 ('worst pain I have ever felt') at the other end. The placebo generally had no effect on pain. By contrast, metkephamid and meperidine had begun to reduce pain by 1/2 h with peak analgesic effect usually at 1 h. (From Calimlim et al., 1982, with permission.)

414

these side effects suggested that the pharmacological properties of metkephamid are different from those of standard narcotic analgesics. Metkephamid has high affinity for both the μ and δ receptors but little or no affinity for the $\varkappa$ receptor. Thus, metkephamid appeared to be an efficacious analgesic with a decreased potential for physical dependence and respiratory depression, and significant advantage for use in obstetric analgesia. Unfortunately, during the human placental transport trials, metkephamid apparently produced a precipitous hypotension in a proportion of the target population, obstetric patients (M. Hynes, personal communication). For this reason clinical trials with metkephamid have been terminated.

Enkephalinase (Enk'ase) inhibitors

Enk'ase is the trivial name given to the neutral metalloendopeptidase (EC 3.4.24.11) that cleaves either methionine- or leucine-enkephalin at the glycinylphenylalanine amide bond. Since endogenous enkephalins have been implicated in the control of nociceptive information in the central nervous system (CNS), and since the limiting factor affecting enkephalin's action is its enzymatic break-down, it has been proposed that inhibitors of Enk'ase would have analgesic effects. This strategy of enzyme inhibition to achieve therapeutic utility has been used in several other areas, including monoamine oxidase inhibitors for depression and angiotensin converting enzyme inhibitors for hypertension.

Currently, the only Enk'ase inhibitors that have had sufficient research from which to draw conclusions are thiorphan (Roques et al., 1980) and its analogs (e.g. acetorphan; Lecomte et al., 1986). These drugs have been shown to produce naloxone-reversible analgesia in animal models of pain such as the mouse low-temperature hot-plate test (Fig. 4; see also Roques et al., 1980) and the mouse writhing test (Chaillet et al., 1983), and to potentiate stress-induced analgesia in rats (Chipkin et al., 1982). The clinical potential of thiorphan is

considered to be limited by its poor bioavailability and short duration of action.

Clinical studies with Enk'ase inhibitors have been less than extensive, but some data do exist which directly relate to the ability of Enk'ase inhibitors to be analgesic in man. For example, Enk'ase has been found to exist in human brain (Arregui et al., 1979) and particularly in areas associated with the transmission of nociceptive information (e.g. the PAG and the dorsal horn of the spinal cord). Additionally, Enk'ase has been identified in human CSF (Hazato et al., 1983; Lantz and Terenius, 1985) and plasma (Johnson et al., 1985). Thus, it has been established that the enzyme exists in humans at sites where enkephalin has been found and that the enzyme functions identically to Enk'ase from other species.

Thiorphan was evaluated in a double-blind study of headache and nausea associated with myelography (Floras et al., 1983) using an intravenous infusion of 150 mg in 250 ml of isotonic glucose for 30 min prior to the lumbar puncture. The results showed that thiorphan significantly inhibited both the headache and nausea typically

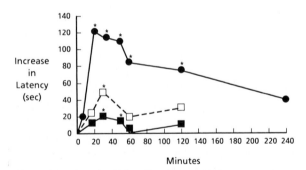

Fig. 4. Potentation of analgesic activity by thiorphan in the mouse hot plate (55°C) test. The graphs show the increase in latency to escape jump over the latency in the presence of saline (□), morphine (■, 0.5 mg/kg) and Tyr-D-Ala-Gly-Phe-Met-NH$_2$ (●, 10 mg/kg) produced by thiorphan (30 μg) injected intracerebroventricularly. Saline, morphine and the enkephalin were injected subcutaneously immediately prior to injection of thiorphan at time 0. The abscissa is in min after injection. *, significant at least at the $p < 0.05$ level.

seen with this procedure, but did not alter respiration, blood pressure or heart rate. This study is notable because thiorphan showed an analgesic effect despite its poor pharmacokinetic profile, and this suggests that Enk'ase inhibitors can produce clinically relevant antinociception at reasonable doses (roughly 3 mg/kg i.v.).

The only other human study that has been done with a selective Enk'ase inhibitor was done by Willer et al. (1986), using electrical stimulation of the sural nerve to experimentally induce pain. The drug in this case was acetorphan (GB52), and it was given intravenously at a dose of 2.5 mg/kg by infusion over 30 min. Using a small sample (n = 7), these authors were unable to show an analgesic effect in this model. However, this is not entirely unexpected since brief, noxious stimuli such as used in this study are known not to be suppressed by Enk'ase inhibitors in infra-human species (e.g. thiorphan does not block the rat tail-flick reflex; Chipkin et al., 1982). Indeed, this study highlights the concept that, in the future, discrete pain syndromes may be targetted with selective analgesics.

Several studies have appeared on other compounds purported to inhibit enkephalin breakdown. For example, D-phenylalanine was thought to have some beneficial effects in human pain (Ehrenpreis et al., 1981); but, this drug has never been shown to inhibit enkephalin degradation at relevant concentrations ($< 10^{-6}$ M). Likewise, the angiotensin-converting enzyme inhibitor captopril has been reported to block enkephalin break-down and produce analgesia in headache sufferers (Sicuteri, 1981). However, captopril does not inhibit Enk'ase, does not produce analgesia in animal models (Chipkin et al., 1981), and it is not probable that the clinical effect occurs through this mechanism. More likely, the antihypertensive actions of captopril contributed to the analgesia seen, since changes in blood pressure would affect headache. It is worth noting that in rats thiorphan had no effect on blood pressure (Baum et al., 1983). Alternatively, captopril may be altering the metabolism of another opioid peptide that is currently unidentified.

The future in this field is dependent upon the discovery of potent, orally active drugs suitable for large scale clinical investigations.

Conclusion

More than a decade after the discovery of the endogenous opioids we do not yet have the therapeutic breakthrough hoped for, but the game is not over yet. δ-Mediated analgesia has been demonstrated and this may not be encumbered by the traditional problems of morphine, particularly dependence liability. Intrathecal opioid peptides may have some advantages for limited use, particularly in obstetrics or in cases of morphine tolerance in chronic pain states. A tightly binding but labile peptide analog with short circulating life may have significant advantage for intrathecal use. The first enkephalin analogs, particularly metkephamid, showed some promise as systemic analgesics, but these have been discontinued because of unexpected side effects. A new orally active opioid dipeptide is being developed toward potential clinical trial (Hammond et al., 1987) as are several potent new enkephalinase inhibitors (e.g. Chipkin et al., 1987). The activities of the next 2 to 5 years will tell us whether this new generation of candidate drugs based on the endogenous opioids will be more successful than the first generation described here, at providing new treatments for pain.

Whether or not a new opioid-related approach to pain treatment derives from our increased understanding of the multiple opioid systems, the descending control systems discussed in this symposium offer new opportunities for providing unique non-opioid management of pain.

References

Akil, H., Watson, S.J., Young, E., Lewis, M.E., Khachaturian, H. and Walker, J.M. (1984) Endogenous opioids: biology and function. *Annu. Rev. Neurosci.,* 7: 223–255.

Arregui, A., Lee, C-M., Emson, P.C. and Iversen, L.L. (1979) Separation of human brain angiotensin-converting enzyme

416

from enkephalin-degrading activity. *Eur. J. Pharmacol.,* 59: 141 – 144.

Baum, T., Becker, F.T., Sybertz, E.J., Sabin, C. and Desiderio, D.M. (1983) 'Enkephalinase A' inhibition by thiorphan: central and peripheral cardiovascular effects. *Eur. J. Pharmacol.,* 94: 85 – 91.

Bloomfield, S.S., Barden, T.P., and Mitchell, J. (1983) Metkephamid and meperidine analgesia after postepisiotomy. *Clin. Pharmacol. Ther.,* 34: 240 – 247.

Broccardo, M., Erspamer, V., Falconieri-Erspamer, G., Improta, G., Linari, G., Melchiorri, P. and Montecucchi P.C. (1981) Pharmacological data on dermorphins, a new class of potent opioid peptides from amphibian skin. *Br. J. Pharmacol.,* 73: 625 – 631.

Calimlim, J.F., Wardell, W.M., Sriwatanakul, K., Lasagna, L., and Cox, C. (1982) Analgesic efficacy of parenteral metkephamid acetate in treatment of post-operative pain. *Lancet,* 1: 1374 – 1375.

Chaillet, P., Marcais-Collardo, H., Constentin, J., Yi, C.C., DeLaBaume, S. and Schwartz, J.-C. (1983) Inhibition of enkephalin metabolism by and antinociceptive activity of bestatin, an aminopeptidase inhibitor. *Eur. J. Pharmacol.,* 86: 329 – 336.

Chipkin, R.E. (1986) Inhibitors of enkephalinase: The next generation of analgesics. *Drugs of the Future,* 11, 593 – 606.

Chipkin, R.E., Iorio, L.C., Barnett, A., Berger, J. and Billard, W. (1982) In vitro and in vivo effects of thiorphan: an inhibitor of enkephalinase A. In E. Costa and M. Trabucchi (Eds.), *Regulatory Peptides: From Molecular Biology to Function,* Raven Press, New York, pp. 235 – 241.

Chipkin, R.E., Billard, W., Ahn, H.S., Sybertz, E.J. and Iorio, L.C. (1983) In vitro and in vivo activities of enkephalinase and angiotensin converting enzyme inhibitions: relationship of enzyme inhibition to analgesic and cardiovascular effects. In S. Ehrenpreis and F. Sicuteri (Eds.), *Degradation of Endogenous Opioids: Its Relevance in Human Pathology and Therapy,* Raven Press, New York, pp. 91 – 105.

Chipkin, R.E., Berger, J.G., Peters, M., Lutranyi, M., Billard, W., Iorio, L. and Barnett, A. (1987) SCH34826, the first orally active enkephalinase inhibitor analgesic. *Pain,* Suppl. 4.

Floras, P., Bidabé, A.-M., Caillé, J.-M. Simonnet, G., LeComte, J.-M. and Sabathié (1983) Double-blind study of effects of enkephalinase inhibitor on adverse reactions to myelography. *Am. J. Neuroradiol.,* 4: 653 – 655.

Frederickson, R.C.A. (1984) Endogenous opioids and related derivatives. In M. Kuhar and G. Pasternak (Eds.), *Analgesics: Neurochemical, Behavioral and Clinical Perspectives,* Raven Press, New York, pp. 9 – 68.

Frederickson, R.C.A. (1986) Endorphins-development of the therapeutic utility of enkephalin analogues. In R.C.A. Frederickson, H.C. Hendrie, J.N. Hingten and M.H. Aprison (Eds.), *Neuroregulation of Autonomic, Endocrine and Immune Systems, Neuronal Control of Bodily Function:*

Basic and Clinical Aspects, Vol. 1, Martinus-Nijhof, Boston, pp. 421 – 442.

Frederickson, R.C.A., Smithwick, E.L. and Henry, D.P. (1980) Opioid peptides as brain neurotransmitters with therapeutic potential: basic and clinical studies. In: C. Ajmone-Marsan and W.Z. Traczyk (Eds.), *Neuropeptides and Neural Transmission.* Raven Press, New York, pp. 227 – 235.

Frederickson, R.C.A., Smithwick, E.L., Shuman, R. and Bemis, K.G. (1981) Metkephamid, a systemically active analog of methionine-enkephalin with potent opioid δ-receptor activity. *Science* 211: 603 – 604.

Frederickson, R.C.A., Parli, C.J., DeVane, G.W. and Hynes, M.D. (1982) Preclinical pharmacology of metkephamid (LY127623), a metenkephalin analogue. In: L.S. Harris, (Ed.), *NIDA Research Monograph, Vol. 43.* pp. 150 – 156.

Gacel, G., Fournie-Zaluski, M.C., Fellion, E. and Roques, B.P. (1981) Evidence of the preferential involvement of μ receptors in analgesia using enkephalins highly selective for peripheral μ or δ receptors. *J. Med. Chem.,* 24: 1119 – 1124.

Goodman, R.R., Snyder, S.H., Kuhar, M.J. and Young, W.S. III. (1980) Differentiation of delta-opiate and mu-opiate receptor localizations by light microscopic autoradiography. *Proc. Natl. Acad. Sci. USA,* 77: 6239 – 6243.

Hammond, D., Mazur, R., Hansen, D., Pilipauskas, D., Bloss, J. and Drower, E. (1987) Analgesic activity of SC-39566. *Pain,* Suppl. 4, p. 5253.

Hazato, T., Shimamura, M., Katayama, T., Kasama, A., Nishioka, S. and Kaya, K. (1983) Enkephalin degrading enzymes in cerebrospinal fluid. *Life Sci.,* 33: 443 – 448.

Holland, D.R., Frederickson, R.C.A., Su, K.S.E. and Parli, C.J. (1986) Bioavailability of .the opioid peptide, Metkephamid. In R.C.A. Frederickson, H.C. Hendrie, J.N. Hingten and M.H. Aprison (Eds.), *Neuroregulation of Autonomic, Endocrine and Immune Systems, Neuronal Control of Bodily Function: Basic and Clinical Aspects, Vol. 1,* Martinus-Nijhof, Boston, pp. 421 – 442.

Hylden, J.L.K. and Wilcox, G.L. (1983) Intrathecal opioids block a spinal action of substance P in mice: functional importance of both μ- and δ-receptors. *Eur. J. Pharmacol.,* 86: 95 – 98.

Hynes, M.D. and Frederickson, R.C.A. (1982) Cross-tolerance studies distinguish morphine- and metkephamid-induced analgesia. *Life Sci.,* 31: 1201 – 1204.

Johnson, A.R., Coalson, J.J., Ashton, J., Larumbride, M. and Erdose, E.G. (1985) Neutral endopeptidase in serum samples from patients with adult respiratory distress syndrome. *Am. Rev. Resp. Dis.,* 132: 1262 – 1267.

Krames, F.S., Wilkie, D.J. and Gershow, J. (1986) Intrathecal D-Ala^2-D-Leu^5-enkephalin (DADL) restores analgesia in a patient analgetically tolerant to intrathecal morphine sulfate. *Pain,* 24: 205 – 209.

Lantz, I. and Terenius, L. (1985) Degradation of enkephalins in human CSF. *Alcohol Drug Res.,* 5: 175.

Lecomte, J.-M., Costentin, J., Vlaiculescu, A., Chaillet, P., Marcais-Collado, H., Llorens-Cortes, C., Lebayer, M. and Schwartz, J.-C. (1986) Pharmacological properties of acetorphan, a parenterally active 'Enkephalinase' inhibitor. *J. Pharmacol. Exp. Ther.,* 237: 937 – 944.

Miglecz, E., Szekely, J.I. and Dumai-Kovacs, Z. (1979) Comparison of tolerance development and dependence capacities of morphine, β-endorphin and [D-Met^2, Pro^5]enkephalinamide. *Psychopharmacology,* 62: 29 – 34.

Moulin, D.E., May, M.B., Kaiko, R.F., Inturrisi, C.E., Naggard, J., Yaksh, T.L. and Foley, K.M. (1985) The analgesic efficacy of intrathecal D-Ala^2-D-Leu^5-enkephalin in cancer patients with chronic pain. *Pain,* 23: 213 – 221.

Moulin, D.E., Inturrissi, C. and Foley, K. (1986) Cerebrospinal fluid pharmacokinetics of intrathecal morphine sulfate and D-Ala^2,D-Leu^5-enkephalin. *Ann. Neurol.,* 20: 218 – 222.

Onofrio, B.M. and Yaksh, T.L. (1983) Intrathecal delta-receptor ligand produces analgesia in man. *Lancet,* i: 1386 – 1387.

Oyama, T., Jin, T., Yamaya, R., Ling, N. and Guillemin, R., (1980a) Profound analgesic effects of β-endorphin in man. *Lancet,* Jan. 19: 112 – 124.

Oyama, T., Matsuki, A., Taneichi, T., Ling, N. and Guillemin, R. (1980b) β-endorphin in obstetric analgesia. *Am. J. Obstet. Gynecol.,* 137: 613 – 616.

Pasternak, G.W., Gintzler, A.R., Houghter, R.A., Ling, G.S.F., Goodman, R.R., Spiegel, K., Nishimura, S., Johnson, N. and Recht, L.D. (1983) Biochemical and pharmacological evidence for opioid receptor multiplicity in the central nervous system. *Life Sci.,* 33: 167 – 173.

Roques, B.P., Fournie-Zaluski, M.C., Soroca, E., Lecomte, J.M., Malfroy, B., Llorens, C. and Schwartz, J.C. (1980) The enkephalinase inhibitor thiorphan shows antinociceptive activity in mice. *Nature,* 288: 286 – 288.

Sandrini, G., Degli Uberti, E.C., Salvadori, S., Margutti, A., Trasforini, G., Tomatis, R., Nappi, G. and Pansini, R. (1986) Demorphin inhibits spinal nociceptive flexion reflex in humans. *Brain Res.,* 371: 364 – 367.

Sicuteri, F. (1981) Enkephalinase inhibition relieves pain syndromes of central dysnociception (migraine and related headache). *Cephalalgia,* 1: 229 – 232.

Szekely, J.I., Török, Karczag, I., Tolna, J. and Till, M. (1986) Effects of D-Met^2,Pro^5-enkephalinamide on pain tolerance and some cognitive functions in man. *Psychopharmacology* 89: 409 – 413.

Tseng, L.F. (1982) Tolerance and cross-tolerance to morphine after chronic spinal DADL infusion. *Life Sci.,* 31: 987 – 992.

Tung, A.S. and Yaksh, T.L. (1982) In vivo evidence for multiple opiate receptors mediating analgesia in the rat spinal cord. *Brain Res.,* 247: 75 – 83.

Vaught, J.L., Mathiasen, J.R. and Raffa, R.B. (1987) Utilization of μ opioid receptor deficient mice proves δ opioid receptor mediated analgesia: differentiation between spinal and supraspinal receptor mechanisms. *Pain,* Suppl. 4: p. 5248.

Wei, E.T. (1981) Enkephalin analogs and physical dependence. *J. Pharmacol. Exp. Ther.,* 216: 12 – 18.

Wei, E.T. and Loh, H.H. (1976) Physical dependence on opiate-like peptides. *Science,* 193: 1262 – 1263.

Willer, J.C., Roby A. and Ernst M. (1986) The enkephalinase inhibitor, GB52, does not affect nociceptive flexion reflexes nor pain sensation in humans. *Neuropharmacology,* 25: 819 – 822.

H.L. Fields and J.-M. Besson (Eds.)
Progress in Brain Research, Vol. 77
© 1988 Elsevier Science Publishers B.V. (Biomedical Division)

CHAPTER 31

Significance of opioid peptides and other potential markers of neuropeptide systems in cerebrospinal fluid

Lars Terenius

Department of Pharmacology, Uppsala University, Uppsala, Sweden

Introduction

Peptidergic pathways constitute a large body of the central and peripheral nervous systems. This extends to the sensory pathways activated by nociceptor stimulation and to pathways modulating their input at the spinal level as reviewed in several chapters of this volume. This chapter deals with these pathways only indirectly. It addresses the question whether activity in peptidergic pathways can be assessed by analyzing the content of neuropeptides, as well as other potential markers of neuropeptide systems, in the cerebrospinal fluid (CSF). Specifically, the value of CSF measurements for defining the role of neuropeptides in pain, particularly clinically relevant pain, will be considered. The chapter will balance obvious limitations of the approach, such as the difficulty of attributing levels of peptides or other markers to individual pathways, with advantages such as the applicability to human disease. Obviously, conditions such as chronic pain, maybe year-long with psychologic or psychiatric overlays, are hard to reproduce experimentally in animals. Because of the complex nature of the phenomena under consideration, the chapter covers both basic methodological issues and empirically found correlations to human pathology, in some detail.

Basic aspects

The CSF compartment

The CSF is in constant exchange with the extracellular fluid of the central nervous system (CNS). Substances released from central neurons and escaping metabolic breakdown will therefore appear in CSF. Most neuropeptides so far identified in CNS tissue can also be demonstrated in CSF (Wood, 1982). For practical purposes a very simple kinetic model can be set up for CSF levels of a neuropeptide or other marker (Fig. 1). It is assumed that the CSF level depends on the (a) rate of formation and (b) rate of release, as well as (c) rate of dilution and (d) metabolism in the CSF compartment itself. Each of these processes will be considered separately. The rate of formation of the neuropeptide in the nerve terminal defines the products available for release. As will be discussed below, formation of a particular peptide is a process occurring in consecutive steps, and depending on the rate of formation, the level and relative proportion of different peptides from the same system will vary.

Its rate of release is one obvious determinant of a peptide's level in the CSF. The rate of CSF dilution is also an obvious determinant of the CSF

420

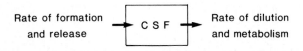

Fig. 1. Kinetic model for the concentration of a neuropeptide or other marker in the CSF compartment.

level. The rate of metabolism within the CSF compartment appears to be of much greater importance for the disappearance of neuropeptides from the CSF than previously thought. Several peptide degrading enzymes occur in substantial amounts in the CSF. Some of these have relevance for levels of peptides under consideration here. These include a dynorphin-converting enzyme cleaving the dynorphin family of peptides, dynorphin A, dynorphin B and α-neoendorphin into Leu-enkephalin-Arg[6], the common N-terminus of these peptides (Nyberg et al., 1985a), and later found to occur in considerable quantities in bovine spinal cord (in preparation). This enzyme seems to require sequences with pairs of basic amino acids. Also present in human CSF is endopeptidase-24.11 (commonly called enkephalinase) which cleaves the enkephalins into Tyr-Gly-Gly and Phe-Met(Leu), respectively. It cleaves substance P at the $9-10$ and other bonds with even higher affinity (Matsas et al., 1984). This enzyme occurs in CSF (Hazato et al., 1983) but has not been studied systematically or quantitatively. It may be less important in the CSF compartment than angiotensin-converting enzyme (ACE), which in addition to angiotensin I shows high affinity for enkephalyl hexapeptides and heptapeptides. ACE is a dicarboxypeptidase inactivating the hexapeptides by generation of a tetrapeptide and releasing enkephalin from heptapeptides. The enkephalins show more than 10-fold higher metabolic stability in the CSF than the enkephalyl hexapeptides (Lantz and Terenius, 1985). There are also several aminopeptidases in CSF which degrade enkephalins (Hazato et al., 1985). However, these enzymes have not been well characterized with regard to biochemical properties or substrate specificity.

Substance P is degraded by several CSF enzymes. Probably the major enzyme is an endopeptidase cleaving the $7-8$ and to a lesser extent, the $8-9$ bonds. This enzyme was first isolated from CSF (Nyberg et al., 1984) and later found to be present in bovine spinal cord (in preparation). Incidentally, the conversion of substance P to substance P$(1-7)$ seems to be the major metabolic route in most CNS areas and particularly in the hypothalamus, medulla and spinal cord (Sakurada et al., 1985). Postproline-cleaving enzymes are also present in CSF (unpublished) and would generate C-terminal substance P fragments which are commonly recognized by antisera used in radioimmunoassay (Rimón et al., 1984). In addition, there are reports of a paradoxical increase in substance P levels in CSF with time (Berrettini et al., 1985). This could be explained by the presence of α-amidating activity in CSF (Wand et al., 1985; Vaeroy et al., in preparation) transforming the substance P-Gly[12] precursor into substance P.

Apparently, the simple scheme of Fig. 1 contains several confounding variables of which metabolism in the CSF compartment is a major contributor.

CSF is normally only accessible in the human through a lumbar puncture. Ventricular-lumbar gradients are known to exist for monoamine transmitter metabolites. These gradients may be due primarily to active transport processes which occur in the choroid plexus and other structures. It is not likely that comparable processes are important for the elimination of peptides from the CSF compartment (Wood, 1982). Negating the existence of gradients is the report by Facchinetti et al. (1987), who found β-endorphin levels to be comparable in ventricular and lumbar CSF. Unpublished studies from this laboratory have also failed to demonstrate marked gradients of substance P. In the context of this chapter, with its focus on pain and pain modulation, spinal processes are of particular importance, and, if anything, contributions from the spinal cord should be favored in the lumbar CSF sample.

Several studies actually show that neuropeptides are released into spinal CSF by afferent stimulation. Thus, Yaksh et al. (1980) found that stimulation of C/A delta fibers in the anesthetized cat, releases substance P into the CSF. Using the same preparation, in the cat and the rat, opioid peptide release also increased markedly. Here, the whole cascade of opioid peptides was measured by receptor assay, and several components increased 10-fold or more. These peptides derived mainly from proenkephalin, with smaller contributions from prodynorphin (Yaksh et al., 1983). In rabbits, given electrical acupuncture sufficient to elevate thresholds to a thermal pain stimulus, intrathecal antisera to enkephalin partially reversed the acupuncture effect (Han et al., 1984), suggesting a humoral mediation of the acupuncture effect. Finally, in humans, Sjölund et al. (1977) studied the acute effects of low-frequency transcutaneous nerve stimulation (TENS) on the release of opioid peptides measured by receptor assay. The area of stimulation was segmentally related to the area of pain. Only in patients who received stimulation over low spinal segments (low back pain) did the lumbar CSF analyses show an increase of opioid peptides; in patients with trigeminal neuralgia and given facial stimulation, no increase was observed.

Neuropeptide biosynthesis

The basic steps in the biosynthesis of neuropeptides are common to all systems. The peptides derive from much larger precursors, prohormones, which usually have more than 200 amino acids and are biologically inert. These prohormones are synthesized, like other proteins, at the ribosomal level by translation of the appropriate mRNA, which of course in turn is transcribed from a DNA segment. Like other eukaryotic genes, the neuropeptide precursor genes are spliced and alternative splicing may occur, generating different RNA transcripts from a single gene. This occurs in the preprotachykinin A gene coding for the substance P precursor which can form an α-transcript with only one neuropeptide, substance P, or a β-transcript with substance P plus an analogous neuropeptide, neurokinin A (also called substance

K). Both transcripts are known in nerve tissue (Nawa et al., 1983).

The events taking place during the biochemical conversion of the prohormone into different neuropeptides are of particular interest in the present context. The current view is that the prohormone is packed into vesicles together with enzymes capable of releasing the active neuropeptide (processing enzymes) or transforming a primary processing product into the active neuropeptide (converting enzymes). The vesicles are transported via axonal flow towards the nerve terminus. During the transport or at the arrival in the nerve terminus, the enzymatic conversions take place. Various peptidases, either vesicular or present in the cytoplasm of the synthesizing cell, in the extracellular space or even in other cells, may metabolically cleave the neuropeptides into biologically active or inactive metabolites. This scheme of metabolic transformations is summarized in Fig. 2.

Conventionally, functional importance has been ascribed to few well-defined products of a neuropeptide system. However, it is becoming obvious that metabolic conversions may not only change the potency of the product but also its biologic profile. An example is the metabolic transformation of substance P to its (1 − 7) fragment. This probably occurs in the nerve endings since, at least in the spinal cord, the enzyme sediments with

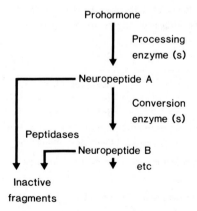

Fig. 2. Outline of the biosynthesis and degradation of neuropeptides. By stepwise transformations several biologically active neuropeptides, A, B, etc., may be released.

synaptosomes (Fried et al., in preparation). Thus, substance P(1 – 7) is also a normal product of pro-tachykinin A neurons. This may have functional consequences, since the pharmacology of substance P(1 – 7) is quite distinct from that of its parent compound (Table I). Another example is the prodynorphin system, where conversion of prodynorphin peptides to Leu-enkephalin-Arg[6] changes the receptor selectivity from μ to δ receptor preference (Paterson et al., 1983). This conversion is probably partly pathway-specific and prominent in, e.g. striatonigral prodynorphin neurons (Zamir et al., 1984; Christensson-Nylander et al., 1986). Analysis of CSF samples can indirectly be of assistance in the definition of which peptide species are actually released from a particular system, as will be discussed below.

The principles of neuropeptide biosynthesis outlined in Fig. 2 suggest that investigations of CSF samples should not only be directed to certain neuropeptides but also to different precursors and fragments as well as to processing or converting enzymes. It is not unlikely that the synaptic vesicles in peptidergic neurons contain precursors at various stages of processing, neuropeptides, neuropeptide fragments, as well as the enzymes. By exocytosis, the total vesicular content may be

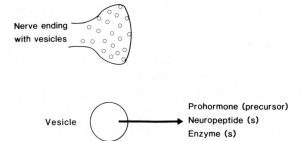

Fig. 3. Schematic representation of a nerve terminal with its vesicles, and one vesicle. It is suggested that by exocytosis, such a vesicle releases not only neuropeptides but also precursors and various enzymes.

released and eventually reach the CSF (Fig. 3). This mechanism may explain the presence of peptidases in CSF and, more importantly, explain why CSF levels of these enzymes are far above those expected from their very minute contribution to total protein in the CNS. From a technical point of view, such enzymes may be very robust markers, probably not subject to metabolic changes which they, however, inflict on peptide species.

Opioid peptides in the CSF

The opioid peptides constitute a big family with their roots in three separate prohormones (and genes), proenkephalin, prodynorphin and pro-opiomelanocortin. Each prohormone is pluripotent, i.e. capable of releasing several different biologically active molecules. The opioid peptides have the same N-terminal core sequence, Tyr-Gly-Gly-Phe-X, where X = Met or = Leu, being necessary for activity. The peptides commonly attributed to these systems are listed in Table II. Several of these peptides have also been identified in CSF by radioimmunoassay, although their chemical identity with the standards has not been proven (Table II). There are discrepancies between CNS content and CSF concentrations of these peptides. For instance, the enkephalins constitute the main opioid peptides in the CNS while their levels in the CSF are relatively low. This may be a reflec-

TABLE I

Selected biological effects of substance P (SP) and its N-terminal (1 – 7) fragment (the peptides were microinjected intracerebroventricularly into rats)

Behavioral test	Biological effect	
	SP	SP (1 – 7)
Hot plate	analgesia	analgesia
Blood pressure (baro-receptor reflex)	lowered	lowered
Agressive behavior (provocation)	inhibited	inhibited
Grooming behavior	increased	inhibited

(From Hall and Stewart, 1983; Hall et al., 1987.)

TABLE II

Opioid peptides deriving from the three opioid prohormones and assayed in human CSF (Means ± SEM are given for 5 to 6 samples)

Prohormone/peptide	No. of amino acids	No. in precursor[a]	Concentration (fmol/ml CSF)
Proopiomelanocortin			
β-endorphin	31	1	21 ± 6
Proenkephalin			
Met-enkephalin-Arg^6-Phe^7	7	1	23 ± 2
Met-enkephalin-Lys^6/Arg^6	6	6	170 ± 30
Met-enkephalin	5	6	51 ± 11
Prodynorphin			
dynorphin A	17	1	9.3 ± 2
dynorphin B	13	1	< 1
Leu-enkephalin-Arg^6	6	3	41 ± 8
Proenkephalin or prodynorphin			
Leu-enkephalin	5	1/3	11 ± 2

[a] Maximum theoretical number.
(From Nyberg et al., 1986.)

tion of rapid breakdown in the nerve tissue or by extracellular enzymes.

A more general way to measure opioid peptides in CSF is by receptor assay. Surprisingly, this procedure identifies more than 10-fold higher levels than accounted for by radioimmunoassays. This has prompted us to investigate the chemical nature of the peptides measured by the receptor assay (Nyberg and Terenius, 1984; Nyberg et al., 1986). The major part of the peptides elutes in two fractions on chromatography on a Sephadex G10 column, Fraction I with peptides of approximately 1 000 – 2 000 dalton and considerably basic in nature, and Fraction II with enkephalyl peptides in the 600 – 1 000 dalton interval. As will be described below, measurement of Fraction I and Fraction II peptides has been used extensively in various studies in humans. The receptor assay is analogous to the use of an antagonist (naloxone) as a probe, but does not identify the active peptide.

To obtain a better view of the total output from the opioid system into the CSF, a method was devised where peptide material was degraded by trypsin which releases enkephalyl hexapeptides from every potential processing product of the proenkephalin or prodynorphin systems (Nyberg et al., 1986). Importantly, the trypsin treatment generates products which can be identified as to the precursor they are derived from (Table III). Thus, any proenkephalin-derived peptide with an intact enkephalyl sequence will generate Met-enkephalin-Arg^6 or -Lys^6 or Leu-enkephalin-Lys^6. From prodynorphin, only Leu-enkephalin-Arg^6 can be generated, which is unique for this prohor-

TABLE III

Peptides which derive by trypsin degradation of proenkephalin or prodynorphin

Prohormone	Peptide	No. in prohormone
Proenkephalin	Leu-enkephalin-Lys^6	1
	Met-enkephalin-Arg^6	3
	Met-enkephalin-Lys^6	3
Prodynorphin	Leu-enkephalin-Arg^6	3

mone. By assay of Met-enkephalin-Arg[6]/Lys[6] and Leu-enkephalin-Arg[6] after trypsin treatment, one may therefore obtain a very good measure of the total output; contributions from pro-opiomelanocortin would not interfere since trypsin treatment would generate a longer enkephalyl peptide. Quite surprisingly, this procedure reveals that molecules from the size of the prohormones to the enkephalyl peptides are present in CSF (Table IV).

Thus, two independent methods, radioreceptor assay and radioimmunoassay of 'tryptides' (peptides released by trypsin treatment) show that a cascade of molecules at different stages of processing and conversion are released into the CSF. The larger peptides may have other properties than those commonly anticipated, higher metabolic stability (perhaps explaining their relatively high levels in CSF), and different receptor profile ($\varkappa$ versus δ receptor selectivity).

TABLE IV

Peptides related to proenkephalin and prodynorphin grouped according to molecular weight

Prohormone	Estimated molecular weight (dalton)	Concentration (femto-equivalents/ml CSF[a])
Proenkephalin	25 000	30
	15 000	23
	9 000	26
	1 300	9
	700[b]	25
Prodynorphin	20 000	2
	10 000	4
	5 000	9
	3 000	10
	1 500	13
	700[b]	5

[a] Met-enkephalin-Lys[6]/Arg[6] for proenkephalin; Leu-enkephalin-Arg[6] for prodynorphin.
[b] Hexapeptide.

Substance P in CSF

Radioimmunoassay has been used to measure CSF levels of substance P. It has been assumed that the immunoactive material is authentic substance P. However, chromatographic characterization suggests that the main components are C-terminal (3 – 11 or 5 – 11) fragments (Rimon et al., 1984). In addition, the N-terminal fragment, substance P (1 – 7) is present (Rimon et al., 1984). The presence of fragments, but undetectable levels of the parent peptide suggest that the metabolic conversion (fragmentation of substance P in the synaptic area or in CSF) is very efficient. It has also been possible to demonstrate large molecular weight precursor forms of substance P in CSF (unpublished) using enzyme treatment followed by radioimmunoassay of substance P(1 – 7), as described by Nyberg et al. (1985b). In terms of CSF analysis, substance P poses far less technical problems than the opioid peptides.

The endopeptidase generating substance P(1 – 7) and to a lesser extent substance P(1 – 8) may also be a marker of activity in protachykinin neurons. Immunohistochemical analysis of this or a related enzyme shows close association with protachykinin-containing primary afferents (Probert and Hanley, 1987).

Peptide system markers in CSF of patients with pain

The opioid system in chronic pain

The earliest studies of opioid peptides in the CSF of patients with pain used receptor assay. Prior to the assay, the CSF sample was fractionated to yield Fraction I and II (Terenius and Wahlström, 1975). This procedure, applied to CSF samples from patients with chronic pain (of more than 6 months' duration) and depression, revealed very marked differences. In patients with chronic neurogenic pain (neuralgia, causalgia etc.) Fraction I levels were very low, frequently below the range found in healthy volunteers. Patients who had chronic pain but no objective signs of organic lesion and who scored high neuroticism, therefore termed idiopathic, showed significantly higher Fraction I levels than controls (Almay et al., 1978). Patients with major depressive disorder also showed high Fraction I levels (Ågren et al., 1985). The discriminatory power of Fraction I analysis for identifying neurogenic versus idiopathic pain is very high (Almay et al., 1985). Puig et al. (1982) also observed low opioid peptide levels in patients with chronic lumbar disc pain, using a bioassay. Radioimmunoassay procedures for β-endorphin also indicate low levels in patients with chronic organic, supposedly neurogenic pain (Tsubokawa et al., 1983; Black et al., 1986). Studies on other specific opioid peptides are too few for any conclusions to be drawn.

A chronic pain condition represents a therapeutic failure. Particularly, chronic neurogenic pain represents a considerable challenge since patients show resistance to common analgesics and are poor placebo responders. Acupuncture, TENS and other non-pharmacological techniques have given at least partial symptom relief where other therapies have failed. Several studies indicate that acupuncture and the related techniques increase activity in opioid systems (Han and Terenius, 1984). There is evidence that patients with neurogenic pain respond better to TENS than those with other chronic pain conditions (e.g. Eriksson et al., 1979). Since low frequency TENS causes acute release of opioid peptides measured by receptor assay (Sjölund et al., 1977), and acupuncture has been reported to release Met-enkephalin-like material (Clement-Jones et al., 1979), it is likely that these treatments activate the opioid peptide systems, which would be particularly significant in conditions with low endorphinergic activity. It is frequently claimed that high frequency TENS treatment does not operate through opioid peptide release. This is probably true in a short-time perspective and with a single treatment session (cf. Terenius, 1981). However, repeated treatment over a week apparently 'normalizes' the low Fraction I levels with essentially

TABLE V

Levels of opioid peptides in CSF of patients with chronic pain measured in radioreceptor assay (Met-enkephalin equivalents pmol/ml CSF; mean ± SEM) before treatment, and 1 week after daily treatments with high-frequency TENS

Subjects	n	Before treatment	Change with treatment
Neurogenic pain	11	0.21 ± 0.13	0.69 ± 0.15[a]
Idiopathic pain	7	1.04 ± 0.38	0.16 ± 0.24
Responders[b]	5		0.71 ± 0.25[c]
Non-responders	12		0.40 ± 0.17

[a] $p < 0.001$ (Student's t test).
[b] Remaining responders (20–100%) at 3 months and continuing treatment.
[c] $p < 0.05$ (Student's t test).
(From Almay et al., 1985.)

no influences on the levels in idiopathic cases (Table V).

Adaptations of the opioid systems, particularly in late pregnancy and parturition

It is well known that there are great differences in the pain sensitivity of various individuals. One possible explanation is varying effectiveness of pain modulation by opioid peptides. Parturition only exists in species of late evolutionary origin. It involves very strong pain (and stress). From a teleological point of view, it would be of advantage if pain modulation was more effective at the end of pregnancy.

Radioimmunoassay of β-endorphin in CSF from women at term pregnancy revealed no difference from non-pregnant women (Datta et al., 1982; Lyrenäs et al., 1987). Also dynorphin A levels showed no significant difference. However, it was observed that women who chose epidural anesthesia to supplement self-administered nitrous oxide:oxygen (60:40) during parturition had lower dynorphin A levels. No difference was, however, observed for β-endorphin (Table VI). Also other potential markers of the prodynorphin system have been measured at term pregnancy. The levels of a dynorphin-converting enzyme are significantly lower ($p < 0.01$) than in non-pregnant controls (6.8 $\pm$ 3.8, $n = 11$ vs. 11.7 $\pm$ 2.6, $n = 10$ units/ml CSF). As a corollary, levels of Leu-enkephalin-Arg^6-containing polypeptides were significantly higher (1.8 $\pm$ 0.3 vs 1.5 $\pm$ 0.4; $p < 0.05$). Enkephalin-like peptides measured by receptor assay and Met-enkephalin-Arg^{6}Phe^7 were significantly higher in women in late pregnancy than in controls (Terenius et al., 1987). At least by receptor assay, the elevated levels were maintained several days after parturition.

Finally, studies have been addressing the general question why individuals differ so much in pain sensitivity. An indirect, and probably objective measure of pain sensitivity is the demand for a strong analgesic following major surgery. By the invention of self-administration technology, a nearly ideal system is available. Individual patients asked to self-administer a strong analgesic during the postoperative period quite accurately 'titrate' the injections so that a pseudo-steady-state of plasma meperidine is reached. This steady-state plasma level may be taken as a measure of a 'pain level'. If the plasma level is compared with the preoperative opioid peptide level (Fraction I measured by receptor assay), an inverse and significant ($p < 0.01$) relationship is observed (Tamsen et al., 1980, 1982). This suggests that low CSF opioid peptide levels signify low opioid peptide activity and that a subject with low levels 'compensates' by self-administering more analgesic than one with higher levels.

The data presented in this section may allow speculation on the adaptability of the opioid peptide systems. They are consonant with studies in experimental animals; e.g. pregnant rats show elevated pain thresholds (Gintzler, 1980). With recent methodological developments and parallel measurements of several potential markers, more definite statements could be made. The available data, as incomplete as they may be, indicate that CSF analysis may give information not easily obtained by other techniques.

The substance P system in chronic pain

Measurement of substance P in CSF has been performed entirely with radioimmunoassay. Even if the measured activity is not the authentic peptide, there is little doubt that the radioimmunoassay measures substance P fragments (see above). Low levels of substance P have been reported in peripheral neuropathy and autonomic dysfunction (Nutt et al., 1980), whereas it has been reported that patients with arachnoiditis and severe pain tend to have higher levels than controls (Hosobuchi et al., 1982). Other severe chronic pain conditions are usually accompanied with low levels. Sicuteri et al. (1985) reported very low levels in patients with cluster headache. In a relatively large series of patients, Almay et al. (unpublished) found substance P levels to be lower than control, particularly in neurogenic pain (Table VII). Interestingly, treatment with high frequency TENS for a week 'normalizes' these levels (Almay et al., 1985). On the other hand, patients with fibromyalgia show substance P levels above those in controls. Levels are particularly high in patients who are frequent smokers (Table VIII). However, the levels of substance P could not be related to

TABLE VI

Peptide levels in the CSF of parturient women who chose or did not choose epidural anesthesia during parturition (means $\pm$ SEM)

Epidural anesthesia	n	Peptide (fmol/ml)	
		β-endorphin	dynorphin A
No	6	6.5 $\pm$ 0.16	9.8 $\pm$ 0.13
Yes	10	5.4 $\pm$ 0.13	5.9 $\pm$ 0.14[a]

[a] $p < 0.05$ (Student's t test).

TABLE VII

Immunoreactive substance P in CSF of healthy volunteers and patients with chronic pain syndromes (mean ± SEM; $F = 5.35$, $p < 0.01$)

Subjects	n	Substance P (fmol/ml CSF)
Healthy volunteers	35	9.6 ± 1.7
Chronic pain, neurogenic	23	6.0 ± 2.8
Chronic pain, idiopathic	37	7.2 ± 2.7

TABLE VIII

Substance P levels in CSF of patients with fibromyalgia (mean ± SEM)

Subjects	n	Substance P (fmol/ml CSF)
Fibromyalgia	30	36.1 ± 2.7
Fibromyalgia and smoker	19	40.1 ± 2.7
Fibromyalgia and non-smoker	11	29.2 ± 4.9[a]

[a] Different from smokers ($p < 0.01$).

clinical characteristics such as disease duration or pain complaint (Vaeroy et al. 1988).

Critique

The CSF studies reviewed have given some insight into the dynamics of peptidergic neurons. Enzymatic transformations may be progressing even at the level of the synapse. As a consequence, the 'signal' from a peptidergic neuron is complex and covers molecules of different sizes and chemical structures, some of which have biological activity. If they have biologic activity, this activity may not be the same for all products. This could explain why empirically the receptor assay, which provides a global index of total opioids available, has been found to provide correlations to clinically relevant variables. Studies of CSF constituents also point to the importance of certain enzymes which critically transform peptide species. These enzymes may be more robust markers of activity in particular peptidergic pathways than the neuropeptides, provided their distribution is parallel. At least one enzyme, a substance P endopeptidase (Probert and Hanley, 1987) may have this property.

Presently, it is hard to see that measurement of neuropeptides or other markers of neuropeptide systems in CSF will become a routine diagnostic procedure. Limitations are both ethical, even if conditions are severe and chronic, and practical (technical). The situation may change, however, if measurements of peptide-transforming enzymes (which require less than 1 ml CSF) turn out to be discriminative in the taxonomy of pain.

Perhaps more importantly, the observation that certain enzymes may be altered in various chronic pain conditions, provides potential targets for pharmacologic agents which may increase the release of pain modulatory neuropeptides in their natural environment.

References

Ågren, A. and Terenius, L. (1985) Hallucinations in patients with major depression. *J. Affect. Disord.,* 9: 25 – 34.

Almay, B.G.L., Johansson, F., Von Knorring, L., Terenius, L. and Wahlström, A. (1978) Endorphins in chronic pain. I. Differences in CSF endorphin levels between organic and psychogenic pain syndromes. *Pain,* 5: 153 – 162.

Almay, B.G.L., Johansson, F., Von Knorring, L., Sakurada, T. and Terenius, L. (1985) Long-term high frequency transcutaneous electrical nerve stimulation (hi-TNS) in chronic pain. Clinical response and effects on CSF-endorphins, monoamine metabolites, substance P-like immunoreactivity (SPLI) and pain measures *J. Psychosomat. Res.,* 29: 247 – 257.

Berrettini, W.H., Rubinow, D.R., Nurnberger, J.I. Jr., Simmons-Alling, S., Post, R.M. and Gershon, E.S. (1985) CSF substance P immunoreactivity in affective disorders. *Biol. Psychiat.,* 20: 965 – 970.

Black, P. McL., Ballentine, H.T. Jr., Carr, D.B., Beal, M.F. and Martin, J.B. (1986) Beta-endorphin and somatostatin concentrations in the ventricular cerebrospinal fluid of patients with affective disorders. *Biol. Psychiat.,* 21: 1075 – 1077.

Christensson-Nylander, I., Herrera-Marschitz, M., Staines, W., Hökfelt, T., Terenius, L., Ungerstedt, U., Cuello, C., Oertel, W.H. and Goldstein, M. (1986) Striato-nigral dynorphin and substance P pathways in the rat. I: Biochemical and immunohistochemical evidence. *Exp. Brain Res.,* 64: 169 – 192.

Clement-Jones V., Besser, G.M., Lowry, P.J., McLoughlin, L., Rees, L.H. and Wen, H.L. (1979) Acupuncture in heroin addicts: changes in met-enkephalin and beta-endorphin in blood and cerebrospinal fluid. *Lancet,* ii, 380 – 383.

Datta, S., Steinbrok, R.A., Carr, D.B., Naulty, J.S. and Lee, C. (1982) Plasma and cerebrospinal fluid endorphin levels during pregnancy. *Anesthesiology,* 57: A380.

Eriksson, M.B.E., Sjölund, B.H. and Nielzén, S. (1979) Longterm results of peripheral conditioning stimulation as an analgesic measure in chronic pain. *Pain,* 6: 335 – 347.

Facchinetti, F., Petraglia, F., Cicero, S., Nappi, G., Valentini, M. and Genazzani, A.R. (1987) No gradient exists between lumbar and ventricular cerebrospinal fluid betaendorphin. *Neurosci. Lett.,* 77: 349 – 352.

Ginzler, A.R. (1980) Endorphin-mediated increases in pain threshold during pregnancy. *Science,* 210: 193 – 195.

Hall, M.E. and Stewart, J. (1983) Substance P and behavior; opposite effects of N-terminal and C-terminal fragments. *Peptides,* 4: 763 – 768.

Hall, M.E., Miley, F.B. and Stewart, J.M. (1987) Modulation of blood pressure by substance P: opposite effects of N- and C-terminal fragments on anesthetized rats. *Life Sci.,* 40: 1909 – 1914.

Han, J.S. and Terenius, L. (1982) Neurochemical basis of acupuncture analgesia. *Annu. Rev. Pharmacol. Toxicol.,* 22: 193 – 220.

Hazato, T., Kasama, A., Katayama, T., Kaya, K., Nishioka, S, and Shimamura, M. (1983) Enkephalin degrading enzymes in cerebrospinal fluid. *Life Sci.,* 33: 443 – 448.

Hazato, T., Katayama, T., Komuro, T. and Shimamura, M. (1985) Partial purification of two distinct enkephalindegrading aminopeptidases from human cerebrospinal fluid. *Biochem. Int.* 10: 813 – 819.

Hosobuchi, Y., Emson, P.C. and Iversen, L.L. (1982) Elevated cerebrospinal fluid substance P in arachnoiditis is reduced by systemic administration of morphine. *Adv. Biochem. Psychopharmacol.,* 33: 497 – 500.

Lantz, I. and Terenius, L. (1985) High enkephalyl peptide degradation, due to angiotensin-converting enzyme-like activity in human CSF. *FEBS Lett.,* 193: 31 – 34.

Lyrenäs, S., Nyberg, F., Lutsch, H., Lindberg, B. and Terenius, L. (1987) Cerebrospinal fluid dynorphin and β-endorphin in late pregnancy and six months after delivery. *Acta Endocrinol.,* 115: 253 – 258.

Matsas, R., Kenny, A.J. and Turner, A.J. (1984) The metabolism of neuropeptides. The hydrolysis of peptides, including enkephalins, tachykinins and their analogues, by endopeptidase-24.11. *Biochem. J.* 223: 433 – 440.

Nawa, H., Hirose, T., Inayama, S., Nakanishi, S. and Takashima, H. (1983) Nucleotide sequences of cloned cDNAs for two types of bovine brain substance P precursor. *Nature,* 306, 32 – 36.

Nutt, J.G., Mroz, E.A., Leeman, S.E., Williams, A.C., Engel, W.K. and Chase, T.N. (1980) Substance P in human cerebrospinal fluid: reductions in peripheral neuropathy and autonomic dysfunction. *Neurology.* 30: 1280 – 1285.

Nyberg, F. and Terenius, L. (1985) Identification of high molecular weight enkephalin precursor forms in human cerebrospinal fluid. *Neuropeptides,* 5: 537 – 540.

Nyberg, F., Le Grevés, P., Sundqvist, C. and Terenius, L. (1984) Characterization of substance P $(1-7)$ and $(1-8)$ generating enzyme in human cerebrospinal fluid. *Biochem. Biophys. Res. Commun.* 125: 244 – 250.

Nyberg, F., Nordström, K. and Terenius, L. (1985a) Endopeptidase in human cerebrospinal fluid which cleaves proenkephalin B opioid peptides at consecutive basic amino acids. *Biochem. Biophys. Res. Commun.,* 131: 1069 – 1074.

Nyberg, F., Le Grevés, P. and Terenius, L. (1985b) Identification of substance P precursor forms in human brain tissue. *Proc. Natl. Acad. Sci. USA,* 82: 3921 – 3924.

Nyberg, F., Nylander I. and Terenius, L. (1986) Enkephalin-containing polypeptides in human cerebrospinal fluid. *Brain Res.,* 371: 278 – 286.

Paterson, S.J., Robson, L.E. and Kosterlitz H.W. (1983) Classification of opioid receptors. *Br. Med. Bull.,* 39: 31 – 36.

Probert, L. and Hanley, M.R. (1987) The immunocytochemical localisation of substance P degrading enzyme within the rat spinal cord. *Neurosci. Lett.,* 78, 132 – 137.

Puig, M.M., Laorden, M.L., Miralles, F.S. and Olaso, M.J. (1982) Endorphin levels in cerebrospinal fluid of patients with postoperative and chronic pain. *Anesthesiology,* 57: 1 – 4.

Rimón, R., Le Grevés, P., Nyberg, F., Heikkilä, L., Salema, L. and Terenius, L. (1984) Elevation of substance P-like peptides in the CSF of psychiatric patients. *Biol. Psychiat.,* 19: 509 – 516.

Sakurada, T., Le Grevés, P., Stewart, J. and Terenius, L. (1985) Measurement of substance P metabolites in rat CNS. *J. Neurochem.,* 44: 718 – 722.

Sicuteri, F., Caleri, D., Fanciullacci, M., Geppetti, P., Renzi, D. and Spillantini, M.G. (1985) Substance P mechanism in cluster headache: evaluation in plasma and cerebrospinal fluid. *Cephalalgia,* 5: 143 – 149.

Sjölund, B., Terenius, L. and Eriksson, M. (1977) Increased cerebrospinal fluid levels of endorphins after electroacupuncture. *Acta Physiol. Scand.,* 100: 382 – 384.

Tamsen, A., Hartvig, P., Dahlström, B., Wahlström, A. and Terenius, L. (1980) Endorphins and on-demand pain relief. *Lancet,* i: 769 – 770.

Tamsen, A., Sakurada, T., Wahlström, A., Terenius, L. and Hartvig, P. (1982) Postoperative demand for analgesics in relation to individual levels of endorphins and substance P in cerebrospinal fluid. *Pain,* 13: 171 – 183.

Terenius, L. (1981) Endorphins and pain. *Front. Horm. Res.,* 8: 162 – 177.

Terenius, L. and Wahlström, A. (1975) Morphine-like ligand for opiate receptors in human CSF. *Life Sci.,* 16: 1759 – 1764.

Terenius, L., Lyrenäs, S., Lutsch, H., Lindström, L., Nyberg, F. and Lindberg, B. (1987) Opioid peptides at term pregnancy in the early puerperium and in postpartum psychosis. In D. Nerozzi, F.K. Goodwin and E. Costa (Eds.), *Hypothalamic Dysfunction in Neuropsychiatric Disorders,* Raven Press, New York, pp. 201 – 209.

Tsubokawa, T., Hirayama, T., Katayama, Y., Sibuya, H. and Yamamoto, T. (1984) Thalamic relay nucleus stimulation for relief of intractable pain. Clinical results and beta-endorphin immunoreactivity in the cerebrospinal fluid. *Pain,* 18: 115 – 126.

Vaeroy, H., Helle, R., Forre, O., Kåss, E. and Terenius, L. (1988) Elevated CSF levels of substance P and high incidence of Raynaud phenomenon in patients with fibromyalgia: new features for diagnosis. *Pain,* 32, 21 – 26.

Wand, G.S., Ney, R.L., Mains, R.E. and Eipper, B.A. (1985) Characterization of peptide alpha-amidation activity in human cerebrospinal fluid and central nervous system tissue. *Neuroendocrinology,* 41: 482 – 489.

Wood, J.H. (1982) Neuroendocrinology of cerebrospinal fluid: Peptides, steroids, and other hormones. *Neurosurgery,* 11: 293 – 305.

Yaksh, T.L., Jessell, T.M., Gamse, R., Mudge, A.W. and Leeman, S.E. (1980) Intrathecal morphine inhibits substance P release from mammalian spinal cord. *Nature,* 286: 155 – 156.

Yaksh, T.L., Terenius, L., Nyberg, F., Jhamandas, K. and Wang, J.-Y. (1983) Studies on the release by somatic stimulation from rat and cat spinal cord of active materials which displace dihydromorphine in an opiate-binding assay. *Brain Res.,* 268: 119 – 128.

Zamir, N., Palkovitz, M., Weber, E., Mezey, E. and Brownstein, M.J. (1984) A dynorphinergic pathway of Leu-enkephalin production in substantia nigra. *Nature,* 307: 643 – 645.

H.L. Fields and J.-M. Besson (Eds.)
Progress in Brain Research, Vol. 77
© 1988 Elsevier Science Publishers B.V. (Biomedical Division)

CHAPTER 32

In vivo and *in vitro* release of central neurotransmitters in relation to pain and analgesia

M. Hamon[a], S. Bourgoin[a], D. Le Bars[b] and F. Cesselin[a]

[a]*INSERM U. 288, Neurobiologie Cellulaire et Fonctionnelle, Faculté de Médecine Pitié-Salpêtrière, 91, Boulevard de l' Hôpital, 75634 Paris Cedex 13 and* [b]*INSERM U. 161, Unité de Recherches de Neurophysiologie Pharmacologique, 2 rue d'Alésia, 75014 Paris, France,*

Introduction

Ten years after the observation by Jessell and Iversen (1977) that opiate agonists exert a negative influence on the release of substance P (SP) from slices of the rat trigeminal nucleus, the situation regarding neurotransmitter release and the transfer and control of pain messages in the CNS is still far from being solved. Originally, simple concepts were proposed in which some neurotransmitters (notably SP) are exclusively involved in the transfer of pain messages whereas others (such as endogenous opioids and serotonin, 5HT) participate in negative controls of these messages, such as the one conveyed by bulbospinal pathways. However, extensive studies on the release of various neurotransmitters at different levels critically involved in pain and analgesia, particularly the dorsal horn of the spinal cord, have shown that this view is no longer valid. Indeed, noxious stimuli can trigger the release not only of SP but also of met-enkephalin (ME) and 5HT. Furthermore both noxious and analgesic stimulations can increase the release of a given neurotransmitter, i.e. 5HT, within the same central area (i.e. the dorsal horn of the spinal cord). Finally, although it was originally proposed that analgesia can reasonably be expected from the administration of 'enkephalinase' inhibitors since such a treatment would

result in the protection of endogenous opioids, it was then demonstrated that the same treatment also protects SP.

These few examples illustrate how studies on neurotransmitter release can lead to a critical reconsideration of commonly accepted views regarding the transfer and control of pain messages. However, these studies also led to the development of new concepts, and the present review is an attempt to show how in vivo and in vitro investigations on neurotransmitter release have contributed to present knowledge of the central mechanisms of pain and analgesia.

I. Central neurotransmitter release in relation to pain

A. *Effects of acute noxious stimuli*

The presence of SP in primary afferent fibres of small diameter within the dorsal roots, and the excitatory action of this neuropeptide on spinal neurons responding to noxious stimuli were the first indirect evidence for its participation in the transfer of pain messages at the level of the dorsal horn (see references in Matsumura et al., 1985). A more direct demonstration was then made by Yaksh et al. (1980) who reported that stimulation of the sciatic nerve at a high intensity to activate small diameter fibres induces a marked increase of SP release in spinal cord superfusates in anaesthetized cats. More recently, Brodin et al. (1987) succeeded in measuring SP release directly at the level of the dorsal horn thanks to the local implantation of a microdialysis probe in pentobarbital anaesthetized cats. Thus, they could confirm that high intensity stimulation of the sciatic nerve induces a local release of SP in the dorsal horn, not only on the stimulated side, but also to a lesser extent on the contralateral side.

Duggan (this volume) has used an antibody-coated microelectrode to show significant release in specific laminae of the dorsal horn of SP-like immunoreactivity by noxious stimuli.

Further investigations on the release of SP were made using an implanted push-pull cannula. For instance, Kuraishi et al. (1983, 1985) showed that noxious mechanical stimuli applied to the skin markedly enhance the release of SP within the dorsal horn in anaesthetized rabbits, and Yonehara et al. (1986) reported that electrical stimulation of the lower incisor pulp induces a marked increase in SP release within the trigeminal nucleus caudalis in the same species.

All these observations clearly support that various kinds of noxious stimuli can trigger the release of SP (and probably other neurokinins) at the trigeminal and spinal relays of nociceptive pathways.

In addition to SP, other neuropeptides (possibly colocalized with SP in the same ganglion cells) exist in primary afferent fibres of small diameter, and noxious stimuli should also trigger their release notably at the spinal level. Indeed, for vasoactive intestinal peptide (VIP) and cholecystokinin (or possibly calcitonin-gene-related peptide; see Ju et al., 1986), Yaksh et al. (1982) could observe a marked enhancement of their release in spinal cord superfusates during bilateral electrical stimulation of the sciatic nerve at high, but not low, intensity in chloralose-urethane anaesthetized cats.

However, it is not only those contained in primary afferent fibres, but also the neurotransmitters of other neuronal systems such as the endogenous opioids mainly from local interneurons and 5HT from descending bulbospinal pathways that are affected by acute noxious stimuli. Thus, Yaksh and Elde (1981) reported that high intensity stimulation of peripheral nerves (i.e. the infraorbital and sciatic nerves) as well as the intraarterial injection of bradykinin resulted in marked enhancement of the release of ME-like immunoreactive material (MELM) in spinal and ventricular perfusates in chloralose-urethane anaesthetized cats. Similarly tooth-pulp stimulation has been shown to increase the concentration of MELM in the cisternal CSF in halothane anaesthetized cats (Cesselin et al., 1982). Whether MELM originating from the nucleus reticularis gigantocellularis contributed to this effect is an interesting possibility, as Kuraishi et al. (1984) observed that the local release of MELM could be triggered by various noxious stimuli (formalin injection into hindpaws, tail heating) in anaesthetized animals.

So far, the exact nature of the opioid peptides which can be released at the spinal level by nociceptive stimulation has not yet been completely elucidated. According to Yaksh et al. (1983), α-neoendorphin, dynorphin(1 − 13) and ME-Lys[6] and/or ME-Arg[6] accounted for most of the endorphinergic material released in spinal cord superfusates during high intensity stimulation of the sciatic nerve in cats. However, ME itself can also be detected in spinal cord superfusates from anaesthetized rats submitted to various noxious stimuli (Cesselin et al., 1985a). Furthermore, the heptapeptide ME-Arg[6]-Phe[7] (Tang et al., 1983), the octapeptide ME-Arg[6]-Gly[7]-Leu[8] (Iadarola et al., 1986) and even larger opioid peptides (derived from the proenkephalins A and B) are likely to be released from the spinal cord of animals submitted to noxious stimuli.

Since Tyce and Yaksh (1981) showed that high intensity stimulation of the sciatic nerve also markedly enhanced the release of 5HT in spinal superfusates, it could be postulated that the (paradoxical) increased outflow of opioids which was observed under the same condition results from some excitatory influence of the activated descending 5HT projections impinging on enkephalinergic interneurons (Glazer and Basbaum, 1984). Alternatively, since SP stimulates the release of ME, ME-Arg[6]-Phe[7] and ME-Arg[6]-Gly[7]-Leu[8] from the rat spinal cord both in vitro and in vivo (Del Rio et al., 1983; Tang et al. 1983; Cesselin et al., 1984a), the increased release of this peptide from excited primary afferent fibres may be responsible for the enhanced outflow of the opioids in animals submitted to noxious stimuli. According to these hypotheses, 5HT antagonists and/or SP antagonists should prevent the stimulatory influence of nociceptive stimulation on the release of opioid peptides, at least at the spinal level. Unfortunately, such experiments have not been performed yet (indeed, no SP antagonist acting on central receptors is presently available), and the above-mentioned functional interactions between SP-, 5HT- and opioid-containing neurons are still purely hypothetical. Nevertheless, the two hypotheses mentioned above have important functional correlates since the involvement of descending serotoninergic projections would imply a non-

segmental control of MELM release, whereas that of primary afferent SP-containing fibres would correspond to a local segmental control of the peptide release. Interestingly, evidence for the existence of both segmental and non-segmental regulation of MELM release has recently been obtained in halothane-anaesthetized rats submitted to various kinds of noxious stimuli. Thus, tail immersion into a water bath at 52°C resulted in a marked increase in the spinal release of MELM, and this effect persisted after transection of the cord at the cervical level (Cesselin et al., 1985b). Therefore, segmental mechanisms are very probably responsible for the increased release of MELM induced by thermal noxious stimulation. In contrast, mechanical noxious stimuli trigger the spinal release of MELM through non-segmental mechanisms since an increased peptide outflow occurs only in the spinal zone which does not receive the nociceptive inputs (Table I). For instance, noxious pinching of the muzzle increased the release of MELM within the lumbar area but not the cervicotrigeminal area, whereas in contrast, hindpaw pinching affected the peptide release at the cervicotrigeminal level but not at the lumbar level (Le Bars et al., 1987a). Fur-

TABLE I

Effects of noxious mechanical stimuli on the release of MELM from the lumbar area or the cervicotrigeminal area of the rat spinal cord

MELM (pg/0.5 ml)

noxious stimulation	lumbar area	(%)	cervicotrigeminal area	(%)
None	2.45 ± 0.10	(100)	3.85 ± 0.29	(100)
Muzzle pinching	4.13 ± 0.17[a]	(169)	4.53 ± 0.45	(118)
Forepaw pinching	3.38 ± 0.38[a]	(138)	4.17 ± 0.51	(108)
Hindpaw pinching	2.66 ± 0.42	(109)	6.87 ± 0.90[a]	(178)
Tail pinching	3.41 ± 0.25*	(139)	5.91 ± 0.50[a]	(154)

Superfusion of the spinal cord in halothane-anaesthetized rats was restricted to either the lumbar area or the cervicotrigeminal area as described by Le Bars et al. (1987a). Noxious pinches were applied repetitively for 30 min to the muzzle, the forepaw, the hindpaw or the tail, and MELM in superfusate fractions (0.5 ml/5 min) collected during the stimulation was measured using a specific radioimmunoassay (Cesselin et al., 1985a). Each value is the mean ± SEM of at least six independent determinations. Figures in parentheses are the percentages relative to control values (when no stimulation was applied).
[a] $p < 0.05$ when compared to MELM release in non-stimulated rats.

thermore, cervical transection of the spinal cord (Cesselin et al., 1985b) as well as the bilateral lesions of the dorsolateral funiculi (Le Bars et al., 1987b) completely prevented the stimulatory influence of muzzle pinching upon the spinal release of MELM. Such differences in the characteristics of MELM release due to thermal and mechanical stimuli indicate that distinct neuronal mechanisms underlie the responses to different kinds of noxious stimuli, in agreement with previous pharmacological observations (see for instance Salt and Hill, 1983; Schmauss and Yaksh, 1984).

Interestingly, Le Bars et al. (1979) have described 'diffuse noxious inhibitory controls' (DNIC) which consist of heterosegmental inhibition of convergent neurons within the dorsal horn in animals submitted to noxious stimuli. According to these authors, the contrast between the increased electrical activity of convergent neurons within the spinal segment impinged on by the excited primary afferent fibres, and the reduction in cell activity due to DNIC in other segments might contribute to the signalling of pain at the spinal level (Dickenson et al., 1981). Comparison of these electrophysiological data with those concerning MELM release has suggested that DNIC were in fact triggered – at least partly – by opioidergic systems. Indeed naloxone treatment markedly reduces DNIC (Le Bars et al., 1981). Furthermore, DNIC as well as MELM release (induced by noxious mechanical stimulation) can no longer be evoked following the bilateral lesion of the dorsolateral funiculi (Le Bars et al., 1987b). Accordingly, although it cannot be excluded that MELM which is released at the spinal level by noxious stimuli might participate in some endogenous pain control mechanism (particularly when segmental processes are concerned), it is reasonable to propose that it may also contribute to the integration of pain messages conveyed from the periphery to supraspinal centres. Although controversial, this concept has experimental support, and may explain the paradoxical analgesic effect of low doses of the opiate antagonist naloxone in animals (Dickenson et al., 1981).

Obviously, the dorsal horn of the spinal cord or the caudal part of the trigeminal nucleus are not the only synaptic relays in the transmission of nociceptive signals. Investigations on putative neurotransmitter release triggered by noxious stimuli must also be carried out at supraspinal levels, notably within thalamic nuclei (rich in enkephalinergic terminals and cell bodies, see Conrath et al., 1986; Covenas et al., 1986), and the cerebral cortex. For instance, Hudson et al. (1985) noted that noxious pinching of the tail induced a marked increase of acetylcholine release within the parietal cortex in halothane anaesthetized rabbits. Future work should, therefore, address the supraspinal relay nuclei for nociception. The recently developed microdialysis technique (Brodin et al., 1987), differential pulse voltammetry (Rivot et al., 1982), and the more established push-pull cannula technique (Bourgoin et al., 1982) are in fact well adapted to the measurement of neurotransmitter release within discrete brain nuclei.

B. Effects of chronic pain

Extensive studies of the commonly accepted chronic pain model, i.e. polyarthritis induced by intradermal injection of complete Freund's adjuvant in rats, have led to the discovery of highly significant alterations in neurotransmitter release, particularly at the level of the spinal cord. Thus, Oku et al. (1987) noted a significant increase in the 'spontaneous' release of SP within the dorsal lumbar horn of rats 2 to 3 weeks after the induction of polyarthritis. Furthermore, passive movements of the inflamed ankle joint evoked a significant elevation of the peptide outflow (as expected from an acute noxious stimulation, see I, A), while a similar non-nociceptive movement of the non-inflamed joint was ineffective (Oku et al., 1987).

Although no direct measurement of 5HT release has been made so far in arthritic rats, Godefroy et al. (1987) have found a marked acceleration of 5HT synthesis in the dorsal part of the spinal cord which was probably coupled to an increased release of the indoleamine in these animals. Similarly, evidence has recently been provided for an acceleration of dynorphin synthesis in the spinal cord of arthritic rats (Höllt et al., 1987) which might suggest that the release of this opioid peptide is affected in a parallel manner. However, preliminary direct measurement of dynorphin release from the spinal cord apparently revealed a decrease instead of the expected increase in arthritic rats (Przewlocka et al., 1986), showing that data on the synthesis of a given neurotransmitter cannot be systematically extrapolated to the release process. In this respect, the best evidence is provided by the enkephalinergic system since the increased levels of ME within the spinal cord of arthritic rats (Cesselin et al., 1980) are clearly associated with a marked reduction in the local 'spontaneous' release of MELM in these animals (Cesselin et al., 1985b; Bourgoin et al., 1988). Nevertheless, as already observed in control rats (see I,A), acute noxious stimulation (i.e. movements of the inflamed hindpaws) produced a significant acceleration of MELM release in polyarthritic rats (Bourgoin et al., 1988).

In view of the negative influence of enkephalins upon SP release at the level of the dorsal horn (Mauborgne et al., 1987), it can be speculated that the tonic elevation of SP release observed in arthritic rats (Oku et al., 1987) results, at least partly, from a sustained reduction in MELM release. However, the origin of the latter change is presently unknown.

Interestingly, measurements in the CSF of chronic suffering patients also revealed reduced levels of endorphins (Almay et al., 1978, 1980) and MELM (Simonnet et al., 1986) when compared to controls. However, the relevance of such observations to the physiology of pain is still a matter of debate as pain alleviation by chronic chlorimipramine treatment was not associated with any significant rise of CSF MELM levels in such patients (Bourgoin et al., 1987b). Furthermore, normal CSF levels of MELM (Cesselin et al., 1984b) and β-endorphin (Dehen et al., 1986) have been found in patients with congenital insensitivity to pain.

In conclusion, investigations on neurotransmitter release show that acute and chronic pain involve different neuronal mechanisms since spinal SP- and ME-containing systems are both activated by acute noxious stimuli, but exhibit opposite changes during chronic pain.

II. Central neurotransmitter release in relation to analgesia

A. Effects of morphine and other opiates

An abundant literature has been devoted to the possible direct effects of morphine and other opioid compounds on the in vitro release of various neurotransmitters from slices and synaptosomes, and only those concerning the neurotransmitters clearly involved in pain signalling and control will be briefly reviewed.

Generally, morphine and other opiates exert a negative influence upon neurotransmitter release (see for instance Loh et al., 1976; Subramanian et al., 1977; Arbilla and Langer, 1978), and such an effect is specially relevant when it concerns SP and other neuroactive molecules participating in the transfer of nociceptive messages. Thus, Jessell and Iversen (1977) first reported that morphine and other opiates inhibit the release of SP from the rat trigeminal nucleus, which led to the concept of presynaptic inhibition of SP-containing primary afferent fibres as being − at least partly − responsible for their analgesic action. The negative influence of opiates upon SP release was then found in cultures of dorsal root ganglion sensory neurons (Mudge et al., 1979), and confirmed in vivo by Yaksh et al. (1980) who noted a marked inhibition by intrathecal morphine of the spinal release of SP induced by high intensity stimulation of the sciatic nerve in anaesthetized cats. Obviously this effect of opiates has a particular importance regarding pain control mechanisms, since it takes place at critical levels such as the trigeminal nucleus and the dorsal horn of the spinal cord (see Kuraishi et al., 1983; Hirota et al., 1985; Lembeck and Donnerer, 1985; Mauborgne et al., 1987). However, it must be emphasized that the same negative influence of opiates upon SP release has also been found in the hypothalamus (Micevych et al., 1982) and the substantia nigra (Bourgoin et al., 1987b; Mauborgne et al., unpublished observations).

Recently, the problem of the opiate control of SP release from the dorsal lumbar cord was reinvestigated in our laboratory on account of the well-known heterogeneity of specific receptors mediating opiate actions in the CNS. In agreement with others (Jessell and Iversen, 1977; Lembeck and Donnerer, 1985), we found that opiate agonists reduce the K^+-induced release of SP-like immunoreactive material (SPLI) provided they act selectively on the δ class of opiate receptors. Surprisingly, mu agonists such as DAGO, FK-33824 and even morphine (in the presence of the selective δ antagonist ICI-154129) increased the K^+-induced release of SPLI from slices of the dorsal lumbar cord (Mauborgne et al., 1987). In contrast, the $\varkappa$ agonist U 50488H did not affect SPLI overflow (Mauborgne et al., unpublished observations), an observation in keeping with the failure of dynorphin (which also acts preferentially on $\varkappa$ opiate receptors) to inhibit noxious stimuli induced SP release from rabbit dorsal horn (Hirota et al., 1985).

Since SP-containing fibres within the dorsal horn are heterogeneous, we postulated that the paradoxical stimulatory effect of μ agonists resulted (may be via an interneuron) from a possible action of these drugs on SP-containing interneurons or descending bulbospinal fibres instead of primary afferent fibres (Mauborgne et al., 1987). In order to further verify this hypothesis, we then used another model for exploring selectively the influence of various opiate agonists on the release of SP from primary afferent fibres. Indeed capsaicin selectively excites primary afferent fibres and elicits a Ca^{2+}-dependent release of SP from slices of the dorsal half of the rat spinal cord (Lembeck and Donnerer, 1985). As illustrated in Fig. 1, the δ agonist deltakephalin (DTLET) markedly reduced the capsaicin-induced release of SP, strongly suggesting that the spinal analgesic action of δ agonists involves a direct presynaptic

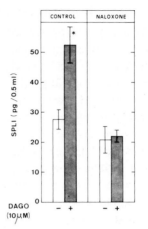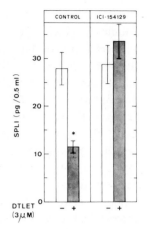

Fig. 1. Modulation through μ and δ opiate receptors of capsaicin-induced release of substance P-like immunoreactive material (SPLI) from the dorsal zone of the rat lumbar enlargement. Slices of the dorsal zone of the lumbar enlargement were continuously superfused with an artificial CSF at a flow rate of 0.5 ml/2 min, and SPLI was assayed in the collected fractions (0.5 ml). The addition of capsaicin (0.5 μM) to the superfusing fluid for 8 min (i.e. four fractions) induced a marked Ca^{2+}-dependent release of SPLI which could be further enhanced by the μ agonist DAGO (10 μM) or, in contrast, significantly reduced by the δ agonist DTLET (3 μM). As expected from the involvement of specific opiate receptors, the μ antagonist naloxone (1 μM) prevented the stimulatory action of DAGO, and the δ antagonist ICI-154129 (10 μM) the inhibitory action of DTLET. Each bar is the mean $\pm$ SEM of SPLI contents (in pg SP equivalents/0.5 ml) in 32–40 separate fractions collected during tissue superfusion with capsaicin and various opiates as indicated on the Fig. * $p < 0.001$, when compared to SPLI release due to capsaicin in the absence of opiates (– on the abscissa).

inhibition of primary afferent fibres (see Porreca et al., 1984). In contrast, the stimulation of μ opiate receptors by DAGO elicited a marked enhancement of SP release due to capsaicin (Fig. 1). As clearly illustrated in Fig. 1, both effects were mediated by specific receptors since they could be totally prevented by the selective δ antagonist ICI-154129 and μ antagonist naloxone, respectively. Although such results would suggest that analgesia due to the intrathecal administration of μ agonists does not involve a presynaptic inhibition of primary afferent fibres by these drugs, care must be taken before drawing any definitive conclusion.

Indeed capsaicin induces the release of other neuroactive molecules at the spinal level (i.e. those contained in primary afferent fibres of small diameter, for instance calcitonin-gene-related peptide, Saria et al., 1986; but also MELM, see Yaksh and Elde, 1981), and complex neuronal interactions, involving possibly interneurons, probably take place in spinal cord slices exposed to this drug. Therefore it cannot be completely excluded at present that, under these particular conditions, the stimulatory effect of μ agonists upon SP release from the dorsal half of the rat spinal cord may correspond to an indirect effect mediated through an interneuron impinging on primary afferent fibres.

Regarding serotoninergic systems, morphine treatment exerts a general stimulatory effect which results in an increased release of 5HT not only at the spinal level (Bardon and Ruckebusch, 1984), but also in the cerebral cortex and caudate nucleus (Aiello-Malmberg et al., 1979). Since morphine does not directly enhance the in vitro release of the indoleamine from spinal cord slices (Bourgoin et al., 1981; Bineau-Thurotte et al., 1984) and synaptosomes (Monroe et al., 1986), it can be proposed that the activation of descending serotoninergic fibres originates from a supraspinal site of action of the drug. Indeed Yaksh and Tyce (1979) demonstrated that the microinjection of morphine (5 μg) into the periaqueductal gray evoked the release of 5HT in spinal superfusates, and Pycock et al. (1981) reported a naloxone-reversible stimulatory effect of morphine on the in vitro release of 5HT from slices of the rat periaqueductal gray. Obviously, numerous other potential supraspinal sites of action exist for morphine and other opiates, but it can be assumed that the periaqueductal gray is probably of critical importance for the opiate-induced activation of descending bulbospinal serotoninergic neurons and associated analgesia in mammals (see Le Bars, 1988).

Another relevant observation regarding morphine-induced analgesia and neurotransmitter release is the negative effect of this drug on the cortical release of acetylcholine evoked by sensory stimulation in rats (Coutinho-Netto et al., 1982).

Indeed noxious stimulation also markedly increases acetylcholine outflow within the cerebral cortex (Hudson et al., 1985), and it can be speculated that some negative influence of morphine upon the cholinergic system might well contribute to reduce the sensation of pain.

To conclude this section, it must be emphasized that opiates can also influence the release of opioid peptides with important functional correlates regarding their analgesic effect. Thus, Tseng (1986) has reported that the intracerebroventricular administration of β-endorphin increases the release of MELM from the spinal cord, and that this effect contributes to its analgesic action in rats. In contrast, superfusion of the spinal cord with morphine (0.5 mM) produced a significant reduction in the local release of MELM normally evoked by high intensity stimulation of the sciatic nerve in anaesthetized cats (Jhamandas et al., 1984). Further studies should tell whether or not such morphine-induced effects are related to the well-known tolerance and dependence to opiates.

B. Effects of other analgesic compounds

On account of the analgesic properties of opioid peptides injected directly into the CSF or selected brain nuclei, attempts have been made to develop new analgesic treatments (at least in animals) which would enhance the concentration of the endogenous opioids at the level of their specific receptors, i.e. in the extracellular fluid. Thus, systematic examination of the effects of various neuroactive substances upon the release of MELM from the dorsal half of the rat lumbar cord revealed that both SP (and particularly its sulfoxide derivative) and cholecystokinin 1–8 (CCK 8) (Cesselin et al., 1984a) exert a stimulatory effect. Interestingly, the intrathecal injection of these two peptides has occasionally been shown to depress nociceptive responses in a naloxone-reversible manner in rats (Doi and Jurna, 1981; Jurna and Zetler, 1981). However, neither SP nor CCK 8 can seriously be proposed for analgesic therapy, as conflicting data show that SP usually exerts hyperalgesic effects by the intrathecal route in awake rats (Masumura et al., 1985), and that CCK 8 may act as an endogenous opiate antagonist within the CNS (Faris et al., 1983).

Another means to increase the extracellular concentration of endogenous opioid peptides at critical sites for the control of nociceptive messages within the CNS may consist of blocking their degradation by the peptidases. In this respect, much effort has been devoted to the identification of the various enzymes involved in the catabolism of enkephalins, and then to the development of selective inhibitors.

Three enzymes, namely aminopeptidase M, dipeptidylaminopeptidase and 'enkephalinase' (membrane metalloendopeptidase, EC 3.4.24.11), were shown to be responsible for the physiological degradation of ME in brain and spinal tissues (see Schwartz et al., 1985). Highly potent inhibitors have subsequently been developed, such as bestatin for aminopeptidase M, thiorphan and phosphoramidon for 'enkephalinase', and kelatorphan for the three enzymes, and their administration resulted in marked analgesia in rodents (Schwartz et al., 1985). Furthermore, in vitro as well as in vivo, these drugs were able to increase the outflow of MELM, notably at the level of the spinal cord (Cesselin et al., 1985b; Bourgoin et al., 1986). However, more recent investigations revealed that these inhibitors also protect other neuropeptides such as SP and CCK 8 from enzymatic degradation, and produce a significant elevation in their outflow from brain slices (Bourgoin et al., 1987b; Fig. 2). Therefore, the following sequence: administration of peptidase inhibitors → increased extracellular concentration of enkephalins → analgesia, is undoubtedly an oversimplified interpretation. Indeed, neuropeptidases are largely non-specific (for instance 'enkephalinase' destroys not only enkephalins but also SP, see Matsas et al., 1983) and it is thus not possible to act selectively on only one neuropeptide or even one class of neuropeptides (such as opioids, neurokinins, etc.) with a given inhibitor. Nevertheless, a compound like kelatorphan is a potent analgesic in rodents

(Fournié-Zaluski et al., 1984), and thorough investigations on its actual mechanism of action in vivo should contribute to a better knowledge of the physiology of nociception.

Other pharmacological treatments known to alleviate pain in human have been explored in

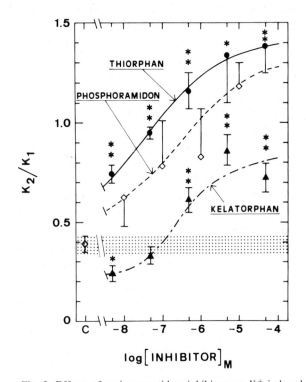

Fig. 2. Effects of various peptidase inhibitors on K^+-induced overflow of SPLI from slices of the rat substantia nigra. Tissues were depolarized twice (K_1, K_2) by 30 mM K^+ for 8 min in the course of a continuous superfusion with artificial CSF (flow rate: 1 ml/4 min), and K^+-induced overflow was estimated by measuring the SPLI contents of collected superfusate fractions. In the absence of drugs, the ratio of SPLI overflow due to the 2nd K^+ pulse to that due to the first, i.e. K_2/K_1 (ordinate), was equal to 0.39 ± 0.03 (mean $\pm$ SEM, $n = 15$). Significant increases in this ratio were noted when the 2nd K^+ pulse took place while tissues were superfused with thiorphan ($\bullet$, 5 nM – 50 μM), phosphoramidon ($\diamond$, 10 nM – 10 μM) or kelatorphan ($\blacktriangle$, 0.5 μM – 50 μM). Accordingly the peptidase inhibitors markedly enhanced K^+-induced SPLI overflow, as expected from the blockade of enzymes normally involved in the degradation of endogenous SP. Each point is the mean $\pm$ SEM of at least four separate determinations. * $p < 0.005$, ** $p < 0.001$ when compared with K_2/K_1 in the absence of drugs (C on the abscissa).

TABLE II

Stimulatory effect of porcine and salmon calcitonins on K^+-induced release of ^{3}H-5HT from slices of the rat dorsal lumbar enlargement

^{3}H-5HT release – K_2/K_1	
Control	0.539 ± 0.028
Porcine calcitonin 1 μM	0.789 ± 0.070[a]
Salmon calcitonin 1 μM	0.759 ± 0.065[a]

Slices of the dorsal zone of the rat lumbar enlargement were incubated with ^{3}H-5HT (50 nM), and then continuously superfused at 37°C with an artificial CSF. Tissues were depolarized twice (K_1, K_2) by 30 mM K^+ in the course of the experiment, and porcine or salmon calcitonin (1 μM) was added to the superfusing fluid 12 min before the second K^+ pulse. The ratio of ^{3}H-5HT release evoked by K_2 over that due to K_1 (K_2/K_1) is the mean $\pm$ SEM of at least 10 separate determinations.
[a] $p < 0.01$ when compared to K_2/K_1 in the absence of calcitonin ('control').

animals regarding their possible effect on neurotransmitter release, and we would like to focus on two of them to end this section: calcitonin and antidepressants. It is well established that numerous antidepressants inhibit the reuptake of monoamines, notably 5HT, by nerve endings, and there is evidence which indicates that the analgesic effect of these drugs depends primarily on the resulting increase in extracellular monoamines in the CNS (references in Le Bars, 1988). However, the opiate antagonist naloxone can abolish the antinociceptive effects of antidepressants (Reichenberg et al., 1985), and the chronic administration of these drugs significantly affects enkephalinergic systems within the spinal cord in rats (Hamon et al., 1987). Direct investigation of the release of enkephalins at selected sites within the CNS would be particularly helpful for a more complete understanding of the mechanism of analgesic action of antidepressants.

Studies of the neurochemical effects of porcine and salmon calcitonins on in vitro neurotransmitter release from various brain regions and the spinal cord revealed that endogenous opioids were probably not involved in their analgesic action since the release of MELM remained unaffected by these two peptides (Cesselin et al., 1985c). Similarly, SP release from spinal cord slices was unchanged by the two calcitonins. In contrast, that of ^{3}H-5HT previously taken up by spinal tissues could be significantly increased by salmon as well as porcine calcitonins (Table II). Since selective lesion of serotoninergic neurons by 5,7-dihydroxytryptamine prevents calcitonin-induced behavioural effects (Clementi et al., 1985), a 5HT releasing action is probably involved in the central mechanism of calcitonin-induced analgesia in rats. Indeed an increased ^{3}H-5HT release due to salmon calcitonin was only found at the spinal level, as neither hippocampal nor hypothalamic ^{3}H-5HT release was affected by the peptide (Cesselin et al., 1985c).

C. Effects of physical analgesic treatments

Electrical stimulation of periventricular and periaqueductal gray matter has been shown to induce pain relief not only in animals but also in humans, and the hypothesis of some analgesic substance being released at critical sites within the CNS upon such stimulation is logical. Indeed, this hypothesis found support as soon as it appeared that naloxone could reverse the stimulation-induced analgesia in animals (Oliveras et al., 1977) and in humans (Hosobushi et al., 1977). Two groups (Akil et al., 1978; Hosobushi et al., 1979) then succeeded in showing the appearance of β-endorphin-like immunoreactive material in ventricular CSF of patients under analgesic electrical stimulation . . . until Dionne et al. (1984) provided evidence that these results are artifact. Indeed, these authors demonstrated that the contrast medium injected into the ventricles directly interferes with the β-endorphin radioimmunoassay, and that β-endorphin levels in CSF are not directly associated with pain relief (Dionne et al., 1984).

Similarly, no direct evidence has been reported so far of the release of an opioid peptide at selected levels of the CNS in animals submitted to central analgesic electrical stimulation. In fact, all authors do not agree about the reversal by naloxone of such analgesia (see Yaksh et al., 1976).

Electroacupuncture is also a well-known technique for alleviating pain in humans, and evidence has been provided for a marked activation of endorphinergic systems by this treatment, since Sjölund et al. (1977) showed increased levels of endogenous opioids in the CSF of stimulated patients. Similarly, indirect evidence exists for the release of ME and possibly ME-Arg[6]-Phe[7] within the spinal cord of rats under electroacupuncture (see Chou et al., 1984). However, more direct investigations are needed in order to demonstrate that electroacupuncture increases the release of endogenous opioids at critical levels within the CNS. For instance, He et al. (1985) reported increased release of opioids (measured by a radioreceptor assay) from the head of the caudate nucleus in rabbits under electroacupuncture, but the relevance of such observation to the pain-alleviating effect of the treatment has not been established clearly.

In contrast with the unclear situation regarding the possible release of opioids, much more convincing evidence has been provided about the releasing effects of central stimulation upon monoamines, notably 5HT and noradrenaline (NA) at the spinal level. In particular, Hammond et al. (1985) demonstrated that electrical stimulation of the nucleus raphe magnus and nucleus reticularis paragigantocellularis markedly increases the efflux of 5HT and NA from the spinal cord. Similarly, Rivot et al. (1982) provided direct evidence of an increased extracellular concentration of 5-hydroxyindoles (detected by differential pulse voltammetry) in the dorsal horn of rats electrically stimulated at the level of the nucleus raphe magnus. There is, therefore, little doubt − if any − that analgesia triggered by the direct electrical stimulation of selected brain stem nuclei is associated with the release of monoamines, notably 5HT (see Le Bars, 1988), at the spinal level.

III. Conclusions and future trends

So far, direct measurement of neurotransmitter release in relation to pain and analgesia has concerned monoamines, particularly 5HT, and some neuropeptides, particularly the opioids and SP, at the level of the spinal cord. Only partial information exists regarding the effects of noxious stimuli and analgesic treatments on the release of other neurotransmitters (e.g. excitatory amino acids and GABA) at the spinal level and at supraspinal regions relaying or controlling the nociceptive transmission. Obviously, future investigations should concern these unexplored fields in order to have a more complete view of the neurochemical events occurring in the neuronal circuits involved in pain and analgesia.

However, even at the restricted level of the spinal relay of nociceptive pathways the situation is far from being clear, in spite of extensive investigations on selected neuroactive substances such as 5HT, SP and ME. Indeed, none of these substances can be considered as a pure 'nociceptive' or 'analgesic' neurotransmitter. For instance, SP can be released from different neuronal populations (primary afferent fibres, local interneurons, descending bulbospinal neurons), and act through different classes of specific receptors to trigger various biological responses. Obviously SP which is released from the mixed bulbospinal SP-5HT-containing neurons is not functionally equivalent to that released from primary afferent fibres. Therefore, care should be taken in order to really identify which neuroactive molecule has been measured (for instance which opioid peptide) and from which neuronal population it originates. With such conditions being fulfilled, significant progress can be expected from studies on neurotransmitter release in relation to pain and analgesia. For instance, recent reports have described the presence of various types of neurotransmitter receptors on the primary afferent fibres entering the dorsal horn (Carstens et al., 1987; Howe et al., 1987; Patterson and Hanley, 1987), and investigations on their possible involvement in the presynaptic control of SP release should provide fruitful information regarding nociception.

Acknowledgements

Original data reported in this review have been obtained thanks to the support of INSERM, DRET and Ciba-Geigy Ltd.

References

Aiello-Malmberg, P., Bartolini, A., Bartolini, R. and Galli, A. (1979) Effects of morphine, physostigmine and raphe nuclei stimulation on 5-hydroxytryptamine release from the cerebral cortex of the cat. *Br. J. Pharmacol.*, 65: 547 – 555.

Akil, H., Richardson, D.E., Barchas, J.D. and Li, C.H. (1978) Appearance of β-endorphin-like immunoreactivity in human ventricular cerebrospinal fluid upon analgesic electrical stimulation. *Proc. Natl. Acad. Sci. USA*, 75: 5170 – 5172.

Almay, B.G.L., Johansson, F., Von Knorring, L., Terenius, L. and Wahlström, A. (1978) Endorphin in chronic pain. I. Difference in CSF endorphin levels between organic and psychogenic pain syndromes. *Pain*, 5: 153 – 162.

Almay, B.G.L, Johansson, F., Von Knorring, L., Sedvall, G. and Terenius, L. (1980) Relationships between CSF levels of endorphins and monoamine metabolites in chronic pain patients. *Psychopharmacology*, 67: 139 – 142.

Arbilla, S. and Langer, S.Z. (1978) Morphine and β-endorphin inhibit release of noradrenaline from cerebral cortex but not of dopamine from rat striatum. *Nature*, 271: 559 – 561.

Bardon, T. and Ruckebusch, M. (1984) Changes in 5-HIAA and 5-HT levels in lumbar CSF following morphine administration to conscious dogs. *Neurosci. Lett.*, 49: 147 – 151.

Bineau-Thurotte, M., Godefroy, F., Weil-Fugazza, J. and Besson, J.M. (1984) The effect of morphine on the potassium evoked release of tritiated 5-hydroxytryptamine from spinal cord slices in the rat. *Brain Res.*, 291: 293 – 299.

Bourgoin, S., Cesselin, F., Artaud, F. and Hamon, M. (1981) In vitro release of met-enkephalin and ^{3}H-serotonin from the dorsal part of the lumbar cord in rats. *Pain*, Suppl. 1: 20.

Bourgoin, S., Cesselin, F., Artaud, F., Glowinski, J. and Hamon, M. (1982) In vivo modulations by GABA-related drugs of met-enkephalin release in basal ganglia of the cat brain. *Brain Res.*, 248: 321 – 330.

Bourgoin, S., Le Bars, D., Artaud, F., Clot, A.M.,

Bouboutou, R., Fournié-Zaluski, M.C., Roques, B.P., Hamon, M. and Cesselin, F. (1986) Effects of kelatorphan and other peptidase inhibitors on the in vitro and in vivo release of methionine-enkephalin-like material from the rat spinal cord. *J. Pharmacol. Exp. Ther.*, 238: 360 – 366.

Bourgoin, S., Cesselin, F., Gozlan, H., Fattaccini, C.M., Tran, M.A., Montastruc, J.L., Rascol, A, and Hamon, M. (1987a) Chronic chlorimipramine does not reverse the reduction of cerebrospinal fluid met-enkephalin-like immunoreactivity in chronic pain patients. *Clin. Neuropharmacol.*, 10: 434 – 442.

Bourgoin, S., Mauborgne, A., Benoliel, J.J., Hirsch, M., Hamon, M. and Cesselin, F. (1987b) 'Enkephalinase' is involved in the degradation of endogenous met-enkephalin, substance P and cholecystokinin in the rat CNS. In S. Tuček (Ed.), *Synaptic Transmitters and Receptors,* Academia, Praha, and John Wiley & Sons Ltd., Chichester, pp. 215 – 221.

Bourgoin, S., Le Bars, D., Clot, A.M., Hamon, M. and Cesselin, F. (1988) Spontaneous and evoked release of met-enkephalin-like material from the spinal cord of arthritic rats in vivo. *Pain*, 32: 107 – 114.

Brodin, E., Linderoth, B., Gazelius, B. and Ungerstedt, U. (1987) In vivo release of substance P in cat dorsal horn studied with microdialysis. *Neurosci. Lett.*, 76: 357 – 362.

Carstens, E., Gilly, H., Schreiber, H. and Zimmermann, M. (1987) Effects of midbrain stimulation and iontophoretic application of serotonin, noradrenaline, morphine and GABA on electrical thresholds of afferent C- and A-fibre terminals in cat spinal cord. *Neuroscience*, 21: 395 – 406.

Cesselin, F., Montastruc, J.L., Gros, C., Bourgoin, S. and Hamon, M. (1980) Met-enkephalin levels and opiate receptors in the spinal cord of chronic suffering rats. *Brain Res.*, 191: 289 – 293.

Cesselin, F., Oliveras, J.L., Bourgoin, S., Sierralta, F., Michelot, R., Besson, J.M. and Hamon, M. (1982) Increased levels of met-enkephalin-like material in the CSF of anaesthetized cats after tooth pulp stimulation. *Brain Res.*, 237: 325 – 338.

Cesselin, F., Bourgoin, S., Artaud, F. and Hamon, M. (1984a) Basic and regulatory mechanisms of in vitro release of met-enkephalin from the dorsal zone of the rat spinal cord. *J. Neurochem.*, 43: 763 – 773.

Cesselin, F., Bourgoin, S., Hamon, M., Artaud, F., Testut, M.F., Rascol, A. and Montastruc, J.L. (1984b) Normal CSF levels of met-enkephalin-like material in a case of naloxone-reversible congenital insensitivity to pain. *Neuropeptides*, 4: 217 – 225.

Cesselin, F., Le Bars, D., Bourgoin, S., Gozlan, H., Clot, A.M., Besson, J.M. and Hamon, M. (1985a) Spontaneous and evoked release of methionine-enkephalin-like material from the rat spinal cord in vivo. *Brain Res.*, 339: 305 – 313.

Cesselin, F., Bourgoin, S., Artaud, F., Gozlan, H., Le Bars, D., Clot, A.M., Besson, J.M. and Hamon, M. (1985b) The release of met-enkephalin-like material at the spinal level. In vivo and in vitro studies. In: J.M. Besson and Y. Lazorthes (Eds.), *Spinal Opioids and the Relief of Pain*, INSERM, 127: 241–264.

Cesselin, F., Bourgoin, S., Mauborgne, A., Caulin, F. and Hamon, M. (1985c) Médiation possible par la sérotonine de l'action analgésique de la calcitonine. *J. Pharmacol. (Paris),* 16: 468.

Chou, J., Tang, J., Del Rio, J., Yang, H.-Y.T. and Costa, E. (1984) Action of peptidase inhibitors on methionine[5]-enkephalin-arginine[6]-phenylalanine[7] (YGGFMRF) and methionine[5]-enkephalin (YGGFM) metabolism and on electroacupuncture antinociception. *J. Pharmacol. Exp. Ther.,* 230: 349–352.

Clementi, G., Amico-Roxas, M., Rapisarda, E., Caruso, A., Prato, A., Trombadore, S., Priolo, G. and Scapagnini, U. (1985) The analgesic activity of calcitonin and the central serotonergic system. *Eur. J. Pharmacol.,* 108: 71–75.

Conrath, M., Covenas, R., Romo, R., Chéramy, A., Bourgoin, S. and Hamon, M. (1986) Distribution of met-enkephalin immunoreactive fibres in the thalamus of the cat. *Neurosci. Lett.,* 65: 299–303.

Coutinho-Netto, J., Abdul-Ghani, A.S. and Bradford, H.F. (1982) Morphine suppression of neurotransmitter release evoked by sensory stimulation in vivo. *Biochem. Pharmacol.,* 31: 1019–1023.

Covenas, R., Romo, R., Chéramy, A., Cesselin, F. and Conrath, M. (1986) Immunocytochemical study of enkephalin-like cell bodies in the thalamus of the cat. *Brain Res* 377: 355–361.

Dehen, H., Amsallem, B., Colas-Linhart, N. and Cambier, J. (1986) Betaendorphine du liquide céphalo-rachidien au cours de l'insensibilité congénitale à la douleur. *Rev. Neurol. (Paris),* 142: 541–544.

Del Rio, J., Naranjo, J.R., Yang, H.-Y.T. and Costa, E. (1983) Substance P-induced release of met-[5]enkephalin from striatal and periaqueductal gray slices. *Brain Res.,* 279: 121–126.

Dickenson, A.H., Le Bars, D. and Besson, J.M. (1981) Endogenous opiates and nociception: a possible functional role in both pain inhibition and detection as revealed by intrathecal naloxone. *Neurosci. Lett.,* 24: 161–164.

Dionne, R.A., Mueller, G.P., Young, R.F. Greenberg, R.P., Hargreaves, K.M., Gracely, R. and Dubner, R. (1984) Contrast medium causes the apparent increase in β-endorphin levels in human cerebrospinal fluid following brain stimulation. *Pain,* 20: 313–321.

Doi, T. and Jurna, I. (1981) Intrathecal substance P depresses the tail flick response – Antagonism by naloxone. *Naunyn-Schmiedeb. Arch. Pharmacol.,* 317: 135–139.

Faris, P.L., Komisaruk, B.R., Watkins, L.R. and Mayer, D.J. (1983) Evidence for the neuropeptide cholecystokinin as an antagonist of opiate analgesia. *Science,* 219: 311–312.

Fournié-Zaluski, M.C., Chaillet, P., Bouboutou, R., Coulaud, A., Cherot, P., Waksman, G., Costentin, J. and Roques,

B.P. (1984) Analgesic effects of kelatorphan, a new highly potent inhibitor of multiple enkephalin degrading enzymes. *Eur. J. Pharmacol.,* 102: 525–528.

Glazer, E.J. and Basbaum, A.I. (1984) Axons which take up [3H]serotonin are presynaptic to enkephalin immunoreactive neurones in cat dorsal horn. *Brain Res.,* 298: 386–391.

Godefroy, F., Weil-Fugazza, J. and Besson, J.M. (1987) Complex temporal changes in 5-hydroxytryptamine synthesis in the central nervous system induced by experimental polyarthritis in the rat. *Pain,* 28: 223–238.

Hammond, D.L., Tyce, G.M. and Yaksh, T.L. (1985) Efflux of 5-hydroxytryptamine and noradrenaline into spinal cord superfusates during stimulation of the rat medulla. *J. Physiol. (Lond.),* 359: 151–162.

Hamon, M., Gozlan, H., Bourgoin, S., Benoliel, J.J., Mauborgne, A., Taquet, H., Cesselin, F. and Mico, J.A. (1987) Opioid receptors and neuropeptides in the CNS in rats treated chronically with amoxapine or amitriptyline. *Neuropharmacology,* 26: 531–539.

He, L., Lu, R., Zhuang, S., Zhang, X. and Pan, X. (1985) Possible involvement of opioid peptides of caudate nucleus in acupuncture analgesia. *Pain,* 23: 83–93.

Hirota, N., Kuraishi, Y., Hino, Y., Sato, Y., Satoh, M. and Takagi, H. (1985) Met-enkephalin and morphine but not dynorphin inhibit noxious stimuli-induced release of substance P from rabbit dorsal horn in situ. *Neuropharmacology,* 24: 567–570.

Höllt, V., Haarmann, I., Millan, M.J. and Herz, A. (1987) Prodynorphin gene expression is enhanced in the spinal cord of chronic arthritic rats. *Neurosci. Lett.,* 73: 90–94.

Hosobuchi, Y., Adams, J.E. and Linchitz, R. (1977) Pain relief by electrical stimulation of the central gray matter in humans and its reversal by naloxone. *Science,* 197: 183–186.

Hosobuchi, Y., Rossier, J., Bloom, F.E. and Guillemin, R. (1979) Stimulation of human periaqueductal gray for pain relief increases immunoreactive β-endorphin in ventricular fluid. *Science,* 203: 279–281.

Howe, J.R., Yaksh, T.L. and Go, V.L.W. (1987) The effect of unilateral dorsal root ganglionectomies or ventral rhizotomies on α_2-adrenoceptor binding to, and the substance P, enkephalin, and neurotensin content of, the cat lumbar spinal cord. *Neuroscience,* 21: 385–394.

Hudson, D.M., Jenden, D.J., Scremin, O.U. and Sonnenschein, R.R. (1985) Cortical acetylcholine efflux with hypercapnia and nociceptive stimulation. *Brain Res.,* 338: 267–272.

Iadarola, M.J., Tang, J., Costa, E. and Yang, H.-Y.T. (1986) Analgesic activity and release of [met[5]]enkephalin-arg[6]-gly[7]-leu[8] from rat spinal cord in vivo. *Eur. J. Pharmacol.,* 121: 39–48.

Jessell, T.M. and Iversen, L.L. (1977) Opiate analgesics inhibit substance P release from rat trigeminal nucleus. *Nature,* 268: 549–551.

Jhamandas, K., Yaksh, T.L. and Go, V.L.M. (1984) Acute and

chronic morphine modifies the in vivo release of methionine-enkephalin-like immunoreactivity from the cat spinal cord and brain. *Brain Res.,* 297: 91 – 103.

Ju, G., Hökfelt, T., Fischer, J.A., Frey, P., Rehfeld, J.F. and Dockray, G.J. (1986) Does cholecystokinin-like immunoreactivity in rat primary sensory neurones represent calcitonin gene-related peptide? *Neurosci. Lett.,* 68: 305 – 310.

Jurna, I. and Zetler, G. (1981) Antinociceptive effect of centrally administered caerulein and cholecystokinin octapeptide (CCK-8). *Eur. J. Pharmacol.,* 73: 323 – 331.

Kuraishi, Y., Hirota, N., Sugimoto, M., Satoh, M. and Takagi, H. (1983) Effects of morphine on noxious stimuli-induced release of substance P from rabbit dorsal horn in vivo. *Life Sci.,* 33 (Suppl. 1): 693 – 696.

Kuraishi, Y., Sugimoto, M., Hamada, T., Kayanoki, Y. and Takagi, H. (1984) Noxious stimuli and met-enkephalin release from nucleus reticularis gigantocellularis. *Brain Res. Bull.,* 12: 123 – 127.

Kuraishi, Y., Hirota, N., Sato, Y., Kaneko, S., Satoh, M. and Takagi, H. (1985) Noradrenergic inhibition of the release of substance P from the primary afferents in the rabbit spinal dorsal horn. *Brain Res.,* 359: 177 – 182.

Le Bars, D. (1988) Serotonin and pain. In: N.N. Osborne and M. Hamon (Eds.), *Neuronal Serotonin,* John Wiley & Sons Ltd, Chichester, pp. 171 – 229.

Le Bars, D., Dickenson, A.H. and Besson, J.M. (1979) Diffuse noxious inhibitory controls (DNIC). I. Effects on dorsal horn convergent neurones in the rat. *Pain,* 6: 283 – 304.

Le Bars, D., Chitour, D., Kraus, E., Dickenson, A.H. and Besson, J.M. (1981) Effect of naloxone upon diffuse noxious inhibitory controls (DNIC) in the rat. *Brain Res.,* 204: 387 – 402.

Le Bars, D., Bourgoin, S., Clot, A.M., Hamon, M. and Cesselin, F. (1987a) Noxious mechanical stimuli increase the release of met-enkephalin-like material heterosegmentally in the rat spinal cord. *Brain Res.,* 402: 188 – 192.

Le Bars, D., Bourgoin, S., Villanueva, L., Clot, A.M., Hamon, M. and Cesselin, F. (1987b) Involvement of the dorsolateral funiculi in the spinal release of met-enkephalin-like material triggered by heterosegmental noxious mechanical stimuli. *Brain Res.,* 412: 190 – 195.

Lembeck, F. and Donnerer, J. (1985) Opioid control of the primary afferent substance P fibres. *Eur. J. Pharmacol.,* 114: 241 – 246.

Loh, H.H., Brase, D.A., Sampath-Khanna, S., Mar, J.B., Way, E.L. and Li, C.H. (1976) β-endorphin in vitro inhibition of striatal dopamine release. *Nature,* 264: 567 – 568.

Matsas, R., Fulcher, I.S., Kenny, A.J. and Turner, A.J. (1983) Substance P and [Leu]enkephalin are hydrolyzed by an enzyme in pig caudate synaptic membranes that is identical with the endopeptidase of kidney microvilli. *Proc. Natl. Acad. Sci. USA,* 80: 3111 – 3115.

Matsumura, H., Sakurada, T., Hara, A., Sakurada, S. and

Kisara, K. (1985) Characterization of the hyperalgesic effect induced by intrathecal injection of substance P. *Neuropharmacology,* 24: 421 – 426.

Mauborgne, A., Lutz, O., Legrand, J.C., Hamon, M. and Cesselin, F. (1987) Opposite effects of δ and μ opioid receptor agonists on the in vitro release of substance P-like material from the rat spinal cord. *J. Neurochem.* 48: 529 – 537.

Micevych, P.E., Yaksh, T.L. and Go, V.L.W. (1982) Opiate-mediated inhibition of the release of cholecystokinin and substance P, but not neurotensin from cat hypothalamic slices. *Brain Res.,* 250: 283 – 289.

Monroe, P.J., Michaux, K. and Smith, D.J. (1986) Evaluation of the direct actions of drugs with a serotonergic link in spinal analgesia on the release of [^{3}H]serotonin from spinal cord synaptosomes. *Neuropharmacology,* 25: 261 – 265.

Mudge, A.W., Leeman, S.E. and Fischbach, G.D. (1979) Enkephalin inhibits release of substance P from sensory neurons in culture and decreases action potential duration. *Proc. Natl. Acad. Sci. USA,* 76: 526 – 530.

Oku, R., Satoh, M. and Takagi, H. (1987) Release of substance P from spinal dorsal horn is enhanced in polyarthritic rats. *Neurosci. Lett.,* 74: 315 – 319.

Oliveras, J.L., Hosobuchi, Y., Redjemi, F., Guibaud, G. and Besson, J.M. (1977) Opiate antagonist, naloxone, strongly reduces analgesia induced by stimulation of a raphe nucleus (centralis inferior). *Brain Res.,* 120: 221 – 229.

Patterson, S.I. and Hanley, M.R. (1987) Autoradiographic evidence for β-adrenergic receptors on capsaicin-sensitive primary afferent terminals in rat spinal cord. *Neurosci. Lett.,* 78: 17 – 21.

Porreca, F., Mosberg, H.I., Hurst, R., Hruby, V.J. and Burks, T.F. (1984) Roles of mu, delta and kappa opioid receptors in spinal and supraspinal mediation of gastrointestinal transit effects and hot-plate analgesia in the mouse. *J. Pharmacol. Exp. Ther.,* 230: 341 – 348.

Przewlocka, B., Lason, W. and Przewlocki, R. (1986) The release of opioid peptides from the rat spinal cord. In S. Tuček, S. Stipek, F. Stastany and J. Krivanek (Eds.), *Molecular Basis of Neural Function.* Eur. Soc. Neurochemistry, p. 243.

Pycock, C.J., Burns, S. and Morris, R. (1981) In vitro release of 5-hydroxytryptamine and γ-amino-butyric acid from rat periaqueductal grey and raphe dorsalis region produced by morphine or an enkephalin analogue. *Neurosci. Lett.,* 22: 313 – 317.

Reichenberg, K., Gaillard-Plaza, G. and Montastruc, J.L. (1985) Influence of naloxone on the antinociceptive effects of some antidepressant drugs. *Arch. Int. Pharmacodyn. Ther.,* 275: 78 – 84.

Rivot, J.P., Chiang, C.Y. and Besson, J.M. (1982) Increase of serotonin metabolism within the dorsal horn of the spinal cord during nucleus raphe magnus stimulation, as revealed by in vivo electrochemical detection. *Brain Res.,* 238:

117 – 126.

Salt, T.E. and Hill, R.G. (1983) Pharmacological differentiation between responses of rat medullary dorsal horn neurons to noxious mechanical and noxious thermal cutaneous stimuli. *Brain Res., 263*: 167 – 171.

Saria, A., Gamse, R., Petermann, J., Fisher, J.A., Theodorsson-Norheim, E. and Lundberg, J.M. (1986) Simultaneous release of several tachykinins and calcitonin-gene-related peptide from rat spinal cord slices. *Neurosci. Lett., 63*: 310 – 314.

Schmauss, C. and Yaksh, T.L. (1984) In vitro studies on spinal opiate receptor systems mediating antinociception. II. Pharmacological profiles suggesting a differential association of mu, delta and kappa receptors with visceral, chemical and cutaneous thermal stimuli in the rat. *J. Pharmacol. Exp. Ther., 228*: 1 – 12.

Schwartz, J.C., Costentin, J. and Lecomte, J.M. (1985) Pharmacology of enkephalinase inhibitors. *Trends Pharmacol. Sci., 6*: 472 – 476.

Simonnet, G., Taquet, H., Floras, P., Caille, J.M., Legrand, J.C., Vincent, J.D. and Cesselin, F. (1986) Simultaneous determination of radio-immuno-assayable methionine-enkephalin and radioreceptor-active opioid peptides in CSF of chronic pain suffering and non-suffering patients. *Neuropeptides, 7*: 229 – 240.

Sjölund, B., Terenius, L. and Ericksson, M. (1977) Increased cerebrospinal fluid levels of endorphins after electroacupuncture. *Acta Physiol. Scand., 100*: 382 – 384.

Subramanian, N., Mitznegg, P., Sprügel, W., Domschke, S., Wünsch, E. and Demling, L. (1977) Influence of enkephalin on K^+-evoked efflux of putative neurotransmitters in rat brain. Selective inhibition of acetylcholine and dopamine release. *Naunyn-Schmiedeb. Arch. Pharmacol., 299*: 163 – 165.

Tang, J., Chou, J., Yang, H.-Y.T. and Costa, E. (1983) Substance P stimulates the release of met[5]-enkephalin-arg[6]-phe[7] and met[5]-enkephalin from rat spinal cord. *Neurophar-*

macology 22: 1147 – 1150.

Tseng, L.-F. (1986) Stereoselective effect of β-endorphin on the production of analgesia and the spinal release of met-enkephalin in rats. *J. Pharmacol. Exp. Ther., 239*: 160 – 165.

Tyce, G.M. and Yaksh, T.L. (1981) The release of serotonin and noradrenaline from cat spinal cord in vivo by somatosensory stimulation: description of an intrinsic modulatory system. *J. Physiol. (Lond.), 314*: 513 – 528.

Yaksh, T.L. and Elde, R.P. (1981) Factors governing release of methionine enkephalin-like immunoreactivity from mesencephalon and spinal cord of the cat in vivo. *J. Neurophysiol., 46*: 1056 – 1075.

Yaksh, T.L. and Tyce, G.M. (1979) Microinjection of morphine into the periaqueductal gray evokes the release of serotonin from spinal cord. *Brain Res., 171*: 176 – 181.

Yaksh, T.L., Young, J.C. and Rudy, T.A. (1976) An inability to antagonize with naloxone the elevated nociceptive thresholds resulting from electrical stimulation of the mesencephalic central grey. *Life Sci., 18*: 1193 – 1198.

Yaksh, T.L., Jessell, T.M., Gamse, R., Mudge, A.W. and Leeman, S.E. (1980) Intrathecal morphine inhibits substance P release from mammalian spinal cord in vivo. *Nature, 286*: 155 – 157.

Yaksh, T.L., Abay, E.O.II and Go, V.L.W. (1982) Studies on the location and release of cholecystokinin and vasoactive intestinal peptide in rat and cat spinal cord. *Brain Res., 242*: 279 – 290.

Yaksh, T.L., Terenius, L., Nyberg, F., Jhamandas, K. and Wang, J.Y. (1983) Studies on the release by somatic stimulation from rat and cat spinal cord of active materials which displace dihydromorphine in an opiate-binding assay. *Brain Res., 268*: 119 – 128.

Yonehara, N., Shibutani, T., Tsai, H.-Y. and Inoki, R. (1986) Effects of opioids and opioid peptides on the release of substance P-like material induced by tooth pulp stimulation in the trigeminal nucleus caudalis of the rabbit. *Eur. J. Pharmacol., 129*: 209 – 216.

Subject Index

Supraspinal facilitation, 193
Supraspinal inhibition, 193
Sympathetic afferent, 240
Sympathetic cell group, 77
Synapses, axonic, 199
Synergistic interaction, 389

Tachycardia, 241
Tail flick reflex, 7, 10, 11, 162, 170, 195, 196, 201, 229, 230, 246 – 255, 325, 330, 331, 334, 350, 373 – 386, 415
Task-related response, 219
Tectum, 146
TENS, 425
Tetracaine, 319
Thalamic pain, 178, 179
Thalamic pulvinar nucleus, 222
Thalamotomy, 176
Thalamus, 4, 16, 17, 41, 42, 217, 263, 264
Thermal paresthesia, 184
Thermal task, 214, 215 – 221
  innocuous, 215
  noxious, 215
Thermoreceptor, 2
Thiorphan, 414, 415, 438
Third ventricle, 396
Thoracic intermediolateral cell group, 69
Thyrotropin-releasing hormone (TRH), 107, 111, 113, 115, 119 – 124, 129, 136, 259
Tibial nerve, 196, 202
Tomography
  computer-aided (CAT), 190, 228
  positron emission, 228
Tonic descending control system, 13
Tonic descending inhibition, 6 – 10, 19, 193 – 204, 209, 210, 324, 386
Tonic response, 220
Tooth pulp, 143
Transcutaneous electrical nerve stimulation, 239 – 241
Transmitter substance, 185
Tricyclic antidepressant, 170
Trigeminal brain stem complex, 159, 225
Trigeminal nucleus caudalis, 281, 284, 287, 432, 434, 435
Trigeminal subnucleus oralis, 150, 214
Trigeminal system, 143, 225
Trypan blue, 315
Trypsin, 423, 424
Tryptamine, 316, 317
L-Tryptophan, 170, 184, 186

Unmyelinated axon, 8, 131

Unmyelinated fiber, 194
Unmyelinated primary afferent, 201, 202, 203
^{14}C-Urea, 317

Vagotomized preparation, 241
Vagus nerve, 240
Vasoactive intestinal peptide (VIP), 108, 109, 115, 119, 124, 186, 432
Vasodilation, 353, 354
Vasopressinergic fiber, 78
Ventral funiculus, 18, 19, 20, 68, 69
Ventral horn, 53, 62, 63, 85, 136, 137, 261
Ventral medulla, 39
Ventral parabrachial nucleus, 54
Ventral posterior lateral nucleus, 4, 17, 18
Ventral tegmental area, 141
Ventral tegmental area of Tsai, 70, 79, 80
Ventricular catheter, 396
Ventriculography, 165 – 168
Ventrobasal thalamus, 42, 228
Ventrolateral funiculus, 19, 21, 58, 62, 63, 69
Ventrolateral medulla, 8 – 10, 196, 202 – 204
Ventrolateral periaqueductal gray, 32, 38, 42
Ventrolateral pontine tegmentum, 361
Ventrolateral quadrants, 283
Ventrolateral reticular formation, 95
Ventromedial funiculus, 285
Ventromedial medulla (VMM), 37, 149, 152, 361, 366
Vesicles
  dense core, 133, 134
  oval agranular, 132, 133
Vestibulospinal tract, 6
Visceral alerting response, 203, 204
Visceral receptor, 17
Visceral stimulus, 16
Viscus, distention, 373
Visual analogue scale, 184
Visual fixation, 220
Visual system, 218
Visual task, 214, 215 – 221
Vocalization threshold, 144, 283, 302, 303, 373, 378

Wind up results, 240
Withdrawal response, 378, 386, 387
Writhing response, 373, 379

Yohimbine, 201, 230, 251, 330, 359 – 364

Zimelidine, 331
Zwitterion, 341